# THE DEVELOPING
# HUMAN
## CLINICALLY ORIENTED EMBRYOLOGY

### KEITH L. MOORE

Recipient of the inaugural **Henry Gray/Elsevier Distinguished Educator Award** in 2007—the American Association of Anatomists' highest award for excellence in human anatomy education at the medical/dental, graduate, and undergraduate levels of teaching; the **Honored Member Award of the American Association of Clinical Anatomists (1994)** for significant contributions to the field of clinically relevant anatomy; and the **J.C.B. Grant Award of the Canadian Association of Anatomists (1984)** "in recognition of meritorious service and outstanding scholarly accomplishments in the field of anatomical sciences." In 2008 Professor Moore was inducted as a **Fellow of the American Association of Anatomists.** The rank of Fellow honors distinguished AAA members who have demonstrated excellence in science and in their overall contributions to the medical sciences. In 2012 Dr. Moore received an **Honorary Doctor of Science** degree from The Ohio State University; The **Queen Elizabeth II Diamond Jubilee Medal** honoring significant contributions and achievements by Canadians; and the **Benton Adkins Jr. Distinguished Service Award** for an outstanding record of service to the American Association of Clinical Anatomists.

### T.V.N. (VID) PERSAUD

Recipient of the **Henry Gray/Elsevier Distinguished Educator Award** in 2010—the American Association of Anatomists' highest award for excellence in human anatomy education at the medical/dental, graduate, and undergraduate levels of teaching; the **Honored Member Award of the American Association of Clinical Anatomists (2008)** for significant contributions to the field of clinically relevant anatomy; and the **J.C.B. Grant Award of the Canadian Association of Anatomists (1991)** "in recognition of meritorious service and outstanding scholarly accomplishments in the field of anatomical sciences." In 2010 Professor Persaud was inducted as a **Fellow of the American Association of Anatomists.** The rank of Fellow honors distinguished AAA members who have demonstrated excellence in science and in their overall contributions to the medical sciences. In 2003 Dr. Persaud was a recipient of the **Queen Elizabeth II Golden Jubilee Medal,** presented by the Government of Canada for "significant contribution to the nation, the community, and fellow Canadians."

### MARK G. TORCHIA

Recipient of the **Norman and Marion Bright Memorial Medal and Award** and the **Silver Medal** of the Chemical Institute of Canada in 1990 for outstanding contributions. In 1993 he was awarded the **TIMEC Medical Device Champion Award.** In 2008 and in 2014 Dr. Torchia was a nominee for the **Manning Innovation Awards,** for innovation talent. Dr. Torchia's most cherished award has been the **Award for Teaching Excellence** in 2011 from the Faculty of Medicine, University of Manitoba, and being asked to address the graduating class of 2014.

# THE DEVELOPING
# HUMAN
## CLINICALLY ORIENTED EMBRYOLOGY

*10th Edition*

## Keith L. Moore,
### BA, MSc, PhD, DSc, FIAC, FRSM, FAAA
Professor Emeritus, Division of Anatomy, Department of Surgery
Former Professor and Chair, Department of Anatomy and Associate Dean for Basic Medical Sciences
Faculty of Medicine, University of Toronto, Toronto, Ontario, Canada
Former Professor and Head of Anatomy, Faculty of Medicine, University of Manitoba, Winnipeg, Manitoba, Canada

## T.V.N. (Vid) Persaud,
### MD, PhD, DSc, FRCPath (Lond.), FAAA
Professor Emeritus and Former Head, Department of Human Anatomy and Cell Science
Professor of Pediatrics and Child Health
Associate Professor of Obstetrics, Gynecology, and Reproductive Sciences, Faculty of Medicine,
University of Manitoba, Winnipeg, Manitoba, Canada
Professor of Anatomy, St. George's University, Grenada, West Indies

## Mark G. Torchia,
### MSc, PhD
Associate Professor and Director of Development, Department of Surgery
Associate Professor, Department of Human Anatomy and Cell Sciences
Director, Centre for the Advancement of Teaching and Learning, University of Manitoba,
Winnipeg, Manitoba, Canada

## ELSEVIER

# ELSEVIER

1600 John F. Kennedy Blvd.
Ste 1800
Philadelphia, PA 19103-2899

Previous editions copyrighted 2013, 2008, 2003, 1998, 1993, 1988, 1982, 1977, and 1973.

**Library of Congress Cataloging-in-Publication Data**
Moore, Keith L., author.
  The developing human : clinically oriented embryology / Keith L. Moore, T.V.N. (Vid) Persaud, Mark G. Torchia.—10th edition.
    p. ; cm.
  Includes bibliographical references and index.
  ISBN 978-0-323-31338-4 (pbk. : alk. paper)—ISBN 978-0-323-31347-6 (international edition : alk. paper)
  I. Persaud, T. V. N., author.  II. Torchia, Mark G., author.  III. Title.
  [DNLM:  1. Embryology. QS 604]
  QM601
  612.6′4018—dc23
                        2015001490

*Content Strategist:* Meghan Ziegler
*Senior Content Development Specialist:* Jennifer Ehlers
*Publishing Services Manager:* Patricia Tannian
*Senior Project Manager:* Kristine Feeherty
*Design Direction:* Margaret Reid

*The cover images show a magnetic resonance image of a 27-week-old fetus in the uterus (Courtesy Dr. Deborah Levine, Beth Israel Deaconess Medical Center, Boston, Massachusetts). The photograph of the baby (Kennedy Jackson) was taken 7 days after her birthday. She is wrapped in a knitted cocoon that symbolizes the uterus.*

Printed in the United States of America

Last digit is the print number:  9  8  7  6  5  4  3  2  1

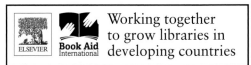

### In Loving Memory of Marion

*My best friend, wife, colleague, mother of our five children and grandmother of our nine grandchildren, for her love, unconditional support, and understanding. Wonderful memories keep you ever near our hearts.*

—*KLM and family*

### For Pam and Ron

*I should like to thank my eldest daughter, Pam, who assumed the office duties previously carried out by her mother, Marion. She has also been helpful in so many other ways (e.g., reviewing the text). I am also grateful to my son-in-law, Ron Crowe, whose technical skills have helped me utilize the new technology when I was improving this book.*

—*KLM*

### For Gisela

*My lovely wife and best friend, for her endless support and patience; our three children—Indrani, Sunita, and Rainer (Ren)—and grandchildren (Brian, Amy, and Lucas).*

—*TVNP*

### For Barbara, Muriel, and Erik

*Nothing could ever mean more to me than each of you. Thank you for your support and your love.*

—*MGT*

### For Our Students and Their Teachers

*To our students: We hope you will enjoy reading this book, increase your understanding of human embryology, pass all of your exams, and be excited and well prepared for your careers in patient care, research, and teaching. You will remember some of what you hear, much of what you read, more of what you see, and almost all of what you experience.*

*To their teachers: May this book be a helpful resource to you and your students.*
*We appreciate the numerous constructive comments we have received over the years from both students and teachers. Your remarks have been invaluable to us in improving this book.*

## CONTRIBUTORS

### David D. Eisenstat, MD, MA, FRCPC
Professor, Departments of Pediatrics, Medical Genetics
and Oncology, Faculty of Medicine and Dentistry,
University of Alberta; Director, Division of Pediatric
Immunology, Hematology, Oncology, Palliative Care,
and Environmental Health, Department of Pediatrics,
Stollery Children's Hospital and the University of
Alberta; Inaugural Chair, Muriel and Ada Hole Kids
with Cancer Society Chair in Pediatric Oncology,
Edmonton, Alberta, Canada

### Jeffrey T. Wigle, PhD
Principal Investigator, Institute of Cardiovascular
Sciences, St. Boniface Hospital Research Centre;
Associate Professor, Department of Biochemistry and
Medical Genetics, University of Manitoba, Winnipeg,
Manitoba, Canada

## CLINICAL REVIEWERS

### Albert E. Chudley, MD, FRCPC, FCCMG
Professor, Department of Pediatrics and Child Health;
Professor, Department of Biochemistry and Medical
Genetics, University of Manitoba, Winnipeg,
Manitoba, Canada

### Michael Narvey, MD, FRCPC, FAAP
Section Head, Neonatal Medicine, Health Sciences
Centre and St. Boniface Hospital; Associate Professor
of Pediatrics and Child Health, University of
Manitoba, Winnipeg, Manitoba, Canada

## FIGURES AND IMAGES (SOURCES)

We are grateful to the following colleagues for the clinical
images they have given us for this book and also for
granting us permission to use figures from their published
works:

### Steve Ahing, DDS
Faculty of Dentistry, University of Manitoba, Winnipeg,
Manitoba, Canada
*Figure 19-20F*

### Franco Antoniazzi, MD
Department of Pediatrics, University of Verona,
Verona, Italy
*Figure 20-4*

### Dean Barringer and Marnie Danzinger
*Figure 6-7*

### †Volker Becker, MD
Pathologisches Institut der Universität, Erlangen,
Germany
*Figures 7-18 and 7-21*

### J.V. Been, MD
Department of Pediatrics, Maastricht University
Medical Centre, Maastricht, The Netherlands
*Figure 10-7C*

### Beryl Benacerraf, MD
Diagnostic Ultrasound Associates, P.C., Boston,
Massachusetts, USA
*Figures 13-29A, 13-35A, and 13-37A*

### Kunwar Bhatnagar, MD
Department of Anatomical Sciences and Neurobiology,
School of Medicine University of Louisville,
Louisville, Kentucky, USA
*Figures 9-33, 9-34, and 19-10*

†Deceased.

**David Bolender, MD**
Department of Cell Biology, Neurobiology, and
  Anatomy, Medical College of Wisconsin, Milwaukee,
  Wisconsin, USA
  *Figure 14-14BC*

**Dr. Mario João Branco Ferreira**
Servico de Dermatologia, Hospital de Desterro, Lisbon,
  Portugal
  *Figure 19-5A*

**Albert E. Chudley, MD, FRCPC, FCCMG**
Department of Pediatrics and Child Health, Section of
  Genetics and Metabolism, Children's Hospital,
  University of Manitoba, Winnipeg, Manitoba,
  Canada
  *Figures 4-6, 9-38, 11-19AB, 11-28A, 12-24, 12-42, 12-43,
  14-11, 15-6, 16-13DE, 16-14, 16-15, 17-14, 17-33, 17-36,
  18-20, 18-21, 18-23, 19-9, 20-3, 20-5, 20-6CD, 20-7, 20-8,
  20-13, 20-14, 20-17, and 20-19A*

**Blaine M. Cleghorn, DMD, MSc**
Faculty of Dentistry, Dalhousie University, Halifax,
  Nova Scotia, Canada
  *Figures 19-19 and 19-20A-E*

**Dr. M.N. Golarz De Bourne**
St. George's University Medical School, True Blue,
  Grenada
  *Figure 11-21*

**Heather Dean, MD, FRCPC**
Department of Pediatrics and Child Health, University
  of Manitoba, Winnipeg, Manitoba, Canada
  *Figures 12-28 and 20-18*

**Marc Del Bigio, MD, PhD, FRCPC**
Department of Pathology (Neuropathology), University
  of Manitoba, Winnipeg, Manitoba, Canada
  *Figures 17-13, 17-29 (inset), 17-30BC, 17-32B, 17-37B,
  17-38, 17-40, and 17-42A*

**David D. Eisenstat, MD, MA, FRCPC**
Manitoba Institute of Cell Biology, Department of
  Human Anatomy and Cell Science, University of
  Manitoba, Winnipeg, Manitoba, Canada
  *Figure 17-2*

**Vassilios Fanos, MD**
Department of Pediatrics, University of Verona,
  Verona, Italy
  *Figure 20-4*

**João Carlos Fernandes Rodrigues, MD**
Servico de Dermatologia, Hospital de Desterro, Lisbon,
  Portugal
  *Figure 19-5B*

**Frank Gaillard, MB, BS, MMed**
Department of Radiology, Royal Melbourne Hospital,
  Australia
  *Figures 4-15 and 9-19B*

**Gary Geddes, MD**
Lake Oswego, Oregon, USA
  *Figure 14-14A*

**Barry H. Grayson, MD, and Bruno L. Vendittelli, MD**
New York University Medical Center, Institute of
  Reconstructive Plastic Surgery, New York,
  New York, USA
  *Figure 9-40*

**Christopher R. Harman, MD, FRCSC, FACOG**
Department of Obstetrics, Gynecology, and
  Reproductive Sciences, Women's Hospital and
  University of Maryland, Baltimore, Maryland, USA
  *Figures 7-17 and 12-23*

**†Jean Hay, MSc**
Department of Anatomy, University of Manitoba,
  Winnipeg, Manitoba, Canada
  *Figure 17-25*

**Blair Henderson, MD**
Department of Radiology, Health Sciences Centre,
  University of Manitoba, Winnipeg, Manitoba,
  Canada
  *Figure 13-6*

**Lyndon M. Hill, MD**
Magee-Women's Hospital, Pittsburgh, Pennsylvania, USA
  *Figures 11-7 and 12-14*

**†Klaus V. Hinrichsen, MD**
Medizinische Fakultät, Institut für Anatomie,
  Ruhr-Universität Bochum, Bochum, Germany
  *Figures 5-12A, 9-2, and 9-26*

**Dr. Jon and Mrs. Margaret Jackson**
  *Figure 6-9B*

---

†Deceased.

**Evelyn Jain, MD, FCFP**
Breastfeeding Clinic, Calgary, Alberta, Canada
*Figure 9-24*

**John A. Jane, Sr., MD**
David D. Weaver Professor of Neurosurgery,
Department of Neurological Surgery, University of
Virginia Health System, Charlottesville, Virginia, USA
*Figure 14-12*

**Robert Jordan, MD**
St. George's University Medical School, True Blue,
Grenada
*Figures 6-6B and 7-25*

**Linda J. Juretschke, MD**
Ronald McDonald Children's Hospital, Loyola
University Medical Center, Maywood, Illinois, USA
*Figure 7-31*

**Dagmar K. Kalousek, MD**
Department of Pathology, University of British
Columbia, Children's Hospital, Vancouver, British
Columbia, Canada
*Figures 8-11AB, 11-14A, 12-12C, 12-16, and 20-6AB*

**E.C. Klatt, MD**
Department of Biomedical Sciences, Mercer University
School of Medicine, Savannah, Georgia, USA
*Figure 7-16*

**Wesley Lee, MD**
Division of Fetal Imaging, William Beaumont Hospital,
Royal Oak, Michigan, USA
*Figures 13-20 and 13-30A*

**Deborah Levine, MD, FACR**
Departments of Radiology and Obstetric &
Gynecologic Ultrasound, Beth Israel Deaconess
Medical Center, Boston, Massachusetts, USA
*Figures 6-8, 6-15, 8-10, 9-43CD, 17-35B, and cover image
(magnetic resonance image of 27-week fetus)*

**E.A. (Ted) Lyons, OC, MD, FRCPC, FACR**
Departments of Radiology, Obstetrics & Gynecology,
and Human Anatomy & Cell Science, Division of
Ultrasound, Health Sciences Centre, University of
Manitoba, Winnipeg, Manitoba, Canada
*Figures 3-7, 3-9, 4-1, 4-13, 5-19, 6-1, 6-10, 6-12, 7-23,
7-26, 7-29, 11-19CD, 12-45, and 13-3*

**Margaret Morris, MD, FRCSC, MEd**
Professor of Obstetrics, Gynaecology, and Reproductive
Sciences, Women's Hospital and University of
Manitoba, Winnipeg, Manitoba, Canada
*Figure 12-46*

**Stuart C. Morrison, MD**
Section of Pediatric Radiology, The Children's Hospital,
Cleveland Clinic, Cleveland, Ohio, USA
*Figures 7-13, 11-20, 17-29E, and 17-41*

**John B. Mulliken, MD**
Children's Hospital Boston, Harvard Medical School,
Boston, Massachusetts, USA
*Figure 9-42*

**W. Jerry Oakes, MD**
Children's Hospital Birmingham, Birmingham,
Alabama, USA
*Figure 17-42B*

**†Dwight Parkinson, MD**
Departments of Surgery and Human Anatomy &
Cell Science, University of Manitoba, Winnipeg,
Manitoba, Canada
*Figure 17-14*

**Maulik S. Patel, MD**
Consultant Pathologist, Surat, India
*Figure 4-15*

**Dr. Susan Phillips**
Department of Pathology, Health Sciences Centre,
Winnipeg, Manitoba, Canada
*Figure 18-6*

**Srinivasa Ramachandra, MD**
*Figure 9-13A*

**†Dr. M. Ray**
Department of Human Genetics, University of
Manitoba, Winnipeg, Manitoba, Canada
*Figure 20-12B*

**Martin H. Reed, MD, FRCPC**
Department of Radiology, University of Manitoba and
Children's Hospital, Winnipeg, Manitoba, Canada
*Figure 11-27*

---

†Deceased.

**Gregory J. Reid, MD, FRCSC**
Department of Obstetrics, Gynecology, and
  Reproductive Sciences, University of Manitoba,
  Women's Hospital, Winnipeg, Manitoba, Canada
  *Figures 9-43AB, 11-18, 12-39, 13-12, and 14-9*

**Michael and Michele Rice**
  *Figure 6-9A*

**Dr. S.G. Robben**
Department of Radiology, Maastricht University
  Medical Centre, Maastricht, The Netherlands
  *Figure 10-7C*

**Prem S. Sahni, MD**
Formerly of the Department of Radiology, Children's
  Hospital, Winnipeg, Manitoba, Canada
  *Figures 8-11C, 10-7B, 10-13, 11-4C, 11-28B, 12-16,
  12-17, 12-19, 14-10, 14-15, and 16-13C*

**Dr. M.J. Schuurman**
Department of Pediatrics, Maastricht University
  Medical Centre, Maastricht, The Netherlands
  *Figure 10-7C*

**P. Schwartz and H.M. Michelmann**
University of Goettingen, Goettingen, Germany
  *Figure 2-13*

**Joseph R. Siebert, MD**
Children's Hospital and Regional Center, Seattle,
  Washington, USA
  *Figures 7-32, 13-36, 16-13B, and 17-16*

**Bradley R. Smith, MD**
University of Michigan, Ann Arbor, Michigan, USA
  *Figures 5-16C, 5-17C, 5-20C, 8-6B, 9-3A (inset), 14-13,
  and 18-18B*

**Gerald S. Smyser, MD**
Formerly of the Altru Health System, Grand Forks,
  North Dakota, USA
  *Figures 9-20, 13-45, 17-24, 17-32A, 17-34, 17-37A,
  and 18-24*

**Pierre Soucy, MD, FRCSC**
Division of Pediatric Surgery, Children's Hospital of
  Eastern Ontario, Ottawa, Ontario, Canada
  *Figures 9-10, 9-11, and 18-22*

**Dr. Y. Suzuki**
Achi, Japan
  *Figure 16-13A*

**R. Shane Tubbs, PhD**
Children's Hospital Birmingham, Birmingham,
  Alabama, USA
  *Figure 17-42B*

**Edward O. Uthman, MD**
Consultant Pathologist, Houston/Richmond,
  Texas, USA
  *Figure 3-11*

**Jeffrey T. Wigle, PhD**
Department of Biochemistry and Medical Genetics,
  University of Manitoba, Winnipeg, Manitoba,
  Canada
  *Figure 17-2*

**Nathan E. Wiseman, MD, FRCSC**
Pediatric Surgeon, Children's Hospital, Winnipeg,
  Manitoba, Canada
  *Figure 11-17A*

**M.T. Zenzes**
In Vitro Fertilization Program, Toronto Hospital,
  Toronto, Ontario, Canada
  *Figure 2-17A*

# Preface

We have entered an era of achievement in the fields of molecular biology, genetics, and clinical embryology, perhaps like no other. The sequencing of the human genome has been achieved and several mammalian species, as well as the human embryo, have been cloned. Scientists have created and isolated human embryonic stem cells, and their use in treating certain intractable diseases continues to generate widespread debate. These remarkable scientific developments have already provided promising directions for research in human embryology, which will have an impact on medical practice in the future.

The 10th edition of *The Developing Human* has been thoroughly revised to reflect current understanding of some of the molecular events that guide development of the embryo. This book also contains more *clinically oriented material* than previous editions; these sections are set as blue boxes to differentiate them from the rest of the text. In addition to focusing on clinically relevant aspects of embryology, we have revised the Clinically Oriented Problems with brief answers and added more case studies online that emphasize the importance of embryology in modern medical practice.

This edition follows the official international list of embryologic terms (*Terminologia Embryologica*, Georg Thieme Verlag, 2013). It is important that physicians and scientists throughout the world use the same name for each structure.

This edition includes numerous new color photographs of embryos (normal and abnormal). Many of the illustrations have been improved using three-dimensional renderings and more effective use of colors. There are also many new diagnostic images (ultrasound and magnetic resonance image) of embryos and fetuses to illustrate their three-dimensional aspects. *An innovative set of 18 animations* that will help students understand the complexities of embryologic development now comes with this book. When one of the animations is especially relevant to a passage in the text, the icon has been added in the margin. Maximized animations are available to teachers who have adopted *The Developing Human* for their lectures (consult your Elsevier representative).

The coverage of **teratology** (studies concerned with birth defects) has been increased because the study of abnormal development of embryos and fetuses is helpful in understanding risk estimation, the causes of birth defects, and how malformations may be prevented. Recent advances in the molecular aspects of developmental biology have been highlighted (in *italics*) throughout the book, especially in those areas that appear promising for clinical medicine or have the potential for making a significant impact on the direction of future research.

We have continued our attempts to provide an easy-to-read account of human development before birth and during the neonatal period (1 to 28 days). Every chapter has been thoroughly reviewed and revised to reflect new findings in research and their clinical significance.

The chapters are organized to present a systematic and logical approach to embryo development. The first chapter introduces readers to the scope and importance of embryology, the historical background of the discipline, and the terms used to describe the stages of development. The next four chapters cover embryonic development, beginning with the formation of gametes and ending with the formation of basic organs and systems. The development of specific organs and systems is then described in a systematic manner, followed by chapters dealing with the highlights of the fetal period, the placenta and fetal membranes, the causes of human birth defects, and common signaling pathways used during development. At the end of each chapter there are summaries of key features, which provide a convenient means of ongoing review. There are also references that contain both classic works and recent research publications.

*Keith L. Moore*
*T.V.N. (Vid) Persaud*
*Mark G. Torchia*

# Acknowledgments

*The Developing Human* is widely used by medical, dental, and many other students in the health sciences. The suggestions, constructive criticisms, and comments we received from instructors and students around the world have helped us improve this 10th edition.

When learning embryology, the illustrations are an essential feature to facilitate both understanding of the subject and retention of the material. Many figures have been improved, and newer clinical images replace older ones.

We are indebted to the following colleagues (listed alphabetically) for either critical reviewing of chapters, making suggestions for improvement of this book, or providing some of the new figures: Dr. Steve Ahing, Faculty of Dentistry, University of Manitoba, Winnipeg; Dr. Albert Chudley, Departments of Pediatrics & Child Health and Biochemistry & Medical Genetics, University of Manitoba, Winnipeg; Dr. Blaine M. Cleghorn, Faculty of Dentistry, Dalhousie University, Halifax, Nova Scotia; Dr. Frank Gaillard, Radiopaedia.org, Toronto, Ontario; Dr. Ray Gasser, Faculty of Medicine, Louisiana State University Medical Center, New Orleans; Dr. Boris Kablar, Department of Anatomy and Neurobiology, Dalhousie University, Halifax, Nova Scotia; Dr. Sylvia Kogan, Department of Ophthalmology, University of Manitoba, Winnipeg, Manitoba; Dr. Peeyush Lala, Faculty of Medicine, Western University, Ontario, London, Ontario; Dr. Deborah Levine, Beth Israel Deaconess Medical Center, Boston, Massachusetts; Dr. Marios Loukas, St. George's University, Grenada; Dr. Stuart Morrison, Department of Radiology, Cleveland Clinic, Cleveland, Ohio; Professor Bernard J. Moxham, Cardiff School of Biosciences, Cardiff University, Cardiff, Wales; Dr. Michael Narvey, Department of Pediatrics and Child Health, University of Manitoba, Winnipeg, Manitoba; Dr. Drew Noden, Department of Biomedical Sciences, Cornell University, College of Veterinary Medicine, Ithaca, New York; Dr. Shannon Perry, School of Nursing, San Francisco State University, California; Dr. Gregory Reid, Department of Obstetrics, Gynecology, and Reproductive Sciences, University of Manitoba, Winnipeg; Dr. L. Ross, Department of Neurobiology and Anatomy, University of Texas Medical School, Houston, Texas; Dr. J. Elliott Scott, Departments of Oral Biology and Human Anatomy & Cell Science, University of Manitoba, Winnipeg; Dr. Brad Smith, University of Michigan, Ann Arbor, Michigan; Dr. Gerald S. Smyser, formerly of the Altru Health System, Grand Forks, North Dakota; Dr. Richard Shane Tubbs, Children's Hospital, Birmingham, Alabama; Dr. Ed Uthman, Clinical Pathologist, Houston/Richmond, Texas; and Dr. Michael Wiley, Division of Anatomy, Department of Surgery, Faculty of Medicine, University of Toronto, Toronto, Ontario. The new illustrations were prepared by Hans Neuhart, President of the Electronic Illustrators Group in Fountain Hills, Arizona.

The stunning collection of animations of developing embryos was produced in collaboration with Dr. David L. Bolender, Associate Professor, Department of Cell Biology, Neurobiology, and Anatomy, Medical College of Wisconsin. We would like to thank him for his efforts in design and in-depth review, as well as his invaluable advice. Our special thanks go to Ms. Carol Emery for skillfully coordinating the project.

At Elsevier, we are indebted to Ms. Meghan K. Ziegler, Content Strategist, for her continued interest and encouragement, and we are especially thankful to Ms. Kelly McGowan, Content Development Specialist, for her invaluable insights and many helpful suggestions. Their unstinting support during the preparation of this new edition was greatly appreciated. Finally, we should also like to thank Ms. Kristine Feeherty, Project Manager; Ms. Maggie Reid, Designer; Ms. Amy Naylor, Art Buyer; and Ms. Thapasya Ramkumar, Multimedia Producer, at Elsevier for nurturing this book to completion. This new edition of *The Developing Human* is the result of their dedication and technical expertise.

*Keith L. Moore*
*T.V.N. (Vid) Persaud*
*Mark G. Torchia*

# Contents

# Introduction to Human Development

**H**uman development is a continuous process that begins when an **oocyte** (ovum) from a female is fertilized by a **sperm** (spermatozoon) from a male (Fig. 1-1). Cell division, cell migration, programmed cell death (apoptosis), differentiation, growth, and cell rearrangement transform the fertilized oocyte, a highly specialized, totipotent cell, a **zygote**, into a multicellular human being. Most changes occur during the embryonic and fetal periods; however, important changes occur during later periods of development: neonatal period (first 4 weeks), infancy (first year), childhood (2 years to puberty), and adolescence (11 to 19 years). Development does not stop at birth; other changes, in addition to growth, occur after birth (e.g., development of teeth and female breasts).

## DEVELOPMENTAL PERIODS

It is customary to divide human development into **prenatal** (before birth) and **postnatal** (after birth) periods. The development of a human from fertilization of an oocyte to birth is divided into two main periods, **embryonic** and **fetal**. The main changes that occur prenatally are illustrated in the Timetable of Human Prenatal Development (see Fig. 1-1). Examination of the timetable reveals that the most *visible* advances occur during the third to eighth weeks— the embryonic period. During the fetal period, differentiation and growth of tissues and organs occur and the rate of body growth increases.

## Stages of Embryonic Development

Early development is described in stages because of the variable period it takes for embryos to develop certain morphologic characteristics. Stage 1 begins at fertilization and embryonic development ends at stage 23, which occurs on day 56 (see Fig. 1-1). A **trimester** is a period of 3 months, one third of the 9-month period of gestation. The most critical stages of development occur during the first trimester (13 weeks), when embryonic and early fetal development is occurring.

## Postnatal Period

This is the period occurring after birth. Explanations of frequently used developmental terms and periods follow.

## Infancy

This is the period of extrauterine life, roughly the first year after birth. An **infant** age 1 month or younger is called a **neonate**. Transition from intrauterine to extrauterine existence requires many critical changes, especially in the cardiovascular and respiratory systems. If neonates survive the first crucial hours after birth, their chances of living are usually good. The body grows rapidly during infancy; total length increases by approximately one half and weight is usually tripled. By 1 year of age, most infants have six to eight teeth.

## Childhood

This is the period between infancy and puberty. The primary (deciduous) teeth continue to appear and are later replaced by the secondary (permanent) teeth. During early childhood, there is active ossification (formation of bone), but as the child becomes older, the rate of body growth slows down. Just before puberty, however, growth accelerates—the **prepubertal growth spurt**.

## Puberty

This is the period when humans become functionally capable of procreation (reproduction). Reproduction is

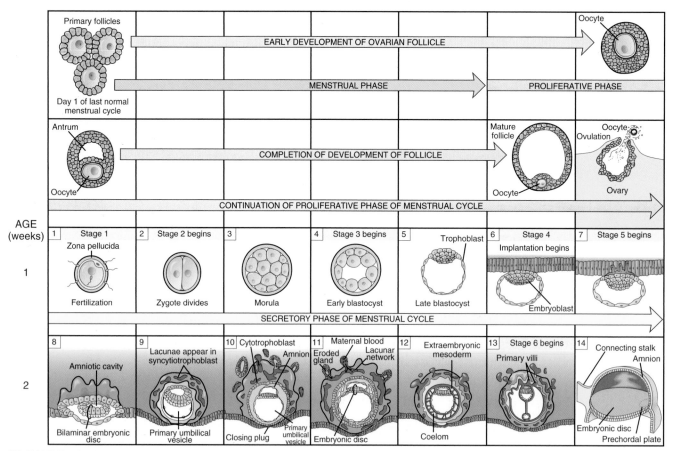

**FIGURE 1−1** Early stages of development. Development of an ovarian follicle containing an oocyte, ovulation, and the phases of the menstrual cycle are illustrated. Human development begins at fertilization, approximately 14 days after the onset of the last normal menstrual period. Cleavage of the zygote in the uterine tube, implantation of the blastocyst in the endometrium (lining) of the uterus, and early development of the embryo are also shown. The alternative term for the umbilical vesicle is the yolk sac; this is an inappropriate term because the human vesicle does not contain yolk.

AGE (weeks)

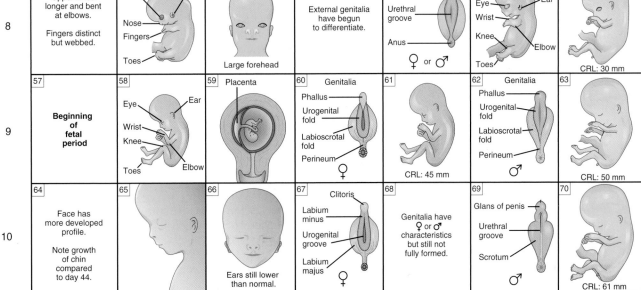

**FIGURE 1–1, cont'd**

the process by which organisms produce children. In **females,** the first signs of puberty may be after age 8; in **males,** puberty commonly begins at age 9.

## Adulthood

Attainment of full growth and maturity is generally reached between the ages of 18 and 21 years. Ossification and growth are virtually completed during early adulthood (21 to 25 years).

## SIGNIFICANCE OF EMBRYOLOGY

**Clinically oriented embryology** refers to the study of embryos; the term generally means prenatal development of embryos, fetuses, and neonates (infants aged 1 month and younger). **Developmental anatomy** refers to the structural changes of a human from fertilization to adulthood; it includes embryology, fetology, and postnatal development. **Teratology** is the division of embryology and pathology that deals with abnormal development (birth defects). This branch of embryology is concerned with various genetic and/or environmental factors that disturb normal development and produce birth defects (see Chapter 20).

**Clinically oriented embryology:**

- Bridges the gap between prenatal development and obstetrics, perinatal medicine, pediatrics, and clinical anatomy
- Develops knowledge concerning the beginnings of life and the changes occurring during prenatal development
- Builds an understanding of the causes of variations in human structure
- Illuminates clinically oriented anatomy and explains how normal and abnormal relations develop
- Supports the research and application of stem cells for treatment of certain chronic diseases

Knowledge that physicians have of normal development and the causes of birth defects is necessary for giving the embryo and fetus the best possible chance of developing normally. Much of the modern practice of obstetrics involves **applied embryology.** Embryologic topics of special interest to *obstetricians* are oocyte and sperm transport, ovulation, fertilization, implantation, fetal-maternal relations, fetal circulation, critical periods of development, and causes of birth defects.

In addition to caring for the mother, physicians guard the health of the embryo and fetus. The significance of embryology is readily apparent to *pediatricians* because some of their patients have birth defects resulting from maldevelopment, such as diaphragmatic hernia, spina bifida cystica, and congenital heart disease.

**Birth defects cause most deaths during infancy.** Knowledge of the development of structure and function is essential for understanding the physiologic changes that occur during the neonatal period (first 4 weeks) and for helping fetuses and neonates in distress. Progress in surgery, especially in the fetal, perinatal, and pediatric age groups, has made knowledge of human development even more clinically significant. *Surgical treatment of fetuses is now possible in some situations.* The understanding and correction of most defects depend on knowledge of normal development and the deviations that may occur. An understanding of common congenital birth defects and their causes also enables physicians, nurses, and other health-care providers to explain the developmental basis of birth defects, often dispelling parental guilt feelings.

Health-care professionals who are aware of common birth defects and their embryologic basis approach unusual situations with confidence rather than surprise. For example, when it is realized that the renal artery represents only one of several vessels originally supplying the embryonic kidney, the frequent variations in the number and arrangement of renal vessels are understandable and not unexpected.

## HISTORICAL GLEANINGS

*If I have seen further, it is by standing on the shoulders of giants.*
– Sir Isaac Newton, English mathematician, 1643–1727

This statement, made more than 300 years ago, emphasizes that each new study of a problem rests on a base of knowledge established by earlier investigators. The theories of every age offer explanations based on the knowledge and experience of investigators of the period. Although we should not consider them final, we should appreciate rather than scorn their ideas. People have always been interested in knowing how they developed and were born and why some embryos and fetuses develop abnormally. Ancient people developed many answers to the reasons for these birth defects.

### Ancient Views of Human Embryology

Egyptians of the Old Kingdom, approximately 3000 BC, knew of methods for incubating birds' eggs, but they left no records. **Akhnaton** (Amenophis IV) praised the sun god Aton as the creator of the germ in a woman, maker of the seed in man, and giver of life to the son in the body of his mother. The ancient Egyptians believed that the soul entered the infant at birth through the placenta.

A brief Sanskrit treatise on **ancient Indian embryology** is thought to have been written in 1416 BC. This scripture of the Hindus, called **Garbha Upanishad,** describes ancient views concerning the embryo. It states:

*From the conjugation of blood and semen (seed), the embryo comes into existence. During the period favorable for conception, after the sexual intercourse, (it) becomes a Kalada (one-day-old embryo). After remaining seven nights, it becomes a vesicle. After a fortnight it becomes a spherical mass. After a month it becomes a firm mass. After two months the head is formed. After three months the limb regions appear.*

**Greek scholars** made many important contributions to the science of embryology. The first recorded embryologic studies are in the books of **Hippocrates of Cos,** the famous Greek physician (circa 460–377 BC), who is regarded as the *father of medicine.* In order to understand how the human embryo develops, he recommended:

*Take twenty or more eggs and let them be incubated by two or more hens. Then each day from the second to that of hatching, remove an egg, break it, and examine it. You will find exactly as I say, for the nature of the bird can be likened to that of man.*

**Aristotle of Stagira** (circa 384–322 BC), a Greek philosopher and scientist, wrote a treatise on embryology in which he described development of the chick and other embryos. Aristotle promoted the idea that the embryo developed from a formless mass, which he described as a "less fully concocted seed with a nutritive soul and all bodily parts." This embryo, he thought, arose from menstrual blood after activation by male semen.

**Claudius Galen** (circa 130–201 AD), a Greek physician and medical scientist in Rome, wrote a book, *On the Formation of the Foetus*, in which he described the development and nutrition of fetuses and the structures that we now call the allantois, amnion, and placenta.

The **Talmud** contains references to the formation of the embryo. The Jewish physician **Samuel-el-Yehudi,** who lived during the second century AD, described six stages in the formation of the embryo from a "formless, rolled-up thing" to a "child whose months have been completed." Talmud scholars believed that the bones and tendons, the nails, the marrow in the head, and the white of the eyes, were derived from the father, "who sows the white," but the skin, flesh, blood, and hair were derived from the mother, "who sows the red." These views were according to the teachings of both Aristotle and Galen.

## Embryology in the Middle Ages

The growth of science was slow during the medieval period, but a few high points of embryologic investigation undertaken during this time are known to us. It is cited in the **Quran** (seventh century AD), the Holy Book of Islam, that human beings are produced from a mixture of secretions from the male and female. Several references are made to the creation of a human being from a *nutfa* (small drop). It also states that the resulting organism settles in the womb like a seed, 6 days after its beginning. Reference is made to the leech-like appearance of the early embryo. Later the embryo is said to resemble a "chewed substance."

**Constantinus Africanus of Salerno** (circa 1020–1087 AD) wrote a concise treatise entitled *De Humana Natura.* Africanus described the composition and sequential development of the embryo in relation to the planets and each month during pregnancy, a concept unknown in antiquity. Medieval scholars hardly deviated from the **theory of Aristotle**, which stated that the embryo was derived from menstrual blood and semen. Because of a lack of knowledge, drawings of the fetus in the uterus often showed a fully developed infant frolicking in the womb (Fig. 1-2).

## The Renaissance

**Leonardo da Vinci** (1452–1519) made accurate drawings of dissections of pregnant uteri containing fetuses

**FIGURE 1–2** A-G, Illustrations from Jacob Rueff's *De Conceptu et Generatione Hominis* (1554) showing the fetus developing from a coagulum of blood and semen in the uterus. This theory was based on the teachings of Aristotle, and it survived until the late 18th century. *(From Needham J: A history of embryology, ed 2, Cambridge, United Kingdom, 1934, Cambridge University Press; with permission of Cambridge University Press, England.)*

(Fig. 1-3). He introduced the quantitative approach to embryology by making measurements of prenatal growth.

It has been stated that the embryologic revolution began with the publication of William Harvey's book *De Generatione Animalium* in 1651. **Harvey** believed that the male seed or sperm, after entering the womb or uterus, became metamorphosed into an egg-like substance from which the embryo developed. Harvey (1578–1657) was greatly influenced by one of his professors at the University of Padua, **Fabricius of Acquapendente**, an Italian anatomist and embryologist who was *the first to study embryos from different species of animals*. Harvey examined chick embryos with simple lenses and made many new observations. He also studied the development of the fallow deer; however, when unable to observe early developmental stages, he concluded that embryos were secreted by the uterus. **Girolamo Fabricius** (1537–1619) wrote two major embryologic treatises, including one entitled *De Formato Foetu* (The Formed Fetus), which contained many illustrations of embryos and fetuses at different stages of development.

Early microscopes were simple but they opened an exciting new field of observation. In 1672, **Regnier de**

**FIGURE 1-3** Reproduction of Leonardo da Vinci's drawing made in the 15th century showing a fetus in a uterus that has been incised and opened.

**FIGURE 1-4** Copy of a 17th-century drawing of a sperm by Hartsoeker. The miniature human being within it was thought to enlarge after the sperm entered an ovum. Other embryologists at this time thought the oocyte contained a miniature human being that enlarged when it was stimulated by a sperm.

**Graaf** observed small chambers in the rabbit's uterus and concluded that they could not have been secreted by the uterus. He stated that they must have come from organs that he called ovaries. Undoubtedly, the small chambers that de Graaf described were blastocysts (see Fig. 1-1). He also described follicles which were called graafian follicles; they are now called vesicular ovarian follicles.

**Marcello Malpighi**, studying what he believed was unfertilized hen's eggs in 1675, observed early embryos. As a result, he thought the egg contained a miniature chick. A young medical student in Leiden, **Johan Ham van Arnheim**, and his countryman **Anton van Leeuwenhoek**, using an improved microscope in 1677, *first observed human sperms*. However, they misunderstood the sperm's role in fertilization. They thought the sperm contained a miniature preformed human being that enlarged when it was deposited in the female genital tract (Fig. 1-4).

**Caspar Friedrich Wolff** refuted both versions of the preformation theory in 1759, after observing that parts of the embryo develop from "globules" (small spherical bodies). He examined unincubated eggs but could not see the embryos described by Malpighi. He proposed the layer concept, whereby division of what we call the zygote produces layers of cells (now called the **embryonic disc**) from which the embryo develops. His ideas formed the basis of the theory of **epigenesis**, which states that "development results from growth and differentiation of specialized cells." These important discoveries first appeared in Wolff's doctoral dissertation *Theoria Generationis*. He also observed embryonic masses of tissue that partly contribute to the development of the urinary and genital systems—wolffian bodies and wolffian ducts—now called the mesonephros and mesonephric ducts, respectively (see Chapter 12).

The preformation controversy ended in 1775 when **Lazzaro Spallanzani** showed that both the oocyte and sperm were necessary for initiating the development of a new individual. From his experiments, including artificial insemination in dogs, he concluded that the sperm was the fertilizing agent that initiated the developmental processes. **Heinrich Christian Pander** discovered the three germ layers of the embryo, which he named the blastoderm. He reported this discovery in 1817 in his doctoral dissertation.

**Etienne Saint Hilaire** and his son, **Isidore Saint Hilaire**, made the first significant studies of abnormal development in 1818. They performed experiments in animals that were designed to produce birth defects, initiating what we now know as the science of teratology.

**Karl Ernst von Baer** described the oocyte in the ovarian follicle of a dog in 1827, approximately 150 years after the discovery of sperms. He also observed cleaving zygotes in the uterine tube and blastocysts in the uterus. He contributed new knowledge about the origin of tissues and organs from the layers described earlier by Malpighi and Pander. **Von Baer** formulated two important embryologic concepts, namely, that corresponding stages of embryonic development and that general characteristics precede specific ones. His significant and far-reaching contributions resulted in his being regarded as the *father of modern embryology*.

**Matthias Schleiden** and **Theodor Schwann** were responsible for great advances being made in embryology when they *formulated the cell theory* in 1839. This concept stated that the body is composed of cells and cell products. The cell theory soon led to the realization that the embryo developed from a single cell, the **zygote**, which underwent many cell divisions as the tissues and organs formed.

**Wilhelm His** (1831–1904), a Swiss anatomist and embryologist, developed improved techniques for fixation, sectioning, and staining of tissues and for reconstruction of embryos. His method of graphic reconstruction paved the way for producing current three-dimensional, stereoscopic, and computer-generated images of embryos.

**Franklin P. Mall** (1862–1917), inspired by the work of Wilhelm His, began to collect human embryos for scientific study. Mall's collection forms a part of the **Carnegie Collection of embryos** that is known throughout the world. It is now in the National Museum of Health and Medicine in the Armed Forces Institute of Pathology in Washington, DC.

**Wilhelm Roux** (1850–1924) pioneered analytic experimental studies on the physiology of development in amphibia, which was pursued further by **Hans Spemann** (1869–1941). For his discovery of the phenomenon of primary induction—how one tissue determines the fate of another—Spemann received the Nobel Prize in 1935. Over the decades, scientists have been isolating the substances that are transmitted from one tissue to another, causing induction.

**Robert G. Edwards** and **Patrick Steptoe** pioneered one of the most revolutionary developments in the history of human reproduction: the technique of **in vitro fertilization**. These studies resulted in the birth of Louise Brown, the first "test tube baby," in 1978. Since then, many millions of couples throughout the world, who were considered infertile, have experienced the birth of their children because of this new reproductive technology.

## GENETICS AND HUMAN DEVELOPMENT

In 1859, **Charles Darwin** (1809–1882), an English biologist and evolutionist, published his book *On the Origin of Species*, in which he emphasized the hereditary nature of variability among members of a species as an important factor in evolution. **Gregor Mendel**, an Austrian monk, developed the principles of heredity in 1865, but medical scientists and biologists did not understand the significance of these principles in the study of mammalian development for many years.

**Walter Flemming** observed chromosomes in 1878 and suggested their probable role in fertilization. In 1883, **Eduard von Beneden** observed that mature germ cells have a reduced number of chromosomes. He also described some features of meiosis, the process whereby the chromosome number is reduced in germ cells.

**Walter Sutton** (1877–1916) and **Theodor Boveri** (1862–1915) declared independently in 1902 that the behavior of chromosomes during germ cell formation and fertilization agreed with Mendel's principles of inheritance. In the same year, **Garrod** reported alcaptonuria (a genetic disorder of phenylalanine-tyrosine metabolism) as the *first example of mendelian inheritance* in human beings. Many geneticists consider **Sir Archibald Garrod** (1857–1936) the *father of medical genetics*. It was soon realized that the zygote contains all the genetic information necessary for directing the development of a new human being.

**Felix von Winiwarter** reported the first observations on human chromosomes in 1912, stating that there were 47 chromosomes in body cells. **Theophilus Shickel Painter** concluded in 1923 that 48 was the correct number, a conclusion that was widely accepted until 1956, when **Joe Hin Tjio** and **Albert Levan** reported finding only 46 chromosomes in embryonic cells.

**James Watson** and **Francis Crick** deciphered the molecular structure of DNA in 1953, and in 2000, the *human genome was sequenced*. The biochemical nature of the genes on the 46 human chromosomes has been decoded. Chromosome studies were soon used in medicine in a number of ways, including clinical diagnosis, chromosome mapping, and prenatal diagnosis.

Once the normal chromosomal pattern was firmly established, it soon became evident that some persons with congenital birth defects had an abnormal number of chromosomes. A new era in medical genetics resulted from the demonstration by **Jérôme Jean Louis Marie Lejeune** and associates in 1959 that infants with **Down syndrome** (**trisomy 21**) have 47 chromosomes instead of the usual 46 in their body cells. It is now known that chromosomal aberrations are a significant cause of birth defects and embryonic death (see Chapter 20).

In 1941, **Sir Norman Gregg** reported an "unusual number of cases of cataracts" and other birth defects in infants whose mothers had contracted rubella (caused by the **rubella virus**) in early pregnancy. For the first time, concrete evidence was presented showing that the development of the human embryo could be adversely affected by an environmental factor. Twenty years later, **Widukind Lenz** and **William McBride** reported rare limb deficiencies and other severe birth defects, induced by the sedative **thalidomide**, in the infants of mothers who had ingested the drug. The **thalidomide tragedy** alerted the public and health-care providers to the potential hazards of drugs, chemicals, and other environmental factors during pregnancy (see Chapter 20).

Sex chromatin was discovered in 1949 by **Dr. Murray Barr** and his graduate student **Ewart (Mike) Bertram** at Western University in London, Ontario, Canada. Their research revealed that the nuclei of nerve cells of female cats had sex chromatin and that cats that did not have sex chromatin were males. The next step was to determine if a similar phenomenon existed in human neurons. **Keith L. Moore**, who joined Dr. Barr's research group in 1950, discovered that sex chromatin patterns existed in somatic cells of humans and many representatives of the animal kingdom. He also developed a **buccal smear sex chromatin test** that is used clinically. This research forms the basis of several techniques currently used worldwide for the screening and diagnosis of human genetic conditions.

## MOLECULAR BIOLOGY OF HUMAN DEVELOPMENT

Rapid advances in the field of molecular biology have led to the application of sophisticated techniques (e.g., recombinant DNA technology, RNA genomic hybridization, chimeric models, transgenic mice, and stem cell manipulation). These techniques are now widely used in research laboratories to address such diverse problems as the genetic regulation of morphogenesis, the temporal and regional expression of specific genes, and how cells are committed to form the various parts of the embryo. For the first time, we are beginning to understand how, when, and where selected genes are activated and expressed in the embryo during normal and abnormal development (see Chapter 21).

The first mammal, a sheep named **Dolly**, was cloned in 1997 by **Ian Wilmut** and his colleagues using the technique of somatic cell nuclear transfer. Since then, other animals have been successfully cloned from cultured differentiated adult cells. Interest in human cloning has generated considerable debate because of social, ethical, and legal implications. Moreover, there is concern that cloning may result in neonates with birth defects and serious diseases.

*Human embryonic stem cells are pluripotential,* capable of self-renewal and able to differentiate into specialized cell types. The isolation and reprogrammed culture of human embryonic stem cells hold great potential for the treatment of chronic diseases, including amyotrophic lateral sclerosis, Alzheimer disease, and Parkinson disease as well as other degenerative, malignant, and genetic disorders (see National Institute of Health Guidelines on Human Stem Cell Research, 2009).

## HUMAN BIOKINETIC EMBRYOLOGY

In the middle of the last century a series of precise reconstructions were made of the surface ectoderm and all organs and cavities within human embryos at representative stages of development. They provided holistic views of human development and revealed new findings on the movements that occur from one stage to the next (Blechschmidt and Gasser, 1978). Because all movement is caused by force (biokinetics), the forces acting where specific tissues arise were discovered to take place simultaneously at every level of magnification, in the cell membrane all the way to the surface of the embryo. The movements and forces bring about differentiation that begins on the outside of the cell and then moves to the inside to react with the nucleus. The nucleus responds to various stimuli at particular times and in specific ways. Specific movements and forces act as regions differentiate. The forces act in regions named *metabolic fields*. New terms were needed to describe the unique forces acting in each field. Eight late metabolic fields were discovered where specific tissues differentiate from either mesenchyme or epithelium. The name of each field and the specific tissue that arises are as follows: condensation = mesenchymal condensation; contusion = precartilage; distussion = cartilage; dilation = muscle; retension = fibrous tissue; detraction = bone; corrosion = epithelial breakdown; and parathelial loosening = glands. The movements and forces begin at fertilization and continue throughout life (e.g., the cell membrane of the fertilized oocyte [ovum] moves inward, marking the beginning of cleavage).

## DESCRIPTIVE TERMS IN EMBRYOLOGY

The English equivalents of the standard Latin forms of terms are given in some cases, such as sperm (spermatozoon). The Federative International Committee on Anatomical Terminology does not recommend the use of **eponyms** (a word derived from someone's name), but they are commonly used clinically; hence, they appear in parentheses, such as uterine tube (fallopian tube). In anatomy and embryology, several terms relating to position and direction are used and reference is made to various planes of the body. All descriptions of the adult are based on the assumption that the body is erect, with the upper limbs by the sides and the palms directed anteriorly (Fig. 1-5A). This is the **anatomical position.**

The terms *anterior* or *ventral* and *posterior* or *dorsal* are used to describe the front or back of the body or limbs and the relations of structures within the body to one another. When describing embryos, the terms *ventral* and *dorsal* are used (see Fig. 1-5B). *Superior* and *inferior* are used to indicate the relative levels of different structures (see Fig. 1-5A). For embryos, the terms *cranial* (or *rostral*) and *caudal* are used to denote relationships to the head and caudal eminence (tail), respectively (see Fig. 1-5B). Distances from the center of the body or the source or attachment of a structure are designated as *proximal* (nearest) or *distal* (farthest). In the lower limb, for example, the knee is proximal to the ankle and distal to the hip.

The *median plane* is an imaginary vertical plane of section that passes longitudinally through the body. *Median sections* divide the body into right and left halves (see Fig. 1-5C). The terms *lateral* and *medial* refer to structures that are, respectively, farther from or nearer to the median plane of the body. A *sagittal plane* is any vertical plane passing through the body that is parallel to the median plane (see Fig. 1-5C). A *transverse (axial) plane* refers to any plane that is at right angles to both the median and coronal planes (see Fig. 1-5D). A *frontal (coronal) plane* is any vertical plane that intersects the median plane at a right angle (see Fig. 1-5E) and divides the body into anterior or ventral and posterior or dorsal parts.

## CLINICALLY ORIENTED PROBLEMS

* What sequence of events occurs during puberty? Are the events the same in males and females? At what age does presumptive puberty occur in males and females?
* How do the terms *embryology* and *teratology* differ?
* What is the difference between the terms *egg, ovum, ovule, gamete,* and *oocyte*?

Discussion of these problems appears in the Appendix at the back of the book.

**FIGURE 1–5** Drawings illustrating descriptive terms of position, direction, and planes of the body. **A,** Lateral view of an adult in the anatomical position. **B,** Lateral view of a 5-week embryo. **C** and **D,** Ventral views of a 6-week embryo. **E,** Lateral view of a 7-week embryo. In describing development, it is necessary to use words denoting the position of one part to another or to the body as a whole. For example, the vertebral column (spine) develops in the dorsal part of the embryo and the sternum (breast bone) develops in the ventral part of the embryo.

## BIBLIOGRAPHY AND SUGGESTED READING

Allen GE: Inducers and "organizers": Hans Spemann and experimental embryology, *Hist Philos Life Sci* 15:229, 1993.

Anon (Voices): Stem cells in translation, *Cell* 153:1177, 2013.

Blechschmidt E, Gasser RF: *Biokinetics and biodynamics of human differentiation: principles and applications,* Springfield, Illinois, 1978, Charles C. Thomas. (Republished Berkeley, California, 2012, North Atlantic Books.)

Chen KG, Mallon BS, Mckay RD, et al: Human pluripotent stem cell culture: considerations for maintenance, expansion, and therapeutics, *Cell Stem Cell* 14:13, 2014.

Churchill FB: The rise of classical descriptive embryology, *Dev Biol (N Y)* 7:1, 1991.

Daughtry B1, Mitalipov S: Concise review: parthenote stem cells for regenerative medicine: genetic, epigenetic, and developmental features, *Stem Cells Transl Med* 3:290, 2014.

Dunstan GR, editor: *The human embryo: Aristotle and the Arabic and European traditions*, Exeter, United Kingdom, 1990, University of Exeter Press.

Gasser R: *Atlas of human embryos*, Hagerstown, Md, 1975, Harper & Row.

Hopwood N: A history of normal plates, tables and stages in vertebrate embryology, *Int J Dev Biol* 51:1, 2007.

Horder TJ, Witkowski JA, Wylie CC, editors: *A history of embryology*, Cambridge, 1986, Cambridge University Press.

Hovatta O, Stojkovic M, Nogueira M, et al: European scientific, ethical and legal issues on human stem cell research and regenerative medicine, *Stem Cells* 28:1005, 2010.

Kohl F, von Baer KE: 1792–1876. Zum 200. Geburtstag des "Vaters der Embryologie, *Dtsch Med Wochenschr* 117:1976, 1992.

Leeb C, Jurga M, McGuckin C, et al: New perspectives in stem cell research: beyond embryonic stem cells, *Cell Prolif* 44(Suppl 1):9, 2011.

Meyer AW: *The rise of embryology*, Stanford, California, 1939, Stanford University Press.

Moore KL, Persaud TVN, Shiota K: *Color atlas of clinical embryology*, ed 2, Philadelphia, 2000, Saunders.

Murillo-Gonzalés J: Evolution of embryology: a synthesis of classical, experimental, and molecular perspectives, *Clin Anat* 14:158, 2001.

Needham J: *A history of embryology*, ed 2, Cambridge, United Kingdom, 1959, Cambridge University Press.

Nusslein-Volhard C: *Coming to life: how genes drive development*, Carlsbad, Calif, 2006, Kales Press.

O'Rahilly R: One hundred years of human embryology. In Kalter H, editor: *Issues and reviews in teratology*, vol 4, New York, 1988, Plenum Press.

O'Rahilly R, Müller F: *Developmental stages in human embryos*, Washington, DC, 1987, Carnegie Institution of Washington.

Persaud TVN, Tubbs RS, Loukas M: *A history of human anatomy*, ed 2, Springfield, Ill, 2014, Charles C. Thomas.

Pinto-Correia C: *The ovary of Eve: egg and sperm and preformation*, Chicago, 1997, University of Chicago Press.

Slack JMW: *Essential developmental biology*, ed 3, Hoboken, NJ, 2012, Wiley-Blackwell.

Slack JMW: *Stem cells: a very short introduction*, Oxford, United Kingdom, 2012, Oxford University Press.

Smith A: Cell biology: potency unchained, *Nature* 505:622, 2014.

Streeter GL: Developmental horizons in human embryos: description of age group XI, 13 to 20 somites, and age group XII, 21 to 29 somites, *Contrib Embryol Carnegie Inst* 30:211, 1942.

Zech NH, Preisegger KH, Hollands P: Stem cell therapeutics—reality versus hype and hope, *J Assist Reprod Genet* 28:287, 2011.

# First Week of Human Development

*He who sees things grow from the beginning will have the finest view of them.*

—Aristotle, 384–322 BC

**H**uman development begins at fertilization when a sperm fuses with an oocyte to form a single cell, the **zygote**. This highly specialized, *totipotent cell* (capable of giving rise to any cell type) marks the beginning of each of us as a unique individual. The zygote, just visible to the unaided eye, contains chromosomes and genes that are derived from the mother and father. The zygote divides many times and becomes progressively transformed into a multicellular human being through cell division, migration, growth, and differentiation.

## GAMETOGENESIS

Gametogenesis (gamete formation) is the process of formation and development of specialized generative cells, **gametes** (oocytes/sperms) from bipotential precursor cells. This development, involving the **chromosomes** and **cytoplasm** of the gametes, prepares these sex cells for fertilization. During **gametogenesis**, the chromosome number is reduced by half and the shape of the cells is altered (Fig. 2-1). A chromosome is defined by the presence of a **centromere**, the constricted portion of a chromosome. Before DNA replication in the S phase of the cell cycle, chromosomes exist as single-chromatid chromosomes (Fig. 2-2). A **chromatid** (one of a pair of chromosome strands) consists of parallel DNA strands. After DNA replication, chromosomes are double-chromatid chromosomes.

The sperm and oocyte (male and female gametes) are highly specialized sex cells. Each of these cells contains half the number of chromosomes (haploid number) that are present in somatic (body) cells. The number of chromosomes is reduced during **meiosis**, a special type of cell division that occurs only during **gametogenesis**. Gamete maturation is called spermatogenesis in males and oogenesis in females. The timing of events during meiosis differs in the two sexes.

## MEIOSIS

Meiosis is a special type of cell division that involves two meiotic cell divisions (see Fig. 2-2); diploid germ cells give rise to **haploid gametes** (sperms and oocytes).

The **first meiotic division** is a reduction division because the chromosome number is reduced from diploid to haploid by pairing of homologous chromosomes in **prophase** (first stage of meiosis) and their segregation at **anaphase** (stage when the chromosomes move from the equatorial plate). Homologous chromosomes, or **homologs** (one from each parent), pair during prophase and separate during anaphase, with one representative of each pair randomly going to each pole of the meiotic spindle (see Fig. 2-2*A* to *D*). The spindle connects to the chromosome at the **centromere** (the constricted part of the chromosome) (see Fig. 2-2*B*). At this stage, they are double-chromatid chromosomes.

*The X and Y chromosomes are not homologs*, but they have homologous segments at the tips of their short arms. They pair in these regions only. By the end of the first meiotic division, each new cell formed (**secondary oocyte**) has the haploid chromosome number, that is, half the number of chromosomes of the preceding cell. This separation or disjunction of paired homologous chromosomes is the physical basis of segregation, the separation of **allelic genes** (may occupy the same locus on a specific chromosome) during meiosis.

The **second meiotic division** (see Fig. 2-1) follows the first division without a normal interphase (i.e., without an intervening step of DNA replication). Each double-chromatid chromosome divides, and each half, or chromatid, is drawn to a different pole. Thus, the haploid number of chromosomes (23) is retained and each daughter cell formed by meiosis has one representative of each chromosome pair (now a single-chromatid chromosome). The second meiotic division is similar to an ordinary mitosis except that the chromosome number of the cell entering the second meiotic division is haploid.

Meiosis:

- Provides constancy of the chromosome number from generation to generation by reducing the chromosome number from diploid to haploid, thereby producing haploid gametes
- Allows random assortment of maternal and paternal chromosomes between the gametes
- Relocates segments of maternal and paternal chromosomes by crossing over of chromosome segments, which "shuffles" the genes and produces a recombination of genetic material

## ABNORMAL GAMETOGENESIS

Disturbances of meiosis during gametogenesis, such as nondisjunction (Fig. 2-3), result in the formation of chromosomally abnormal gametes. If involved in fertilization, these gametes with numeric chromosome abnormalities cause abnormal development, as occurs in infants with Down syndrome (see Chapter 20).

## SPERMATOGENESIS

Spermatogenesis is the sequence of events by which spermatogonia (primordial germ cells) are transformed into mature sperms; this maturation process begins at puberty (see Fig. 2-1). **Spermatogonia** are dormant in the seminiferous tubules of the testes during the fetal and postnatal periods (see Fig. 2-12). They increase in number during puberty. After several mitotic divisions, the spermatogonia grow and undergo changes.

Spermatogonia are transformed into **primary spermatocytes**, the largest germ cells in the seminiferous tubules of the testes (see Fig. 2-1). Each primary spermatocyte subsequently undergoes a reduction division—*the first meiotic division*—to form two haploid **secondary spermatocytes**, which are approximately half the size of primary spermatocytes. Subsequently, the secondary spermatocytes undergo a second meiotic division to form four **haploid spermatids**, which are approximately half the size of secondary spermatocytes (see Fig. 2-1). The spermatids (cells in a late stage of development of sperms) are gradually transformed into four **mature sperms** by a process known as **spermiogenesis** (Fig. 2-4). The entire process, which includes spermiogenesis, takes approximately 2 months. When spermiogenesis is complete, the sperms enter the lumina of the seminiferous tubules (see Fig. 2-12).

**Sertoli cells** lining the seminiferous tubules support and nurture the germ cells (sex cells—sperms/oocytes) and are involved in the regulation of spermatogenesis. Sperms are transported passively from the **seminiferous tubules** to the epididymis, where they are stored and become functionally mature during puberty.

## NORMAL GAMETOGENESIS

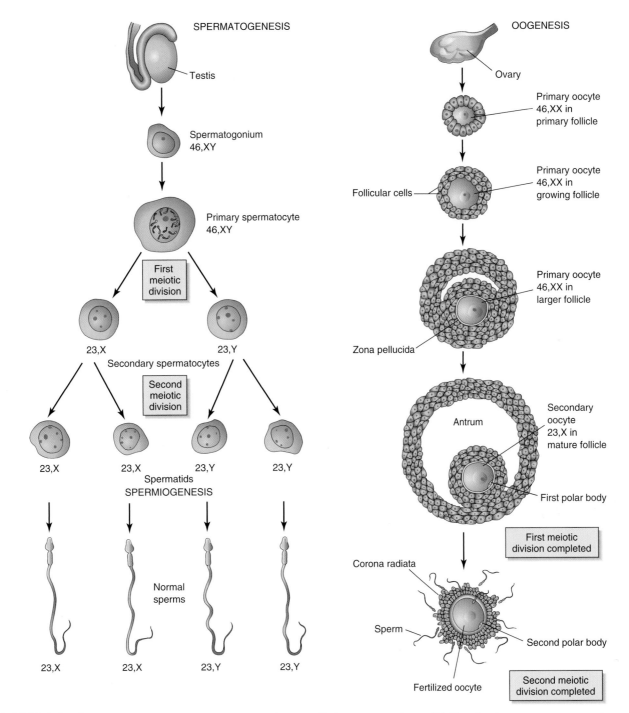

**FIGURE 2-1** Normal gametogenesis: conversion of germ cells into gametes (sex cells). The drawings compare spermatogenesis and oogenesis. Oogonia are not shown in this figure, because they differentiate into primary oocytes before birth. The chromosome complement of the germ cells is shown at each stage. The number designates the total number of chromosomes, including the sex chromosome(s) shown after the comma. *Notes: (1) Following the two meiotic divisions, the diploid number of chromosomes, 46, is reduced to the haploid number, 23. (2) Four sperms form from one primary spermatocyte, whereas only one mature oocyte results from maturation of a primary oocyte. (3) The cytoplasm is conserved during oogenesis to form one large cell, the mature oocyte (see Fig. 2-5C). The polar bodies are small nonfunctional cells that eventually degenerate.*

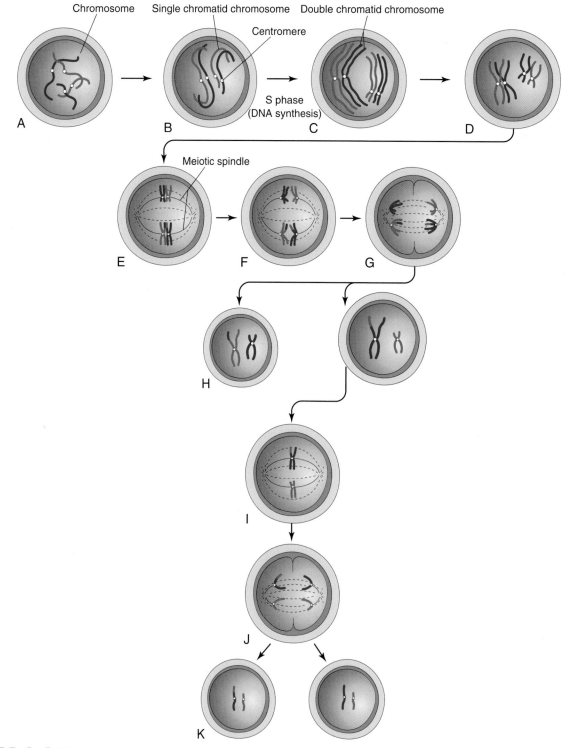

**FIGURE 2–2** Diagrammatic representation of meiosis. Two chromosome pairs are shown. **A** to **D**, Stages of prophase of the first meiotic division. The homologous chromosomes approach each other and pair; each member of the pair consists of two chromatids. Observe the single crossover in one pair of chromosomes, resulting in the interchange of chromatid segments. **E**, Metaphase. The two members of each pair become oriented on the meiotic spindle. **F**, Anaphase. **G**, Telophase. The chromosomes migrate to opposite poles. **H**, Distribution of parental chromosome pairs at the end of the first meiotic division. **I** to **K**, Second meiotic division. It is similar to mitosis except that the cells are haploid.

## ABNORMAL GAMETOGENESIS

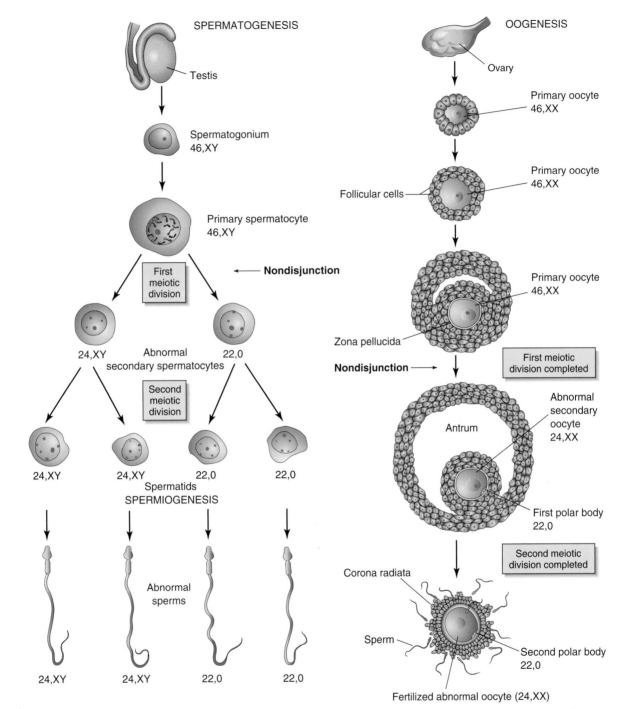

**FIGURE 2–3** Abnormal gametogenesis. The drawings show how nondisjunction (failure of one or more pairs of chromosomes to separate at the meiotic stage) results in an abnormal chromosome distribution in gametes. Although nondisjunction of sex chromosomes is illustrated, a similar defect may occur in autosomes (any chromosomes other than sex chromosomes). When nondisjunction occurs during the first meiotic division of spermatogenesis, one secondary spermatocyte contains 22 autosomes plus an X and a Y chromosome and the other one contains 22 autosomes and no sex chromosome. Similarly, nondisjunction during oogenesis may give rise to an oocyte with 22 autosomes and 2 X chromosomes (as shown), or it may result in one with 22 autosomes and no sex chromosome.

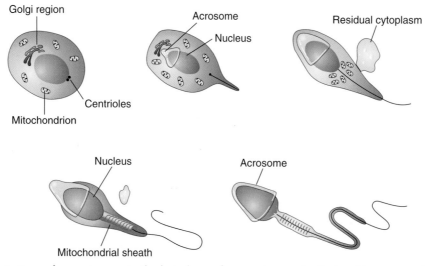

**FIGURE 2-4** Illustrations of spermiogenesis, the last phase of spermatogenesis. During this process, the rounded spermatid is transformed into an elongated sperm. Note the loss of cytoplasm (see Fig. 2-5C), development of the tail, and formation of the acrosome. The acrosome, derived from the Golgi region *(first drawing)* of the spermatid, contains enzymes that are released at the beginning of fertilization to assist the sperm in penetrating the corona radiata and zona pellucida surrounding the secondary oocyte.

**FIGURE 2-5** Male and female gametes (sex cells). A, The main parts of a human sperm (×1250). The head, composed mostly of the nucleus, is partly covered by the cap-like acrosome, an organelle containing enzymes. The tail of the sperm consists of three regions, the middle piece, principal piece, and end piece. B, A sperm drawn to approximately the same scale as the oocyte. C, A human secondary oocyte (×200), surrounded by the zona pellucida and corona radiata.

The **epididymis** is an elongated coiled duct (see Fig. 2-12). The epididymis is continuous with the **ductus deferens,** which transports the sperms to the urethra (see Fig. 2-12).

**Mature sperms** are free-swimming, actively motile cells consisting of a head and a tail (Fig. 2-5A). The *neck of the sperm* is the junction between the head and tail. The *head of the sperm* forms most of the bulk of the sperm and contains the nucleus. The anterior two thirds of the head is covered by the **acrosome,** a cap-like saccular organelle containing several enzymes (see Figs. 2-4 and 2-5A). When released, the enzymes facilitate dispersion of follicular cells of the **corona radiata** and sperm penetration of the **zona pellucida** during fertilization (see Figs. 2-5A and C and 2-13A and B).

The tail of the sperm consists of three segments: middle piece, principal piece, and end piece (see Fig. 2-5A). The tail provides the motility of the sperm that assists its transport to the site of fertilization. The *middle piece* contains **mitochondria**, which provide *adenosine triphosphate*, necessary to support the energy required for motility.

Many genes and molecular factors are implicated in spermatogenesis. For example, recent studies indicate that proteins of the *Bcl-2 family* are involved in the maturation of germ cells, as well as their survival at different stages. At the molecular level, *HOX* genes influence microtubule dynamics and the shaping of the head of the sperm and formation of the tail. For normal spermatogenesis, the Y chromosome is essential; microdeletions result in defective spermatogenesis and infertility.

## OOGENESIS

Oogenesis is the sequence of events by which **oogonia** (primordial germ cells) are transformed into mature oocytes. All oogonia develop into primary oocytes before birth; no oogonia develop after birth. Oogenesis continues to **menopause**, which is the permanent cessation of the menstrual cycle (see Figs. 2-7 and 2-11).

### Prenatal Maturation of Oocytes

During early fetal life, oogonia proliferate by **mitosis** (reproduction of cells), a special type of cell division (see Fig. 2-2). **Oogonia** (primordial sex cells) enlarge to form **primary oocytes** before birth; for this reason, no oogonia are shown in Figures 2-1 and 2-3. As the oocytes form, connective tissue cells surround them and form a single layer of flattened, **follicular cells** (see Fig. 2-8). The primary oocyte enclosed by this layer of cells constitutes a **primordial follicle** (see Fig. 2-9A). As the primary oocyte enlarges during puberty, the follicular epithelial cells become cuboidal in shape and then columnar, forming a **primary follicle** (see Fig. 2-1).

The primary oocyte is soon surrounded by a covering of amorphous, acellular, glycoproteinaceous material, the **zona pellucida** (see Figs. 2-8 and 2-9B). Scanning electron microscopy of the surface of the zona pellucida reveals a regular mesh-like appearance with intricate fenestrations. Primary oocytes begin the first meiotic divisions before birth (see Fig. 2.3), but completion of **prophase** (see Fig. 2-2A to D) does not occur until adolescence (beginning with puberty). The follicular cells surrounding the primary oocytes secrete a substance, **oocyte maturation inhibitor**, which keeps the meiotic process of the oocyte arrested.

### Postnatal Maturation of Oocytes

Beginning during puberty, usually one ovarian follicle matures each month and **ovulation** (release of oocyte from the ovarian follicle) occurs (see Fig. 2-7), except when oral contraceptives are used. The long duration of the first meiotic division (up to 45 years) may account in part for the relatively high frequency of **meiotic errors**, such as nondisjunction (failure of paired chromatids of a chromosome to dissociate), that occur with increasing maternal age. The **primary oocytes** in suspended prophase (dictyotene) are vulnerable to environmental agents such as radiation.

*No primary oocytes form after birth*, in contrast to the continuous production of primary spermatocytes (see Fig. 2-3). The primary oocytes remain dormant in ovarian follicles until puberty (see Fig. 2-8). As a follicle matures, the primary oocyte increases in size, and shortly before ovulation, the primary oocyte completes the first meiotic division to give rise to a **secondary oocyte** (see Fig. 2-10A and B) and the first polar body. Unlike the corresponding stage of spermatogenesis, however, the division of **cytoplasm** is unequal. The secondary oocyte receives almost all the cytoplasm (see Fig. 2-1), and the **first polar body** receives very little. The polar body is a small cell destined for degeneration.

At ovulation, the nucleus of the secondary oocyte begins the second meiotic division, but it progresses only to metaphase (see Fig. 2-2E), when division is arrested. If a sperm penetrates the secondary oocyte, the second meiotic division is completed, and most cytoplasm is again retained by one cell, the fertilized oocyte (see Fig. 2-1). The other cell, the **second polar body**, is also formed and will degenerate. As soon as the polar bodies are extruded, maturation of the oocyte is complete.

There are approximately 2 million primary oocytes in the ovaries of a neonate, but most of them regress during childhood so that by adolescence no more than 40,000 primary oocytes remain. Of these, only approximately 400 become secondary oocytes and are expelled at ovulation during the reproductive period. Very few of these oocytes, if any, are fertilized. The number of oocytes that ovulate is greatly reduced in women who take oral contraceptives because the hormones in them prevent ovulation from occurring.

## COMPARISON OF GAMETES

The gametes (oocytes/sperms) are **haploid cells** (have half the number of chromosomes) that can undergo **karyogamy** (fusion of nuclei of two sex cells). The oocyte is a massive cell compared with the sperm and it is immotile, whereas the microscopic sperm is highly motile (see Fig. 2-5A). The oocyte is surrounded by the **zona pellucida** and a layer of follicular cells, the **corona radiata** (see Fig. 2-5C).

With respect to **sex chromosome constitution**, there are *two kinds of normal sperms*: 23,X and 23,Y, whereas there is only one kind of secondary oocyte: 23,X (see Fig. 2-1). By convention, the number 23 is followed by a comma and an X or Y to indicate the sex chromosome constitution; for example, 23,X indicates that there are 23 chromosomes in the complement, consisting of 22 **autosomes** (chromosomes other than sex chromosomes) and 1 sex chromosome (X in this case). The difference in the sex chromosome complement of sperms forms the basis of primary sex determination.

## ABNORMAL GAMETES

The ideal biologic maternal age for reproduction is from 20 to 35 years. The likelihood of chromosomal abnormalities in an embryo gradually increases as the mother ages. In older mothers, there is an *appreciable risk of Down syndrome* (trisomy 21) or other form of trisomy in the infant (see Chapter 20). The likelihood of a fresh gene mutation (change in DNA) also increases with age. The older the parents are at the time of conception, the more likely they are to have accumulated mutations that the embryo might inherit.

During gametogenesis, homologous chromosomes sometimes fail to separate, a pathogenic process called **nondisjunction**; as a result, some gametes have 24 chromosomes and others only 22 (see Fig. 2-3). If a gamete with 24 chromosomes unites with a normal one with 23 chromosomes during fertilization, a zygote with 47 chromosomes forms (see Chapter 20, Fig. 20-2). This condition is called **trisomy** because of the presence of three representatives of a particular chromosome, instead of the usual two. If a gamete with only 22 chromosomes unites with a normal one, a zygote with 45 chromosomes forms. This condition is called **monosomy** because only one representative of the particular chromosome pair is present. For a description of the clinical conditions associated with numeric disorders of chromosomes, see Chapter 20.

As many as 10% of sperms ejaculated are grossly abnormal (e.g., with two heads), but it is believed that these abnormal sperms do not fertilize oocytes due to their lack of normal motility. Most morphologically abnormal sperms are unable to pass through the mucus in the cervical canal. Measurement of forward progression is a subjective assessment of the quality of sperm movement. Such sperms are not believed to affect fertility unless their number exceeds 20%. Although some oocytes have two or three nuclei, these cells die before they reach maturity. Similarly, some ovarian follicles contain two or more oocytes, but this phenomenon is rare.

## UTERUS, UTERINE TUBES, AND OVARIES

A brief description of the structure of the uterus, uterine tubes, and ovaries is presented as a basis for understanding reproductive ovarian cycles and implantation of blastocysts (Figs. 2-6 and 2-7, and see Fig. 2-19).

### Uterus

The uterus is a thick-walled, pear-shaped muscular organ, averaging 7 to 8 cm in length, 5 to 7 cm in width at its superior part, and 2 to 3 cm in wall thickness. The uterus consists of two major parts (see Fig. 2-6A and B): the body, the superior two thirds, and the **cervix**, the cylindric inferior one third.

The **body of the uterus** narrows from the **fundus**, the rounded superior part of the body, to the **isthmus**, the 1-cm-long constricted region between the body and cervix (see Fig. 2-6A). The **cervix of the uterus** is its tapered vaginal end that is nearly cylindric in shape. The lumen of the cervix, the **cervical canal**, has a constricted opening at each end. The **internal os** (opening) of the uterus communicates with the cavity of the uterine body, and the **external os** communicates with the vagina (see Fig. 2-6A and B).

The walls of the body of the uterus consist of three layers (see Fig. 2-6B):

- Perimetrium, the thin external layer
- Myometrium, the thick smooth muscle layer
- Endometrium, the thin internal layer

The **perimetrium** is a peritoneal layer that is firmly attached to the **myometrium** (see Fig. 2-6B). During the *luteal (secretory) phase* of the menstrual cycle, three layers of the endometrium can be distinguished microscopically (see Fig. 2-6C):

- A thin, **compact layer** consisting of densely packed connective tissue around the necks of the uterine glands
- A thick, **spongy layer** composed of edematous (having large amounts of fluid) connective tissue containing the dilated, tortuous bodies of the uterine glands
- A thin, **basal layer** containing the blind ends of the uterine glands
- At the peak of its development, the **endometrium** is 4 to 5 mm thick (see Fig. 2-6B and C). The basal layer of the endometrium has its own blood supply and is not sloughed off during **menstruation** (see Fig. 2-7). The compact and spongy layers, known collectively as the *functional layer*, disintegrate and are shed during menstruation and after **parturition** (delivery of a fetus).

### Uterine Tubes

The **uterine tubes**, approximately 10 cm long and 1 cm in diameter, extend laterally from the horns of the uterus (see Fig. 2-6A and B). Each tube opens at its proximal end into the horn of the uterus and into the peritoneal cavity at its distal end. For descriptive purposes, the uterine tube is divided into four parts: **infundibulum, ampulla, isthmus,** and **uterine part** (see Fig. 2-6B). One of the tubes carries an oocyte from one of the ovaries; the tubes also carry sperms entering from the uterus to reach the fertilization site, the **ampulla** (see Figs. 2-6B and 2-20). The uterine tube also conveys the cleaving zygote to the uterine cavity.

### Ovaries

The **ovaries** are almond-shaped reproductive glands located close to the lateral pelvic walls on each side of the uterus. The ovaries produce oocytes (see Fig. 2-6B) and estrogen and progesterone, the hormones responsible

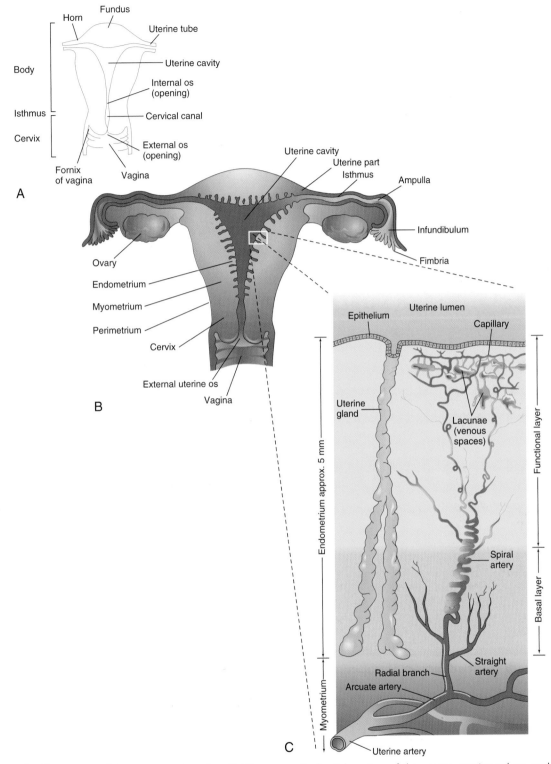

**FIGURE 2–6** A, Parts of the uterus and vagina. B, Diagrammatic frontal section of the uterus, uterine tubes, and vagina. The ovaries are also shown. C, Enlargement of the area outlined in B. The functional layer of the endometrium is sloughed off during menstruation.

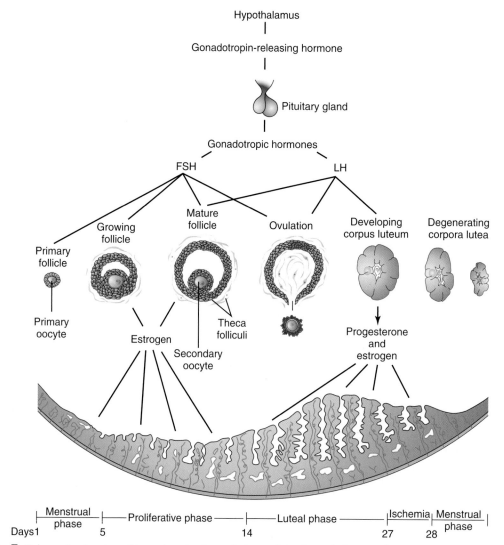

**FIGURE 2–7** Schematic drawings illustrating the interrelations of the hypothalamus of the brain, pituitary gland, ovaries, and endometrium. One complete menstrual cycle and the beginning of another are shown. Changes in the ovaries, the *ovarian cycle*, are induced by the gonadotropic hormones (follicle-stimulating hormone [FSH] and luteinizing hormone [LH]). Hormones from the ovaries (estrogens and progesterone) then promote cyclic changes in the structure and function of the endometrium, the *menstrual cycle*. Thus, the cyclic activity of the ovary is intimately linked with changes in the uterus. The ovarian cycles are under the rhythmic endocrine control of the pituitary gland, which in turn is controlled by the gonadotropin-releasing hormone produced by neurosecretory cells in the hypothalamus.

for the development of secondary sex characteristics and regulation of pregnancy.

## FEMALE REPRODUCTIVE CYCLES

Commencing at puberty (10 to 13 years of age), females undergo reproductive cycles (sexual cycles), involving activities of the **hypothalamus** of the brain, pituitary gland, ovaries, uterus, uterine tubes, vagina, and mammary glands (see Fig. 2-7). These monthly cycles prepare the reproductive system for pregnancy.

A *gonadotropin-releasing hormone* is synthesized by neurosecretory cells in the hypothalamus. This hormone is carried by a capillary network, the **portal hypophyseal circulation** (hypophyseal portal system), to the anterior lobe of the pituitary gland. The hormone stimulates the

release of two hormones produced by this gland that act on the ovaries:

- **Follicle-stimulating hormone** (FSH) stimulates the development of ovarian follicles and the production of estrogen by the follicular cells.
- **Luteinizing hormone** (LH) serves as the "trigger" for ovulation (release of a secondary oocyte) and stimulates the follicular cells and corpus luteum to produce progesterone.
- These hormones also induce growth of the ovarian follicles and the endometrium.

## OVARIAN CYCLE

FSH and LH produce cyclic changes in the ovaries— the **ovarian cycle** (see Fig. 2-7)—development of follicles

(Fig. 2-8), **ovulation** (release of an oocyte from a mature follicle), and **corpus luteum formation.** During each cycle, FSH promotes growth of several primordial follicles into 5 to 12 primary follicles (Fig. 2-9A); however, only one primary follicle usually develops into a **mature follicle** and ruptures through the surface of the ovary, expelling its oocyte (Fig. 2-10).

**FIGURE 2–8** Photomicrograph of a human primary oocyte in a secondary follicle, surrounded by the zona pellucida and follicular cells. The mound of tissue, the cumulus oophorus, projects into the antrum. *(From Bloom W, Fawcett DW: A textbook of histology, 10th ed, Philadelphia, 1975, Saunders. Courtesy L. Zamboni.)*

## Follicular Development

Development of an ovarian follicle (see Figs. 2-8 and 2-9) is characterized by:

- Growth and differentiation of a primary oocyte
- Proliferation of follicular cells
- Formation of the zona pellucida
- Development of the theca folliculi

As the **primary follicle** increases in size, the adjacent connective tissue organizes into a capsule, the **theca folliculi** (see Fig. 2-7). This theca soon differentiates into two layers, an internal vascular layer and glandular layer, the **theca interna,** and a capsule-like layer, the **theca externa.** Thecal cells are thought to produce an **angiogenesis factor** that promotes growth of blood vessels in the theca interna, which provide nutritive support for follicular development. The follicular cells divide actively, producing a stratified layer around the oocyte (see Fig. 2-9B). The ovarian follicle soon becomes oval and the oocyte eccentric in position. Subsequently, fluid-filled spaces appear around the follicular cells, which coalesce to form a single large cavity, the **antrum,** which contains **follicular fluid** (see Figs. 2-8 and 2-9B). After the antrum forms, the ovarian follicle is called a vesicular or **secondary follicle.**

The primary oocyte is pushed to one side of the follicle, where it is surrounded by a mound of follicular cells, the **cumulus oophorus,** that projects into the antrum (see Fig. 2-9B). The follicle continues to enlarge until it reaches maturity and produces a swelling (follicular stigma) on the surface of the ovary (see Fig. 2-10A).

The early development of ovarian follicles is induced by FSH, but final stages of maturation require LH as well. Growing follicles produce **estrogen,** a hormone that regulates development and function of the reproductive organs. The vascular theca interna produces **follicular**

**FIGURE 2–9** Micrographs of the ovarian cortex. A, Several primordial follicles (P) are visible (×270). Observe that the primary oocytes are surrounded by follicular cells. B, Secondary ovarian follicle. The oocyte is surrounded by granulosa cells of the cumulus oophorus (×132). The antrum can be clearly seen. *(From Gartner LP, Hiatt JL: Color textbook of histology, 2nd ed, Philadelphia, 2001, Saunders.)*

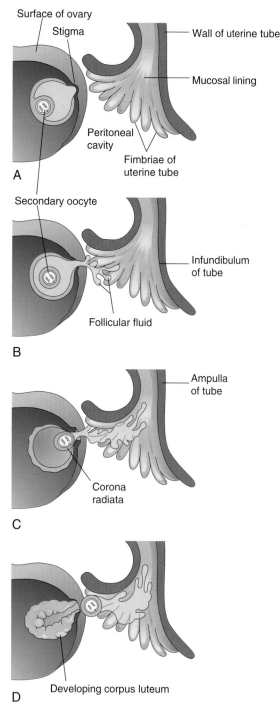

A

B

C

D

Surface of ovary
Stigma
Wall of uterine tube
Mucosal lining
Peritoneal cavity
Fimbriae of uterine tube
Secondary oocyte
Infundibulum of tube
Follicular fluid
Ampulla of tube
Corona radiata
Developing corpus luteum

**FIGURE 2–10** A–D, Illustrations of ovulation. Note that fimbriae of the infundibulum of the uterine tube are closely applied to the ovary. The finger-like fimbriae move back and forth over the ovary and "sweep" the oocyte into the infundibulum. When the stigma (swelling) ruptures, the secondary oocyte is expelled from the ovarian follicle with the follicular fluid. After ovulation, the wall of the follicle collapses and is thrown into folds. The follicle is transformed into a glandular structure, the corpus luteum.

**fluid** and some estrogen (see Fig. 2-10*B*). Its cells also secrete androgens that pass to the follicular cells (see Fig. 2-8), which, in turn, convert them into estrogen. Some estrogen is also produced by widely scattered groups of stromal secretory cells, known collectively as the **interstitial gland of the ovary.**

## Ovulation

Around the middle of the ovarian cycle, the ovarian follicle, under the influence of FSH and LH, undergoes a sudden **growth spurt**, producing a cystic swelling or bulge on the surface of the ovary. A small avascular spot, the **stigma**, soon appears on this swelling (see Fig. 2-10*A*). Before ovulation, the secondary oocyte and some cells of the cumulus oophorus detach from the interior of the distended follicle (see Fig. 2-10*B*).

Ovulation is triggered by a **surge of LH production** (Fig. 2-11). Ovulation usually follows the LH peak by 12 to 24 hours. The LH surge, elicited by the high estrogen level in the blood, appears to cause the stigma to balloon out, forming a vesicle (see Fig. 2-10*A*). The stigma soon ruptures, expelling the secondary oocyte with the follicular fluid (see Fig. 2-10*B* to *D*). Expulsion of the oocyte is the result of intrafollicular pressure, and possibly by contraction of smooth muscle in the theca externa (sheath) owing to stimulation by prostaglandins.

*Mitogen-activated protein kinases 3 and 1 (MAPK 3/1), also known as extracellular signal-regulated kinases 1 and 2 (ERK1/2), in ovarian follicular cells seem to regulate signaling pathways that control ovulation. Plasmins and matrix metalloproteins appear also to play a role in controlling rupture of the follicle.* The expelled secondary oocyte is surrounded by the **zona pellucida** (see Fig. 2-8) and one or more layers of follicular cells, which are radially arranged as the **corona radiata** (see Fig. 2-10*C*), forming the oocyte–cumulus complex. The LH **surge** also seems to induce resumption of the first meiotic division of the primary oocyte. Hence, mature ovarian follicles contain secondary oocytes (see Fig. 2-10*A* and *B*). The zona pellucida (see Fig. 2-8) is composed of three glycoproteins (ZPA, ZPB, and ZPC), which usually form a network of filaments with multiple pores. Binding of the sperm to the zona pellucida (sperm–oocyte interactions) is a complex and critical event during fertilization (see Fig. 2-13*A* and *B*.)

## Corpus Luteum

Shortly after ovulation, the walls of the ovarian follicle and theca folliculi collapse and are thrown into folds (see Fig. 2-10*D*). Under LH influence, they develop into a glandular structure, the **corpus luteum**, which secretes progesterone and some estrogen, causing the endometrial glands to secrete and prepare the endometrium for implantation of the blastocyst (see Figs. 2-7 and 2-10).

*If the oocyte is fertilized*, the corpus luteum enlarges to form a **corpus luteum of pregnancy** and increases its hormone production. Degeneration of the corpus luteum is prevented by **human chorionic gonadotropin,** a hormone secreted by the syncytiotrophoblast of the blastocyst (see Fig. 2-19*B*). The corpus luteum of pregnancy

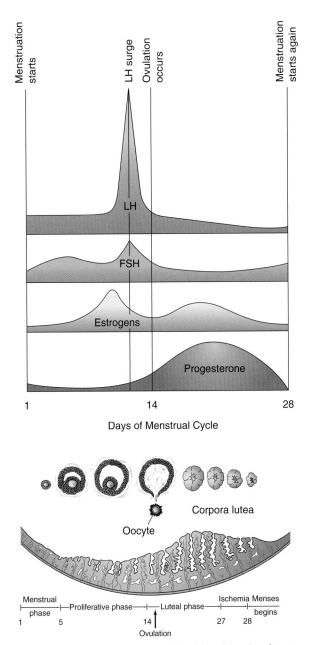

**FIGURE 2–11** Illustration of the blood levels of various hormones during the menstrual cycle. Follicle-stimulating hormone *(FSH)* stimulates the ovarian follicles to develop and produce estrogens. The level of estrogens rises to a peak just before the luteinizing hormone *(LH)* surge. Ovulation normally occurs 24 to 36 hours after the LH surge. If fertilization does not occur, the blood levels of circulating estrogens and progesterone fall. This hormone withdrawal causes the endometrium to regress and menstruation to start again.

## MITTELSCHMERZ AND OVULATION

A variable amount of abdominal pain, **mittelschmerz** (German *mittel*, mid + *schmerz*, pain), accompanies ovulation in some women. In these cases, ovulation results in slight bleeding into the peritoneal cavity, which results in sudden constant pain in the lower abdomen. Mittelschmerz may be used as a secondary indicator of ovulation, but there are better primary indicators, such as elevation of basal body temperature.

## ANOVULATION

Some women do not ovulate (cessation of ovulation, or **anovulation**) because of an inadequate release of gonadotropins. In some of these women, ovulation can be induced by the administration of gonadotropins or an ovulatory agent such as clomiphene citrate. This drug stimulates the release of pituitary gonadotropins (FSH and LH), resulting in maturation of several ovarian follicles and multiple ovulations. The incidence of a multiple pregnancy increases significantly when ovulation is induced. Rarely do more than seven embryos survive.

white scar tissue in the ovary, called a **corpus albicans**. Ovarian cycles terminate at **menopause**, the permanent cessation of menstruation due to ovarian failure. Menopause usually occurs between the ages of 48 and 55 years. The endocrine, somatic (body), and psychological changes occurring at the termination of the reproductive period are called the **climacteric**.

## MENSTRUAL CYCLE

The menstrual cycle is the time during which the oocyte matures, is ovulated, and enters the uterine tube. The hormones produced by the ovarian follicles and corpus luteum (estrogen and progesterone) produce cyclic changes in the endometrium (see Fig. 2-11). These monthly changes in the internal layer of the uterus constitute the **endometrial cycle**, commonly referred to as the **menstrual cycle** (period) because menstruation (flow of blood from the uterus) is an obvious event.

*The endometrium is a "mirror" of the ovarian cycle* because it responds in a consistent manner to the fluctuating concentrations of gonadotropic and ovarian hormones (see Figs. 2-7 and 2-11). The average menstrual cycle is 28 days, with day 1 of the cycle designated as the day on which menstrual flow begins. Menstrual cycles normally vary in length by several days. In 90% of women, the length of the cycles ranges between 23 and

remains functionally active throughout the first 20 weeks of pregnancy. By this time, the placenta has assumed the production of estrogen and progesterone necessary for the maintenance of pregnancy (see Chapter 7).

*If the oocyte is not fertilized*, the corpus luteum involutes and degenerates 10 to 12 days after ovulation (see Fig. 2-7). It is then called a **corpus luteum of menstruation**. The corpus luteum is subsequently transformed into

35 days. Almost all these variations result from alterations in the duration of the proliferative phase of the menstrual cycle (see Fig. 2-11).

## ANOVULATORY MENSTRUAL CYCLES

The typical menstrual cycle, illustrated in Figure 2-11, is not always realized, because the ovary may not produce a mature follicle and so ovulation does not occur. In anovulatory cycles, the endometrial changes are minimal; the proliferative endometrium develops as usual, but ovulation does not occur and no corpus luteum forms. Consequently, the endometrium does not progress to the luteal phase; it remains in the proliferative phase until menstruation begins. Anovulatory cycles may result from ovarian hypofunction. The estrogen, with or without progesterone, in oral contraceptives (birth control pills) acts on the hypothalamus and pituitary gland, resulting in inhibition of secretion of gonadotropin-releasing hormone, FSH, and LH, the secretion of which is essential for ovulation to occur.

## Phases of Menstrual Cycle

Changes in the estrogen and progesterone levels cause cyclic changes in the structure of the female reproductive tract, notably the endometrium. The menstrual cycle is a continuous process; each phase gradually passes into the next one (see Fig. 2-11).

### Menstrual Phase

The functional layer of the uterine wall (see Fig. 2-6C) is sloughed off and discarded with the menstrual flow, or **menses** (monthly bleeding), which usually lasts 4 to 5 days. The blood discharged from the vagina is combined with small pieces of endometrial tissue. After menstruation, the eroded endometrium is thin (see Fig. 2-11).

### Proliferative Phase

This phase, lasting approximately 9 days, coincides with the growth of ovarian follicles and is controlled by estrogen secreted by the follicles. There is a two- to three-fold increase in the thickness of the endometrium and in its water content during this phase of repair and proliferation (see Fig. 2-11). Early during this phase, the surface epithelium reforms and covers the endometrium. The glands increase in number and length and the spiral arteries elongate (see Fig. 2-6).

### Luteal Phase

The luteal (secretory phase), lasting approximately 13 days, coincides with the formation, functioning, and growth of the corpus luteum. The progesterone produced by the corpus luteum stimulates the glandular epithelium to secrete a glycogen-rich material. The glands become wide, tortuous, and saccular, and the endometrium thickens because of the influence of progesterone and estrogen

from the corpus luteum (see Figs. 2-7 and 2-11) and because of increased fluid in the connective tissue. As the **spiral arteries** grow into the superficial compact layer, they become increasingly coiled (see Fig. 2-6C). The venous network becomes complex, and large **lacunae** (venous spaces) develop. Direct arteriovenous anastomoses are prominent features of this stage.

*If fertilization does not occur:*

- The corpora lutea degenerate.
- Estrogen and progesterone levels fall and the secretory endometrium enters an ischemic phase.
- Menstruation occurs (see Fig. 2-7).

### Ischemia

Ischemia occurs when the oocyte is not fertilized; spiral arteries constrict (see Fig. 2-6C), giving the endometrium a pale appearance. This constriction results from the decreasing secretion of hormones, primarily progesterone, by the degenerating corpora lutea (see Fig. 2-11). In addition to vascular changes, the hormone withdrawal results in the stoppage of glandular secretion, a loss of interstitial fluid, and a marked shrinking of the endometrium. Toward the end of the ischemic phase, the spiral arteries become constricted for longer periods. This results in **venous stasis** (congestion and slowing of circulation in veins) and patchy **ischemic necrosis** (death) in the superficial tissues. Eventually, rupture of damaged vessel walls follows and blood seeps into the surrounding connective tissue. Small pools of blood form and break through the endometrial surface, resulting in bleeding into the uterine cavity and through the vagina. As small pieces of the endometrium detach and pass into the uterine cavity, the torn ends of the arteries bleed into the cavity, resulting in a loss of 20 to 80 ml of blood. Eventually, over 3 to 5 days, the entire compact layer and most of the spongy layer of the endometrium are discarded in the **menses** (see Fig. 2-11). Remnants of the spongy and basal layers remain to undergo regeneration during the subsequent *proliferative phase* of the endometrium. It is obvious from the previous descriptions that the cyclic hormonal activity of the ovary is intimately linked with cyclic histologic changes in the endometrium.

*If fertilization occurs:*

- Cleavage of the zygote and blastogenesis (formation of a blastocyst) begin.
- The blastocyst begins to implant in the endometrium on approximately the sixth day of the luteal phase (see Fig. 2-19A).
- Human chorionic gonadotropin, a hormone produced by the syncytiotrophoblast (see Fig. 2-19B), keeps the corpora lutea secreting estrogens and progesterone.
- The luteal phase continues and menstruation does not occur.

### Pregnancy

If pregnancy occurs, the menstrual cycles cease and the endometrium passes into a pregnancy phase. With the termination of pregnancy, the ovarian and menstrual cycles resume after a variable period (usually 6 to 10 weeks if the woman is not breast-feeding her baby).

Except during pregnancy, the reproductive cycles normally continue until menopause.

## TRANSPORTATION OF GAMETES

### 1 Oocyte Transport

The secondary oocyte is expelled at ovulation from the ovarian follicle with the escaping follicular fluid (see Fig. 2-10C and D). During ovulation, the fimbriated end of the uterine tube becomes closely applied to the ovary. The finger-like processes of the tube, **fimbriae**, move back and forth over the ovary. The sweeping action of the fimbriae and fluid currents produced by the cilia (motile extensions) of the mucosal cells of the fimbriae "sweep" the secondary oocyte into the funnel-shaped **infundibulum** of the uterine tube (see Fig. 2-10B). The oocyte then passes into the **ampulla** of the tube (see Fig. 2-10C), mainly as the result of **peristalsis** (movements of the wall of the tube characterized by alternate contraction and relaxation), which causes the oocyte to pass toward the uterus.

### Sperm Transport

The reflex ejaculation of semen may be divided into two phases:

- **Emission**: Semen passes to the prostatic part of the urethra through the ejaculatory ducts after peristalsis (peristaltic movements) of the ductus deferens (Fig. 2-12); emission is a sympathetic response.
- **Ejaculation**: Semen is expelled from the urethra through the external urethral orifice; this results from closure of the vesical sphincter at the neck of the bladder, contraction of the urethral muscle, and contraction of the bulbospongiosus muscles.

The sperms are rapidly transported from the epididymis to the urethra by peristaltic contractions of the thick muscular coat of the **ductus deferens** (see Fig. 2-12). The accessory sex glands, that is, the **seminal glands** (vesicles), **prostate**, and **bulbourethral glands**, produce secretions that are added to the sperm-containing fluid in the ductus deferens and urethra.

From 200 to 600 million sperms are deposited around the external os of the uterus and in the fornix of the vagina during intercourse (see Fig. 2-6A and B). The sperms pass through the cervical canal by movements of their tails (see Fig. 2-5A). The enzyme *vesiculase*, produced by the prostate gland, assists with reducing the viscosity (liquification) of a seminal fluid coagulum that forms shortly after ejaculation. When ovulation occurs, the cervical mucus increases in amount and becomes less viscid (sticky), making it more favorable for sperm transport.

Passage of sperms through the uterus into the uterine tubes results mainly from muscular contractions of the walls of these organs. **Prostaglandins** (physiologically active substances) in the semen are thought to stimulate uterine motility at the time of intercourse and assist in the movement of sperms to the site of fertilization in the ampulla of the uterine tube. **Fructose**, secreted by the seminal glands, is an energy source for the sperms in the semen.

The volume of **ejaculate** (sperms mixed with secretions from the accessory sex glands) averages 3.5 ml, with a range of 2 to 6 ml. The sperms move 2 to 3 mm per minute, but the speed varies with the pH of the

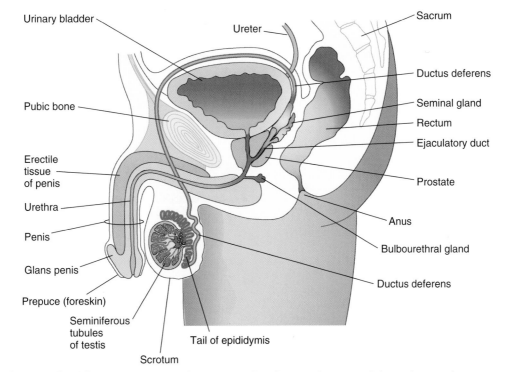

**FIGURE 2–12** Sagittal section of the male pelvis showing the parts of the male reproductive system.

environment. The sperms are nonmotile during storage in the epididymis (see Fig. 2-12) but become motile in the ejaculate. They move slowly in the acid environment of the vagina but move more rapidly in the alkaline environment of the uterus. It is not known how long it takes sperms to reach the fertilization site in the ampulla of the uterine tube (see Figs. 2-10C and 2-20), but the time of transport is probably short. **Motile sperms** have been recovered from the ampulla 5 minutes after their deposition near the external uterine os (see Fig. 2-6B). Some sperms, however, take as long as 45 minutes. Approximately 200 sperms reach the fertilization site; however, most sperms degenerate and are absorbed in the female genital tract.

## MATURATION OF SPERMS

Freshly ejaculated sperms are unable to fertilize an oocyte. Sperms must undergo a period of conditioning, or **capacitation**, lasting approximately 7 hours. During this period, a glycoprotein coat and seminal proteins are removed from the surface of the sperm **acrosome** (see Figs. 2-4 and 2-5A). The membrane components of the sperms are extensively altered. **Capacitated sperms** show no morphologic changes, but they are more active. Sperms are usually capacitated while they are in the uterus or uterine tubes by substances secreted by these parts of the female genital tract. During **in vitro fertilization**, capacitation is induced by incubating the sperms in a defined medium for several hours (see Fig. 2-15). Completion of capacitation permits the acrosome reaction to occur.

The **acrosome** of the capacitated sperm binds to a glycoprotein (ZP3) on the zona pellucida (Fig. 2-13A and B). Studies have shown that the sperm plasma membrane, calcium ions, prostaglandins, and progesterone play a critical role in the **acrosome reaction**. This reaction of sperms must be completed before the sperms can fuse with the oocyte. When capacitated sperms come into contact with the **corona radiata** surrounding a secondary oocyte (see Fig. 2-13A and B), they undergo complex molecular changes that result in the development of perforations in the acrosome. Multiple point fusions of the **plasma membrane** of the sperm and the external **acrosomal membrane** occur. Breakdown of the membranes at these sites produces apertures (openings). The changes induced by acrosome reaction are associated with the release of enzymes, including hyaluronidase and acrosin, from the acrosome that facilitate fertilization. *Capacitation and acrosome reaction appear to be regulated by a tyrosine kinase, src kinase.*

## VIABILITY OF GAMETES

Studies on early stages of development indicate that **human oocytes** are usually fertilized within 12 hours after ovulation. In vitro observations have shown that the oocyte cannot be fertilized after 24 hours and that it degenerates shortly thereafter. Most **human sperms** probably do not survive for more than 48 hours in the female genital tract. **After ejaculation**, sperms that pass through

## MALE FERTILITY

During evaluation of male fertility, an analysis of semen is made. Sperms account for less than 10% of the semen. The remainder of the ejaculate consists of secretions of the seminal glands, prostate, and bulbourethral glands. There are usually more than 100 million sperms per milliliter of semen in the ejaculate of normal males. Although there is much variation in individual cases, men whose semen contains 20 million sperms per milliliter, or 50 million in the total specimen, are more likely to be fertile. A man with fewer than 10 million sperms per milliliter of semen is less likely to be fertile, especially when the specimen contains immotile and abnormal sperms. For high fertility probability, 50% of sperms should be motile after 2 hours and some should be motile after 24 hours. Male infertility may result from a low sperm count, poor sperm motility, medications and drugs, endocrine disorders, exposure to environmental pollutants, cigarette smoking, abnormal sperms, or obstruction of a genital duct, as in the ductus deferens (see Fig. 2-12). Male infertility is detectable in 30% to 50% of involuntary childless couples.

## VASECTOMY

The most effective method of permanent contraception in men is vasectomy, surgical removal of all or part of the ductus deferens (vas deferens). Following vasectomy, there are no sperms in the semen or ejaculate, but the volume is essentially the same. Reversal of vasectomy is technically feasible by microsurgical techniques; however, the success rate is variable.

## DISPERMY AND TRIPLOIDY

Although several sperms penetrate the corona radiata and zona pellucida (Fig. 2-14A), usually only one sperm enters the oocyte and fertilizes it. Two sperms may participate in fertilization during an abnormal process known as **dispermy**, resulting in a zygote with an extra set of chromosomes. **Triploid conceptions** account for approximately 20% of chromosomally abnormal spontaneous abortions. Triploid embryos (69 chromosomes) may appear normal, but they nearly always abort or die shortly after birth.

**FIGURE 2–13** Acrosome reaction and sperm penetrating an oocyte. The detail of the area outlined in **A** is given in **B**. 1, Sperm during capacitation, a period of conditioning that occurs in the female reproductive tract. 2, Sperm undergoing the acrosome reaction, during which perforations form in the acrosome. 3, Sperm digesting a path through the zona pellucida by the action of enzymes released from the acrosome. 4, Sperm after entering the cytoplasm of the oocyte. Note that the plasma membranes of the sperm and oocyte have fused and that the head and tail of the sperm enter the oocyte, leaving the sperm's plasma membrane attached to the oocyte's plasma membrane. **C**, Scanning electron microscopy of an unfertilized human oocyte showing relatively few sperms attached to the zona pellucida. **D**, Scanning electron microscopy of a human oocyte showing penetration of the sperm (arrow) into the zona pellucida.

the cervix enter the uterus. Some sperms are stored in folds of the *cervical crypts* and are gradually released and pass along the body of the uterus into the uterine tubes. The short-term storage of sperms in the crypts provides a gradual release of sperms and thereby increases the chances of fertilization. Sperms and oocytes can be frozen and stored for many years and can be used for *in vitro fertilization.*

## SEQUENCE OF FERTILIZATION

The usual site of fertilization is in the ampulla of the uterine tube (see Figs. 2-6B and 2-20). If the oocyte is not fertilized here, it slowly passes along the tube to the body of the uterus, where it degenerates and is resorbed. Although fertilization may occur in other parts of the tube, it does not occur in the body of the uterus. Chemical

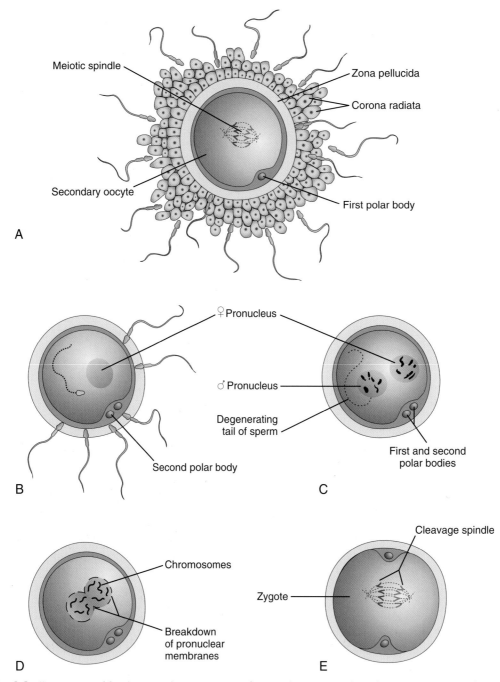

**FIGURE 2–14** Illustrations of fertilization, the procession of events beginning when the sperm contacts the secondary oocyte's plasma membrane and ending with the intermingling of maternal and paternal chromosomes at metaphase of the first mitotic division of the zygote. **A,** Secondary oocyte surrounded by several sperms, two of which have penetrated the corona radiata. (Only 4 of the 23 chromosome pairs are shown.) **B,** The corona radiata is not shown. A sperm has entered the oocyte, and the second meiotic division has occurred, causing a mature oocyte to form. The nucleus of the oocyte is now the female pronucleus. **C,** The sperm head has enlarged to form the male pronucleus. This cell, now called an ootid, contains the male and female pronuclei. **D,** The pronuclei are fusing. **E,** The zygote has formed; it contains 46 chromosomes, the diploid number.

signals (attractants), secreted by the oocyte and surrounding follicular cells, guide the **capacitated sperms** (sperm chemotaxis) to the oocyte.

Fertilization is a complex sequence of coordinated molecular events that begins with contact between a sperm and an oocyte (see Fig. 2-13A and B) and ends with the intermingling of maternal and paternal chromosomes at metaphase of the first mitotic division of the **zygote,** a unicellular embryo (see Fig. 2-14E).

Defects at any stage in the sequence of these events may cause the death of the zygote. The fertilization process takes approximately 24 hours. Transgenic and gene knockout studies in animals have shown that carbohydrate-binding molecules and gamete-specific proteins on the surface of the sperms are involved in sperm–egg recognition and union.

## Phases of Fertilization

As it has been stated, fertilization is a sequence of coordinated events (see Figs. 2-13 and 2-14):

- **Passage of a sperm through the corona radiata.** Dispersal of the follicular cells of the corona radiata surrounding the oocyte and zona pellucida appears to result mainly from the action of the enzyme *hyaluronidase* released from the **acrosome of the sperm** (see Fig. 2-5A), but the evidence of this is not unequivocal. Tubal mucosal enzymes also appear to assist the dispersal. Movements of the tail of the sperm are also important in its penetration of the corona radiata (see Fig. 2-13A).
- **Penetration of the zona pellucida.** Passage of a sperm through the zona pellucida is the important phase in the initiation of fertilization. Formation of a pathway also results from the action of enzymes released from the acrosome. The enzymes esterase, acrosin, and neuraminidase appear to cause **lysis** (dissolution or loosening) of the zona pellucida, thereby forming a path for the sperm to enter the oocyte. The most important of these enzymes is **acrosin**, a proteolytic enzyme.
- Once the sperm penetrates the zona pellucida, a **zona reaction**, a change in the properties of the zona pellucida, occurs that makes it impermeable to other sperms. The composition of this extracellular glycoprotein coat changes after fertilization. The zona reaction is believed to result from the action of lysosomal enzymes released by cortical granules near the plasma membrane of the oocyte. The contents of these granules, which are released into the **perivitelline space** (see Fig. 2-13A), also cause changes in the plasma membrane that make it impermeable to other sperms.
- **Fusion of cell membranes of the oocyte and sperm.** The plasma or cell membranes of the oocyte and sperm fuse and break down in the area of fusion. The head and tail of the sperm enter the cytoplasm of the oocyte (see Fig. 2-13A and B), but the sperm's cell membrane (plasma membrane) and mitochondria remain behind.
- **Completion of the second meiotic division of the oocyte and formation of the female pronucleus.** Penetration of the oocyte by a sperm activates the oocyte into completing the second meiotic division and forming a **mature oocyte** and a second polar body (see Fig. 2-14B). Following decondensation of the maternal chromosomes, the nucleus of the mature oocyte becomes the female pronucleus.
- **Formation of the male pronucleus.** Within the cytoplasm of the oocyte, the nucleus of the sperm enlarges to form the male pronucleus (see Fig. 2-14C), and the tail of the sperm degenerates. Morphologically, the male and female pronuclei are indistinguishable. During growth of the pronuclei, they replicate their DNA-1 n (haploid), 2 c (two chromatids). The oocyte containing the two haploid pronuclei is called an **ootid,** the nearly mature oocyte after the first meiotic divisions have been completed (see Fig. 2-14C).

- **As the pronuclei fuse into a single diploid aggregation of chromosomes, the ootid becomes a zygote.** The chromosomes in the zygote become arranged on a cleavage spindle (see Fig. 2-14E) in preparation for cleavage of the zygote (see Fig. 2-16).
- *The zygote is genetically unique* because half of its chromosomes came from the mother and half from the father. The zygote contains a new combination of chromosomes that is different from those in the cells of either of the parents. This mechanism forms the basis of **biparental inheritance** and variation of the human species. Meiosis allows independent assortment of maternal and paternal chromosomes among the germ cells (see Fig. 2-2). **Crossing over of chromosomes**, by relocating segments of the maternal and paternal chromosomes, "shuffles" the genes, thereby producing a recombination of genetic material. *The embryo's chromosomal sex is determined at fertilization* by the kind of sperm (X or Y) that fertilizes the oocyte. Fertilization by an X-bearing sperm produces a 46,XX zygote, which develops into a female, whereas fertilization by a Y-bearing sperm produces a 46,XY zygote, which develops into a male.

## Fertilization

- Stimulates the penetrated oocyte to complete the second meiotic division
- Restores the normal diploid number of chromosomes (46) in the zygote
- Results in variation of the human species through mingling of maternal and paternal chromosomes
- Determines the chromosomal sex of the embryo
- Causes metabolic activation of the **ootid** (nearly mature oocyte) and initiates cleavage of the zygote

## PRESELECTION OF EMBRYO'S SEX

Because X and Y sperms are formed in equal numbers, the expectation is that the sex ratio at fertilization (primary sex ratio) would be 1.00 (100 males per 100 females). It is well known, however, that there are more male neonates than female neonates born in all countries. In North America, for example, the sex ratio at birth (secondary sex ratio) is approximately 1.05 (105 boys per 100 girls). Various microscopic techniques have been developed in an attempt to separate X and Y sperms (gender selection) using:

- The differential swimming abilities of the X and Y sperms
- Different speed of migration of sperms in an electric field
- Differences in the appearance of X and Y sperms
- DNA difference between X (2.8% more DNA) and Y sperms

The use of a selected sperm sample in artificial insemination may produce the desired sex.

## ASSISTED REPRODUCTIVE TECHNOLOGIES

### In Vitro Fertilization and Embryo Transfer

In vitro fertilization (IVF) of oocytes and transfer of cleaving zygotes into the uterus have provided an opportunity for many women who are sterile (e.g., owing to tubal occlusion) to have children. In 1978, Robert G. Edwards and Patrick Steptoe pioneered IVF, one of the most revolutionary developments in the history of human reproduction. Their studies resulted in the birth of the first "test tube baby," Louise Brown. Since then, several million children have been born after an IVF procedure. The steps involved during IVF and embryo transfer are as follows (Fig. 2-15):

- Ovarian follicles are stimulated to grow and mature by the administration of clomiphene citrate or gonadotropin (superovulation).
- Several mature oocytes are aspirated from mature ovarian follicles during laparoscopy. Oocytes can also be removed by an ultrasonography-guided needle inserted through the vaginal wall into the ovarian follicles.
- The oocytes are placed in a Petri dish containing a special culture medium and capacitated sperms.
- Fertilization of the oocytes and cleavage of the zygotes are monitored microscopically for 3 to 5 days.
- Depending on the mother's age, one to three of the resulting embryos (four-cell to eight-cell stage, or early blastocysts) are transferred by introducing a catheter through the vagina and cervical canal into the uterus. Any remaining embryos are stored in liquid nitrogen for later use.
- The patient lies supine (face upward) for several hours. The chances of multiple pregnancies are higher following IVF, as is the incidence of spontaneous abortion.

### Cryopreservation of Embryos

Early embryos resulting from IVF can be preserved for long periods by freezing them in liquid nitrogen with a cryoprotectant (e.g., glycerol or dimethyl sulfoxide [DMSO]). Successful transfer of four- to eight-cell embryos and blastocysts to the uterus after thawing is now a common practice. The longest period of **sperm cryopreservation** that resulted in a live birth was reported to be 21 years.

### Intracytoplasmic Sperm Injection

A sperm can be injected directly into the cytoplasm of a mature oocyte. This technique has been successfully used for the treatment of couples for whom IVF failed, or in cases where there are too few sperms available.

### Assisted In Vivo Fertilization

A technique enabling fertilization to occur in the uterine tube is called **gamete intrafallopian (intratubal) transfer**. It involves superovulation (similar to that used for IVF), oocyte retrieval, sperm collection, and laparoscopic placement of several oocytes and sperms into the uterine tubes. Using this technique, fertilization occurs in the ampulla, its usual location.

### Surrogate Mothers

Some women produce mature oocytes but are unable to become pregnant, for example, a woman who has had her uterus excised (**hysterectomy**). In these cases, IVF may be performed and the embryos transferred to another woman's uterus for fetal development and delivery.

Several studies have reported a higher incidence of birth defects, including embryonal tumors and chromosomal (molecular) changes (gene mutations), in children conceived as a result of assisted reproductive technologies. Long-term follow-up and evaluation of these children will provide guidance for parents and physicians.

# CLEAVAGE OF ZYGOTE

*Cleavage consists of repeated mitotic divisions of the zygote*, resulting in a rapid increase in the number of cells (blastomeres). These embryonic cells become smaller with each successive cleavage division (Figs. 2-16 and 2-17). Cleavage occurs as the zygote passes along the uterine tube toward the uterus (see Fig. 2-20). During cleavage, the zygote is within the zona pellucida (see Fig. 2-17A). Division of the zygote into blastomeres begins approximately 30 hours after fertilization. Subsequent cleavage divisions follow one another, forming progressively smaller blastomeres (see Fig. 2-16D to F). After the nine-cell stage, the blastomeres change their shape and tightly align themselves against each other to form a compact ball of cells (see Fig. 2-16D). This phenomenon, **compaction**, is probably mediated by cell-surface–adhesion glycoproteins. Compaction permits greater cell-to-cell interaction and is a prerequisite for segregation of the internal cells that form the **embryoblast (inner cell mass)** of the blastocyst (see Fig. 2-16E and F). *Hippo signaling plays an essential role in segregating the embryoblast from the trophoblast.* When there are 12 to 32 blastomeres, the developing human is called a **morula**. Internal cells of the morula are surrounded by trophoblastic cells. The morula forms approximately 3 days after fertilization as it enters the uterus (see Figs. 2-16D and 2-20).

Uterus   Uterine tube

Ovary

Hormonal stimulation of mature oocyte
formation, resulting in several mature follicles

Collection of oocytes from follicles
with aspirator during laparoscopy

Placement of oocytes in Petri dish with
capacitated sperms; in vitro fertilization
of oocytes

Cleavage of zygotes in
culture medium until four- to
eight-cell stages are reached

Speculum in vagina

Uterus    Bladder

Transfer of one or two cleaving embryos into
uterine cavity by way of a catheter inserted
through the vagina and cervical canal

Catheter

Rectum

**FIGURE 2-15** In vitro fertilization and embryo transfer procedures.

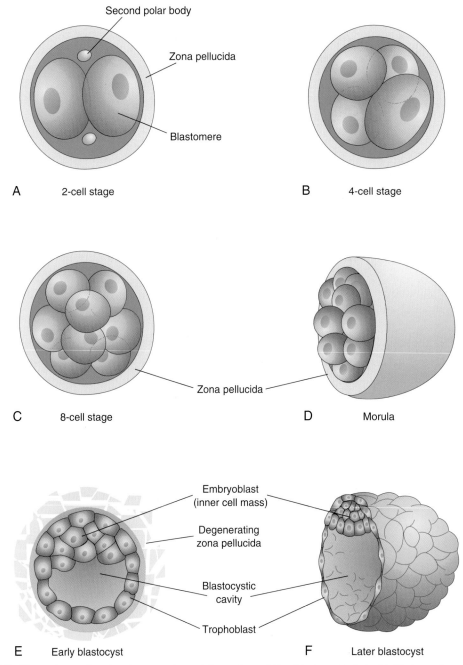

**FIGURE 2–16** Illustrations of a cleaving zygote and formation of the blastocyst. **A** to **D**, Various stages of cleavage of the zygote. The period of the morula begins at the 12-cell to 16-cell stage and ends when the blastocyst forms. **E** and **F**, Sections of blastocysts. The zona pellucida has disappeared by the late blastocyst stage (5 days). The second polar bodies shown in **A** are small, nonfunctional cells. Cleavage of the zygote and formation of the morula occur as the dividing zygote passes along the uterine tube. Blastocyst formation occurs in the uterus. Although cleavage increases the number of blastomeres, note that each of the daughter cells is smaller than the parent cells. As a result, there is no increase in the size of the developing embryo until the zona pellucida degenerates. The blastocyst then enlarges considerably (**F**).

Corona radiata
(composed of follicular cells)

Blastomere

Polar body
(nonfunctional cell)

Degenerating sperm

Zona pellucida

Sperm

**FIGURE 2–17** A, Two-cell-stage of a cleaving zygote developing in vitro. Observe that it is surrounded by many sperms. B, In vitro fertilization, two-cell-stage human embryo. The zona pellucida has been removed. A small rounded polar body *(pink)* is still present on the surface of a blastomere (artificially colored, scanning electron microscopy, ×1000). C, Three-cell-stage human embryo, in vitro fertilization (scanning electron microscopy, ×1300). D, Eight-cell-stage human embryo, in vitro fertilization (scanning electron microscopy, ×1100). Note the rounded large blastomeres with several sperms attached. *(D, From Makabe S, Naguro T, Motta PM: Three-dimensional features of human cleaving embryo by ODO method and field emission scanning electron microscopy. In Motta PM: Microscopy of reproduction and development: a dynamic approach, Rome, 1997, Antonio Delfino Editore.)*

## MOSAICISM

If nondisjunction (failure of a chromosome pair to separate) occurs during an early cleavage division of a zygote, an embryo with two or more cell lines with different chromosome complements is produced. Individuals who have numeric mosaicism are **mosaics**; for example, a zygote with an additional chromosome 21 might lose the extra chromosome during an early division of the zygote. Consequently, some cells of the embryo would have a normal chromosome complement and others would have an additional chromosome 21. In general, individuals who are mosaic for a given trisomy, such as the mosaic Down syndrome, are less severely affected than those with the usual nonmosaic condition.

## FORMATION OF BLASTOCYST

Shortly after the morula enters the uterus (approximately 4 days after fertilization), a fluid-filled space, the

**blastocystic cavity**, appears inside the morula (see Fig. 2-16E). The fluid passes from the uterine cavity through the zona pellucida to form this space. As fluid increases in the blastocystic cavity, it separates the blastomeres into two parts:

- A thin, outer cell layer, the **trophoblast** (Greek *trophe*, nutrition), which gives rise to the embryonic part of the placenta (see Fig. 2-18)
- A group of centrally located blastomeres, the **embryoblast**, which gives rise to the embryo (see Fig. 2-16F)

**Early pregnancy factor**, an immunosuppressant protein, is secreted by the trophoblastic cells and appears in the maternal serum within 24 to 48 hours after fertilization. Early pregnancy factor forms the basis of a pregnancy test during the first 10 days of development.

During this stage of development, or **blastogenesis**, the conceptus (embryo and its membranes) is called a **blastocyst** (Fig. 2-18). The embryoblast now projects into the blastocystic cavity and trophoblast forms the wall of the blastocyst. After the blastocyst has floated in the uterine secretions for approximately 2 days, the **zona pellucida** gradually degenerates and disappears (see Figs. 2-16E

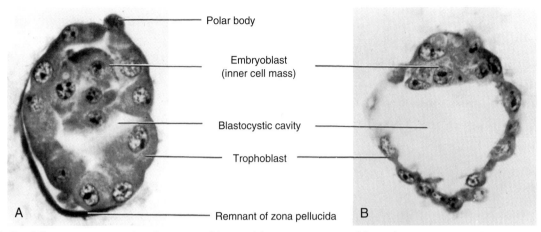

Polar body

Embryoblast
(inner cell mass)

Blastocystic cavity

Trophoblast

A

Remnant of zona pellucida

B

**FIGURE 2–18** Photomicrographs of sections of human blastocysts recovered from the uterine cavity (×600). **A,** At 4 days, the blastocystic cavity is just beginning to form and the zona pellucida is deficient over part of the blastocyst. **B,** At 4.5 days, the blastocystic cavity has enlarged and the embryoblast and trophoblast are clearly defined. The zona pellucida has disappeared. *(From Hertig AT, Rock J, Adams EC: A description of 34 human ova within the first seventeen days of development, Am J Anat 98:435, 1956. Courtesy the Carnegie Institution of Washington.)*

and *F* and 2-18*A*). Shedding of the zona pellucida and hatching of the blastocyst have been observed in vitro. **Shedding of the zona pellucida** permits the blastocyst to increase rapidly in size. While in the uterus, the embryo derives nourishment from secretions of the uterine glands (see Fig. 2-6*C*).

Approximately 6 days after fertilization (day 20 of a 28-day menstrual cycle), the blastocyst attaches to the endometrial epithelium, usually adjacent to the embryonic pole (Fig. 2-19*A*). As soon as it attaches to the **endometrial epithelium**, the trophoblast proliferates rapidly and differentiates into two layers (see Fig. 2-19*B*):

- An inner layer of **cytotrophoblast**
- An outer layer of **syncytiotrophoblast** consisting of a multinucleated protoplasmic mass in which no cell boundaries can be observed

Both intrinsic and extracellular matrix factors modulate, in carefully timed sequences, the differentiation of

the trophoblast. *Transforming growth factor-β regulates the proliferation and differentiation of the trophoblast by interaction of the ligand with type I and type II receptors, serine/threonine protein kinases.* At approximately 6 days, the finger-like processes of syncytiotrophoblast extend through the endometrial epithelium and invade the connective tissue. By the end of the first week, the blastocyst is superficially implanted in the compact layer of the endometrium and is deriving its nourishment from the eroded maternal tissues (see Fig. 2-19*B*). The highly invasive syncytiotrophoblast expands quickly adjacent to the embryoblast, the area known as the **embryonic pole** (see Fig. 2-19*A*). The syncytiotrophoblast produces

## PREIMPLANTATION GENETIC DIAGNOSIS

Preimplantation genetic diagnosis can be carried out 3 to 5 days after IVF of the oocyte (see Fig. 2-15). One or two cells (blastomeres) are removed from the embryo known to be at risk for a single gene defect or chromosomal anomaly. These cells are then analyzed before transfer into the uterus. The sex of the embryo can also be determined from one blastomere taken from a six- to eight-cell dividing zygote, and analyzed by polymerase chain reaction and fluorescence in situ hybridization techniques. This procedure has been used to detect female embryos during IVF in cases in which a male embryo would be at risk of a serious X-linked disorder. The polar body may also be tested for diseases where the mother is the carrier (see Fig. 2-14*A*).

## ABNORMAL EMBRYOS AND SPONTANEOUS ABORTIONS

Many zygotes, morulae, and blastocysts abort spontaneously. Early implantation of the blastocyst is a critical period of development that may fail to occur owing to inadequate production of progesterone and estrogen by the corpus luteum (see Fig. 2-7). Clinicians occasionally see a patient who states that her last menstrual period was delayed by several days and that her last menstrual flow was unusually profuse. Very likely such patients have had early spontaneous abortions. The overall early **spontaneous abortion rate** is thought to be approximately 45%. Early spontaneous abortions occur for a variety of reasons, one being the presence of chromosomal abnormalities. More than half of all known spontaneous abortions occur because of these abnormalities. The early loss of embryos appears to represent a removal of abnormal conceptuses that could not have developed normally, that is, it is a natural screening of embryos without which the incidence of fetuses with birth defects would be far greater.

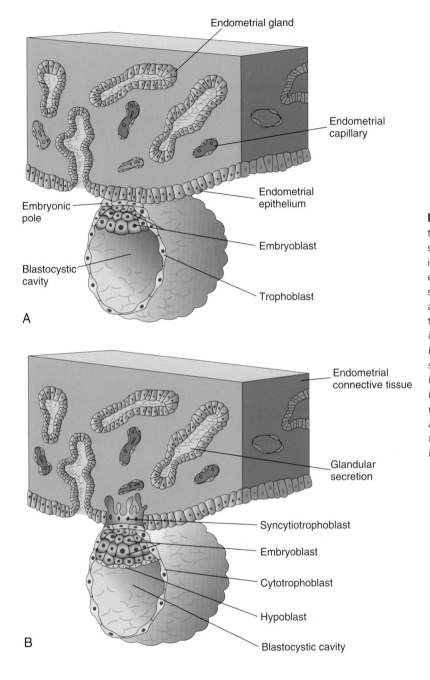

Endometrial gland

Endometrial capillary

Endometrial epithelium

Embryonic pole

Embryoblast

Blastocystic cavity

Trophoblast

A

Endometrial connective tissue

Glandular secretion

Syncytiotrophoblast

Embryoblast

Cytotrophoblast

Hypoblast

Blastocystic cavity

B

**FIGURE 2–19** Attachment of the blastocyst to the endometrial epithelium during the early stages of implantation. **A,** At 6 days, the trophoblast is attached to the endometrial epithelium at the embryonic pole of the blastocyst. **B,** At 7 days, the syncytiotrophoblast has penetrated the epithelium and has started to invade the endometrial connective tissue. *Note: In embryologic studies, the embryo is usually shown with its dorsal surface upward. Because the embryo implants on its future dorsal surface, it would appear upside down if the histologic convention (epithelium upward) were followed. In this book, the histologic convention is followed when the endometrium is the dominant consideration (e.g., Fig. 2-6C), and the embryologic convention is used when the embryo is the center of interest, as in the adjacent illustrations.*

enzymes that erode the maternal tissues, enabling the blastocyst to "burrow" into the endometrium. Endometrial cells also assist to control the depth of penetration of the syncytiotrophoblast. At approximately 7 days, a layer of cells, the **hypoblast** (primary endoderm), appears on the surface of the embryoblast facing the blastocystic cavity (see Fig. 2-19B). Comparative embryologic data suggest that the hypoblast arises by delamination of blastomeres from the embryoblast.

## SUMMARY OF FIRST WEEK

● Oocytes are produced by the ovaries (**oogenesis**) and expelled from them during ovulation (Fig. 2-20). The fimbriae of the uterine tubes sweep the oocyte into the ampulla, where it may be fertilized. Usually only one oocyte is expelled at ovulation.

● Sperms are produced in the testes (**spermatogenesis**) and are stored in the **epididymis** (see Fig. 2-12). Ejaculation of semen results in the deposit of millions of sperms in the vagina. Several hundred sperms pass through the uterus and enter the uterine tubes.

● When an oocyte is contacted by a sperm, it completes the second meiotic division (see Fig. 2-1). As a result, a mature oocyte and a second polar body are formed. The nucleus of the mature oocyte constitutes the female pronucleus (see Fig. 2-14B and C).

● After the sperm enters the oocyte, the head of the sperm separates from the tail and enlarges to become the male pronucleus (see Figs. 2-13 and 2-14C). Fertilization is complete when the male and female

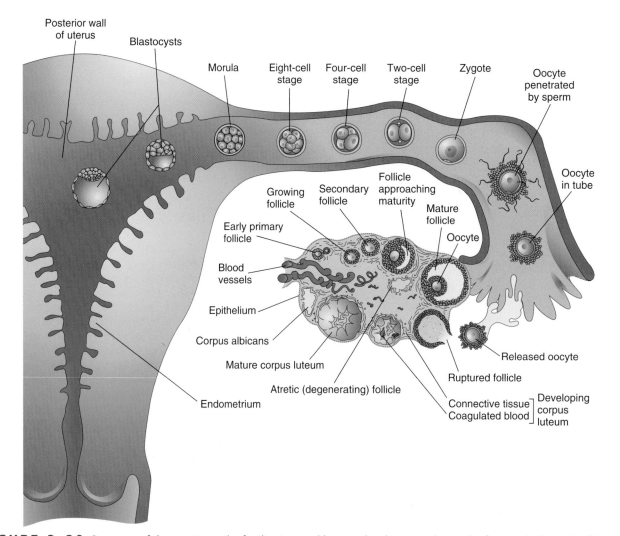

**FIGURE 2–20** Summary of the ovarian cycle, fertilization, and human development during the first week. Stage 1 of development begins with fertilization in the ampulla of the uterine tube and ends when the zygote forms. Stage 2 (days 2 to 3) comprises the early stages of cleavage (from 2 to approximately 32 cells, the morula). Stage 3 (days 4 to 5) consists of the free (unattached) blastocyst. Stage 4 (days 5 to 6) is represented by the blastocyst attaching to the posterior wall of the uterus, the usual site of implantation. The blastocysts have been sectioned to show their internal structure.

pronuclei unite and the maternal and paternal chromosomes intermingle during metaphase of the first mitotic division of the zygote (see Fig. 2-14D and C).

- As it passes along the uterine tube toward the uterus, the zygote undergoes cleavage (a series of mitotic cell divisions) into a number of smaller cells, or blastomeres. Approximately 3 days after fertilization, a ball of 12 or more blastomeres (a morula) enters the uterus (see Fig. 2-20).

- A cavity forms in the morula, converting it into a blastocyst consisting of the embryoblast, a blastocystic cavity, and the trophoblast (see Fig. 2-16D to F). The trophoblast encloses the embryoblast and blastocystic cavity and later forms extraembryonic structures and the embryonic part of the placenta.

- At 4 to 5 days after fertilization, the zona pellucida is shed and the trophoblast adjacent to the embryoblast attaches to the endometrial epithelium (see Fig. 2-16E).

- The trophoblast at the embryonic pole differentiates into two layers, an outer syncytiotrophoblast and an inner cytotrophoblast (see Fig. 2-19B). The syncytiotrophoblast invades the endometrial epithelium and underlying connective tissue. Concurrently, a cuboidal layer of hypoblast forms on the deep surface of the embryoblast. By the end of the first week, the blastocyst is superficially implanted in the endometrium (see Fig. 2-19B).

## CLINICALLY ORIENTED PROBLEMS

- ✳ What is the main cause of numeric aberrations of chromosomes? Define this process. What is the usual result of this chromosomal abnormality?

- ✳ During in vitro cleavage of a zygote, all blastomeres of a morula were found to have an extra set of chromosomes. Explain how this could happen. Can such a morula develop into a viable fetus?

* What is a major cause of (a) female infertility and (b) male infertility?
* Some people have a mixture of cells, some with 46 chromosomes and others with 47 chromosomes (e.g., some persons with Down syndrome). How do mosaics form? Would children with mosaicism and Down syndrome have the same stigmata as other infants with Down syndrome? At what stage of development does mosaicism develop? Can this chromosomal abnormality be diagnosed before birth?
* A young woman asked you about "morning-after pills" (postcoital oral contraceptives). How would you explain to her the action of such medication?
* What is the most common abnormality in early spontaneously aborted embryos?
* Mary, 26 years old, is unable to conceive after 4 years of marriage. Her husband, Jerry, 32 years old, also appears to be in good health. Mary and Jerry consulted their family physician, who referred them to an infertility clinic. How common is infertility in couples? What do you think are likely causes of possible infertility in this couple? What investigation(s) would you recommend first?

Discussion of these problems appears in the Appendix at the back of the book.

## BIBLIOGRAPHY AND SUGGESTED READING

Alfarawati S, Goodall N, Gordon T, et al: Cytogenetic analysis of human blastocysts with the use of FISH, CGH and aCGH: scientific data and technical evaluation, *Hum Reprod* 25(Suppl 1):i41, 2010.

American Society for Reproductive Medicine: Revised guidelines for human embryology and andrology laboratories, *Fertil Steril* 90(Suppl):s45, 2008.

Barratt CLR, Kay V, Oxenham SK: The human spermatozoa—a stripped down but refined machine, *J Biol* 8:63, 2009.

Cameron S: The normal menstrual cycle. In Magowan BA, Owen P, Thomson A, editors: *Clinical obstetrics and gynaecology*, ed 3, Philadelphia, 2014, Saunders.

Chiu PC, Lam KK, Wong RC, et al: The identity of zona pellucida receptor on spermatozoa: an unresolved issue in developmental biology, *Semin Cell Dev Biol* 30:86, 2014.

Clermont Y, Trott M: Kinetics of spermatogenesis in mammals: seminiferous epithelium cycle and spermatogonial renewal, *Physiol Rev* 52:198, 1972.

Duggavathi R, Murphy BD: Ovulation signals, *Science* 324:890, 2009.

Fragouli E, Lenzi M, Ross R, et al: Comprehensive molecular cytogenetic analysis of the human blastocyst stage, *Hum Reprod* 23:2596, 2008.

Frey KA: Male reproductive health and infertility, *Prim Care* 37:643, 2010.

Gadella BM: Dynamic regulation of sperm interactions with the zona pellucida prior to and after fertilisation, *Reprod Fertil Dev* 25:26, 2012.

Gleicher N, Kushnir VA, Barad DH: Preimplantation genetic screening (PGS) still in search of a clinical application: a systematic review, *Reprod Biol Endocrinol* 12:22, 2014.

Gunby J, Bissonnette F, Librach C, et al: Assisted reproductive technologies (ART) in Canada: 2007 results from the Canadian ART Register, *Fertil Steril* 95:542, 2011.

Harper J, editor: *Preimplantation genetic diagnosis*, ed 2, Cambridge, 2009, Cambridge University Press.

Hertig AT, Rock J, Adams EC, et al: Thirty-four fertilized human ova, good, bad, and indifferent, recovered from 210 women of known fertility, *Pediatrics* 23:202, 1959.

Jequier AM: *Male infertility: a clinical guide*, ed 2, Cambridge, 2011, Cambridge University Press.

Jia J, Geng L, Zong Y: Birth defects in assisted reproductive technology and spontaneously conceived children: a meta-analysis, *J Reprod Contracept* 24:237, 2013.

Myers M, Pangas SA: Regulatory roles of transforming growth factor beta family members in folliculogenesis, *WIREs Syst Biol Med* 2:117, 2010.

Nusbaum RL, McInnes RR, Willard HF: *Thompson and Thompson genetics in medicine*, ed 7, Philadelphia, 2007, Saunders.

Quenby S, Brosens JJ: Human implantation: a tale of mutual maternal and fetal attraction, *Biol Reprod* 88:81, 2013.

Robertson SA: Immune regulation of embryo implantation: all about quality control, *J Reprod Immun* 81:113, 2009.

Rock J, Hertig AT: The human conceptus during the first two weeks of gestation, *Am J Obstet Gynecol* 55:6, 1948.

Simpson JL: Birth defects and assisted reproductive technology, *Semin Fetal Neonatal Med* 19:177, 2014.

Steptoe PC, Edwards RG: Birth after implantation of a human embryo, *Lancet* 2:36, 1978.

Weremowicz S, Sandstrom DJ, Morton CC, et al: Fluorescence in situ hybridization (FISH) for rapid detection of aneuploidy: experience in 911 prenatal cases, *Prenat Diagn* 21:262, 2001.

Wilmut I, Schnieke AE, McWhir J, et al: Viable offspring derived from fetal and adult mammalian cells, *Nature* 385:810, 1997.

# Second Week of Human Development

**A**s implantation of the blastocyst occurs, morphologic changes in the embryoblast produce a bilaminar **embryonic disc** composed of epiblast and hypoblast (Fig. 3-1*A*). The **embryonic disc** gives rise to the germ layers that form all the tissues and organs of the embryo. Extraembryonic structures forming during the second week are the amniotic cavity, amnion, umbilical vesicle connecting stalk, and chorionic sac.

## COMPLETION OF IMPLANTATION OF BLASTOCYST

Implantation of the blastocyst is completed during the second week. It occurs during a restricted time period 6 to 10 days after ovulation and fertilization. As the blastocyst implants (see Fig. 3-1), more trophoblast contacts the endometrium and differentiates into two layers:

● An inner layer, the cytotrophoblast, that is mitotically active (i.e., mitotic figures are visible) and forms new cells that migrate into the increasing mass of syncytiotrophoblast, where they fuse and lose their cell membranes
● The syncytiotrophoblast, a rapidly expanding, multinucleated mass in which no cell boundaries are discernible

The erosive **syncytiotrophoblast** invades the endometrial connective tissue, and the blastocyst slowly becomes embedded in the endometrium (Fig. 3-2). **Syncytiotrophoblastic cells** displace endometrial cells at the implantation site. The endometrial cells undergo **apoptosis** (programmed cell death), which facilitates the invasion.

*The molecular mechanisms of implantation involve synchronization between the invading blastocyst and a receptive endometrium. The microvilli of endometrial cells, cell adhesion*

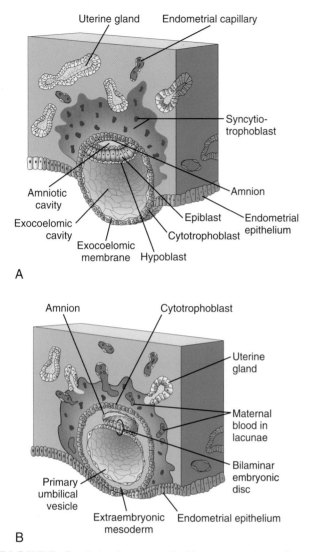

A

B

**FIGURE 3–1** Implantation of a blastocyst in the endometrium. The actual size of the **conceptus** is 0.1 mm, approximately the size of the period at the end of this sentence. **A,** Drawing of a section through a blastocyst partially embedded in the uterine endometrium (approximately 8 days). Note the slit-like amniotic cavity. **B,** Drawing of a section through a blastocyst of approximately 9 days implanted in the endometrium. Note the lacunae appearing in the syncytiotrophoblast.

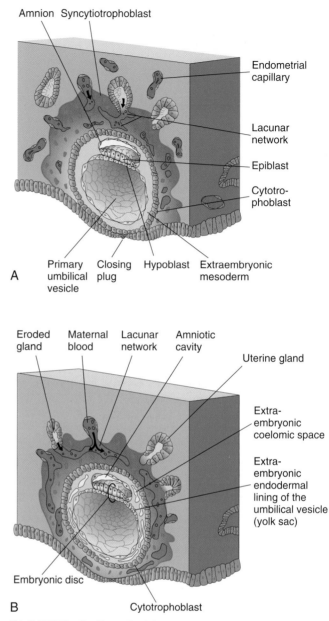

A

B

**FIGURE 3–2** Embedded blastocysts. **A,** 10 days. **B,** 12 days. This stage of development is characterized by communication of the blood-filled lacunar networks. Note in **B** that **coelomic spaces** have appeared in the **extraembryonic mesoderm**, forming the beginning of the **extraembryonic coelom** (cavity).

*molecules (integrins), cytokines, prostaglandins, hormones (human chorionic gonadotropin [hCG] and progesterone), growth factors, and extracellular matrix and enzymes (matrix metalloproteinase and protein kinase A) play a role in making the endometrium receptive.* In addition, the endometrial cells help to modulate the depth of penetration of the syncytiotrophoblast.

The connective tissue cells around the implantation site accumulate glycogen and lipids and assume a polyhedral (many-sided) appearance. Some of these cells, **decidual cells,** degenerate adjacent to the penetrating syncytiotrophoblast. The syncytiotrophoblast engulfs these cells, providing a rich source of embryonic nutrition. The **syncytiotrophoblast** produces a glycoprotein hormone,

**hCG,** which enters the maternal blood via isolated cavities (**lacunae**) in the syncytiotrophoblast (see Fig. 3-1B); hCG maintains the hormonal activity of the corpus luteum in the ovary during pregnancy. The **corpus luteum** is an endocrine glandular structure that secretes estrogen and progesterone to maintain pregnancy (see Chapter 2, Fig. 2-11). Highly sensitive radioimmunoassays are available for detecting hCG, and they form the basis for **pregnancy tests.** Enough hCG is produced by the syncytiotrophoblast at the end of the second week to give a positive pregnancy test, even though the woman is probably unaware that she may be pregnant.

# FORMATION OF AMNIOTIC CAVITY, EMBRYONIC DISC, AND UMBILICAL VESICLE

As implantation of the blastocyst progresses, a small space appears in the embryoblast, which is the primordium of the **amniotic cavity** (see Figs. 3-1*A* and 3-2*B*). Soon, amniogenic (amnion-forming) cells, **amnioblasts**, separate from the epiblast and form the **amnion**, which encloses the amniotic cavity. Concurrently, morphologic changes occur in the **embryoblast** (cluster of cells from which the embryo develops) that result in the formation of a flat, almost circular bilaminar plate of cells, the **embryonic disc**, consisting of two layers (see Fig. 3-2*A* and *B*):

- **Epiblast**, the thicker layer, consisting of high columnar cells related to the amniotic cavity
- **Hypoblast**, consisting of small cuboidal cells adjacent to the exocoelomic cavity

The **epiblast** forms the floor of the amniotic cavity and is continuous peripherally with the amnion. The **hypoblast** forms the roof of the exocoelomic cavity (see Fig. 3-1*A*) and is continuous with the thin **exocoelomic membrane**. This membrane, together with the hypoblast, lines the **primary umbilical vesicle**. The embryonic disc now lies between the amniotic cavity and vesicle (see Fig. 3-1*B*). Cells from the vesicle endoderm form a layer of connective tissue, the **extraembryonic mesoderm** (see Fig. 3-2*A*), which surrounds the amnion and umbilical vesicle. This vesicle and amniotic cavity make morphogenetic movements of the cells of the embryonic disc possible.

As the amnion, embryonic disc, and umbilical vesicle form, **lacunae** (small spaces) appear in the syncytiotrophoblast (see Figs. 3-1*A* and 3-2). The lacunae become filled with a mixture of maternal blood from ruptured endometrial capillaries and cellular debris from eroded uterine glands (see Chapter 2, Fig. 2-6*C*). The fluid in the lacunar spaces, **embryotroph**, passes to the embryonic disc by diffusion and provides nutritive material to the embryo.

The communication of the eroded endometrial capillaries with the lacunae in the syncytiotrophoblast establishes the **primordial uteroplacental circulation**. When maternal blood flows into the **lacunar networks** (see Fig. 3-2*A* and B), oxygen and nutritive substances pass to the embryo. **Oxygenated blood** passes into the lacunae from the **spiral endometrial arteries** (see Chapter 2, Fig. 2-6*C*), and poorly **oxygenated blood** is removed from them through the endometrial veins.

The **10-day conceptus** (embryo and membranes) is completely embedded in the uterine endometrium (see Fig. 3-2*A*). Initially, there is a surface defect in the endometrial epithelium that is soon closed by a **closing plug** of a fibrin coagulum of blood (see Fig. 3-2*A*). By day 12, an almost completely regenerated uterine epithelium covers the closing plug (Fig. 3-3, and see Fig. 3-2*B*). This partially results from signaling by cyclic adenosine monophosphate and progesterone. As the conceptus implants, the endometrial connective tissue cells continue to undergo a transformation, the **decidual reaction**. The cells

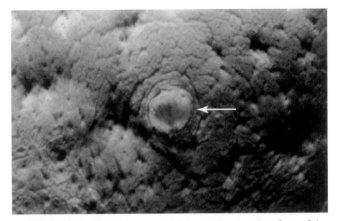

**FIGURE 3–3** Photograph of the endometrial surface of the body of the uterus, showing the implantation site of the 12-day embryo shown in Figure 3-4. The implanted **conceptus** produces a small elevation (*arrow*) (×8). *(From Hertig AT, Rock J: Two human ova of the pre-villous stage, having an ovulation age of about eleven and twelve days respectively, Contrib Embryol Carnegie Inst 29:127, 1941. Courtesy the Carnegie Institution of Washington, DC.)*

swell because of the accumulation of glycogen and lipid in their cytoplasm. The primary function of the decidual reaction is to provide nutrition for the early embryo and an immunologically privileged site for the conceptus.

In a **12-day embryo**, adjacent syncytiotrophoblastic **lacunae** (small spaces) have fused to form **lacunar networks** (Fig. 3-4*B*, and see Fig. 3-2*B*), giving the syncytiotrophoblast a sponge-like appearance. The networks, particularly obvious around the embryonic pole, are the primordia of the **intervillous spaces of the placenta** (see Chapter 7, Fig. 7-5). The endometrial capillaries around the implanted embryo become congested and dilated to form **maternal sinusoids**, thin-walled terminal vessels that are larger than ordinary capillaries (Fig. 3-5*A*). The formation of blood vessels in the endometrial **stroma** (framework of connective tissue) is under the influence of estrogen and progesterone. *Expression of connexin 43 (Cx43), a gap junction protein, plays a critical role in angiogenesis at the implantation site and in maintenance of pregnancy.*

The syncytiotrophoblast erodes the sinusoids, and maternal blood flows freely into the lacunar networks (see Figs. 3-4*B* and 3-8*B*). The trophoblast absorbs nutritive fluid from the lacunar networks, which is transferred to the embryo. *Growth of the bilaminar embryonic disc is slow* compared with growth of the trophoblast (see Figs. 3-1, 3-2, and 3-8*B*). The implanted 12-day embryo produces a minute elevation on the endometrial surface that protrudes into the uterine cavity (see Figs. 3-3 and 3-4).

As changes occur in the trophoblast and endometrium, the extraembryonic mesoderm increases and isolated **extraembryonic coelomic spaces** appear within it (see Figs. 3-2*B* and 3-4*B*). These spaces rapidly fuse to form a large isolated cavity, the **extraembryonic coelom** (see Fig. 3-5*A*). This fluid-filled cavity surrounds the amnion and umbilical vesicle, except where they are attached to the **chorion** (outermost fetal membrane) by

Spongy layer

Compact layer

Embryonic disc

Endometrial glands

Endometrial blood vessels

Endometrial epithelium

Closing plug

A

Embryonic hypoblast

Lacunar network

Cyto-trophoblast

Extra-embryonic coelom

Embryonic epiblast

Amnion

Syncytio-trophoblast

Primary umbilical vesicle (yolk sac)

Extra-embryonic mesoderm

B

**FIGURE 3–4** Embedded blastocyst. **A**, Section through the implantation site of the 12-day embryo described in Figure 3-3. The embryo is embedded superficially in the compact layer of the endometrium (×30). **B**, Higher magnification of the conceptus and uterine endometrium surrounding it (×100). Lacunae (small cavities) containing maternal blood are visible in the syncytiotrophoblast. *(From Hertig AT, Rock J: Two human ova of the pre-villous stage, having an ovulation age of about eleven and twelve days respectively, Contrib Embryol Carnegie Inst 29:127, 1941. Courtesy the Carnegie Institution of Washington, DC.)*

the **connecting stalk** (see Fig. 3-8A and B). As the extra-embryonic coelom forms, the primary umbilical vesicle decreases in size and a smaller **secondary umbilical vesicle** forms (see Fig. 3-5B). This smaller vesicle is formed by extraembryonic endodermal cells that migrate from the hypoblast inside the primary umbilical vesicle (Fig. 3-6). During formation of the secondary umbilical vesicle, a large part of the primary umbilical vesicle is pinched off, leaving a remnant of the vesicle (see Fig. 3-5B). *The umbilical vesicle in humans contains no yolk*; however,

it has important functions—for example, it is the site of origin of primordial germ cells (see Chapter 12). It may also have a role in the selective transfer of nutrients to the embryo.

## DEVELOPMENT OF CHORIONIC SAC

The end of the second week is characterized by the appearance of **primary chorionic villi** (see Fig. 3-5A and

2

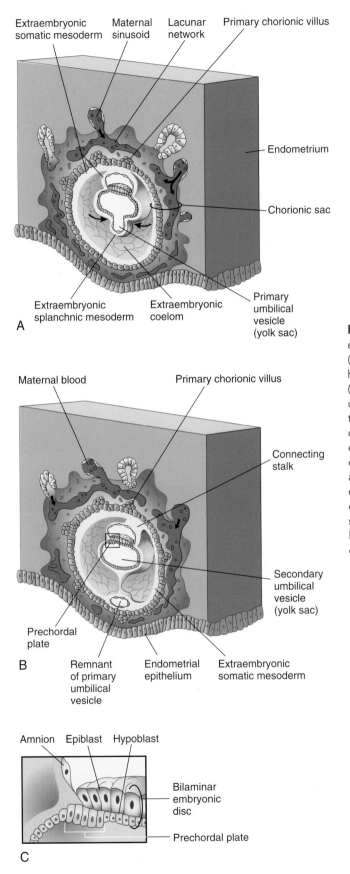

A

B

C

**FIGURE 3–5** Drawings of sections of implanted human embryos, based mainly on the studies of Hertig and colleagues (1956). Observe (1) that the defect in the endometrial epithelium has disappeared; (2) a small secondary umbilical vesicle has formed; (3) a large cavity, the extraembryonic coelom, now surrounds the umbilical vesicle and amnion, except where the amnion is attached to the chorion by the connecting stalk; and (4) the extraembryonic coelom splits the extraembryonic mesoderm into two layers: the extraembryonic somatic mesoderm lining the trophoblast and covering the amnion, and the extraembryonic splanchnic mesoderm around the umbilical vesicle. A, A 13-day embryo, illustrating the decrease in relative size of the primary umbilical vesicle and the early appearance of primary chorionic villi. B, A 14-day embryo, showing the newly formed secondary umbilical vesicle and the location of the prechordal plate in its roof. C, Detail of the prechordal plate outlined in B.

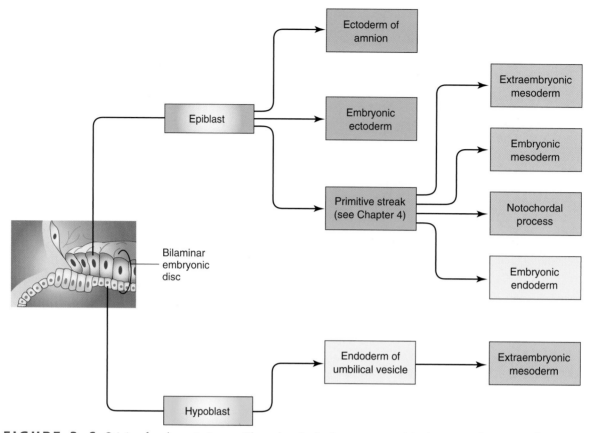

**FIGURE 3-6** Origin of embryonic tissues. The colors in the boxes are used in drawings of sections of embryos.

*B*). The villi (vascular processes of the chorion) form columns with syncytial coverings. The cellular extensions grow into the syncytiotrophoblast. The growth of these extensions is thought to be induced by the underlying **extraembryonic somatic mesoderm**. The cellular projections form **primary chorionic villi** (see Fig. 3-5*A* and *B*), the first stage in the development of the chorionic villi of the **placenta** (fetomaternal organ of metabolic interchange between the embryo and mother).

The **extraembryonic coelom** splits the extraembryonic mesoderm into two layers (see Fig. 3-5*A* and *B*):

- **Extraembryonic somatic mesoderm**, lining the trophoblast and covering the amnion
- **Extraembryonic splanchnic mesoderm**, surrounding the umbilical vesicle

The extraembryonic somatic mesoderm and the two layers of trophoblast form the **chorion** (outermost fetal membrane), which forms the wall of the **chorionic sac** (see Fig. 3-5*A* and *B*). The embryo, amniotic sac, and umbilical vesicle are suspended in this sac by the connecting stalk. (The term *umbilical vesicle* is preferred because the yolk sac does not contain yolk in humans.) The extraembryonic coelom is the primordium of the **chorionic cavity**.

**Transvaginal ultrasonography** (endovaginal sonography) is used for measuring the chorionic sac diameter (Fig. 3-7). This measurement is valuable for evaluating early embryonic development and pregnancy outcome.

A 14-day embryo still has the form of a flat **bilaminar embryonic disc** (Fig. 3-8*B*, and see Fig. 3-5*C*), but the

**FIGURE 3-7** Endovaginal sonogram (sagittal and axial) of an early chorionic sac (5 weeks) (+). The mean chorionic sac diameter is calculated from the three orthogonal measurements (d1, d2, d3). The secondary umbilical vesicle can also be seen on the left image.

hypoblastic cells in a localized area are now columnar and form a thickened circular area, the **prechordal plate** (see Fig. 3-5*B* and *C*). This plate indicates the site of the mouth and is an important organizer of the head region.

**FIGURE 3–8** Photomicrographs of longitudinal sections of an embedded 14-day embryo. Note the large size of the extraembryonic coelom. **A,** Low-power view (×18). **B,** High-power view (×95). The embryo is represented by the bilaminar embryonic disc composed of epiblast and hypoblast. *(From Nishimura H, editor: Atlas of human prenatal histology, Tokyo, Igaku-Shoin, 1983.)*

# IMPLANTATION SITES OF BLASTOCYSTS

Implantation of blastocysts usually occurs in the uterine endometrium in the superior part of the body of the uterus, slightly more often on the posterior wall than on the anterior wall of the uterus (see Fig. 3-10). Implantation of a blastocyst can be detected by **ultrasonography** and highly sensitive **radioimmunoassays of hCG** as early as the end of the second week (Fig. 3-9).

## SUMMARY OF IMPLANTATION

Implantation of the blastocyst in the uterine endometrium begins at the end of the first week (see Chapter 2, Fig. 2-19B) and is completed by the end of the second week (see Fig. 3-2B). The cellular and molecular events relating to implantation are complex. Implantation may be summarized as follows:

- The **zona pellucida degenerates** (day 5). Its disappearance results from enlargement of the blastocyst and degeneration caused by enzymatic lysis. The **lytic enzymes** are released from the acrosomes of sperms that surround and partially penetrate the zona pellucida.
- The **blastocyst adheres** to the endometrial epithelium (day 6).
- The **trophoblast differentiates into two layers**, the syncytiotrophoblast and the cytotrophoblast (day 7).
- The **syncytiotrophoblast erodes endometrial tissues** and the blastocyst begins to embed in the endometrium (day 8).

## EXTRAUTERINE IMPLANTATIONS

Blastocysts sometimes implant outside the uterus (ectopic sites). These implantations result in **ectopic pregnancies**; 95% to 98% of ectopic implantations occur in the uterine tubes, *most often in the ampulla and isthmus* (Figs. 3-9, 3-10, and 3-11, and see Chapter 2, Fig. 2-6B). The incidence of ectopic pregnancy has increased in most countries, ranging from 1 in 80 to 1 in 250 pregnancies, depending partly on the socioeconomic level of the population. In the United States, the frequency of ectopic pregnancy is approximately 2% of all pregnancies; *tubal pregnancy is the main cause of maternal deaths during the first trimester.*

A woman with a **tubal pregnancy** has signs and symptoms of pregnancy. She may also experience abdominal pain and tenderness because of distention of the uterine tube, abnormal bleeding, and irritation of the pelvic peritoneum (**peritonitis**). *The pain may be confused with appendicitis if the pregnancy is in the right uterine tube.* Ectopic pregnancies produce β-human chorionic gonadotropin at a slower rate than normal pregnancies; consequently, β-human chorionic gonadotropin assays may give false-negative results if performed too early. **Transvaginal ultrasonography** is very helpful in the early detection of ectopic tubal pregnancies (see Fig. 3-9).

There are several causes of tubal pregnancy and they are often related to factors that delay or prevent transport of the cleaving zygote into the uterus, for example, by mucosal adhesions in the uterine tube or from blockage of the tube, which is caused by scarring resulting from **pelvic inflammatory disease**. Ectopic tubal pregnancies usually result in rupture of the uterine tube and hemorrhage into the peritoneal cavity during the first 8 weeks, followed by death of the embryo. *Tubal rupture and hemorrhage constitute a threat to the mother's life.* The affected tube and conceptus are usually surgically removed (see Fig. 3-11).

When blastocysts implant in the **isthmus of the uterine tube** (Fig. 3-10D, and see Chapter 2, Fig. 2-6B), the tube tends to rupture early because this narrow part of the tube is relatively unexpandable, and there is often extensive bleeding, probably because of the rich anastomoses between ovarian and uterine vessels in this area. When blastocysts implant in the uterine (intramural) part of the tube (see Fig. 3-10E), they may develop beyond 8 weeks before expulsion occurs. When an intramural uterine tubal pregnancy ruptures, it usually bleeds profusely.

Blastocysts that implant in the ampulla or on the fimbriae of the uterine tube (see Fig. 3-10A, and see Chapter 2, Fig. 2-10A) may be expelled into the peritoneal cavity, where they usually implant in the **rectouterine pouch** (a pocket formed by the deflection of the peritoneum from the rectum to the uterus). In exceptional cases, an **abdominal pregnancy** may continue to full term and the fetus may be delivered alive through a laparotomy. Usually, however, the placenta attaches to abdominal organs (see Fig. 3-10G), which causes considerable intraperitoneal bleeding. *An abdominal pregnancy increases the risk of maternal death from hemorrhage* by a factor of 90 when compared with an intrauterine pregnancy, and seven times more than that for tubal pregnancy. In very unusual cases, an abdominal conceptus (embryo/fetus and membranes) dies and is not detected; the fetus becomes calcified, forming a "stone fetus," or **lithopedion**.

**Heterotopic pregnancies** (simultaneous intrauterine and extrauterine pregnancies) are unusual, occurring in approximately 1 in 8000 to 30,000 naturally conceived pregnancies. The incidence is much higher (approximately 3 in 1000) in women treated with **ovulation induction drugs** as part of assisted reproductive technologies. The ectopic pregnancy is masked initially by the presence of the uterine pregnancy. Usually the ectopic pregnancy can be terminated by surgical removal of the involved uterine tube without interfering with the intrauterine pregnancy (see Fig. 3-11).

*Cervical implantations are unusual* (see Fig. 3-10); in some cases, the placenta becomes firmly attached to fibrous and muscular tissues of the cervix, often resulting in bleeding, which requires subsequent surgical intervention, such as **hysterectomy** (excision of the uterus).

**FIGURE 3–9** A, Frontal section of the uterus and left uterine tube, illustrating an ectopic pregnancy in the ampulla of the tube. B, Ectopic tubal pregnancy. Endovaginal axial sonogram of the uterine fundus and isthmic portion of the right uterine tube. The dark ring-like mass is a 4-week ectopic chorionic sac in the tube.

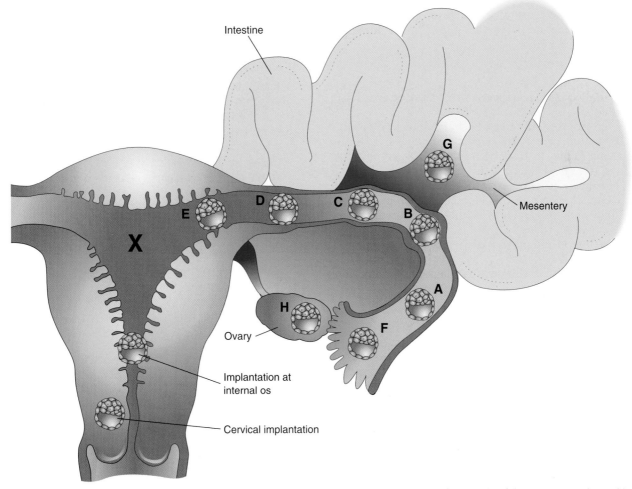

**FIGURE 3–10** Implantation sites of blastocysts. The usual site in the posterior wall of the body of the uterus is indicated by an X. The approximate order of frequency of ectopic implantations is indicated alphabetically (A, most common; H, least common). A to F, tubal pregnancies; G, abdominal pregnancy; H, ovarian pregnancy. Tubal pregnancies are the most common type of ectopic pregnancy. Although appropriately included with uterine pregnancy sites, a cervical pregnancy is often considered to be an ectopic pregnancy.

**FIGURE 3–11** Tubal pregnancy. The uterine tube has been surgically removed and sectioned to show the 5-week-old embryo (10-mm crown–rump length) within the opened chorionic sac (C). *Note the fragments of the amnion (A) and the thin mucosal folds (M) of the uterine tube projecting into the lumen of the tube.*

- **Blood-filled lacunae appear** in the syncytiotrophoblast (day 9).
- The **blastocyst sinks beneath the endometrial epithelium** and the defect is filled by a closing plug (day 10).
- **Lacunar networks form** by fusion of adjacent lacunae (days 10 and 11).
- The **syncytiotrophoblast erodes endometrial blood vessels,** allowing maternal blood to seep in and out of lacunar networks, thereby establishing a uteroplacental circulation (days 11 and 12).
- The **defect in the endometrial epithelium is repaired** (days 12 and 13).
- **Primary chorionic villi develop** (days 13 and 14).

## SUMMARY OF SECOND WEEK

- **Rapid proliferation and differentiation of the trophoblast** occurs as the blastocyst completes implantation in the uterine endometrium.
- The endometrial changes resulting from the adaptation of these tissues in preparation for implantation are known as the **decidual reaction.**
- Concurrently, the **primary umbilical vesicle forms** and **extraembryonic mesoderm** develops. The extraembryonic coelom (cavity) forms from spaces that develop in the extraembryonic mesoderm. The coelom later becomes the **chorionic cavity.**
- The primary umbilical vesicle becomes smaller and gradually disappears as the **secondary umbilical vesicle develops.**

- The amniotic cavity **appears** between the cytotrophoblast and embryoblast.
- The **embryoblast differentiates into a** bilaminar embryonic disc consisting of **epiblast,** related to the amniotic cavity, and **hypoblast,** adjacent to the blastocystic cavity.
- The **prechordal plate develops** as a localized thickening of the hypoblast, which indicates the future cranial region of the embryo and the future site of the mouth; the prechordal plate is also an important organizer of the head region.

## SPONTANEOUS ABORTION OF EMBRYOS AND FETUSES

**Spontaneous abortion** (miscarriage) occurs within the first 12 completed weeks of pregnancy with a frequency of 10% to 20%. Most spontaneous abortions of embryos occur during the first 3 weeks. **Sporadic and recurrent spontaneous abortions** are two of the most common gynecologic problems. The frequency of early spontaneous abortions is difficult to establish because they often occur before a woman is aware that she is pregnant. A spontaneous abortion occurring several days after the first missed period is very likely to be mistaken for a delayed menstruation.

*More than 50% of all known spontaneous abortions result from chromosomal abnormalities.* The higher incidence of early spontaneous abortions in older women probably results from the increasing frequency of **nondisjunction during oogenesis** (see Chapter 2). It has been estimated that 30% to 50% of all zygotes never develop into blastocysts and implant. Failure of blastocysts to implant may result from a poorly developed endometrium; however, in many cases, there are probably lethal chromosomal abnormalities in the embryo. There is a higher incidence of spontaneous abortion of fetuses with neural tube defects, cleft lip, and cleft palate.

## INHIBITION OF IMPLANTATION

The administration of relatively large doses of progestins and/or estrogens (morning-after pills) for several days, beginning shortly after unprotected sexual intercourse, usually does not prevent fertilization but often prevents implantation of the blastocyst. A high dose of **diethylstilbestrol**, given daily for 5 to 6 days, may also accelerate passage of the cleaving zygote along the uterine tube. Normally, the endometrium progresses to the luteal phase of the menstrual cycle as the zygote forms, undergoes cleavage, and enters the uterus. The large amount of estrogen disturbs the normal balance between estrogen and progesterone that is necessary for preparation of the endometrium for implantation.

An **intrauterine device** (IUD) usually interferes with implantation by causing a local inflammatory reaction. Some IUDs contain progesterone, which is slowly released and interferes with the development of the endometrium so that implantation does not usually occur. Other IUDs have a wrap of copper wire. Copper is directly toxic to sperms and also causes uterine endothelial cells to produce substances that are also toxic to sperms.

## CLINICALLY ORIENTED PROBLEMS

### CASE 3–1

*A 22-year-old woman who complained of a severe "chest cold" was sent for a radiograph of her thorax.*

* Is it advisable to examine a healthy female's chest radiographically during the last week of her menstrual cycle?
* Are birth defects likely to develop in her embryo if she happens to be pregnant?

### CASE 3–2

*A woman was given a large dose of estrogen (twice for 1 day) to interrupt a possible pregnancy.*

* If fertilization had occurred, what do you think would be the mechanism of action of this hormone?
* What do laypeople call this type of medical treatment? Is this what the media refer to as the "abortion pill"? If not, explain the method of action of the hormone treatment.
* How early can a pregnancy be detected?

### CASE 3–3

*A 23-year-old woman consulted her physician about severe right lower abdominal pain. She said that she had missed two menstrual periods. A diagnosis of ectopic pregnancy was made.*

* What techniques might be used to confirm this diagnosis?
* What is the most likely site of the extrauterine implantation?
* How do you think the physician would likely treat the condition?

### CASE 3–4

*A 30-year-old woman had an appendectomy toward the end of her menstrual cycle; 8½ months later she had a child with a congenital anomaly of the brain.*

* Could the surgery have produced this child's congenital anomaly? Explain.

### CASE 3–5

*A 42-year-old woman became pregnant after many years of trying to conceive. She was concerned about the healthy development of her baby.*

* What would the physician likely tell her?
* Can women over age 40 have normal babies?
* What tests and diagnostic techniques would likely be performed?

Discussion of these problems appears in the Appendix at the back of the book.

## BIBLIOGRAPHY AND SUGGESTED READING

Basile F, Di Cesare C, Quagliozzi L, et al: Spontaneous heterotopic pregnancy, simultaneous ovarian and intrauterine: a case report, *Case Rep Obstet Gynecol* 509:694, 2012.

Benirschke K: Normal early development. In Creasy RK, Resnik R, Iams JD, et al, editors: *Creasy and Resnik's maternal-fetal medicine: principles and practice*, ed 7, St. Louis, 2014, Saunders.

Bianchi DW, Wilkins-Haug LE, Enders AC, et al: Origin of extraembryonic mesoderm in experimental animals: relevance to chorionic mosaicism in humans, *Am J Med Genet* 46:542, 1993.

Cadmak H, Taylor HS: Implantation failure: treatment and clinical implications, *Hum Reprod Update* 17:242, 2011.

Callen PW: Obstetric ultrasound examination. In Callen PW, editor: *Ultrasonography in obstetrics and gynecology*, ed 5, Philadelphia, 2008, Saunders.

Cole LA: New discoveries on the biology and detection of human chorionic gonadotropin, *Reprod Biol Endocrinol* 7:8, 2009.

Capmas P, Bouyer J, Fernandez H: Treatment of ectopic pregnancies in 2014: new answers to some old questions, *Fertil Steril* 101:615, 2014.

Coulam CB, Faulk WP, McIntyre JA: Spontaneous and recurrent abortions. In Quilligan EJ, Zuspan FP, editors: *Current therapy in obstetrics and gynecology*, vol 3, Philadelphia, 1990, Saunders.

Dickey RP, Gasser R, Olar TT, et al: Relationship of initial chorionic sac diameter to abortion and abortus karyotype based on new growth curves for the 16 to 49 post-ovulation day, *Hum Reprod* 9:559, 1994.

Enders AC, King BF: Formation and differentiation of extraembryonic mesoderm in the rhesus monkey, *Am J Anat* 181:327, 1988.

FitzPatrick DR: Human embryogenesis. In Magowan BA, Owen P, Thomson A, editors: *Clinical obstetrics and gynaecology*, 3rd ed, Philadelphia, 2014, Saunders.

Galliano D, Pellicer A: MicroRNA and implantation, *Fertil Steril* 101:2014, 1531.

Hertig AT, Rock J: Two human ova of the pre-villous stage, having a development age of about seven and nine days respectively, *Contrib Embryol Carnegie Inst* 31:65, 1945.

Hertig AT, Rock J: Two human ova of the pre-villous stage, having a developmental age of about eight and nine days, respectively, *Contrib Embryol Carnegie Inst* 33:169, 1949.

Hertig AT, Rock J, Adams EC: A description of 34 human ova within the first seventeen days of development, *Am J Anat* 98:435, 1956.

Hertig AT, Rock J, Adams EC, et al: Thirty-four fertilized human ova, good, bad, and indifferent, recovered from 210 women of known fertility, *Pediatrics* 23:202, 1959.

Kirk E, Bottomley C, Bourne T: Diagnosing ectopic pregnancy and current concepts in the management of pregnancy of unknown location, *Hum Reprod Update* 20:250, 2014.

Koot YE, Teklenburg G, Salker MS, et al: Molecular aspects of implantation failure, *Biochim Biophys Acta* 1822(12):1943, 2012.

Levine D: Ectopic pregnancy. In Callen PW, editor: *Ultrasonography in obstetrics and gynecology*, ed 5, Philadelphia, 2008, Saunders.

Lindsay DJ, Lovett IS, Lyons EA, et al: Endovaginal sonography: yolk sac diameter and shape as a predictor of pregnancy outcome in the first trimester, *Radiology* 183:115, 1992.

Luckett WP: Origin and differentiation of the yolk sac and extraembryonic mesoderm in presomite human and rhesus monkey embryos, *Am J Anat* 152:59, 1978.

Nogales FF, editor: *The human yolk sac and yolk sac tumors*, New York, 1993, Springer-Verlag.

Quenby S, Brosens JJ: Human implantation: a tale of mutual maternal and fetal attraction, *Biol Reprod* 88:81, 2013.

Saravelos SH, Regan L: Unexplained recurrent pregnancy loss, *Obstet Gynecol Clin North Am* 41:157, 2014.

Streeter GL: Developmental horizons in human embryos. Description of age group XI, 13 to 20 somites, and age group XII, 21 to 29 somites, *Contrib Embryol Carnegie Inst* 30:211, 1942.

Zorn AM, Wells JM: Vertebrate endoderm development and organ formation, *Annu Rev Cell Dev Biol* 25:221, 2009.

# Third Week of Human Development

**R**apid development of the embryo from the **trilaminar embryonic disc** during the third week (see Fig. 4-2*H*) is characterized by:

- Appearance of primitive streak
- Development of notochord
- Differentiation of three germ layers

The third week of development coincides with the week following the first missed menstrual period, that is, 5 weeks after the first day of the last normal menstrual period. *Cessation of menstruation is often the first indication that a woman may be pregnant.* Approximately 5 weeks after the last normal menstrual period, a normal pregnancy can be detected with ultrasonography (Fig. 4-1).

## GASTRULATION: FORMATION OF GERM LAYERS

**Gastrulation** is a formative process by which the three germ layers, which are precursors of all embryonic tissues, and the axial orientation are established in embryos. During gastrulation, the bilaminar embryonic disc is converted into a **trilaminar embryonic disc** (Fig. 4-2*H*). Extensive cell shape changes, rearrangement, movement, and alterations in adhesive properties contribute to the process of gastrulation.

4

**FIGURE 4–1** Ultrasonograph sonogram of a 3.5-week conceptus. Note the secondary umbilical vesicle *(calipers)* and the surrounding trophoblast *(1, bright ring of tissue)*.

## PREGNANCY SYMPTOMS

Frequent symptoms of pregnancy are nausea and vomiting, which may occur by the end of the third week; however, the time of onset of these symptoms varies. *Vaginal bleeding at the expected time of menstruation does not rule out pregnancy*, because sometimes there is some loss of blood from the implantation site of the blastocyst. **Implantation bleeding** results from leakage of blood from the closing plug into the uterine cavity from disrupted **lacunar networks** in the implanted blastocyst (see Chapter 3, Figs. 3-2A and 3-5A). When bleeding is interpreted as menstruation, an error occurs in determining the expected delivery date of the fetus.

Gastrulation is the beginning of **morphogenesis** (development of body form) and is the most significant event occurring during the third week. During this week, the embryo is referred to as a **gastrula**. *Bone morphogenetic proteins and other signaling molecules such as FGFs, Shh (sonic hedgehog), Tgifs, and Wnts play a crucial role in gastrulation.*

Each of the three germ layers (ectoderm, mesoderm, and endoderm) gives rise to specific tissues and organs:

- **Embryonic ectoderm** gives rise to the epidermis, central and peripheral nervous systems, eyes and internal ears, neural crest cells, and many connective tissues of the head.
- **Embryonic endoderm** is the source of the epithelial linings of the respiratory and alimentary (digestive) tracts, including the glands opening into the gastrointestinal tract, and glandular cells of associated organs such as the liver and pancreas.

**Embryonic mesoderm** gives rise to all skeletal muscles, blood cells, the lining of blood vessels, all visceral smooth muscular coats, serosal linings of all body cavities, ducts and organs of the reproductive and excretory systems, and most of the cardiovascular system. In the body (trunk or torso), excluding the head and limbs, it is the source of all connective tissues, including cartilage, bones, tendons, ligaments, dermis, and stroma (connective tissue) of internal organs.

## PRIMITIVE STREAK

The first morphologic sign of gastrulation is the formation of the **primitive streak** on the surface of the **epiblast** of the bilaminar embryonic disc (see Fig. 4-2A, B, and C). By the beginning of the third week, this thickened linear band of epiblast appears caudally in the median plane of the dorsal aspect of the embryonic disc (Fig. 4-3A and B, and see Fig. 4-2C). The primitive streak results from the proliferation and movement of cells of the epiblast to the median plane of the embryonic disc. As soon as the primitive streak appears, it is possible to identify the embryo's craniocaudal axis, cranial and caudal ends, dorsal and ventral surfaces, and right and left sides. As the streak elongates by addition of cells to its caudal end, its cranial end proliferates to form the **primitive node** (see Figs. 4-2E and F and 4-3A and B).

Concurrently, a narrow groove, the **primitive groove**, develops in the primitive streak that is continuous with a small depression in the primitive node, the **primitive pit**. The primitive groove and pit result from the invagination (inward movement) of epiblastic cells, which is indicated by arrows in Figure 4-2E.

Shortly after the primitive streak appears, cells leave its deep surface and form **mesenchyme**, an embryonic connective tissue consisting of small, spindle-shaped cells loosely arranged in an extracellular matrix (intercellular substance of a tissue) of sparse collagen (reticular) fibers (Fig. 4-4B). *Mesenchyme forms the supporting tissues of the embryo*, such as most of the connective tissues of the body and the connective tissue framework of glands. Some mesenchyme forms **mesoblast** (undifferentiated mesoderm), which forms intraembryonic mesoderm (see Fig. 4-2D).

Cells from the **epiblast**, as well as from the primitive node and other parts of the primitive streak, displace the hypoblast, forming **embryonic endoderm** in the roof of the umbilical vesicle (see Fig. 4-2H). The cells remaining in the epiblast form the **embryonic ectoderm**.

*Research data suggest that signaling molecules (nodal factors) of the transforming growth factor-β superfamily induce formation of mesoderm. The concerted action of other signaling molecules (e.g., Wnt3a, Wnt5a, and FGFs) also participates in specifying germ cell layer fates. Moreover, transforming growth factor-β (nodal), a T-box transcription factor (veg T), and the Wnt signaling pathway appear to be involved in specification of the endoderm.*

Mesenchymal cells derived from the primitive streak migrate widely. These pluripotential cells differentiate into diverse types of cells, such as fibroblasts, chondroblasts, and osteoblasts (see Chapter 5). In summary, cells

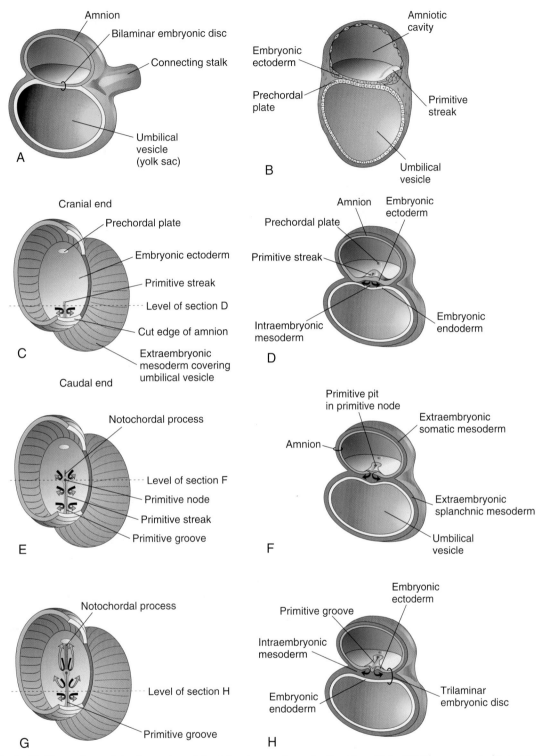

**FIGURE 4–2** Illustrations of the formation of the trilaminar embryonic disc (days 15 to 16). The *arrows* indicate invagination and migration of mesenchymal cells from the primitive streak between the ectoderm and endoderm. C, E, and G, Dorsal views of the trilaminar embryonic disc early in the third week, exposed by removal of the amnion. A, B, D, F, and H, Transverse sections through the embryonic disc. The levels of the sections are indicated in C, E, and G. The prechordal plate, indicating the head region in Figure 4-2C, is indicated by a light blue oval because this thickening of endoderm cannot be seen from the dorsal surface.

**FIGURE 4-3** A, Dorsal view of an embryo approximately 16 days old. B, Drawing of structures shown in A. (*A, From Moore KL, Persaud TVN, Shiota K: Color atlas of clinical embryology, ed 2, Philadelphia, 2000, Saunders.*)

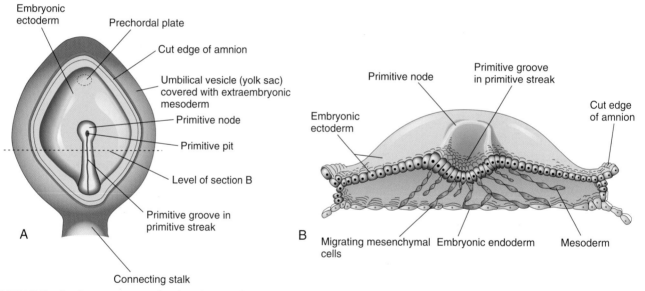

**FIGURE 4-4** A, Drawing of a dorsal view of a 16-day embryo. The amnion has been removed to expose the primitive node, primitive pit, and primitive streak. B, Drawing of the cranial half of the embryonic disc. The trilaminar embryonic disc has been cut transversely to show the migration of mesenchymal cells from the primitive streak to form mesoblast that soon organizes to form the intraembryonic mesoderm. This illustration also shows that most of the embryonic endoderm also arises from the epiblast. Most of the hypoblastic cells are displaced to extraembryonic regions, such as the wall of the umbilical vesicle.

of the epiblast, through the process of gastrulation, give rise to all three germ layers in the embryo, the primordia of all its tissues and organs.

## Fate of Primitive Streak

The primitive streak actively forms mesoderm by the ingression (entrance) of cells until the early part of the fourth week; thereafter, production of mesoderm slows down. The primitive streak diminishes in relative size and becomes an insignificant structure in the sacrococcygeal region of the embryo (Fig. 4-5D). Normally the primitive streak undergoes degenerative changes and disappears by the end of the fourth week.

## NOTOCHORDAL PROCESS AND NOTOCHORD

Some mesenchymal cells migrate through the primitive streak and, as a consequence, acquire mesodermal cell fates. These cells migrate cranially from the primitive node and pit, forming a median cellular cord, the **notochordal process**. This process soon acquires a lumen, the *notochordal canal* (Fig. 4-7C to E). The notochordal process grows cranially between the ectoderm and endoderm until it reaches the **prechordal plate** (see Fig. 4-7A and C), a small circular area of columnar endodermal cells where the ectoderm and endoderm are fused. **Prechordal mesoderm** is a mesenchymal population of neural

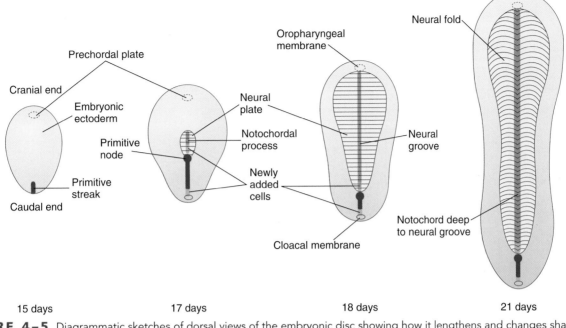

15 days       17 days          18 days        21 days

**FIGURE 4–5** Diagrammatic sketches of dorsal views of the embryonic disc showing how it lengthens and changes shape during the third week. The primitive streak lengthens by addition of cells at its caudal end, and the notochordal process lengthens by migration of cells from the primitive node. The notochordal process and adjacent mesoderm induce the overlying embryonic ectoderm to form the neural plate, the primordium of the central nervous system. Observe that as the notochordal process elongates, the primitive streak shortens. At the end of the third week, the notochordal process is transformed into the notochord.

## SACROCOCCYGEAL TERATOMA

Remnants of the primitive streak may persist and give rise to a **sacrococcygeal teratoma** (Fig. 4-6). A teratoma is a type of germ cell tumor that may be benign or malignant. Because they are derived from pluripotent primitive streak cells, the tumors contain tissues derived from all three germ layers in varying stages of differentiation. These teratomas are the most common tumor in neonates and have an incidence of approximately 1 in 35,000. Most affected infants (80%) are female. The teratomas are usually diagnosed on routine antenatal ultrasonography; most tumors are benign (nonmalignant). They are usually surgically excised promptly, with the prognosis dependent on many factors. A presacral teratoma may cause intestinal (bowel) or urinary obstruction, and surgical excision of such masses can have long-term sequelae in terms of normal function of these same systems.

**FIGURE 4–6** Female infant with a large sacrococcygeal teratoma that developed from remnants of the primitive streak. The tumor, a neoplasm made up of several different types of tissue, was surgically removed.

crest origin, rostral to the notochord. The **prechordal plate** gives rise to the endoderm of the **oropharyngeal membrane**, located at the future site of the oral cavity (Fig. 4-8C). *The prechordal plate serves as a signaling center (Shh and PAX6) for controlling development of cranial structures, including the forebrain and eyes.*

Mesenchymal cells from the primitive streak and notochordal process migrate laterally and cranially, among other mesodermal cells between the ectoderm and endoderm, until they reach the margins of the embryonic disc.

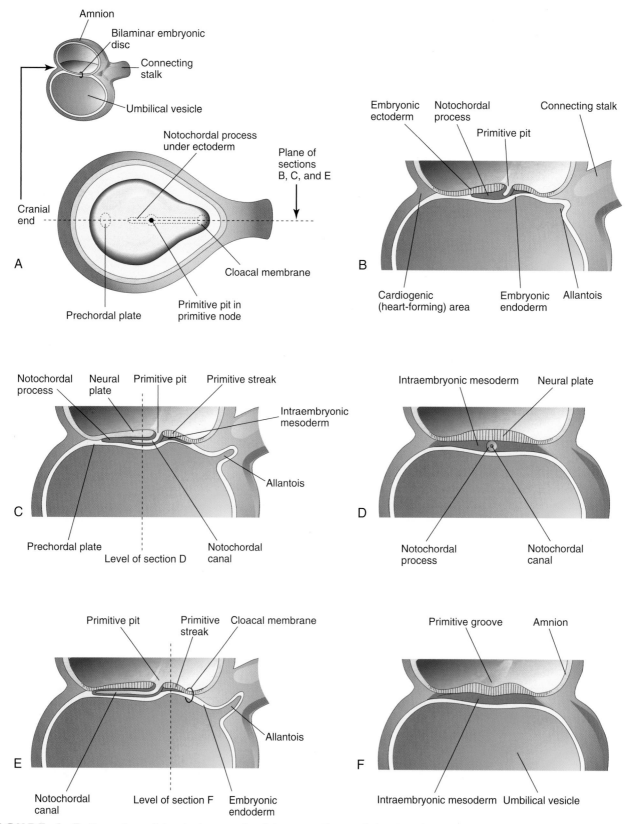

**FIGURE 4–7** Illustrations of developing notochordal process. The small sketch at the upper left is for orientation. **A,** Dorsal view of the embryonic disc (approximately 16 days) exposed by removal of the amnion. The notochordal process is shown as if it were visible through the embryonic ectoderm. **B, C,** and **E,** Median sections at the plane shown in A, illustrating successive stages in the development of the notochordal process and canal. The stages shown in **C** and **E** occur at approximately 18 days. **D** and **F,** Transverse sections through the embryonic disc at the levels shown in **C** and **E.**

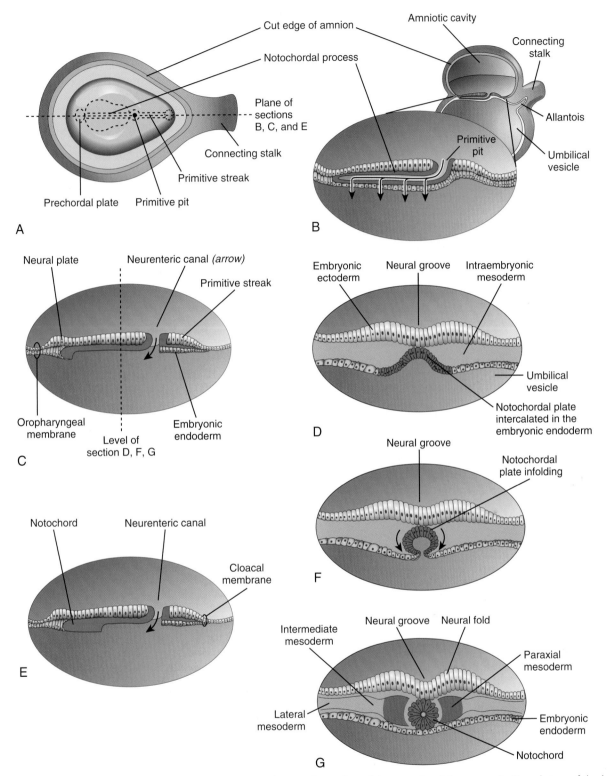

**FIGURE 4–8** Illustrations of notochord development by transformation of the notochordal process. **A,** Dorsal view of the bilaminar embryonic disc at 18 days, exposed by removing the amnion. **B,** Three-dimensional median section of the embryo. **C** and **E,** Similar sections of slightly older embryos. **D, F,** and **G,** Transverse sections of the trilaminar embryonic disc at the levels shown in **C** and **E.**

These cells are continuous with the extraembryonic mesoderm covering the amnion and umbilical vesicle (see Fig. 4-2C and D). Some mesenchymal cells from the primitive streak that have mesodermal fates migrate cranially on each side of the notochordal process and around the prechordal plate (see Fig. 4-4A and C). Here they meet cranially to form cardiogenic mesoderm in the **cardiogenic area**, where the **heart primordium** begins to develop at the end of the third week (see Figs. 4-7B and 4-11B).

Caudal to the primitive streak there is a circular area, the **cloacal membrane**, which indicates the future site of the anus (see Fig. 4-7E). The embryonic disc remains bilaminar here and at the **oropharyngeal membrane** because the embryonic ectoderm and endoderm are fused at these sites, thereby preventing migration of mesenchymal cells between them (see Fig. 4-8C). By the middle of the third week, intraembryonic mesoderm separates the ectoderm and endoderm (see Fig. 4-8D and G) everywhere except

- At the oropharyngeal membrane cranially (see Fig. 4-8C)
- In the median plane cranial to the primitive node (see Fig. 4-4A and B), where the notochordal process is located (see Fig. 4-5)
- At the cloacal membrane caudally (see Fig. 4-7A and E)

Instructive signals from the primitive streak region induce notochordal precursor cells to form the **notochord**, a cellular rod-like structure (see Fig. 4-8E). *The molecular mechanism that induces these cells involves (at least) Shh signaling from the floor plate of the neural tube.*

The **notochord**:

- Defines the primordial longitudinal axis of the embryo and gives it some rigidity
- Provides signals that are necessary for development of axial musculoskeletal structures and the central nervous system (CNS)
- Contributes to the intervertebral discs interposed between the bodies of adjacent vertebrae

Initially, the **notochordal process** elongates by invagination of cells from the primitive pit. An indentation, the **primitive pit**, develops and extends into the notochordal process, forming a **notochordal canal** (see Fig. 4-7C). The notochordal process now becomes a cellular tube that extends cranially from the primitive node to the prechordal plate (see Figs. 4-5 and 4-7A to D). Later, the floor of the notochordal process fuses with the underlying embryonic endoderm (see Fig. 4-7E). These fused layers gradually undergo degeneration, resulting in the formation of openings in the floor of the notochordal process, which brings the notochordal canal into communication with the umbilical vesicle (see Fig. 4-8B). As these openings become confluent, the floor of the notochordal canal disappears (see Fig. 4-8C) and the remains of the notochordal process form the flattened, grooved **notochordal plate** (see Fig. 4-8D). Beginning at the cranial end of the embryo, the notochordal plate cells proliferate and undergo infolding, which creates the **notochord** (see

Fig. 4-8F and G). The proximal part of the notochordal canal persists temporarily as the **neurenteric canal** (see Fig. 4-8C and E), forming a transitory communication between the amniotic and umbilical vesicle cavities. When development of the notochord is complete, the *neurenteric canal normally is obliterated.*

The notochord becomes detached from the endoderm of the umbilical vesicle, the latter once again becoming a continuous layer (see Fig. 4-8G).

The notochord extends from the oropharyngeal membrane to the primitive node (see Fig. 4-5B and D). It degenerates as the bodies of the vertebrae form, but small portions of it persist as the *nucleus pulposus* of each intervertebral disc (see Chapter 14).

*The notochord functions as the primary inductor (signaling center) in the early embryo.* The developing notochord induces the overlying embryonic ectoderm to thicken and form the **neural plate** (see Fig. 4-8C), the primordium of the CNS.

## REMNANTS OF NOTOCHORDAL TISSUE

Both benign and malignant tumors (**chordomas**) may form from vestigial remnants of notochordal tissue. Approximately one third of chordomas occur at the base of the cranium and extend to the nasopharynx. Chordomas grow slowly, and malignant forms infiltrate adjacent bone.

## ALLANTOIS

The allantois appears on approximately day 16 as a small diverticulum (outpouching) from the caudal wall of the umbilical vesicle, which extends into the connecting stalk (see Figs. 4-7B, C, and E and 4-8B). The allantois remains very small, but allantoic mesoderm expands beneath the chorion and forms blood vessels that will serve the placenta. The proximal part of the original allantoic diverticulum persists throughout much of development as a stalk, the **urachus**, which extends from the bladder to the umbilical region (see Chapter 12). The urachus is represented in adults by the **median umbilical ligament**. The blood vessels of the allantoic stalk become **umbilical arteries** (see Fig. 4-12). The intraembryonic part of the umbilical veins has a separate origin.

## NEURULATION: FORMATION OF NEURAL TUBE

The processes involved in the formation of the neural plate and neural folds and closure of the folds to form the neural tube constitute **neurulation**. Neurulation is completed by the end of the fourth week, when closure of the **caudal neuropore** occurs (see Chapter 5, Fig. 5-9A and B).

## ALLANTOIC CYSTS

These cysts, remnants of the extraembryonic portion of the allantois, are usually found between the fetal umbilical vessels; they can be detected by ultrasonography. They are most commonly detected in the proximal part of the umbilical cord, near its attachment to the anterior abdominal wall. The cysts are generally asymptomatic until childhood or adolescence, when they may become infected and inflamed.

## Neural Plate and Neural Tube

As the notochord develops, it induces the overlying embryonic ectoderm, located at or adjacent to the midline, to thicken and form an elongated **neural plate** of thickened epithelial cells (see Fig. 4-7C and D). The neuroectoderm of the plate gives rise to the **CNS**, the brain and spinal cord. **Neuroectoderm** also gives rise to various other structures, for example, the retina. At first, the neural plate corresponds in length to the underlying notochord. It appears rostral (at the head end) to the primitive node and dorsal (posterior) to the notochord and mesoderm adjacent to it (see Fig. 4-5B). As the notochord elongates, the neural plate broadens and eventually extends cranially as far as the **oropharyngeal membrane** (see Figs. 4-5C and 4-8C). Eventually the neural plate extends beyond the notochord.

On approximately the 18th day, the neural plate invaginates along its central axis to form a longitudinal median neural groove, which has neural folds on each side (see Fig. 4-8G). The neural folds become particularly prominent at the cranial end of the embryo and are the first signs of brain development. By the end of the third week, the neural folds have begun to move together and fuse, converting the neural plate into the neural tube, the primordium of the brain vesicles and spinal cord (Figs. 4-9 and 4-10). The neural tube soon separates from the surface ectoderm as the neural folds meet.

Neural crest cells undergo an epithelial to mesenchymal transition and migrate away as the neural folds meet, and the free edges of the surface ectoderm (nonneural ectoderm) fuse so that this layer becomes continuous over the neural tube and the back of the embryo (see Fig. 4-10E and F). Subsequently, the surface ectoderm differentiates into the epidermis. *Neurulation is completed during the fourth week.* Neural tube formation is a complex cellular and multifactorial process involving a cascade of *molecular mechanisms* and extrinsic factors (see Chapter 17).

## Neural Crest Formation

As the neural folds fuse to form the **neural tube**, some neuroectodermal cells lying along the inner margin of each neural fold lose their epithelial affinities and attachments to neighboring cells (see Fig. 4-10). As the neural tube separates from the surface ectoderm, *neural crest cells* form a flattened irregular mass, the **neural crest**, between the neural tube and the overlying surface ectoderm (see Fig. 4-10E). *Wnt/β-catenin signaling activates the GBX2 homeobox gene and is essential for the development of the neural crest.*

The neural crest soon separates into right and left parts that shift to the dorsolateral aspects of the neural tube; here they give rise to the sensory ganglia of the spinal and cranial nerves. Neural crest cells subsequently move both into and over the surface of somites. Although these cells are difficult to identify, special tracer techniques have revealed that neural crest cells disseminate widely, but usually along predefined pathways. *Differentiation and migration of neural crest cells are regulated by molecular interactions of specific genes (e.g., FOXD3, SNAIL2, SOX9, and SOX10), signaling molecules, and transcription factors.*

Neural crest cells give rise to the spinal ganglia (dorsal root ganglia) and ganglia of the autonomic nervous system. The ganglia of cranial nerves V, VII, IX, and X are also partly derived from neural crest cells. In addition to forming ganglion cells, neural crest cells form the neurolemma sheaths of peripheral nerves and contribute to the formation of the **leptomeninges**, the arachnoid mater, and pia mater (see Chapter 17, Fig. 17-10). Neural crest cells also contribute to the formation of pigment cells, the suprarenal medulla, and many other tissues and organs.

Laboratory studies indicate that cell interactions both within the surface epithelium and between it and underlying mesoderm are required to establish the boundaries of the neural plate and specify the sites where epithelial–mesenchymal transformation will occur. *These are mediated by bone morphogenetic proteins and Wnt, Notch, and FGF signaling systems. Also, molecules such as ephrins are important in guiding specific streams of migrating neural crest cells.* Many human diseases result from defective migration and/or differentiation of neural crest cells.

## BIRTH DEFECTS RESULTING FROM ABNORMAL NEURULATION

Because the neural plate, the primordium of the CNS, appears during the third week and gives rise to the neural folds and the beginning of the neural tube, disturbance of neurulation may result in severe birth defects of the brain and spinal cord (see Chapter 17). **Neural tube defects** are among the most common congenital anomalies (see Chapter 17, Fig. 17-12). Available evidence suggests that primary disturbance (e.g., a teratogenic drug; see Chapter 20) affects cell fates, cell adhesion, and the mechanism of neural tube closure. This results in failure of the neural folds to fuse and form the neural tube.

**FIGURE 4–9** Drawings of embryos at 19 to 21 days illustrating development of the somites and intraembryonic coelom. A, C, and E, Dorsal views of the embryo, exposed by removal of the amnion. B, D, and F, Transverse sections through the trilaminar embryonic disc at the levels shown. A, Presomite embryo of approximately 18 days. C, An embryo of approximately 20 days showing the first pair of somites. Part of the somatopleure on the right has been removed to show the coelomic spaces in the lateral mesoderm. E, A three-somite embryo (approximately 21 days) showing the horseshoe-shaped intraembryonic coelom, exposed on the right by removal of part of the somatopleure.

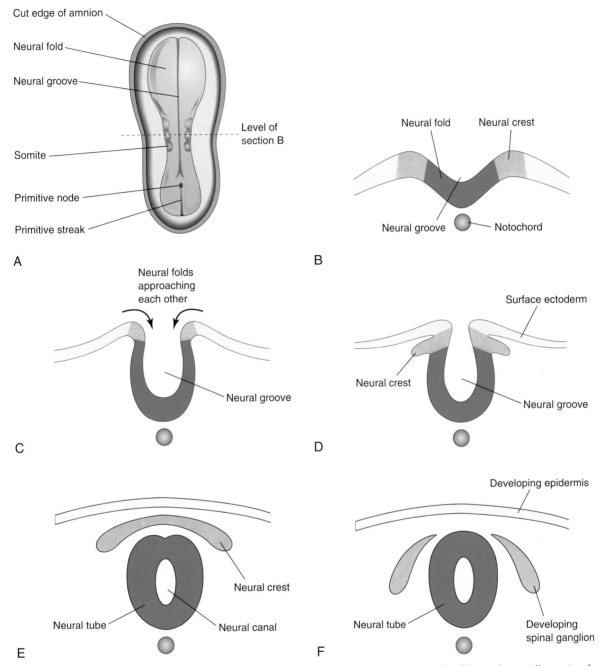

**FIGURE 4–10** A–F, Diagrammatic drawings of transverse sections through progressively older embryos, illustrating formation of the neural groove, neural folds, neural tube, and neural crest. **A,** Dorsal view of an embryo at approximately 21 days.

## DEVELOPMENT OF SOMITES

In addition to the notochord, cells derived from the primitive node form **paraxial mesoderm** (see Figs. 4-9B and 4-10A). Close to the primitive node, this cell population appears as a thick, longitudinal column of cells (see Figs. 4-8G and 4-9B). Each column is continuous laterally with the **intermediate mesoderm**, which gradually thins into a layer of lateral mesoderm. The **lateral mesoderm** is continuous with the extraembryonic mesoderm covering the umbilical vesicle and amnion. Toward the end of the third week, the **paraxial mesoderm** differentiates, condenses, and begins to divide into paired cuboidal bodies, the **somites** (Greek *soma*, body), which form in a craniocaudal sequence.

The blocks of mesoderm are located on each side of the developing neural tube (see Fig. 4-9C to F). About 38 pairs of somites form during the *somite period of human development* (days 20 to 30). The size and shape of the somites are determined by cell–cell interactions. By the end of the fifth week, 42 to 44 pairs of somites are present. The somites form distinct surface elevations on the embryo and are somewhat triangular in transverse sections (see Fig. 4-10A to F). Because the somites are so prominent during the fourth and fifth weeks, they are used as one of several criteria for determining an embryo's age (see Chapter 5, Table 5-1).

Somites first appear in the future occipital region of the head of the embryo (see Fig. 4-9C to F). They soon develop craniocaudally and give rise to most of the *axial skeleton* and associated musculature, as well as to the adjacent dermis of the skin. The first pair of somites appears a short distance caudal to the site at which the otic placode forms (see Fig. 4-9C). Motor axons from the spinal cord innervate muscle cells in the somites, a process that requires the correct guidance of axons from the spinal cord to the appropriate target cells.

*Formation of somites from the paraxial mesoderm involves the expression of NOTCH pathway genes (Notch signaling pathway), HOX genes, and other signaling factors. Moreover, somite formation from paraxial mesoderm is preceded by expression of the forkhead transcription factors FoxC1 and FoxC2 and the craniocaudal segmental pattern of the somites is regulated by the Delta-Notch signaling. A molecular oscillator or clock has been proposed as the mechanism responsible for the orderly sequencing of somites.*

# ▶ DEVELOPMENT OF INTRAEMBRYONIC COELOM

The primordium of the intraembryonic coelom (embryonic body cavity) appears as isolated **coelomic spaces** in the lateral intraembryonic mesoderm and *cardiogenic (heart-forming) mesoderm* (see Fig. 4-9A and C). These spaces soon coalesce to form a single horseshoe-shaped cavity, the **intraembryonic coelom** (see Fig. 4-9D and E), which divides the lateral mesoderm into two layers:

- A somatic or parietal layer of lateral mesoderm located beneath the ectodermal epithelium, which is continuous with the extraembryonic mesoderm covering the amnion
- A splanchnic or visceral layer of lateral mesoderm located adjacent to the endoderm, which is continuous with the extraembryonic mesoderm covering the umbilical vesicle

The *somatic mesoderm* and overlying embryonic ectoderm form the embryonic body wall, or **somatopleure** (see Fig. 4-9F), whereas the splanchnic mesoderm and underlying embryonic endoderm form the embryonic gut, or *splanchnopleure*. During the second month, the intraembryonic coelom is divided into three body cavities: *pericardial cavity, pleural cavities,* and *peritoneal cavity.* For a description of these divisions of the intraembryonic coelom, see Chapter 8.

# EARLY DEVELOPMENT OF CARDIOVASCULAR SYSTEM

At the end of the second week, embryonic nutrition is obtained from the maternal blood by diffusion through the extraembryonic coelom and umbilical vesicle. At the beginning of the third week, blood vessel formation begins in the extraembryonic mesoderm of the umbilical vesicle, connecting stalk, and chorion (Fig. 4-11). **Embryonic blood vessels** begin to develop approximately 2 days later. The early formation of the cardiovascular system is correlated with the urgent need for blood vessels to bring oxygen and nourishment to the embryo from the maternal circulation through the placenta. During the third week, a primordial uteroplacental circulation develops (Fig. 4-12).

## Vasculogenesis and Angiogenesis

The formation of the embryonic vascular system involves two processes, vasculogenesis and angiogenesis. **Vasculogenesis** is the formation of new vascular channels by assembly of individual cell precursors (**angioblasts**). **Angiogenesis** is the formation of new vessels by budding and branching from preexisting vessels. Blood vessel formation in the embryo and extraembryonic membranes during the third week (see Fig. 4-11) begins when mesenchymal cells differentiate into endothelial cell precursors, or angioblasts (vessel-forming cells). Angioblasts aggregate to form isolated angiogenic cell clusters, or **blood islands**, which are associated with the umbilical vesicle or endothelial cords within the embryo. Small cavities appear within the blood islands and **endothelial cords** by confluence of intercellular clefts.

The angioblasts flatten to form endothelial cells that arrange themselves around the cavities in the blood islands to form the endothelium. Many of these endothelium-lined cavities soon fuse to form networks of endothelial channels (vasculogenesis). Additional vessels sprout into adjacent areas by endothelial budding (angiogenesis) and fuse with other vessels. The mesenchymal cells surrounding the primordial **endothelial blood vessels** differentiate into the muscular and connective tissue elements of the vessels.

**Blood cells** develop from specialized endothelial cells (hemangiogenic epithelium) of vessels as they grow on the umbilical vesicle and allantois at the end of the third week (see Fig. 4-11E and F) and later in specialized sites along the dorsal aorta. Progenitor blood cells also arise directly from hemangiopoietic stem cells. Blood formation (hematogenesis) does not begin in the embryo until the fifth week. It occurs first along the aorta and then in various parts of the embryonic mesenchyme, mainly the liver and later in the spleen, bone marrow, and lymph nodes. Fetal and adult erythrocytes are derived from *hematopoietic progenitor cells.*

## Primordial Cardiovascular System

The **heart and great vessels** form from mesenchymal cells in the *cardiogenic area* (see Figs. 4-9A and 4-11B). Paired, longitudinal endothelial-lined channels, or **endocardial heart tubes**, develop during the third week and fuse to form a **primordial heart tube** (see Fig. 4-12). The tubular heart joins with blood vessels in the embryo, connecting the stalk, chorion, and umbilical vesicle to form a **primordial cardiovascular system**. By the end of the third week, the blood is circulating, and *the heart begins to beat on the 21st or 22nd day.*

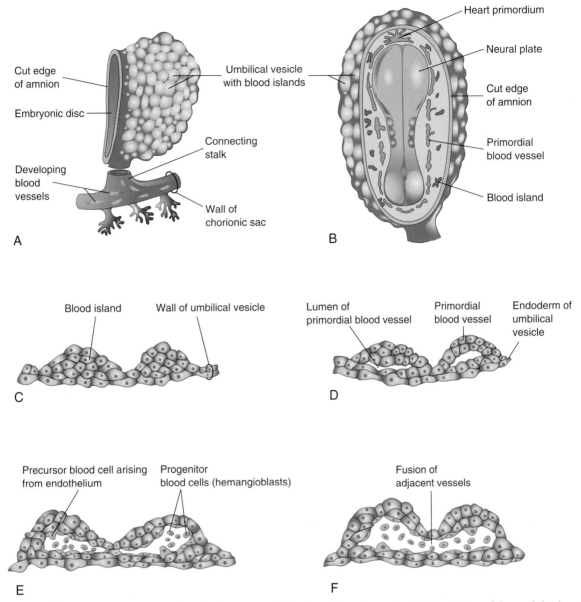

**FIGURE 4–11** Successive stages in the development of blood and blood vessels. **A**, Lateral view of the umbilical vesicle and part of the chorionic sac (approximately 18 days). **B**, Dorsal view of the embryo exposed by removing the amnion (approximately 20 days). **C** to **F**, Sections of blood islands showing progressive stages in the development of blood and blood vessels.

*The cardiovascular system is the first organ system to reach a functional state.* The embryonic heartbeat can be detected using *Doppler ultrasonography* during the fourth week, approximately 6 weeks after the last normal menstrual period (Fig. 4-13).

## DEVELOPMENT OF CHORIONIC VILLI

Shortly after **primary chorionic villi** appear at the end of the second week, they begin to branch. Early in the third week, mesenchyme grows into these villi, forming a core of mesenchymal tissue. The villi at this stage, **secondary chorionic villi**, cover the entire surface of the chorionic sac (Fig. 4-14*A* and *B*). Some mesenchymal cells in the villi soon differentiate into capillaries and blood cells (see Fig. 4-14*C* and *D*). Villi are called **tertiary chorionic villi** when blood vessels are visible in them.

The capillaries in the chorionic villi fuse to form **arteriocapillary networks**, which soon become connected with the embryonic heart through vessels that differentiate in the mesenchyme of the chorion and connecting stalk (see Fig. 4-12). By the end of the third week, embryonic blood begins to flow slowly through the capillaries in the chorionic villi. Oxygen and nutrients in the maternal blood in the **intervillous space** diffuse through the walls of the villi and enter the embryo's blood (see Fig. 4-14*C* and *D*). Carbon dioxide and waste products diffuse from blood in the fetal capillaries through the wall of the chorionic villi into the maternal blood. Concurrently, cytotrophoblastic cells of the chorionic villi proliferate and extend through the syncytiotrophoblast to form

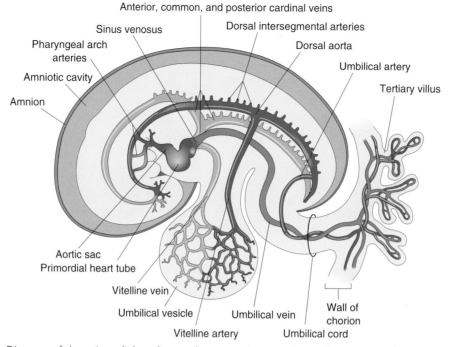

Anterior, common, and posterior cardinal veins

Sinus venosus

Dorsal intersegmental arteries

Pharyngeal arch
arteries

Dorsal aorta

Amniotic cavity

Umbilical artery

Amnion

Tertiary villus

Aortic sac
Primordial heart tube

Vitelline vein

Umbilical vesicle

Umbilical vein

Wall of
chorion

Vitelline artery

Umbilical cord

**FIGURE 4-12** Diagram of the primordial cardiovascular system in an embryo of approximately 21 days, viewed from the left side. Observe the transitory stage of the paired symmetric vessels. Each heart tube continues dorsally into a dorsal aorta that passes caudally. Branches of the aortae are (1) umbilical arteries establishing connections with vessels in the chorion, (2) vitelline arteries to the umbilical vesicle, and (3) dorsal intersegmental arteries to the body of the embryo. Vessels on the umbilical vesicle form a vascular plexus that is connected to the heart tubes by vitelline veins. The cardinal veins return blood from the body of the embryo. The umbilical vein carries oxygenated blood and nutrients to the chorion, which, in turn, provides nourishment to the embryo. The arteries carry poorly oxygenated blood and waste products to the chorionic villi for transfer to the mother's blood.

**FIGURE 4-13** Endovaginal ultrasonogram of a 4-week embryo A, Secondary umbilical vesicle (*calipers*, 2 mm). B, Bright (echogenic) 4-week embryo (*calipers*, 2.4 mm). C, Cardiac activity of 116 beats/min demonstrated with motion mode. The calipers are used to encompass two beats.

an extravillous **cytotrophoblastic shell** (see Fig. 4-14C), which gradually surrounds the chorionic sac and attaches it to the endometrium.

Villi that attach to the maternal tissues through the cytotrophoblastic shell are **stem villi** (anchoring villi). The villi that grow from the sides of the stem villi are **branch villi**. It is through the walls of the branch villi that the main exchange of material between the blood of the mother and embryo takes place. The branch villi (see Chapter 7, Fig. 7-5) are bathed in continually changing maternal blood in the intervillous space (see Fig. 4-14C).

## SUMMARY OF THIRD WEEK

- The **bilaminar embryonic disc** is converted into a **trilaminar embryonic disc** during **gastrulation**. These changes begin with the appearance of the **primitive streak**, which appears at the beginning of the third week as a thickening of the epiblast at the caudal end of the embryonic disc.
- The **primitive streak** results from migration of epiblastic cells to the median plane of the disc. Invagination of epiblastic cells from the primitive streak gives rise

Secondary chorionic villus

Syncytiotrophoblast

Cytotrophoblast

Developing blood vessel

Wall of chorionic sac (primordial placenta)

Endometrium

Mesenchymal core

Cytotrophoblastic shell

Connecting stalk

Tertiary chorionic villus

Intervillous space

Maternal blood

Maternal sinusoid

Connective tissue

Capillaries with fetal blood

**FIGURE 4–14** Diagrams illustrating development of secondary chorionic villi into tertiary chorionic villi. Early formation of the placenta is also shown. **A,** Sagittal section of an embryo (approximately 16 days). **B,** Section of a secondary chorionic villus. **C,** Section of an implanted embryo (approximately 21 days). **D,** Section of a tertiary chorionic villus. The fetal blood in the capillaries is separated from the maternal blood surrounding the villus by the endothelium of the capillaries, embryonic connective tissue, cytotrophoblast, and syncytiotrophoblast.

## ABNORMAL GROWTH OF TROPHOBLAST

Sometimes the embryo dies and the chorionic villi (see Fig. 4-14A) do not complete their development, that is, they do not become vascularized to form **tertiary villi** (see Fig. 4-14C). These degenerating villi form cystic swellings, **hydatidiform moles**, which resemble a grape bunch (Fig. 4-15). The moles exhibit variable degrees of trophoblastic proliferation and produce excessive amounts of **human chorionic gonadotropin**. Some moles develop after spontaneous abortions, and others occur after normal fetal deliveries. Moles develop into malignant trophoblastic lesions, choriocarcinomas, in about 3% to 5% of cases.

**Choriocarcinomas** invariably metastasize (spread) through the bloodstream to various sites such as the lungs, vagina, liver, bone, intestine, and brain.

The main mechanisms for development of **complete hydatidiform moles** follow:

- Fertilization of an empty oocyte (absent or inactive pronucleus) by a sperm, followed by duplication (**monospermic mole**)
- Fertilization of an empty oocyte by two sperms (**dispermic mole**)

Most complete hydatidiform moles are monospermic, and the genetic origin of the nuclear DNA is paternal.

A **partial hydatidiform mole** usually results from fertilization of a normal oocyte by two sperms (**dispermy**).

**FIGURE 4–15** Ultrasound image demonstrating a complete hydatidiform mole. Note numerous small cystic spaces. The "cluster of grapes sign" is a typical feature of a molar pregnancy.

to mesenchymal cells that migrate ventrally, laterally, and cranially between the **epiblast** and **hypoblast**.

- As soon as the primitive streak begins to produce mesenchymal cells, the epiblast is called **embryonic ectoderm**. Some cells of the epiblast displace the hypoblast and form **embryonic endoderm**. Mesenchymal cells produced by the primitive streak soon organize into a third germ layer, the **intraembryonic (embryonic) mesoderm**, occupying the area between the former hypoblast and cells in the epiblast. Cells of the mesoderm migrate to the edges of the embryonic disc, where they join the **extraembryonic mesoderm** covering the amnion and umbilical vesicle.
- At the end of the third week, the embryo is a flat ovoid embryonic disc (see Fig. 4-2H). Mesoderm exists between the ectoderm and endoderm of the disc everywhere except at the **oropharyngeal membrane**, in the median plane occupied by the notochord, and at the **cloacal membrane** (see Fig. 4-8E).
- Early in the third week, mesenchymal cells from the primitive streak form the **notochordal process** between the embryonic ectoderm and endoderm. The notochordal process extends from the primitive node to the **prechordal plate**. Openings develop in the floor of the **notochordal canal**, and they soon coalesce, leaving a **notochordal plate**. This plate infolds to form the **notochord**, the primordial axis of the embryo around which the **axial skeleton** forms (e.g., vertebral column).
- The **neural plate** appears as a thickening of embryonic ectoderm, induced by the developing notochord. A longitudinal **neural groove** develops in the neural plate, which is flanked by **neural folds**. Fusion of the folds forms the **neural tube**, the primordium of the **CNS** (see Figs. 4-9A and 4-10).
- As the neural folds fuse to form the neural tube, neuroectodermal cells form a **neural crest** between the surface ectoderm and neural tube.
- The mesoderm on each side of the notochord condenses to form longitudinal columns of paraxial mesoderm, which, by the end of the third week, give rise to **somites**.
- The **coelom** (cavity) within the embryo arises as isolated spaces in the lateral mesoderm and cardiogenic mesoderm. The **coelomic vesicles** subsequently coalesce to form a single, horseshoe-shaped cavity that eventually gives rise to **body cavities** (see Fig. 4-9E).
- **Blood vessels** first appear in the wall of the umbilical vesicle, allantois, and chorion. They develop within the embryo shortly thereafter. Fetal erythrocytes develop from different hematopoietic precursors.
- The **primordial heart** is represented by paired **endocardial heart tubes**. By the end of the third week, the heart tubes have fused to form a **tubular heart** that is joined to vessels in the embryo, umbilical vesicle, chorion, and connecting stalk to form a **primordial cardiovascular system** (see Fig. 4-12).
- **Primary chorionic villi** become **secondary chorionic villi** as they acquire mesenchymal cores. Before the end of the third week, capillaries develop in the secondary chorionic villi, transforming them into **tertiary chorionic villi** (see Fig. 4-14C). Cytotrophoblastic extensions from the stem villi join to form a **cytotrophoblastic**

**shell** that anchors the chorionic sac to the endometrium.

## CLINICALLY ORIENTED PROBLEMS

### CASE 4–1

*A 30-year-old woman became pregnant 2 months after discontinuing use of oral contraceptives. Approximately 3 weeks later, she had a spontaneous abortion.*

* How do hormones in these contraceptives affect the ovarian and menstrual cycles?
* What might have caused the spontaneous abortion?

### CASE 4–2

*A 25-year-old woman with a history of regular menstrual cycles was 5 days overdue on menses. A menstrual extraction (uterine evacuation) was performed. The tissue removed was examined for evidence of a pregnancy.*

* Would a radioimmune assay have detected pregnancy at this early stage?
* What clinical findings would indicate an early pregnancy?
* What would be the age of the conceptus?

### CASE 4–3

*A woman who had just missed her menstrual period was concerned that a glass of wine she had consumed the week before may have harmed her embryo.*

* What major organ systems undergo early development during the third week?
* What severe congenital anomaly might result from teratogenic factors (see Chapter 20) acting during this period of development?
* What information might you discuss with the patient?

### CASE 4–4

*A female infant had a large tumor situated between her anus and sacrum. A diagnosis of sacrococcygeal teratoma was made, and the mass was surgically removed.*

* What is the probable embryologic origin of this tumor?

* Explain why these tumors often contain various types of tissue derived from all three germ layers.

### CASE 4–5

*A woman with a history of early spontaneous abortions had an ultrasound examination to determine whether her embryo was still implanted.*

* Is ultrasonography helpful in assessing pregnancy during the third week? If so, do special ultrasonographic techniques need to be used?
* What structures might be recognizable?
* If a pregnancy test is negative, is it correct to assume that the woman is not pregnant? Explain.
* Could an extrauterine gestation be present?

Discussion of these problems appears in the Appendix at the back of the book.

## BIBLIOGRAPHY AND SUGGESTED READING

De Val S: Key transcriptional regulators of early vascular development, *Arterioscler Thromb Vasc Biol* 31:1469, 2011.

Dias AS, de Almeida I, Belmonte JM: Somites without a clock, *Science* 343:791, 2014.

Downs KM: The enigmatic primitive streak: prevailing notions and challenges concerning the body axis of mammals, *Bioessays* 31:892, 2009.

Gasser RF: Evidence that some events of mammalian embryogenesis can result from differential growth, making migration unnecessary, *Anat Rec B New Anat* 289B:53, 2006.

Gibb S, Maroto M, Dale JK: The segmentation clock mechanism moves up a notch, *Trends Cell Biol* 20:593, 2010.

Gucciardo L, Uyttebroek A, De Wever I, et al: Prenatal assessment and management of sacrococcygeal teratoma, *Prenat Diagn* 31:678, 2011.

Hall BK: *Bones and cartilage: developmental skeletal biology*, Philadelphia, 2005, Elsevier.

Hur E-M, Zhou F-Q: GSK3 signalling in neural development, *Nature Rev Neurosci* 11:539, 2010.

Jagannathan-Bogdan M, Zon LI: Hematopoiesis, *Development* 140:2463, 2013.

Lewis J, Hanisch A, Holder M: Notch signaling, the segmentation clock, and the patterning of vertebrate somites, *J Biol* 8:44, 2009.

Liu W, Komiya Y, Mezzacappa C, et al: MIM regulates vertebrate neural tube closure, *Development* 138:2035, 2011.

Mayor R, Theveneau E: The neural crest, *Development* 140:2247, 2013.

Piccolo S: Developmental biology: mechanics in the embryo, *Nature* 504:223, 2013.

Satoh N, Tagawa K, Takahasi H: How was the notochord born?, *Evol Dev* 14:56, 2012.

Savage P: Gestational trophoblastic disease. In Magowan BA, Owen P, Thomson A, editors: *Clinical obstetrics and gynaecology*, ed 3, Philadelphia, 2014, Saunders.

Slack JMW: *Essential developmental biology*, ed 2, Oxford, 2006, Blackwell.

Tovar JA: The neural crest in pediatric surgery, *J Pediatr Surg* 42:915, 2007.

Zorn AM, Wells JM: Vertebrate endoderm development and organ formation, *Annu Rev Cell Dev Biol* 25:221, 2009.

# Fourth to Eighth Weeks of Human Development

**A**ll major external and internal structures are established during the fourth to eighth weeks. By the end of this embryonic period, the main organ systems have started to develop. As the tissues and organs form, the shape of the embryo changes, and by the end of this period, the embryo has a distinctly human appearance. Because the tissues and organs are differentiating rapidly, exposure of embryos to teratogens during this period may cause major birth defects. **Teratogens** are agents (such as some drugs and viruses) that produce or increase the incidence of major birth defects (see Chapter 20).

## PHASES OF EMBRYONIC DEVELOPMENT

Human development is divided into three phases, which to some extent are interrelated:

- The first phase is **growth**, which involves cell division and elaboration of cell products.
- The second phase is **morphogenesis**, the development of shape, size, and other features of a particular organ or part or the whole body. Morphogenesis is a complex molecular process controlled by the expression and regulation of specific genes in an orderly sequence. Changes in cell fate, cell shape, and cell movement allow the cells to interact with each other during the formation of tissues and organs.

- The third phase is **differentiation**, during which cells are organized in a precise pattern of tissues and organs that are capable of performing specialized functions.

# ▶ FOLDING OF EMBRYO

5    A significant event in the establishment of body form is folding of the flat trilaminar embryonic disc into a somewhat cylindric embryo (Fig. 5-1). Folding occurs in the median and horizontal planes and results from rapid growth of the embryo. The growth rate at the sides of the embryonic disc fails to keep pace with the rate of growth in the long axis as the embryo increases rapidly in length. Folding at the cranial and caudal ends and sides of the embryo occurs simultaneously. Concurrently, there is relative constriction at the junction of the embryo and umbilical vesicle.

## Folding of Embryo in the Median Plane

Folding of the ends of the embryo produces **head and tail folds** that result in the cranial and caudal regions moving ventrally as the embryo elongates cranially and caudally (see Fig. 5-1$A_2$ to $D_2$).

### Head Fold

At the beginning of the fourth week, the **neural folds** in the cranial region form the **primordium of the brain** (see Fig. 5-1$A_2$ and $B_2$). Initially, the developing brain projects dorsally into the **amniotic cavity**, the fluid-filled cavity inside the **amnion** (the innermost membrane around the embryo). The amniotic cavity contains amniotic fluid and the embryo. Later, the developing forebrain grows cranially beyond the **oropharyngeal membrane** and overhangs the developing heart (Fig. 5-2$B$ and $C$). At the same time, the **septum transversum**, primordial heart, pericardial coelom, and oropharyngeal membrane move onto the ventral surface of the embryo. During folding, part of the endoderm of the **umbilical vesicle** is incorporated into the embryo as the **foregut** (primordium of pharynx, esophagus, and lower respiratory system) (see Fig. 5-2$C$, and also see Chapter 11). The foregut lies between the forebrain and primordial heart, and the **oropharyngeal membrane** separates the foregut from the **stomodeum**, the primordial mouth (see Figs. 5-3$B$ and 5-2$C$).

After folding of the head, the **septum transversum** lies caudal to the heart, where it subsequently develops into the **central tendon of the diaphragm**, the partition between the abdominal and thoracic cavities (see Fig. 5-3$B$, and also see Chapter 8). The head fold also affects the arrangement of the **embryonic coelom** (primordium of the body cavity). Before folding, the coelom consists of a flattened, horseshoe-shaped cavity (see Fig. 5-1$A_1$). After folding, the **pericardial coelom** lies ventral to the heart and cranial to the septum transversum (see Fig. 5-2$B$ and $C$). At this stage, the **intraembryonic coelom** communicates widely on each side with the **extraembryonic coelom** (see Figs. 5-1$A_3$ and 5-3$A$ and $B$).

### Tail Fold

Folding of the caudal end of the embryo results primarily from growth of the distal part of the **neural tube**, the primordium of the spinal cord (Fig. 5-4$A$ and $B$). As the embryo grows, the **caudal eminence** (tail region) projects over the **cloacal membrane**, the future site of the anus (see Figs. 5-3$A$ and 5-4$B$). During folding, part of the endodermal germ layer is incorporated into the embryo as the **hindgut**, the descending colon and rectum (see Fig. 5-4$B$).

The terminal part of the hindgut soon dilates slightly to form the **cloaca**, the rudiment of the urinary bladder and rectum (see Fig. 5-4$B$, and also see Chapters 11 and 12). Before folding, the **primitive streak** lies cranial to the cloacal membrane (see Fig. 5-4$A$); after folding, it lies caudal to it (see Fig. 5-4$B$). The **connecting stalk** (primordium of the umbilical cord) is now attached to the ventral surface of the embryo (see Fig. 5-4$A$), and the **allantois**, or the diverticulum of the umbilical vesicle, is partially incorporated into the embryo (see Fig. 5-4$A$ and $B$).

## Folding of Embryo in the Horizontal Plane

Folding of the sides of the developing embryo produces right and left **lateral folds** (see Fig. 5-1$A_3$ to $D_3$). Lateral folding is produced by the rapidly growing spinal cord and somites. The primordia of the ventrolateral abdominal wall fold toward the median plane, rolling the edges of the **embryonic disc** ventrally and forming a roughly cylindric embryo (see Fig. 5-6$A$). As the **abdominal wall** forms, part of the endoderm germ layer is incorporated into the embryo as the **midgut**, the primordium of the small intestine (see Fig. 5-1$C_2$, and also see Chapter 11).

Initially, there is a wide connection between the midgut and umbilical vesicle (see Fig. 5-1$A_2$); however, after lateral folding, the connection is reduced, forming an **omphaloenteric duct** (see Fig. 5-1$C_2$). The region of attachment of the **amnion** to the ventral surface of the embryo is also reduced to a relatively narrow umbilical region (see Fig. 5-1$D_2$ and $D_3$). As the **umbilical cord** forms from the connecting stalk (see Fig. 5-1$B_2$ and $D_2$), ventral fusion of the lateral folds reduces the region of communication between the intraembryonic and extraembryonic coelomic cavities to a narrow communication (see Fig. 5-1$C_2$). As the amniotic cavity expands and obliterates most of the extraembryonic coelom, the amnion forms the epithelial covering of the umbilical cord (see Fig. 5-1$D_2$).

# GERM LAYER DERIVATIVES

The three germ layers (ectoderm, mesoderm, and endoderm) formed during **gastrulation** (Fig. 5-5) give rise to the primordia of all tissues and organs. The specificity of the germ layers, however, is not rigidly fixed. The cells of each germ layer divide, migrate, aggregate, and differentiate in patterns as they form the various organ systems. The main germ layer derivatives are as follows (see Fig. 5-5):

- **Ectoderm** gives rise to the central nervous system; peripheral nervous system; sensory epithelia of the

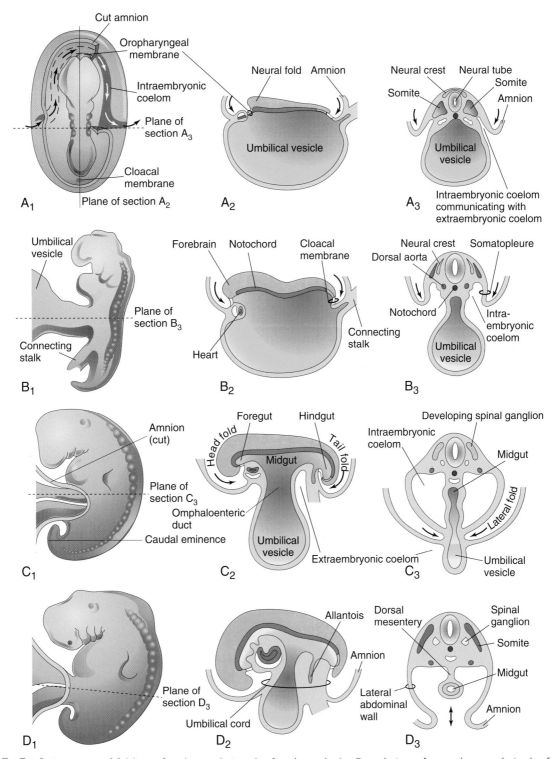

**FIGURE 5–1** Drawings of folding of embryos during the fourth week. **A₁**, Dorsal view of an embryo early in the fourth week. Three pairs of somites are visible. The continuity of the intraembryonic coelom and extraembryonic coelom is illustrated on the right side by removal of a part of the embryonic ectoderm and mesoderm. **B₁, C₁,** and **D₁,** Lateral views of embryos at 22, 26, and 28 days, respectively. **A₂** to **D₂,** Sagittal sections at the plane shown in **A₁**. **A₃** to **D₃,** Transverse sections at the levels indicated in **A₁** to **D₁**.

eyes, ears, and nose; epidermis and its appendages (hair and nails); mammary glands; pituitary gland; subcutaneous glands; and enamel of the teeth. **Neural crest cells,** derived from **neuroectoderm,** the central region of early ectoderm, eventually give rise to or

participate in the formation of many cells types and organs, including cells of the spinal cord, cranial nerves (V, VII, IX, and X), and autonomic ganglia; ensheathing cells of the peripheral nervous system; pigment cells of the dermis; muscles, connective tissues,

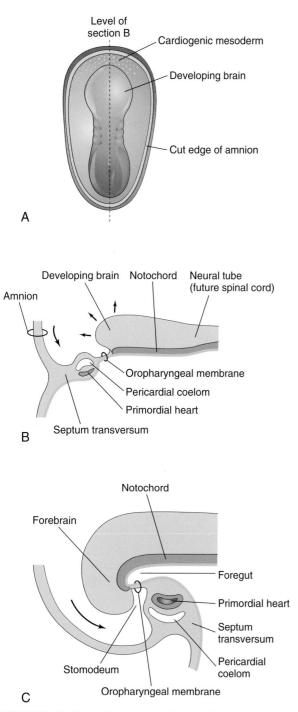

**FIGURE 5–2** Folding of cranial end of embryo. **A,** Dorsal view of embryo at 21 days. **B,** Sagittal section of the cranial part of the embryo at the plane shown in **A.** Observe the ventral movement of the heart in **B** and **C. C,** Sagittal section of an embryo at 26 days. Note that the septum transversum, primordial heart, pericardial coelom, and oropharyngeal membrane have moved onto the ventral surface of the embryo. Observe also that part of the umbilical vesicle is incorporated into the embryo as the foregut.

and bones of pharyngeal arch origin; suprarenal medulla; and **meninges** (coverings) of the brain and spinal cord.

- **Mesoderm** gives rise to connective tissue, cartilage, bone, striated and smooth muscles, heart, blood, and lymphatic vessels; kidneys; ovaries; testes; genital ducts; serous membranes lining the **body cavities** (pericardial, pleural, and peritoneal membranes); spleen; and cortex of the suprarenal glands.
- **Endoderm** gives rise to the epithelial lining of the digestive and respiratory tracts; parenchyma (connective tissue framework) of the tonsils; thyroid and parathyroid glands; thymus, liver, and pancreas; epithelial lining of the urinary bladder and most of the urethra; and epithelial lining of the tympanic cavity, tympanic antrum, and pharyngotympanic tube (see Fig. 5-5).

## CONTROL OF EMBRYONIC DEVELOPMENT

Embryonic development results from genetic plans in the chromosomes. Knowledge of the genes that control human development is increasing (see Chapter 21). Most information about developmental processes has come from studies of other organisms, especially *Drosophila* (fruit flies used extensively in genetic research) and mice because of ethical problems associated with the use of human embryos for laboratory studies.

Most developmental processes depend on a precisely coordinated interaction of genetic and environmental factors. Several control mechanisms guide differentiation and ensure synchronized development, such as tissue interactions, regulated migration of cells and cell colonies, controlled proliferation, and programmed cell death (**apoptosis**). Each system of the body has its own developmental pattern.

*Embryonic development is essentially a process of growth and increasing complexity of structure and function.* Growth is achieved by mitosis (somatic reproduction of cells) together with the production of extracellular matrices (surrounding substances), whereas complexity is achieved through morphogenesis and differentiation. The cells that make up the tissues of very early embryos are pluripotential (i.e., they have the capacity to affect more than one organ or tissue), which under different circumstances are able to follow more than one pathway of development. This broad developmental potential becomes progressively restricted as tissues acquire the specialized features necessary for increasing their sophistication of structure and function. Such restriction presumes that choices must be made to achieve tissue diversification.

Most evidence indicates that these choices are determined not as a consequence of cell lineage, but rather in response to cues from immediate surroundings, including the adjacent tissues. As a result, the architectural precision and coordination that are often required for normal function of an organ appear to be achieved by the interaction of the organ's constituent parts during development.

The interaction of tissues during development is a recurring theme in embryology. The interactions that lead

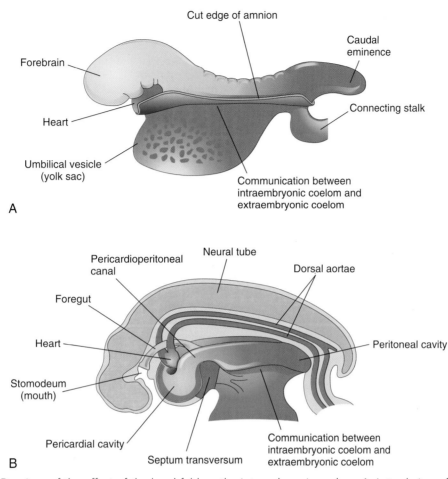

**FIGURE 5–3** Drawings of the effect of the head fold on the intraembryonic coelom. **A,** Lateral view of an embryo (24 to 25 days) during folding, showing the large forebrain, ventral position of the heart, and communication between the intraembryonic and extraembryonic parts of the coelom. **B,** Schematic drawing of an embryo (26 to 27 days) after folding, showing the pericardial cavity ventrally, the pericardioperitoneal canals running dorsally on each side of the foregut, and the intraembryonic coelom in communication with the extraembryonic coelom.

to a change in the course of development of at least one of the interactants are called **inductions**. Numerous examples of such inductive interactions can be found; for example, *during development of the eye,* the optic vesicle induces the development of the lens from the surface ectoderm of the head. When the optic vesicle is absent, the eye fails to develop. Moreover, if the optic vesicle is removed and placed in association with surface ectoderm that is not usually involved in eye development, lens formation can be induced.

Clearly then, development of a lens is dependent on the ectoderm acquiring an association with a second tissue. In the presence of neuroectoderm of the optic vesicle, the surface ectoderm of the head adopts a pathway of development that it would not otherwise have taken. In a similar fashion, many of the morphogenetic tissue movements that play such important roles in shaping the embryo also provide for the changing tissue associations that are fundamental to **inductive tissue interactions**.

The fact that one tissue can influence the *developmental pathway adopted by another tissue* presumes that a signal passes between the two interactants. Analysis of

the molecular defects in mutant strains shows that abnormal tissue interactions occur during embryonic development, and studies of the development of embryos with targeted gene mutations have begun to reveal the molecular mechanisms of induction. The mechanism of signal transfer appears to vary with the specific tissues involved. In some cases, the signal appears to take the form of a diffusible molecule, such as a **sonic hedgehog**, that passes from the inductor to the reacting tissue. In others, the message appears to be mediated through a nondiffusible extracellular matrix that is secreted by the inductor and with which the reacting tissue comes into contact. In still other cases, the signal appears to require that physical contacts occur between the inducing and responding tissues. Regardless of the mechanism of intercellular transfer involved, the signal is translated into an intracellular message that influences the genetic activity of the responding cells.

The signal can be relatively nonspecific in some interactions. The role of the natural inductor in a variety of interactions has been shown to be mimicked by a number of heterologous tissue sources and, in some instances,

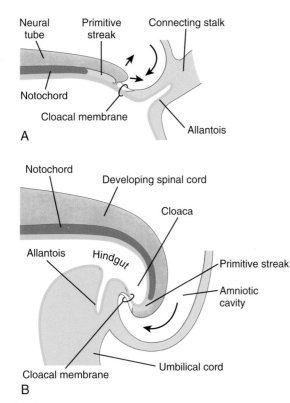

**FIGURE 5-4** Folding of caudal end of the embryo. A, Sagittal section of caudal part of the embryo at the beginning of the fourth week. B, Similar section at the end of the fourth week. Note that part of the umbilical vesicle is incorporated into the embryo as the hindgut and that the terminal part of the hindgut has dilated to form the cloaca. Observe also the change in position of the primitive streak, allantois, cloacal membrane, and connecting stalk.

even by a variety of cell-free preparations. Studies suggest that the specificity of a given induction is a property of the reacting tissue rather than of the inductor. Inductions should not be thought of as isolated phenomena. Often they occur in a sequential fashion that results in the orderly development of a complex structure; for example, following induction of the lens by the optic vesicle, the lens induces the development of the cornea from the surface ectoderm and adjacent mesenchyme. This ensures the formation of component parts that are appropriate in size and relationship for the function of the organ. In other systems, there is evidence that the interactions between tissues are reciprocal. During *development of the kidney*, for instance, the uteric bud (metanephric diverticulum) induces the formation of tubules in the metanephric mesoderm (see Chapter 12). This mesoderm, in turn, induces branching of the diverticulum that results in the development of the collecting tubules and calices of the kidney.

To be competent to respond to an inducing stimulus, the cells of the reacting system must express the appropriate receptor for the specific inducing-signal molecule, the components of the particular **intracellular signal transduction pathway**, and the **transcription factors** that will mediate the particular response. Experimental evidence suggests that the acquisition of competence by the responding tissue is often dependent on its previous interactions with other tissues. For example, the lens-forming response of head ectoderm to the stimulus provided by the optic vesicle appears to be dependent on a previous association of the head ectoderm with the anterior neural plate.

The ability of the reacting system to respond to an inducing stimulus is not unlimited. Most inducible tissues appear to pass through a transient but more or less sharply delimited physiologic state in which they are competent to respond to an inductive signal from the neighboring tissue. Because this state of receptiveness is limited in time, a delay in the development of one or more components in an interacting system may lead to failure of an inductive interaction. Regardless of the signal mechanism employed, inductive systems seem to have the common feature of close proximity between the interacting tissues. Experimental evidence has demonstrated that interactions may fail if the interactants are too widely separated. Consequently, inductive processes appear to be limited in space as well as by time. Because tissue induction plays such a fundamental role in ensuring the orderly formation of precise structures, failed interactions can be expected to have drastic developmental consequences (e.g., birth defects such as absence of the lens).

## HIGHLIGHTS OF FOURTH TO EIGHTH WEEKS

The following descriptions summarize the main developmental events and changes in external form of the embryo during the fourth to eighth weeks. The main criteria for estimating developmental stages in human embryos are listed in Table 5-1.

### Fourth Week

*Major changes in body form occur during the fourth week.* At the beginning, the embryo is almost straight and has 4 to 12 somites that produce conspicuous surface elevations (Fig. 5-6A to D). The **neural tube** is formed opposite the somites, but it is widely open at the rostral and caudal **neuropores** (see Fig. 5-6C and D). By 24 days, the first pharyngeal arches are visible. The **first pharyngeal arch** (mandibular arch) is distinct (Fig. 5-7). The major part of the first arch gives rise to the mandible (lower jaw), and a rostral extension of the arch, the **maxillary prominence**, contributes to the maxilla (upper jaw). The embryo is now slightly curved because of the head and tail folds. The heart produces a large ventral **heart prominence** and pumps blood (see Fig. 5-7). The rostral neuropore is closing.

Three pairs of **pharyngeal arches** are visible at 26 days (Fig. 5-8), and the rostral neuropore is closed. The **forebrain** produces a prominent elevation of the head, and folding of the embryo has given the embryo a C-shaped curvature. **Upper limb buds** are recognizable at day 26 or 27 as small swellings on the ventrolateral body walls (Fig. 5-9). The **otic pits** (primordia of the internal ears) are also visible. Ectodermal thickenings (**lens placodes**), indicating the primordia of the future lenses of the eyes,

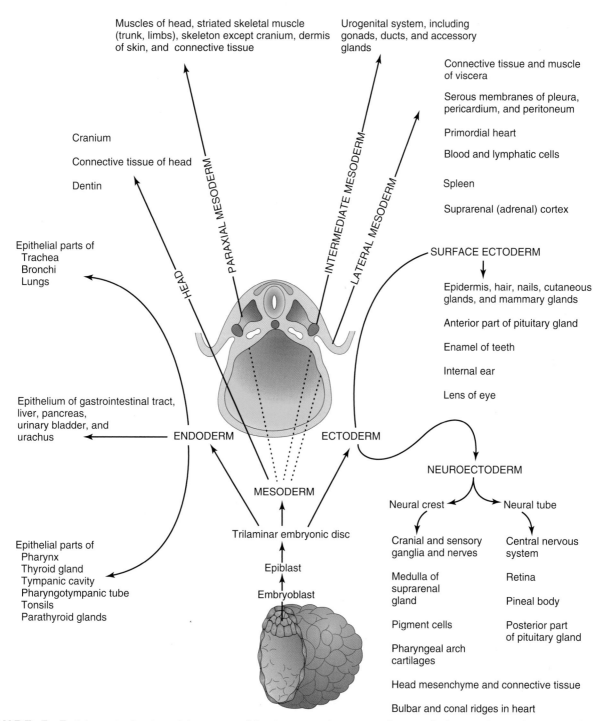

Muscles of head, striated skeletal muscle (trunk, limbs), skeleton except cranium, dermis of skin, and connective tissue

Urogenital system, including gonads, ducts, and accessory glands

Connective tissue and muscle of viscera

Serous membranes of pleura, pericardium, and peritoneum

Primordial heart

Blood and lymphatic cells

Spleen

Suprarenal (adrenal) cortex

Cranium

Connective tissue of head

Dentin

PARAXIAL MESODERM

INTERMEDIATE MESODERM

LATERAL MESODERM

HEAD

SURFACE ECTODERM

Epidermis, hair, nails, cutaneous glands, and mammary glands

Anterior part of pituitary gland

Enamel of teeth

Internal ear

Lens of eye

Epithelial parts of
Trachea
Bronchi
Lungs

Epithelium of gastrointestinal tract, liver, pancreas, urinary bladder, and urachus

ENDODERM

ECTODERM

MESODERM

Trilaminar embryonic disc

Epiblast

Embryoblast

NEUROECTODERM

Neural crest

Neural tube

Cranial and sensory ganglia and nerves

Central nervous system

Medulla of suprarenal gland

Retina

Pineal body

Pigment cells

Posterior part of pituitary gland

Pharyngeal arch cartilages

Head mesenchyme and connective tissue

Bulbar and conal ridges in heart

Epithelial parts of
Pharynx
Thyroid gland
Tympanic cavity
Pharyngotympanic tube
Tonsils
Parathyroid glands

**FIGURE 5–5** Schematic drawing of derivatives of the three germ layers, ectoderm, endoderm, and mesoderm. Cells from these layers contribute to the formation of different tissues and organs.

are visible on the sides of the head (see Fig. 5-9*B*). The fourth pair of pharyngeal arches and lower limb buds are visible by the end of the fourth week. A long tail-like **caudal eminence** is also a characteristic feature (Fig. 5-10, and see Figs. 5-8 and 5-9). Rudiments of many of the organ systems, especially the **cardiovascular system,** are established (Fig. 5-11). By the end of the fourth week, the caudal neuropore is usually closed.

## Fifth Week

*Changes in body form are minor during the fifth week* compared with those that occurred during the fourth week, but growth of the head exceeds that of other regions (Figs. 5-12 and 5-13). Enlargement of the head results mainly from the rapid development of the brain and facial prominences. The face soon contacts the heart prominence. The rapidly growing second pharyngeal arch

**Table 5–1    Criteria for Estimating Developmental Stages in Human Embryos**

| AGE (DAYS) | FIGURE REFERENCE | CARNEGIE STAGE | NUMBER OF SOMITES | LENGTH (mm)* | MAIN EXTERNAL CHARACTERISTICS† |
|---|---|---|---|---|---|
| 20–21 | | 9 | 1–3 | 1.5–3.0 | Flat embryonic disc. Deep neural groove and prominent neural folds. One to three pairs of somites present. Head fold evident. |
| 22–23 | 5–6 | 10 | 4–12 | 1.0–3.5 | Embryo straight or slightly curved. Neural tube forming or formed opposite somites but widely open at rostral and caudal neuropores. First and second pairs of pharyngeal arches visible. |
| 24–25 | 5–7 | 11 | 13–20 | 2.5–4.5 | Embryo curved owing to head and tail folds. Rostral neuropore closing. Otic placodes present. Optic vesicles formed. |
| 26–27 | 5–8 | 12 | 21–29 | 3.0–5.0 | Upper limb buds appear. Rostral neuropore closed. Caudal neuropore closing. Three pairs of pharyngeal arches visible. Heart prominence distinct. Otic pits present. |
| 28–30 | 5–9 5–11 | 13 | 30–35 | 4.0–6.0 | Embryo has C-shaped curve. Caudal neuropore closed. Four pairs of pharyngeal arches visible. Lower limb buds appear. Otic vesicles present. Lens placodes distinct. Tail-like caudal eminence present. |
| 31–32 | 5–12 5–13 | 14 | ‡ | 5.0–7.0 | Lens pits and nasal pits visible. Optic cups present. |
| 33–36 | | 15 | | 7.0–9.0 | Hand plates formed; digital rays visible. Lens vesicles present. Nasal pits prominent. Cervical sinuses visible. |
| 37–40 | | 16 | | 8.0–11.0 | Foot plates formed. Pigment visible in retina. Auricular hillocks developing. |
| 41–43 | 5–14 | 17 | | 11.0–14.0 | Digital rays clearly visible in hand plates. Auricular hillocks outline future auricle of external ear. Trunk beginning to straighten. Cerebral vesicles prominent. |
| 44–46 | | 18 | | 13.0–17.0 | Digital rays clearly visible in foot plates. Elbow region visible. Eyelids forming. Notches between digital rays in the hands. Nipples visible. |
| 47–48 | 5–15 | 19 | | 16.0–18.0 | Limbs extend ventrally. Trunk elongating and straightening. Midgut herniation prominent. |
| 49–51 | | 20 | | 18.0–22.0 | Upper limbs longer and bent at elbows. Fingers distinct but webbed. Notches between digital rays in the feet. Scalp vascular plexus appears. |
| 52–53 | 5–16 | 21 | | 22.0–24.0 | Hands and feet approach each other. Fingers are free and longer. Toes distinct but webbed. |
| 54–55 | | 22 | | 23.0–28.0 | Toes free and longer. Eyelids and auricles of external ears more developed. |
| 56 | | 23 | | 27.0–31.0 | Head more rounded and shows human characteristics. External genitalia still have indistinct appearance. Distinct bulge still present in umbilical cord, caused by herniation of intestines. Caudal eminence (tail) has disappeared. |

*The embryonic lengths indicate the usual range. In stages 9 and 10, the measurement is greatest length; in subsequent stages, crown–rump length measurements are given (see Fig. 5-20).
†Based on Nishimura et al (1974), O'Rahilly and Müller (1987), Shiota (1991), and the Virtual Human Embryo Project (Project Leaders: Dr. Raymond Gasser and Dr. John Cork [http://www.ehd.org/virtual-human-embryo/]).
‡At this and subsequent stages, the number of somites is difficult to determine and so is not a useful criterion.

**FIGURE 5–6** **A,** Dorsal view of a five-somite embryo at Carnegie stage 10, approximately 22 days. Observe the neural folds and deep neural groove. The neural folds in the cranial region have thickened to form the primordium of the brain. **B,** Drawing of structures shown in **A.** Most of the amniotic and chorionic sacs have been cut away to expose the embryo. **C,** Dorsal view of an older eight-somite embryo at Carnegie stage 10. The neural tube is in open communication with the amniotic cavity at the cranial and caudal ends through the rostral and caudal neuropores, respectively. **D,** Diagram of structures shown in **C.** The neural folds have fused opposite the somites to form the neural tube (primordium of spinal cord in this region). (*A and C, From Moore KL, Persaud TVN, Shiota K: Color atlas of clinical embryology, ed 2, Philadelphia, 2000, Saunders.*)

Rostral neuropore closing

Forebrain

1st pharyngeal arch

Amnion

Heart prominence

Somites

Neural tube in region of developing spinal cord

Caudal neuropore

Connecting stalk

(24-day embryo) = 3.5 mm

**FIGURE 5–7** A, Dorsal view of a 13-somite embryo at Carnegie stage 11, approximately 24 days. The rostral neuropore is closing but the caudal neuropore is wide open. **B,** Illustration of the structures shown in A. The embryo is lightly curved because of folding at the cranial and caudal ends. (**A,** *From Moore KL, Persaud TVN, Shiota K:* Color atlas of clinical embryology, *ed 2, Philadelphia, 2000, Saunders.*)

overgrows the third and fourth arches, forming a lateral depression on each side, the **cervical sinus.** Mesonephric ridges indicate the site of the developing mesonephric kidneys (see Fig. 5-13*B*), which, in humans, are interim excretory organs.

## Sixth Week

Embryos in the sixth week show **spontaneous movements,** such as twitching of the trunk and developing limbs. It has been reported that embryos at this stage show **reflex responses to touch.** The upper limbs begin to show regional differentiation as the elbows and large **hand plates** develop (Fig. 5-14). The primordia of the digits (fingers), or **digital rays,** begin to develop in the hand plates.

Development of the lower limbs occurs during the sixth week, 4 to 5 days later than that of the upper limbs. Several small swellings, **auricular hillocks,** develop around the *pharyngeal groove* between the first two pharyngeal arches (see Figs. 5-13 and 5-14*B*). This groove becomes the **external acoustic meatus** (external ear canal). The

auricular hillocks contribute to the formation of the auricle (pinna), the shell-shaped part of the external ear. Largely because retinal pigment has formed, the eyes are now obvious (see Fig. 5-14). The head is now much larger relative to the trunk and is bent over the **heart prominence.** This head position results from bending in the cervical (neck) region. The trunk and neck have begun to straighten, and the intestines enter the extraembryonic coelom in the proximal part of the umbilical cord (see Fig. 5-18). This umbilical herniation is a normal event. The herniation occurs because the abdominal cavity is too small at this age to accommodate the rapidly growing intestine.

## Seventh Week

The limbs undergo considerable change during the seventh week. Notches appear between the **digital rays** (grooves or notches that separate the areas of the hand and foot plates), which clearly indicate the **digits** (fingers or toes; Fig. 5-15). Communication between the

*Text continued on p. 84*

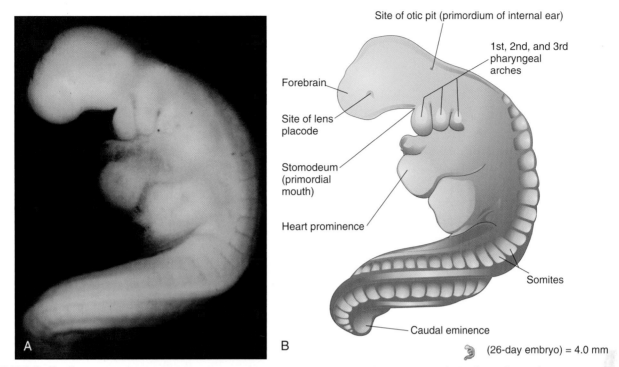

**FIGURE 5–8** **A,** Lateral view of a 27-somite embryo at Carnegie stage 12, approximately 26 days. The embryo is curved, especially its tail-like caudal eminence. Observe the lens placode (primordium of lens of eye) and the otic pit, indicating early development of the internal ear. **B,** Illustration of structures shown in **A.** The rostral neuropore is closed and three pairs of pharyngeal arches are present. (*A, From Nishimura H, Semba R, Tanimura T, Tanaka O: Prenatal development of the human with special reference to craniofacial structures: an atlas, Washington, DC, 1977, National Institutes of Health.*)

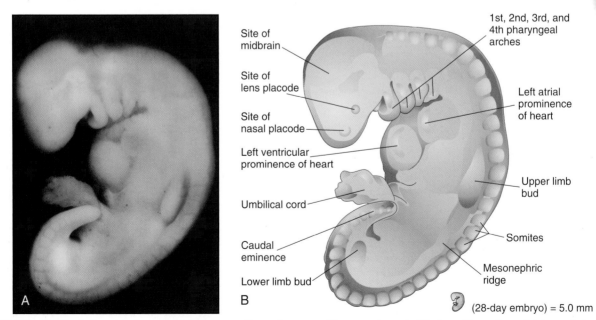

**FIGURE 5–9** **A,** Lateral view of an embryo at Carnegie stage 13, approximately 28 days. The primordial heart is large and divided into a primordial atrium and ventricle. The rostral and caudal neuropores are closed. **B,** Drawing indicating the structures shown in **A.** The embryo has a characteristic C-shaped curvature, four pharyngeal arches, and upper and lower limb buds. (*A, From Nishimura H, Semba R, Tanimura T, Tanaka O: Prenatal development of the human with special reference to craniofacial structures: an atlas, Washington, DC, 1977, National Institutes of Health.*)

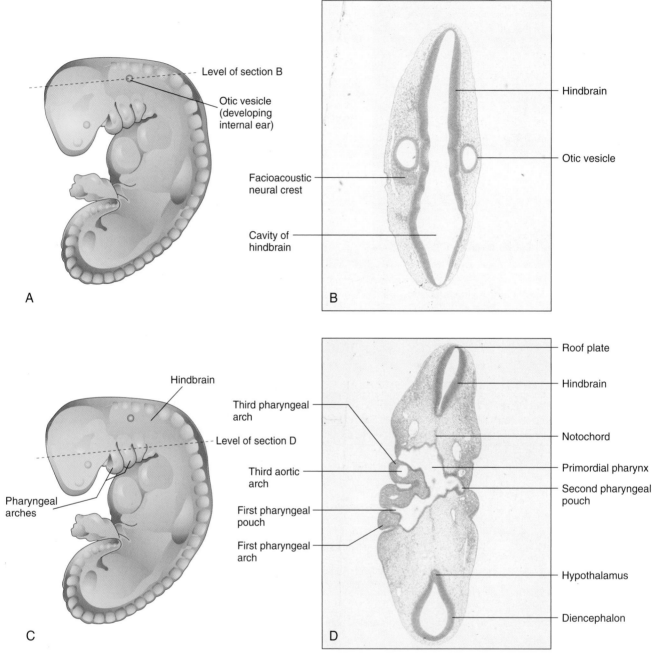

**FIGURE 5-10** A, Drawing of an embryo at Carnegie stage 13, approximately 28 days. B, Photomicrograph of a section of the embryo at the level shown in A. Observe the hindbrain and otic vesicle (primordium of internal ear). C, Drawing of same embryo showing the level of the section in D. Observe the primordial pharynx and pharyngeal arches. (*B and D, From Moore KL, Persaud TVN, Shiota K: Color atlas of clinical embryology, ed 2, Philadelphia, 2000, Saunders.*)

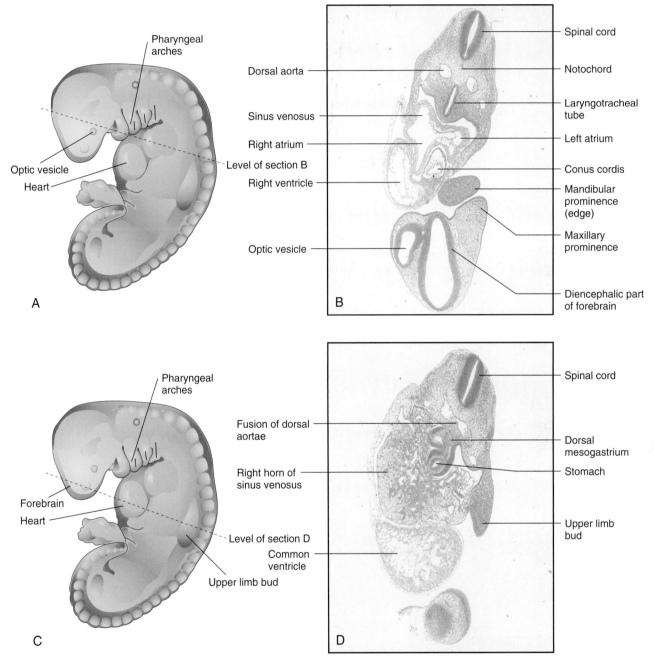

**FIGURE 5–11** **A,** Drawing of an embryo at Carnegie stage 13, approximately 28 days. **B,** Photomicrograph of a section of the embryo at the level shown in **A.** Observe the parts of the primordial heart. **C,** Drawing of the same embryo showing the level of section in **D.** Observe the primordial heart and stomach. *(B and D, From Moore KL, Persaud TVN, Shiota K: Color atlas of clinical embryology, ed 2, Philadelphia, 2000, Saunders.)*

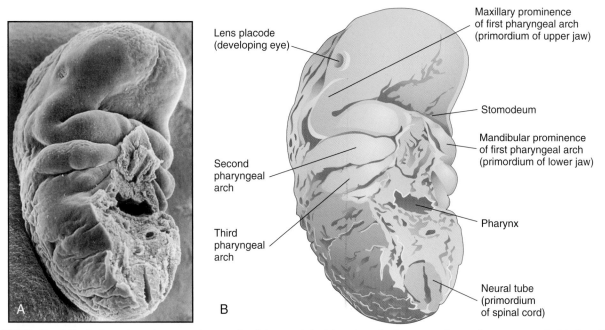

**FIGURE 5–12** A, Scanning electron micrograph of the craniofacial region of a human embryo of approximately 32 days (Carnegie stage 14, 6.8 mm). Three pairs of pharyngeal arches are present. The maxillary and mandibular prominences of the first arch are clearly delineated. Observe the large stomodeum (mouth) located between the maxillary prominences and fused mandibular prominences. B, Drawing of the scanning electron micrograph illustrating the structures shown in A.

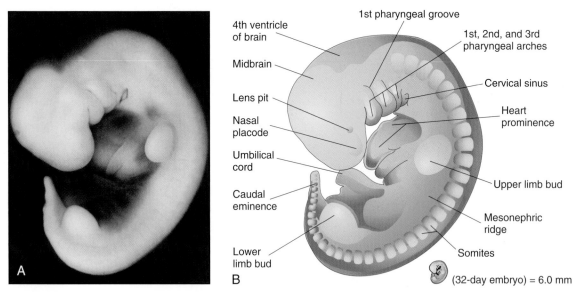

**FIGURE 5–13** A, Lateral view of an embryo at Carnegie stage 14, approximately 32 days. The second pharyngeal arch has overgrown the third arch, forming the **cervical sinus**. The mesonephric ridge indicates the site of the mesonephric kidney, an interim kidney (see Chapter 12). B, Illustration of structures shown in A. (A, From Nishimura H, Semba R, Tanimura T, Tanaka O: Prenatal development of the human with special reference to craniofacial structures: an atlas, Washington, DC, 1977, National Institutes of Health.)

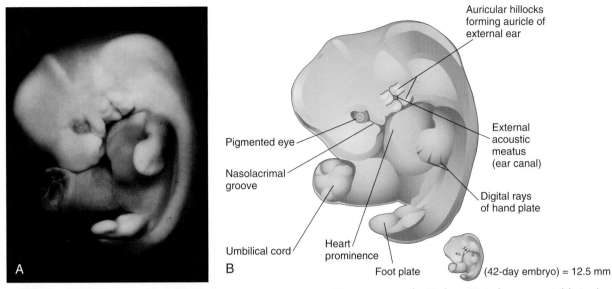

**FIGURE 5–14** **A,** Lateral view of an embryo at Carnegie stage 17, approximately 42 days. Digital rays are visible in the hand plate, indicating the future site of the digits (fingers). **B,** Drawing illustrating structures shown in **A.** The eye, auricular hillocks, and external acoustic meatus are now obvious. (*A, From Moore KL, Persaud TVN, Shiota K: Color atlas of clinical embryology, ed 2, Philadelphia, 2000, Saunders.*)

**FIGURE 5–15** **A,** Lateral view of an embryo at Carnegie stage 19, about 48 days. The auricle and external acoustic meatus are now clearly visible. Note the relatively low position of the developing ear at this stage. Digital rays are now visible in the foot plate. The prominence of the abdomen is caused mainly by the large size of the liver. **B,** Drawing indicating structures shown in **A.** Observe the large hand and notches between the digital rays, which clearly indicate the developing digits (fingers). (*A, From Moore KL, Persaud TVN, Shiota K: Color atlas of clinical embryology, ed 2, Philadelphia, 2000, Saunders.*)

**FIGURE 5-16** A, Lateral view of an embryo at Carnegie stage 21, approximately 52 days. Note that the scalp vascular plexus now forms a characteristic band across the head. The nose is stubby, and the eye is heavily pigmented. B, Illustration of structures shown in A. The fingers are separated, and the toes are beginning to separate. C, A Carnegie stage 20 human embryo, approximately 50 days after ovulation, imaged with optical microscopy (*left*) and magnetic resonance microscopy (*right*). The three-dimensional data set from magnetic resonance microscopy has been edited to reveal anatomic detail from a midsagittal plane. (*A, From Nishimura H, Semba R, Tanimura T, Tanaka O: Prenatal development of the human with special reference to craniofacial structures: an atlas, Washington, DC, 1977, National Institutes of Health; B, From Moore KL, Persaud TVN, Shiota K: Color atlas of clinical embryology, ed 2, Philadelphia, 2000, Saunders.*)

primordial gut and umbilical vesicle is now reduced. The yolk stalk now becomes the **omphaloenteric duct** (see Fig. 5-1C2). By the end of the seventh week, ossification of bones of the upper limbs has begun.

## Eighth Week

At the beginning of this final week of the embryonic period, the digits of the hand are separated but noticeably webbed (Fig. 5-16A and B). Notches are also clearly visible between the digital rays of the feet. The **caudal eminence** is still present but stubby. The **scalp vascular plexus** has appeared and forms a characteristic band around the head. At the end of the eighth week, all regions of the limbs are apparent and the digits have lengthened and are completely separated (Fig. 5-17).

Purposeful limb movements first occur during the eighth week. Primary ossification begins in the **femora** (long bones of the thigh). All evidence of the caudal eminence has disappeared, and both hands and feet approach each other ventrally. At the end of this week, the embryo has distinct **human characteristics** (Fig. 5-18); however, the head is still disproportionately large, constituting almost half of the embryo. The neck is established and

Scalp vascular plexus

Auricle of external ear

Eyelid

Nose

Mouth

Lower jaw

Umbilical cord

Toes separated

A

B

C

5 mm

(56-day embryo) = 29.0 mm

**FIGURE 5–17** A, Lateral view of an embryo at Carnegie stage 23, approximately 56 days (end of embryonic period). The embryo has a distinct human appearance. B, Illustration of structures shown in A. C, A Carnegie stage 23 embryo, approximately 56 days after ovulation, imaged with optical microscopy (*left*) and magnetic resonance microscopy (*right*). (*A, From Nishimura H, Semba R, Tanimura T, Tanaka O: Prenatal development of the human with special reference to craniofacial structures: an atlas, Washington, DC, 1977, National Institutes of Health; B, From Moore KL, Persaud TVN, Shiota K: Color atlas of clinical embryology, ed 2, Philadelphia, 2000, Saunders.*)

the eyelids are more obvious. The eyelids are closing, and by the end of the eighth week, they begin to unite by epithelial fusion. The intestines are still in the proximal portion of the umbilical cord (see Fig. 5-18). Although there are slight sex differences in the appearance of the external genitalia, they are not distinctive enough to permit accurate sexual identification.

## ESTIMATION OF EMBRYONIC AGE

Estimates of the age of embryos *recovered after a spontaneous abortion,* for example, are determined from their external characteristics and measurements of their length (Figs. 5-19 and 5-20, and also see Table 5-1).

*However, size alone may be an unreliable criterion* because some embryos undergo a progressively slower rate of growth before death. Embryos of the third and early fourth weeks are straight (see Fig. 5-20A), so measurements indicate the greatest length. The **crown–rump length** (CRL) is most frequently used for older embryos (14 to 18 weeks) (see Fig. 5-20B). Because no anatomic marker clearly indicates the CRL, one assumes that the longest CRL is the most accurate. Standing height, or **crown–heel length,** is sometimes measured. *The length of an embryo is only one criterion for establishing age.* The **Carnegie Embryonic Staging System** is used internationally; its use enables comparisons to be made between the findings of one person and those of another (see Table 5-1).

Umbilical vesicle (yolk sac)

Chorionic blood vessels

Intestine in umbilical cord

Umbilical cord

Chorionic sac

Chorionic villi

**FIGURE 5–18** Lateral view of an embryo and its chorionic sac at Carnegie stage 23, approximately 56 days. Observe the human appearance of the embryo. Although it may appear to be a male, it may not be possible to estimate sex because the external genitalia of males and females are similar at this stage of the embryonic period (see Chapter 1, Fig. 1-1). *(From Nishimura H, Semba R, Tanimura T, Tanaka O: Prenatal development of the human with special reference to craniofacial structures: an atlas, Washington, DC, 1977, National Institutes of Health.)*

**FIGURE 5–19** Transvaginal sonogram of a 7-week embryo *(calipers, crown–rump length 10 mm)* surrounded by the amniotic membrane within the chorionic cavity *(dark region).*

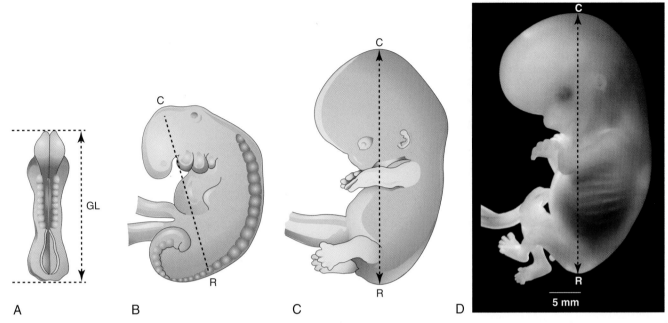

**FIGURE 5–20** Illustrations of methods used to measure the length of embryos. **A,** Greatest length (GL). **B, C,** and **D,** Crown–rump (CR) length. **D,** Photograph of an 8-week-old embryo at Carnegie stage 23.

## ESTIMATION OF GESTATIONAL AND EMBRYONIC AGE

By convention, obstetricians date pregnancy from the presumed first day of the **last normal menstrual period (LNMP)**. This is the gestational age, which in embryology is superfluous because gestation does not begin until fertilization of an oocyte occurs. **Embryonic age** *begins at fertilization, approximately 2 weeks after the* LNMP (see Chapter 1, Fig. 1-1). Fertilization age is used in patients who have undergone in vitro fertilization or artificial insemination (see Chapter 2, Fig. 2-15).

Knowledge of embryonic age is important because it affects clinical management, especially when invasive procedures such as chorionic villus sampling and amniocentesis are necessary (see Chapter 6). In some women, estimation of their gestational age from the menstrual history alone may be unreliable. The probability of error in establishing the LNMP is highest in women who become pregnant after cessation of oral contraception because the interval between discontinuance of hormones and the onset of ovulation is highly variable. In other women, slight uterine bleeding (spotting), which sometimes occurs during implantation of the blastocyst, may be incorrectly regarded by a woman as light menstruation.

Other contributing factors to LNMP unreliability may include **oligomenorrhea** (scanty menstruation), pregnancy in the postpartum period (i.e., several weeks after childbirth), and use of intrauterine devices. Despite possible sources of error, the LNMP is a reliable criterion in most cases. **Ultrasound assessment** of the size of the embryo and chorionic cavity enables clinicians to obtain an accurate estimate of the date of conception (see Fig. 5-19).

The day on which fertilization occurs is the most accurate reference point for estimating age; this is commonly calculated from the estimated time of ovulation because the oocyte is usually fertilized within 12 hours after ovulation. All statements about embryonic age should indicate the reference point used, that is, days after LNMP or after the estimated time of fertilization.

## SUMMARY OF FOURTH TO EIGHTH WEEKS

- At the beginning of the fourth week, *folding in the median and horizontal planes* converts the flat trilaminar embryonic disc into a C-shaped, cylindric embryo. The formation of the head, caudal eminence, and lateral folds is a continuous sequence of events that results in a constriction between the embryo and umbilical vesicle.

- *As the head folds ventrally,* part of the endodermal layer is incorporated into the developing embryonic head region as the **foregut.** Folding of the head region also results in the oropharyngeal membrane and heart being carried ventrally and the developing brain becoming the most cranial part of the embryo.

## ULTRASOUND EXAMINATION OF EMBRYOS

Most women seeking obstetric care have at least one ultrasound examination during their pregnancy for one or more of the following reasons:

- Estimation of gestational age for confirmation of clinical dating
- Evaluation of embryonic growth when intrauterine growth restriction is suspected
- Guidance during chorionic villus or amniotic fluid sampling (see Chapter 6)
- Examination of a clinically detected pelvic mass
- Suspected ectopic pregnancy (see Chapter 3, Fig. 3-9)
- Possible uterine birth defects (see Chapter 12, Fig. 12-44)
- Detection of birth defects

Current data indicate that there are no confirmed biologic effects of diagnostic ultrasonography or MRI evaluation on embryos or fetuses (see Figs. 5-16C, 5-17C, and 5-19).

The size of an embryo in utero can be estimated using ultrasound measurements. **Transvaginal sonography** permits an earlier and more accurate measurement of CRL in early pregnancy (see Fig. 5-19). Early in the fifth week, the embryo is 4 to 7 mm long (see Fig. 5-13). During the sixth and seventh weeks, discrete embryonic structures can be visualized (e.g., parts of limbs) and CRL measurements are predictive of embryonic age with an accuracy of 1 to 4 days. Furthermore, after the sixth week, dimensions of the head and trunk can be obtained and used for assessment of embryonic age. There is, however, considerable variability in early embryonic growth and development. Differences are greatest before the end of the first 4 weeks of development but less so by the end of the embryonic period.

---

- *As the caudal eminence folds ventrally,* part of the endodermal germ layer is incorporated into the caudal end of the embryo as the **hindgut.** The terminal part of the hindgut expands to form the **cloaca.** Folding of the caudal region also results in the cloacal membrane, allantois, and connecting stalk being carried to the ventral surface of the embryo.
- *Folding of the embryo in the horizontal plane* incorporates part of the endoderm into the embryo as the **midgut.**
- The **umbilical vesicle** remains attached to the midgut by a narrow **omphaloenteric duct** (yolk stalk). During folding of the embryo in the horizontal plane, the *primordia of the lateral and ventral body walls are formed.* As the **amnion** expands, it envelops the connecting stalk, omphaloenteric duct, and allantois, thereby forming an epithelial covering for the umbilical cord.
- *The three germ layers differentiate into various tissues and organs,* so that by the end of the embryonic period, the beginnings of *the main organ systems have been established.*
- The external appearance of the embryo is greatly affected by the formation of the brain, heart, liver, somites, limbs, ears, nose, and eyes.
- Because the beginnings of most essential external and internal structures are formed during the fourth to eighth weeks, *this is the most critical period of development.* Developmental disturbances during this period may give rise to major birth defects.
- Reasonable estimates of the age of embryos can be determined from the day of onset of the LNMP, the estimated time of fertilization, ultrasound measurements of the chorionic sac and embryo, and examination of external characteristics of the embryo.

## CLINICALLY ORIENTED PROBLEMS

### CASE 5–1

*A 28-year-old woman who has been a heavy cigarette smoker since her teens was informed that she was in the second month of pregnancy.*

- What would the doctor likely tell the patient about her smoking habit and its possible impacts on the embryo and fetal health?

### CASE 5–2

*A pregnant patient was concerned about what she had read in the newspaper about teratogenic effects of drugs on laboratory animals.*

- Can one predict the possible harmful effects of drugs on the human embryo from studies performed in laboratory animals? Explain.

### CASE 5–3

*A 30-year-old woman was unsure when her LNMP had occurred. She stated that her periods were irregular.*

- What clinical techniques could be used for evaluating embryonic age in this pregnancy?

**CASE 5–4**

*A woman who had just become pregnant told her doctor that she had taken a sleeping pill given to her by a friend. She wondered whether it could harm the development of her baby's limbs.*

* Would a drug known to cause severe limb defects be likely to cause these birth defects if it were taken during the second week? Sixth week? Eighth week?

Discussion of these problems appears in the Appendix at the back of the book.

## BIBLIOGRAPHY AND SUGGESTED READING

Ashe HL, Briscoe J: The interpretation of morphogen gradients, *Development* 133:385, 2006.

Barnea ER, Hustin J, Jauniaux E, editors: *The first twelve weeks of gestation*, Berlin, 1992, Springer-Verlag.

Blechschmidt E, Gasser RF: *Biokinetics and biodynamics of human differentiation: principles and applications*, reprint edition, Berkeley, Calif., 2012, North Atlantic Books.

Callen PW: Obstetric ultrasound examination. In Callen PW, editor: *Ultrasonography in obstetrics and gynecology*, ed 5, Philadelphia, 2008, Saunders.

Dickey RP, Gasser RF: Computer analysis of the human embryo growth curve: differences between published ultrasound findings on living embryos in utero and data on fixed specimens, *Anat Rec* 237:400, 1993.

Dickey RP, Gasser RF: Ultrasound evidence for variability in the size and development of normal human embryos before the tenth post-insemination week after assisted reproductive technologies, *Hum Reprod* 8:331, 1993.

Gasser RF: *Atlas of human embryos*, Baltimore, 1975, Lippincott Williams & Wilkins.

Gasser RF, Cork RJ, Stillwell BJ, et al: Rebirth of human embryology, *Dev Dyn* 243:621, 2014.

Gilbert SF: *Developmental biology*, ed 9, Sunderland, Mass., 2010, Sinauer.

Hardin J, Walston T: Models of morphogenesis: the mechanisms and mechanics of cell rearrangement, *Curr Opin Genet Dev* 14:399, 2004.

Iffy L, Shepard TH, Jakobovits A, et al: The rate of growth in young human embryos of Streeter's horizons XIII and XXIII, *Acta Anat* 66:178, 1967.

Iwarsson E, Malmgren H, Blennow E: Preimplantation genetic diagnosis: twenty years of practice, *Semin Fetal Neonatal Med* 16:74, 2011.

Jirásek JE: *An atlas of human prenatal developmental mechanics: anatomy and staging*, London and New York, 2004, Taylor and Francis.

Kliegman RM: Intrauterine growth restriction. In Martin RJ, Fanaroff AA, Walsh MC, editors: *Fanaroff and Martin's neonatal-perinatal medicine: diseases of the fetus and infant*, ed 8, Philadelphia, 2006, Mosby.

Laing FC, Frates MC, Benson CB: Ultrasound evaluation during the first trimester. In Callen PW, editor: *Ultrasonography in obstetrics and gynecology*, ed 5, Philadelphia, 2008, Saunders.

Moore KL, Persaud TVN, Shiota K: *Color atlas of clinical embryology*, ed 2, Philadelphia, 2000, Saunders.

Nishimura H, Tanimura T, Semba R, et al: Normal development of early human embryos: observation of 90 specimens at Carnegie stages 7 to 13, *Teratology* 10:1, 1974.

O'Rahilly R, Müller F: *Developmental stages in human embryos*, Washington, DC, 1987, Carnegie Institute of Washington.

Persaud TVN, Hay JC: Normal embryonic and fetal development. In Reece EA, Hobbins JC, editors: *Clinical obstetrics: the fetus and mother*, ed 3, Oxford, 2006, Blackwell.

Plaisier M: Decidualization and angiogenesis, *Best Pract Res Clin Obstet Gynaecol* 25:259, 2011.

Pooh RK, Shiota K, Kurjak A: Imaging of the human embryo with magnetic resonance imaging microscopy and high-resolution trans-vaginal 3-dimensional sonography: human embryology in the 21st century, *Am J Obstet Gynecol* 204:77.e1, 2011.

Shiota K: Development and intrauterine fate of normal and abnormal human conceptuses, *Congen Anom* 31:67, 1991.

Steding G: *The anatomy of the human embryo: a scanning electron-microscopic atlas*, Basel, 2009, Karger.

Streeter GL: Developmental horizons in human embryos: description of age group XI, 13 to 20 somites, and age group XII, 21 to 29 somites, *Contrib Embryol Carnegie Inst* 30:211, 1942.

Streeter GL: Developmental horizons in human embryos: description of age group XIII, embryos of 4 or 5 millimeters long, and age group XIV, period of identification of the lens vesicle, *Contrib Embryol Carnegie Inst* 31:27, 1945.

Streeter GL: Developmental horizons in human embryos: description of age groups XV, XVI, XVII, and XVIII, *Contrib Embryol Carnegie Inst* 32:133, 1948.

Streeter GL, Heuser CH, Corner GW: Developmental horizons in human embryos: description of age groups XIX, XX, XXI, XXII, and XXIII, *Contrib Embryol Carnegie Inst* 34:165, 1951.

Whitworth M, Bricker L, Neilson JP, et al: Ultrasound for fetal assessment in early pregnancy, *Cochrane Database Syst Rev* (4):CD007058, 2010.

Yamada S, Samtani RR, Lee ES, et al: Developmental atlas of the early first trimester human embryo, *Dev Dyn* 239:2010, 1585.

Zhang J, Merialdi M, Platt LD, et al: Defining normal and abnormal fetal growth: promises and challenges, *Am J Obstet Gynecol* 202:522, 2010.

# Fetal Period: Ninth Week to Birth

**T**he transformation of an embryo to a fetus is gradual, but the name change is meaningful because it signifies that the embryo has developed into a recognizable human and the primordia of all major systems have formed. Development during the fetal period is primarily concerned with rapid body growth and differentiation of tissues, organs, and systems. A notable change occurring during the fetal period is the relative slowdown in the growth of the head compared with the rest of the body. The rate of body growth during the fetal period is very rapid (Table 6-1), and fetal weight gain is phenomenal during the terminal weeks. Periods of normal continuous growth alternate with prolonged intervals of absent growth.

**Table 6–1    Criteria for Estimating Fertilization Age during the Fetal Period**

| AGE (WEEKS) | CROWN-RUMP LENGTH (mm)* | FOOT LENGTH (mm)* | FETAL WEIGHT (g)† | MAIN EXTERNAL CHARACTERISTICS |
|---|---|---|---|---|
| **Previable Fetuses** | | | | |
| 9 | 50 | 7 | 8 | *Eyelids closing or closed. Head large and more rounded.* External genitalia are not distinguishable as male or female. Some of the small intestines are in the proximal part of umbilical cord. The ears are low set. |
| 10 | 61 | 9 | 14 | *Intestines in abdomen. Early fingernail development.* |
| 12 | 87 | 14 | 45 | *Sex distinguishable externally. Well-defined neck.* |
| 14 | 120 | 20 | 110 | *Head erect. Eyes face anteriorly. Ears are close to their definitive position. Lower limbs well developed. Early toenail development.* |
| 16 | 140 | 27 | 200 | *External ears stand out from head.* |
| 18 | 160 | 33 | 320 | *Vernix caseosa covers skin. Quickening (first movements) felt by mother.* |
| 20 | 190 | 39 | 460 | *Head and body hair (lanugo) visible.* |
| **Viable Fetuses‡** | | | | |
| 22 | 210 | 45 | 630 | *Skin wrinkled, translucent, and pink to red.* |
| 24 | 230 | 50 | 820 | *Fingernails present. Lean body.* |
| 26 | 250 | 55 | 1000 | *Eyelids partially open. Eyelashes present.* |
| 28 | 270 | 59 | 1300 | *Eyes wide open.* Considerable scalp hair sometimes present. Skin slightly wrinkled. |
| 30 | 280 | 63 | 1700 | *Toenails present. Body filling out. Testes descending.* |
| 32 | 300 | 68 | 2100 | *Fingernails reach fingertips. Skin smooth.* |
| 36 | 340 | 79 | 2900 | *Body usually plump. Lanugo (hairs) almost absent. Toenails reach toe tips. Flexed limbs; firm grasp.* |
| 38 | 360 | 83 | 3400 | *Prominent chest; breasts protrude.* Testes in scrotum or palpable in inguinal canals. Fingernails extend beyond fingertips. |

*These measurements are averages and so may not apply to specific cases; dimensional variations increase with age.
†These weights refer to fetuses that have been fixed for approximately 2 weeks in 10% formalin. Fresh specimens usually weigh approximately 5% less.
‡There is no sharp limit of development, age, or weight at which a fetus automatically becomes viable or beyond which survival is ensured, but experience has shown that it is rare for a baby to survive whose weight is less than 500 g or whose fertilization age is less than 22 weeks. Even fetuses born between 26 and 28 weeks have difficulty surviving, mainly because the respiratory system and the central nervous system are not completely differentiated.

## VIABILITY OF FETUSES

*Viability* is defined as the ability of fetuses to survive in the extrauterine environment. Most fetuses weighing less than 500 g at birth do not usually survive. Many full-term, low-birth-weight infants result from **intrauterine growth restriction (IUGR)**. Consequently, if given expert postnatal care, some fetuses weighing less than 500 g may survive; they are referred to as extremely low-birth-weight infants, or **immature infants**.

Most fetuses weighing between 750 and 1500 g usually survive, but complications may occur; they are referred to as **preterm infants**. Each year, approximately 500,000 preterm infants are born in the United States. Many of these infants suffer from severe medical complications or early **mortality** (death). The use of antenatal steroids and the postnatal administration of endotracheal surfactant have greatly lowered the rates of acute and long-term morbidity. *Prematurity is one of the most common causes of morbidity and perinatal death.*

## ESTIMATION OF FETAL AGE

Ultrasound measurements of the **crown–rump length (CRL)** of the fetus are taken to determine its size and probable age and to provide a prediction of the *expected date of delivery*. Fetal head measurements and femur length are also used to evaluate age. In clinical practice, *gestational age is usually timed from the onset of the last normal menstrual period (LNMP)*.

In embryology, **gestational age** based on the LNMP is superfluous because gestation (time of fertilization) does not begin until the oocyte is fertilized, which occurs around the middle of the menstrual cycle. This difference in the use of the term *gestational age* may be confusing; therefore, it is important that the person ordering the ultrasound examination and the ultrasonographer use the embryologic terminology (see Chapter 1, Fig. 1-1, first week).

The **intrauterine period** may be divided into days, weeks, or months (Table 6-2), but confusion arises if it is not stated whether the age is calculated from the onset of the LNMP or from the estimated day of fertilization of the oocyte. Uncertainty about age arises when months are used, particularly when it is not stated whether calendar months (28 to 31 days) or lunar months (28 days) are meant. *Unless otherwise stated, embryologic or fetal age in this book is calculated from the estimated time of fertilization.*

### Trimesters of Pregnancy

Clinically, the gestational period is divided into three trimesters, each lasting 3 months. By the end of the first trimester, one third of the length of the pregnancy, major systems have been developed (see Table 6-1). In the second trimester, the fetus grows sufficiently in size so that good anatomical detail can be visualized during **ultrasonography**. During this period, most major birth defects can be detected using **high-resolution real-time ultrasonography**. By the beginning of the third trimester, the fetus may survive if born prematurely. The fetus reaches a major developmental landmark at 35 weeks and weighs approximately 2500 g; these data are used to define the level of fetal maturity. At 35 weeks, fetuses usually survive if born prematurely.

### Measurements and Characteristics of Fetuses

Various measurements and external characteristics are useful for estimating fetal age (see Table 6-1). CRL is the method of choice for estimating fetal age until the end of the first trimester because there is very little variability in fetal size during this period. In the second and third trimesters, several structures can be identified and measured ultrasonographically, but the most common measurements are **biparietal diameter** (diameter of the head between the two parietal eminences), **head circumference**, abdominal circumference, femur length, and foot length.

Weight is often a useful criterion for estimating age, but there may be a discrepancy between the age and weight, particularly when the mother has had metabolic disturbances such as diabetes mellitus during pregnancy. In these cases, the weight often exceeds values considered normal for the corresponding CRL. Fetal dimensions obtained from ultrasound measurements closely approximate CRL measurements obtained from spontaneously aborted fetuses. Determination of the size of a fetus, especially its head circumference, is helpful to the obstetrician for management of patients.

| Table 6–2 | Comparison of Gestational Time Units and Date of Birth* | | | |
|---|---|---|---|---|
| **REFERENCE POINT** | **DAYS** | **WEEKS** | **CALENDAR MONTHS** | **LUNAR MONTHS** |
| Fertilization | 266 | 38 | 8.75 | 9.5 |
| Last normal menstrual period | 280 | 40 | 9.25 | 10 |

*The common delivery date rule (Nägele's rule) for estimating the expected date of delivery is to count back 3 months from the first day of the last normal menstrual period and add a year and 7 days.

## HIGHLIGHTS OF FETAL PERIOD

There is no formal staging system for the fetal period; however, it is helpful to describe the changes that occur in periods of 4 to 5 weeks.

### Nine to Twelve Weeks

At the beginning of the fetal period (ninth week), the head constitutes approximately half of the CRL of the fetus (Figs. 6-1 and 6-2A). Subsequently, growth in body length accelerates rapidly, so that by the end of 12 weeks, the CRL has almost doubled (Fig. 6-2B and see Table 6-1). Although growth of the head slows down considerably by this time, the head is still disproportionately large compared with the rest of the body (Fig. 6-3).

At 9 weeks, the face is broad, the eyes are widely separated, the ears are low set, and the eyelids are fused (see Fig. 6-2B). By the end of 12 weeks, **primary ossification centers** appear in the skeleton, especially in the cranium (skull) and long bones. Early in the ninth week, the legs are short and the thighs are relatively small (see Fig. 6-2). By the end of 12 weeks, the upper limbs have almost reached their final relative lengths but the lower limbs are still not so well developed, and they are slightly shorter than their final relative lengths.

The **external genitalia** of males and females appear similar until the end of the ninth week. Their mature form is not established until the 12th week. Intestinal coils are clearly visible in the proximal end of the umbilical cord until the middle of the 10th week (see Fig. 6-2B). By the

11th week, the intestines have returned to the abdomen (see Fig. 6-3).

At 9 weeks, the beginning of the fetal period, the liver is the major site of **erythropoiesis** (formation of red blood cells). By the end of 12 weeks, this activity has decreased in the liver and has begun in the spleen. **Urine formation** begins between the 9th and 12th weeks, and urine is discharged through the urethra into the amniotic fluid in the amnionic cavity. The fetus reabsorbs (absorbs again)

**FIGURE 6–1** Ultrasound image of 9-week fetus (11 weeks' gestational age). Note the amnion, amniotic cavity (AC), and chorionic cavity (CC). Crown–rump length, 4.2 cm (calipers).

**FIGURE 6–2** A 9-week fetus in the amniotic sac exposed by removal from the chorionic sac. **A**, Actual size. The remnant of the umbilical vesicle is indicated by an arrow. **B**, Enlarged photograph of the fetus (×2). Note the following features: large head, fused eyelids, cartilaginous ribs, and intestines in umbilical cord (arrow).

**FIGURE 6–3** An 11-week fetus (×1.5). Note its relatively large head and that the intestines are no longer in the umbilical cord.

some amniotic fluid after swallowing it. Fetal waste products are transferred to the maternal circulation by passage across the **placental membrane** (see Chapter 7, Fig. 7-7).

## Thirteen to Sixteen Weeks

Growth is very rapid during this period (Figs. 6-4 and 6-5, and see Table 6-1). By 16 weeks, the head is relatively smaller than the head of a 12-week fetus and the lower limbs have lengthened (Fig. 6-6A). **Limb movements**, which first occur at the end of the embryonic period, become coordinated by the 14th week, but they are too slight to be felt by the mother. However, these movements are visible during ultrasonographic examinations.

**Ossification of the fetal skeleton** is active during this period, and the developing bones are clearly visible on ultrasound images by the beginning of the 16th week. **Slow eye movements** occur at 14 weeks. Scalp hair patterning is also determined during this period. By 16 weeks, the ovaries are differentiated and contain **primordial ovarian follicles**, which contain **oogonia**, or primordial germ cells (see Chapter 12, Fig. 12-31).

*The genitalia of male and female fetuses can be recognized by 12 to 14 weeks.* By 16 weeks, the eyes face anteriorly rather than anterolaterally. In addition, the external ears are close to their definitive positions on the sides of the head.

## Seventeen to Twenty Weeks

Growth slows down during this period, but the fetus still increases its CRL by approximately 50 mm (see Fig. 6-4, Fig. 6-6, and Table 6-1). Fetal movements (**quickening**)

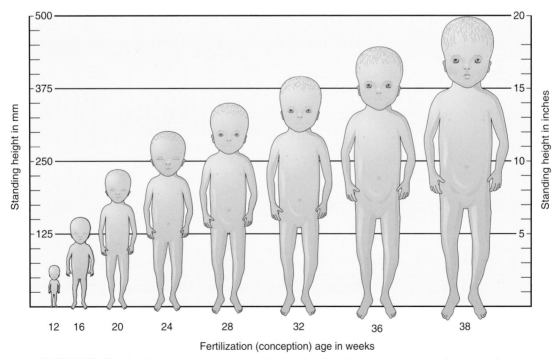

**FIGURE 6–4** Diagram, drawn to scale, illustrating the changes in the size of a human fetus.

**FIGURE 6–5** Enlarged photograph of the head and superior part of the trunk of a 13-week fetus.

**FIGURE 6–6** A, A 17-week fetus. Because there is little subcutaneous tissue and the skin is thin, the blood vessels of the scalp are visible. Fetuses at this age are unable to survive if born prematurely, mainly because their respiratory systems are immature. B, A frontal view of a 17-week fetus. Note that the eyes are closed at this stage. (A, From Moore KL, Persaud TVN, Shiota K: Color atlas of clinical embryology, ed 2, Philadelphia, 2000, Saunders.)

are commonly felt by the mother. The skin is now covered with a greasy, cheese-like material, the **vernix caseosa**. It consists of a mixture of dead epidermal cells and a fatty substance from the fetal sebaceous glands. *The vernix protects the delicate fetal skin from abrasions, chapping, and hardening that result from exposure to the amniotic fluid.* Fetuses are covered with fine, downy hair, **lanugo**, which helps the vernix to adhere to the skin.

Eyebrows and head hair are visible at 20 weeks. **Brown fat** forms during this period and is the site of heat production. This specialized fat, **adipose tissue**, is connective tissue that consists chiefly of fat cells; it is found mostly at the root of the neck, posterior to the sternum, and in the perirenal area. The brown fat produces heat by oxidizing fatty acids.

By 18 weeks, the fetal uterus is formed and canalization of the vagina has begun. Many primordial ovarian follicles containing oogonia are also visible. By 20 weeks, the testes have begun to descend, but they are still located on the posterior abdominal wall, as are the ovaries.

## Twenty-One to Twenty-Five Weeks

Substantial weight gain occurs during this period, and the fetus is better proportioned (Fig. 6-7). The skin is usually wrinkled and more translucent, particularly during the early part of this period. The skin is pink to red because blood in the capillaries is visible. At 21 weeks, rapid eye movements begin, and **blink–startle responses** have been reported at 22 to 23 weeks. The secretory epithelial cells (type II pneumocytes) in the interalveolar walls of the

lung have begun to secrete **surfactant**, a surface-active lipid that maintains the patency of the developing alveoli of the lungs (see Chapter 10).

Fingernails are present by 24 weeks. Although a 22- to 25-week fetus born prematurely may survive if given intensive care (see Fig. 6-7), there is also a chance that it may die because its respiratory system is still immature. The risk for **neurodevelopmental disability** (e.g., mental deficiency) is high in fetuses born before 26 weeks.

## Twenty-Six to Twenty-Nine Weeks

During this period, fetuses usually survive if they are born prematurely and given intensive care (Fig. 6-8B and C). The **lungs and pulmonary vasculature** have developed sufficiently to provide adequate gas exchange. In addition, the central nervous system has matured to the stage where it can direct rhythmic **breathing movements** and control body temperature. The highest rate of neonatal mortality occurs in infants classified as low birth weight (≤2500 g) and very low birth weight (≤1500 g).

**FIGURE 6-7** A 25-week-old normal female neonate weighing 725 g.

The **eyelids** *are open* at 26 weeks, and **lanugo** *(fine downy hair)* and head hair are well developed. Toenails are visible, and considerable subcutaneous fat is under the skin, smoothing out many of the wrinkles. During this period, the quantity of white fat increases to approximately 3.5% of the body weight. The fetal spleen has been an important site of **erythropoiesis** (formation of red blood cells). This ends at 28 weeks, by which time bone marrow has become the major site of erythropoiesis.

## Thirty to Thirty-Four Weeks

The **pupillary reflex** *(change in diameter of the pupil in response to a stimulus caused by light)* can be elicited at 30 weeks. Usually by the end of this period, the skin is pink and smooth and the upper and lower limbs have a chubby appearance. At this age, the quantity of white fat is approximately 8% of the body weight. Fetuses 32 weeks and older usually survive if born prematurely.

## Thirty-Five to Thirty-Eight Weeks

Fetuses born at 35 weeks have a firm grasp and exhibit a spontaneous orientation to light. As term approaches, *the nervous system is sufficiently mature to carry out some integrative functions.* Most fetuses during this "finishing period" are plump (Fig. 6-9B). By 36 weeks, the circumferences of the head and abdomen are approximately equal. After this, the circumference of the abdomen

**FIGURE 6-8** Magnetic resonance images of normal fetuses. **A,** At 18 weeks. **B,** At 26 weeks. **C,** At 28 weeks.

**FIGURE 6-9** Healthy neonates. **A,** At 34 weeks. **B,** At 38 weeks.

**FIGURE 6–10** Ultrasound scan of the foot of a fetus at 19 weeks.

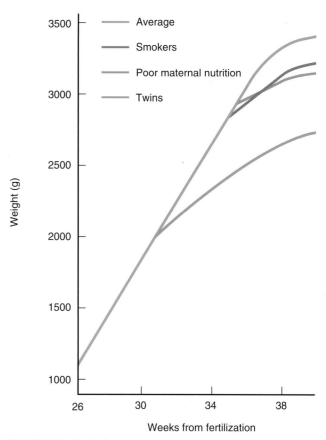

**FIGURE 6–11** Graph showing the rate of fetal growth during the last trimester (3 months). Average refers to neonates in the United States. After 36 weeks, the growth rate deviates from the straight line. The decline, particularly after full term (38 weeks) has been reached, probably reflects inadequate fetal nutrition caused by placental changes. *(Modified from Gruenwald P: Growth of the human fetus. I. Normal growth and its variation, Am J Obstet Gynecol 94:1112, 1966.)*

may be greater than that of the head. The **foot length of fetuses** is usually slightly larger than the femoral length (long bone of the thigh) at 37 weeks, and is an alternative parameter for confirmation of fetal age (Fig. 6-10). There is a slowing of growth as the time of birth approaches (Fig. 6-11).

At full term (38 weeks), most fetuses usually reach a CRL of 360 mm and weigh approximately 3400 g. The amount of white fat is approximately 16% of the body weight. A fetus adds approximately 14 g of fat per day during these last weeks. The thorax (chest) is prominent and the breasts often protrude slightly in both sexes. The testes are usually in the scrotum in full-term male neonates; premature male neonates commonly have undescended testes. Although the head is smaller at full term in relation to the rest of the body than it was earlier in fetal life, it still is one of the largest regions of the fetus. In general, male fetuses are longer and weigh more at birth than females.

## LOW BIRTH WEIGHT

Not all low-birth-weight babies are premature. Approximately one third of those with a birth weight of 2500 g or less are actually small for gestational age. These "small for dates" infants may be underweight because of **placental insufficiency** (see Chapter 7). The placentas are often small or poorly attached and/or have undergone degenerative changes that progressively reduce the oxygen supply and nourishment to the fetus.

It is important to distinguish between **full-term neonates** who have a low birth weight because of IUGR and **preterm neonates** who are underweight because of a shortened gestation (i.e., premature by date). IUGR may be caused by **preeclampsia** (hypertension), smoking or some illicit drugs, multiple gestations (e.g., triplets), infectious diseases, cardiovascular defects, inadequate maternal nutrition, and maternal and fetal hormones. **Teratogens** and genetic factors are also known to cause IUGR (see Chapter 20). Infants with IUGR show a characteristic lack of subcutaneous fat, and their skin is wrinkled, suggesting that white fat has actually been lost.

## EXPECTED DATE OF DELIVERY

The expected date of delivery of a fetus is 266 days or 38 weeks after fertilization, that is, 280 days or 40 weeks after the LNMP (see Table 6-2). Approximately 12% of fetuses are born 1 to 2 weeks after the expected time of birth.

### POSTMATURITY SYNDROME

*Prolongation of pregnancy* for 3 or several weeks beyond the expected date of delivery occurs in 5% to 6% of women. Some infants in such pregnancies develop the **postmaturity syndrome**, which may be associated with *fetal dysmaturity*: absence of subcutaneous fat, wrinkling of the skin, or **meconium** (greenish-colored feces) **staining of the skin**, and, often, excessive weight. Fetuses with this syndrome have an increased risk of mortality. Labor is usually induced when the fetus is postmature.

## FACTORS INFLUENCING FETAL GROWTH

> *By accepting the shelter of the uterus, the fetus also takes the risk of maternal disease or malnutrition and of biochemical, immunological and hormonal adjustment.*
>
> –George W. Corner, renowned American embryologist, 1888 to 1981

Fetuses require substrates (nutrients) for growth and production of energy. Gases and nutrients pass freely to the fetus from the mother through the **placental membrane** (see Chapter 7, Fig. 7-7). **Glucose** is a primary source of energy for fetal metabolism and growth; **amino acids** are also required. These substances pass from the mother's blood to the fetus through the placental membrane. **Insulin** required for the metabolism of glucose is secreted by the fetal pancreas; no significant quantities of maternal insulin reach the fetus because the placental membrane is relatively impermeable to this hormone. Insulin, insulin-like growth factors, human growth hormone, and some small polypeptides (such as somatomedin C) are believed to stimulate fetal growth.

Many factors may affect prenatal growth; they may be maternal, fetal, or environmental factors. Some factors operating throughout pregnancy, such as maternal vascular disease, intrauterine infection, cigarette smoking, and consumption of alcohol, tend to produce *infants with IUGR or small-for-gestational-age (SGA) infants*, whereas factors operating during the last trimester, such as maternal malnutrition, usually produce underweight infants with normal length and head size. The terms "IUGR" and "SGA" are related, but they are not synonymous.

IUGR refers to a process that causes a reduction in the expected pattern of fetal growth as well as fetal growth potential. Constitutionally small-for-gestational-age infants have a birth weight that is lower than a predetermined cutoff value for a particular gestational age (<2 standard deviations below the mean or less than the third percentile). **Severe maternal malnutrition** resulting from a poor-quality diet is known to cause restricted fetal growth (see Fig. 6-11).

Low birth weight has been shown to be a risk factor for many adult conditions, including hypertension, diabetes, and cardiovascular disease. High birth weight due to maternal gestational diabetes is associated with later obesity and diabetes in the offspring.

### Cigarette Smoking

Smoking is a well-established cause of IUGR. The growth rate for fetuses of mothers who smoke cigarettes is less than normal during the last 6 to 8 weeks of pregnancy (see Fig. 6-11). On average, the birth weight of infants whose mothers smoke heavily during pregnancy is 200 g less than normal, and the rate of **perinatal morbidity** is increased when adequate medical care is unavailable. The effect of maternal smoking is greater on fetuses whose mothers also receive inadequate nutrition. Cigarette smoking has also been implicated as a major cause of cleft lip and palate.

### Multiple Pregnancy

Individuals of multiple births usually weigh considerably less than infants resulting from a single pregnancy (see Fig. 6-11). It is evident that the total metabolic requirements of two or more fetuses exceed the nutritional supply available from the placenta during the third trimester.

### Alcohol and Illicit Drugs

Infants born to mothers that drink alcohol often exhibit IUGR as part of the **fetal alcohol syndrome** (see Chapter 20, Fig. 20-17). Similarly, the use of marijuana and other illicit drugs (e.g., cocaine) can cause IUGR and other obstetric complications.

### Impaired Uteroplacental and Fetoplacental Blood Flow

The maternal placental circulation may be reduced by conditions that decrease uterine blood flow (e.g., small chorionic vessels, severe maternal hypotension, and renal disease). Chronic reduction of uterine blood flow can cause fetal starvation resulting in IUGR. Placental dysfunction (e.g., infarction; see Chapter 7) can also cause IUGR.

The net effect of these placental abnormalities is a reduction of the total area for exchange of nutrients between the fetal and maternal bloodstreams. It is very difficult to separate the effect of these placental changes from the effect of reduced maternal blood flow to the placenta. In some instances of chronic maternal disease, the maternal vascular changes in the uterus are primary and placental defects are secondary.

## Genetic Factors and Growth Retardation

It is well established that genetic factors can cause IUGR. Repeated cases of this condition in one family indicate that recessive genes may be the cause of the abnormal growth. Structural and numeric chromosomal aberrations have also been shown to be associated with cases of retarded fetal growth. IUGR is pronounced in infants with Down syndrome and is very characteristic of fetuses with trisomy 18 syndrome (see Chapter 20).

## PROCEDURES FOR ASSESSING FETAL STATUS

**Perinatology** is the branch of medicine that is concerned with the well-being of the fetus and neonate, generally covering the period from approximately 26 weeks after fertilization to 4 weeks after birth. This subspecialty of medicine combines aspects of obstetrics and pediatrics.

### Ultrasonography

Ultrasonography is the primary imaging modality in the evaluation of fetuses because of its wide availability, low cost, quality of images, and lack of known adverse effects. The chorionic sac and its contents may be visualized by ultrasonography during the embryonic and fetal periods. Placental and fetal size, multiple births, abnormalities of placental shape, and abnormal presentations can also be determined.

**Ultrasound scans** give accurate measurements of the biparietal diameter of the fetal cranium (skull), from which close estimates of fetal age and length can be made. Figures 6-10 and 6-12 illustrate how details of the fetus can be observed in these scans. Ultrasound examinations are also helpful for diagnosing abnormal pregnancies at a very early stage. Rapid advances in ultrasonography have made this technique a major tool for prenatal diagnosis of fetal abnormalities. Biopsy of fetal tissues, such as the skin, liver, kidney, and muscle, can be performed with ultrasound guidance.

### Diagnostic Amniocentesis

This is a common invasive prenatal diagnostic procedure, usually performed between 15 and 18 weeks' gestation. **Amniotic fluid** is sampled by inserting a 22-gauge needle through the mother's anterior abdominal and uterine walls into the amniotic cavity by piercing the chorion and amnion (Fig. 6-13A). Because there is relatively little amniotic fluid before the 14th week, amniocentesis is difficult to perform before this time. The amniotic fluid volume is approximately 200 ml, and 15 to 20 ml can be safely withdrawn. Amniocentesis is relatively devoid of risk, especially when the procedure is performed by an experienced physician using real-time ultrasonography guidance for outlining the position of the fetus and placenta.

### DIAGNOSTIC VALUE OF AMNIOCENTESIS

Amniocentesis is a common technique for detecting genetic disorders (e.g., Down syndrome). The common indications for amniocentesis are:

- Advanced maternal age (≥38 years)
- Previous birth of a child with trisomy 21 (see Chapter 20, Fig. 20-6B)
- Chromosome abnormality in either parent
- Women who are carriers of X-linked recessive disorders (e.g., *hemophilia*)
- History of neural tube defects in the family (e.g., spina bifida cystica; see Chapter 17, Fig. 17-15)
- Carriers of inborn errors of metabolism

**FIGURE 6–12** A, Three-dimensional ultrasound (sonogram) of a 28-week fetus showing the face. The surface features are clearly recognizable. B, Photograph of the same neonate, 3 hours after birth.

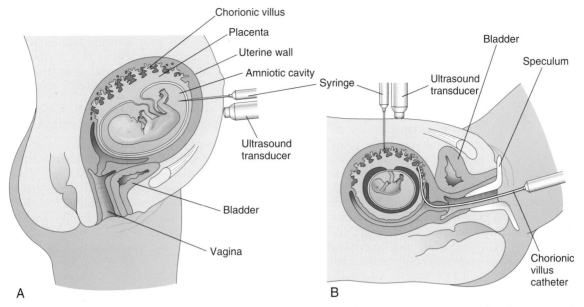

**FIGURE 6–13** A, Illustration of amniocentesis. A needle is inserted through the lower abdominal and uterine walls into the amniotic cavity. A syringe is attached and amniotic fluid is withdrawn for diagnostic purposes. B, Drawing illustrating chorionic villus sampling. Two sampling approaches are illustrated: through the maternal anterior abdominal wall with a needle and through the vagina and cervical canal using a malleable catheter. A speculum is an instrument for exposing the vagina.

## Alpha-Fetoprotein Assay

Alpha-fetoprotein (AFP) is a glycoprotein that is synthesized in the fetal liver, umbilical vesicle, and gut. AFP is found in high concentrations in fetal serum, with levels peaking at 14 weeks after the LNMP. Only small amounts of AFP normally enter the amniotic fluid.

### ALPHA-FETOPROTEIN AND FETAL ANOMALIES

The concentration of AFP is high in the amniotic fluid surrounding fetuses with severe defects of the central nervous system and ventral abdominal wall. The amniotic fluid AFP concentration is measured by immunoassay; when the measurement is known and ultrasonographic scanning is performed, approximately 99% of fetuses with these severe defects can be diagnosed prenatally. When a fetus has an open neural tube defect, the concentration of AFP is also likely to be higher than normal in the maternal serum. The maternal serum AFP concentration is lower than normal when the fetus has Down syndrome (trisomy 21), Edward syndrome (trisomy 18), or other chromosome defects.

## Spectrophotometric Studies

Examination of amniotic fluid by spectrophotometric studies may be used for assessing the degree of **erythroblastosis fetalis**, also called **hemolytic disease of the neonate**. This disease results from destruction of fetal red blood cells by maternal antibodies (see Chapter 7, blue box titled "Hemolytic Disease of the Neonate"). The concentration of bilirubin (and other related pigments) is correlated with the degree of hemolytic disease.

## Chorionic Villus Sampling

Biopsies of trophoblastic tissue (5 to 20 mg) may be obtained by inserting a needle, guided by ultrasonography, through the mother's abdominal and uterine walls (transabdominal insertion) into the uterine cavity (see Fig. 6-13B). Chorionic villus sampling (CVS) can also be performed transcervically by passing a polyethylene catheter through the cervix under guidance by real-time ultrasonography. For assessing the condition of a fetus at risk, the **fetal karyotype** (chromosome characteristics) can be obtained; in this way, using CVS, a diagnosis can be made weeks earlier than would be possible with amniocentesis.

### DIAGNOSTIC VALUE OF CHORIONIC VILLUS SAMPLING

Biopsies of chorionic villi are used for detecting chromosomal abnormalities, inborn errors of metabolism, and X-linked disorders. CVS can be performed at between 10 and 12 weeks of gestation. The rate of fetal loss is approximately 0.5% to 1%, a rate that is slightly higher than the rate with amniocentesis. Reports regarding an increased risk of limb defects after CVS are conflicting. The advantage of CVS over amniocentesis is that it can be carried out sooner, so that the results of chromosomal analysis are available several weeks earlier.

## Cell Cultures and Chromosomal Analysis

The prevalence of chromosomal disorders is approximately 1 in 120 neonates. Fetal sex and chromosomal aberrations can be determined by studying the chromosomes in cultured fetal cells obtained during **amniocentesis**. If conception occurs by means of assisted reproductive technologies, it is possible to obtain fetal cells by performing a biopsy of the maturing blastocyst (Fig. 6-14A and B). These cultures are commonly done when an autosomal abnormality, such as occurs in Down syndrome, is suspected. Knowledge of fetal sex can be useful in diagnosing the presence of severe sex-linked hereditary diseases, such as **hemophilia** (an inherited disorder of blood coagulation) and **muscular dystrophy** (a hereditary progressive degenerative disorder affecting skeletal muscles). Moreover, microdeletions and microduplications, as well as subtelomeric rearrangements, can now

be detected with fluorescence in situ hybridization technology (see Fig. 6-14C and D). **Inborn errors of metabolism in fetuses** can also be detected by studying cell cultures. Enzyme deficiencies can be determined by incubating cells recovered from amniotic fluid and then detecting the specific enzyme deficiency in the cells.

## Noninvasive Prenatal Diagnosis

Down syndrome (trisomy 21) is the most commonly known chromosomal disorder. Children born with this condition have varying degrees of intellectual disabilities. Noninvasive screening for trisomy 21 is based on the isolation of fetal cells in maternal blood and the detection of cell-free DNA and RNA. Such DNA-based diagnostic tests need additional refinement to improve their reliability for the detection of fetal trisomy of chromosomes 13, 18, and 21.

**FIGURE 6–14** A, Microscopic images of human blastocyst with trophectoderm cells (which will form extraembryonic tissues) starting to hatch. B, The trophectoderm cells biopsied with assisted laser cutting. C and D, Fluorescence in situ hybridization images in aneuploidy blastocysts. C, Three dots that have stained green in A indicate the presence of three chromosomes 21 in the sample (46,XX, +21). D, One dot that has stained red in B indicates the presence of only one chromosome 13 in the sample (45,XX, –13.) *(From Liang L, Wang CT, Sun X, et al: Identification of chromosomal errors in human preimplantation embryos with oligonucleotide DNA microarray, PLoS ONE 8:4, 2013.)*

## Fetal Transfusion

Fetuses with **hemolytic disease of the neonate** can be treated by intrauterine blood transfusions. The blood is injected through a needle inserted into the fetal peritoneal cavity. With recent advances in **percutaneous umbilical cord blood sampling**, blood and packed red blood cells can be transfused directly into the umbilical vein for the treatment of fetal anemia due to isoimmunization. The need for fetal blood transfusions is reduced nowadays owing to the treatment of Rh-negative mothers of Rh-positive fetuses with anti-Rh immunoglobulin, which in many cases prevents development of this disease. Fetal transfusion of platelets directly into the umbilical cord vein is carried out for the treatment of alloimmune thrombocytopenia. Also, fetal infusion of drugs in a similar manner for the treatment of a few medical conditions in the fetus has been reported.

## Fetoscopy

Using fiberoptic instruments, external parts of the fetal body may be directly observed. The **fetoscope** is usually introduced through the mother's abdominal and uterine walls into the amniotic cavity. Fetoscopy is usually carried out at 17 to 20 weeks of gestation, but with new approaches, such as **transabdominal thin-gauge embryo fetoscopy**, it is possible to detect certain defects in the embryo or fetus during the first trimester. Because of the higher risk to the fetus compared with other prenatal diagnostic procedures, fetoscopy now has few indications for routine prenatal diagnosis or treatment of the fetus. Fetoscopy combined with laser coagulation is used to treat fetal conditions such as **twin–twin transfusion syndrome**. Fetoscopy has also been used for the release of amniotic bands (see Chapter 7, Fig. 7-21).

## Percutaneous Umbilical Cord Blood Sampling

Fetal blood samples may be obtained directly from the umbilical vein by percutaneous umbilical cord blood sampling, or cordocentesis, for the diagnosis of many fetal abnormal conditions, including aneuploidy, fetal growth restriction, fetal infection, and fetal anemia. Percutaneous umbilical cord blood sampling is usually performed after 18 weeks of gestation under continuous direct ultrasound guidance, which is used to locate the umbilical cord and its vessels. The procedure also permits treating the fetus directly, including transfusion of packed red blood cells for the management of fetal anemia resulting from isoimmunization.

## Magnetic Resonance Imaging

When planning fetal treatment, magnetic resonance imaging (MRI) may be used to provide more information about a defect that has been detected in ultrasonic images. Important advantages of MRI are that it does not use ionizing radiation and it has high soft tissue contrast and resolution (Fig. 6-15).

**FIGURE 6–15** Sagittal magnetic resonance image of the pelvis of a pregnant woman. The fetus is in the breech presentation. Note the brain, eyes, and liver.

## Fetal Monitoring

Continuous fetal heart rate monitoring in high-risk pregnancies is routine and provides information about the oxygenation of the fetus. There are various causes of prenatal fetal distress, such as maternal diseases that reduce oxygen transport to the fetus (e.g., cyanotic heart disease). **Fetal distress** (e.g., indicated by an abnormal heart rate or rhythm) suggests that the fetus is in jeopardy. A noninvasive method of monitoring uses transducers placed on the mother's abdomen.

## SUMMARY OF FETAL PERIOD

- The fetal period begins 8 weeks after fertilization (10 weeks after the LNMP) and ends at birth. It is characterized by *rapid body growth and differentiation of tissues and organ systems*. An obvious change in the fetal period is the relative slowing of head growth compared with that of the rest of the body.
- At the beginning of the *20th week*, **lanugo** (fine downy hair) and head hair appear and the skin is coated with **vernix caseosa (a fatty cheesy substance)**. The eyelids are closed during most of the fetal period, but they begin to reopen at approximately *26 weeks*. At this time, the fetus is usually capable of **extrauterine existence**, mainly because of the maturity of its respiratory system.
- Up to *30 weeks*, the fetus appears reddish and wizened (wrinkled) because of the thinness of its skin and the

**FIGURE 6–16** Fetus at 21 weeks undergoing bilateral ureterostomies, the establishment of openings of the ureters into the bladder. *(From Harrison MR, Globus MS, Filly RA, editors: The unborn patient: prenatal diagnosis and treatment,* ed 2, *Philadelphia, 1994, Saunders.)*

relative absence of subcutaneous fat. Fat usually develops rapidly at 26 to 29 weeks, giving the fetus a *smooth, healthy appearance* (see Fig. 6-9).

- The fetus is less vulnerable to the teratogenic effects of drugs, viruses, and radiation, but these agents may interfere with growth and normal functional development, especially of the brain and eyes.
- The physician can determine whether a fetus has a particular disease or birth defect by using various diagnostic techniques, such as amniocentesis, CVS, ultrasonography, and MRI.
- In selected cases, treatments can be given to the fetus, such as drugs to correct **cardiac arrhythmia** or thyroid disorders. Surgical correction of some birth defects in utero (Fig. 6-16) is also possible (e.g., ureters that do not open into the bladder can be surgically corrected).

## CLINICALLY ORIENTED PROBLEMS

### CASE 6–1

*A woman in the 20th week of a high-risk pregnancy was scheduled for a repeat cesarean section. Her physician wanted to establish an expected date of delivery.*

- ✳ How would an expected date of delivery be established?
- ✳ When would labor likely be induced?
- ✳ How could this be accomplished?

### CASE 6–2

*A 44-year-old pregnant woman was worried that her fetus may have major birth defects.*

- ✳ How could the status of her fetus be determined?
- ✳ What chromosomal abnormality would be most likely?
- ✳ What other chromosomal aberrations might be detected?

### CASE 6–3

*A 19-year-old woman in the second trimester of pregnancy asked a physician whether her fetus was vulnerable to over-the-counter drugs and street drugs. She also wondered about the effect of her heavy drinking and cigarette smoking on her fetus.*

- ✳ What would the physician likely tell her?

### CASE 6–4

*An ultrasound examination of a pregnant woman revealed that her fetus had IUGR.*

- ✳ What factors may cause IUGR? Discuss how these factors might influence fetal growth.
- ✳ Which factors can the mother eliminate? Would removing these factors result in reversal of IUGR?

### CASE 6–5

*A woman in the first trimester of pregnancy who was to undergo amniocentesis expressed concerns about a miscarriage and the possibility of injury to her fetus.*

- ✳ What are the risks of these complications?
- ✳ What procedures are used to minimize these risks?
- ✳ What other technique might be used for obtaining cells for a chromosomal study?

### CASE 6–6

*A pregnant woman is told that she is going to have an AFP test to determine whether there are any birth defects.*

- ✳ What is AFP and where can it be found?
- ✳ What types of fetal defect can be detected by an AFP assay of maternal serum?
- ✳ What is the significance of high and low levels of AFP?

Discussion of these problems appears in the Appendix at the back of the book.

## BIBLIOGRAPHY AND SUGGESTED READING

Anderson MS, Hay WW: Intrauterine growth restriction and the small-for-gestational-age infant. In MacDonald MG, Seshia MMK, Mullett MD, editors: *Avery's neonatology: pathophysiology and management of the newborn*, ed 6, Philadelphia, 2005, Lippincott Williams and Wilkins.

Bloomfield H, Spiroski AM, Harding HE: Fetal growth factors and nutrition, *Semin Fetal Neonatal Med* 18:118, 2013.

Chiu RW, Lo YM: Non-invasive prenatal diagnosis by fetal nucleic acid analysis in maternal plasma: the coming of age, *Semin Fetal Neonatal Med* 16:88, 2011.

Deprest JA, Devlieger R, Srisupundit K, et al: Fetal surgery is a clinical reality, *Semin Fetal Neonatal Med* 15:58, 2010.

Durkin EF, Shaaban A: Commonly encountered surgical problems in the fetus and neonate, *Pediatr Clin North Am* 56:647, 2009.

Filly RA, Feldstein VA: Ultrasound evaluation of normal fetal anatomy. In Callen PW, editor: *Ultrasonography in obstetrics and gynecology*, ed 5, Philadelphia, 2008, Saunders.

Gowen CW Jr: Fetal and neonatal medicine. In Marcdante KJ, Kliegman KJ, editors: *Nelson essentials of pediatrics*, ed 7, Philadelphia, 2015, Saunders.

Hinrichsen KV, editor: *Humanembryologie*, Berlin, 1990, Springer-Verlag.

Jirásel JE: *An atlas of human prenatal developmental mechanics: anatomy and staging*, London and New York, 2004, Taylor and Francis.

Khambalia AZ, Roberts CL, Nguyen M, et al: Predicting date of birth and examining the best time to date a pregnancy, *Int J Gynaecol Obstet* 123:105, 2013.

Kilby M: Prenatal diagnosis. In Magowan BA, Owen P, Thomson A, editors: *Clinical obstetrics and gynaecology*, ed 3, Philadelphia, 2014, Saunders.

Korf BR, Rehm HL: New approaches to molecular diagnosis, *JAMA* 309:2013, 1511.

Levine DA: Growth and development. In Marcdante KJ, Kliegman KJ, editors: *Nelson essentials of pediatrics*, ed 7, Philadelphia, 2015, Saunders.

Moran S, Greene MF, Mello MM: A new era in noninvasive prenatal testing, *N Engl J Med* 369:2164, 2013.

O'Rahilly R, Müller F: *Development stages in human embryos*, Publication 637, Washington, DC, 1987, Carnegie Institution of Washington.

Owen P: Small babies. In Magowan BA, Owen P, Thomson A, editors: *Clinical obstetrics and gynaecology*, ed 3, Philadelphia, 2014, Saunders.

Persaud TVN, Hay JC: Normal embryonic and fetal development. In Reece EA, Hobbins JC, editors: *Clinical obstetrics: the fetus and mother*, ed 3, Malden, Mass., 2006, Blackwell, pp 19–32.

Pooh RK, Shiota K, Kurjak A: Imaging of the human embryo with magnetic resonance imaging microscopy and high-resolution transvaginal 3-dimensional sonography: human embryology in the 21st century, *Am J Obstet Gynecol* 204:77.e1–77.e16, 2011.

Poon LCY, Musci T, Song K: Maternal plasma cell-free fetal and maternal DNA at 11-13 weeks' gestation: relation to fetal and maternal characteristics and pregnancy outcomes, *Fetal Diagn Ther* 33:215, 2013.

Salihu HM, Miranda S, Hill L, et al: Survival of pre-viable preterm infants in the United States: a systematic review and meta-analysis, *Semin Perinatol* 37:389, 2013.

Simpson JL: Cell-free fetal DNA and maternal serum analytes for monitoring embryonic and fetal status, *Fertil Steril* 99:1124, 2013.

Steding G: *The anatomy of the human embryo: a scanning electron-microscopic atlas*, Basel, 2009, Karger.

Streeter GL: Weight, sitting height, head size, foot length and menstrual age of the human embryo, *Contrib Embryol Carnegie Inst* 11:143, 1920.

Whitworth M, Bricker L, Neilson JP, et al: Ultrasound for fetal assessment in early pregnancy, *Cochrane Database Syst Rev* (4):CD007058, 2010.

Zhang J, Merialdi M, Platt LD, et al: Defining normal and abnormal fetal growth: promises and challenges, *Am J Obstet Gynecol* 202:522, 2010.

# Placenta and Fetal Membranes

The placenta and fetal membranes separate the fetus from the **endometrium**, the inner layer of the uterine wall. An interchange of substances, such as nutrients and oxygen, occurs between the maternal and fetal bloodstreams through the placenta. The vessels in the umbilical cord connect the placental circulation with the fetal circulation. The **fetal membranes** include the **chorion, amnion, umbilical vesicle,** and **allantois.**

## PLACENTA

The placenta is the primary site of nutrient and gas exchange between the mother and embryo/fetus. The placenta is a **fetomaternal organ** that has two components (Fig. 7-1):

- A **fetal part** that develops from the chorionic sac, the outermost fetal membrane
- A **maternal part** that is derived from the endometrium, the mucous membrane comprising the inner layer of the uterine wall

**FIGURE 7-1** Development of the placenta and fetal membranes. **A,** Frontal section of the uterus showing elevation of the decidua capsularis by the expanding chorionic sac of a 4-week-old embryo implanted in the endometrium on the posterior wall *(asterisk).* **B,** Enlarged drawing of the implantation site. The chorionic villi were exposed by cutting an opening in the decidua capsularis. **C** to **F,** Sagittal sections of the gravid (pregnant) uterus from weeks 5 to 22 showing the changing relations of the fetal membranes to the decidua. In **F,** the amnion and chorion are fused with each other and the decidua parietalis, thereby obliterating the uterine cavity. Note in **D** to **F** that the chorionic villi persist only where the chorion is associated with the decidua basalis.

*The placenta and umbilical cord form a transport system for substances passing between the mother and embryo/fetus.* Nutrients and oxygen pass from the maternal blood through the placenta to the embryo/fetal blood, and waste materials and carbon dioxide pass from the fetal blood through the placenta to the maternal blood. *The placenta and fetal membranes* perform the following functions and activities: protection, nutrition, respiration, excretion of waste products, and hormone production. Shortly after birth, the placenta and membranes are expelled from the uterus as the **afterbirth.**

## Decidua

The **decidua** is the endometrium of the uterus in a pregnant woman. It is the functional layer of the endometrium that separates from the remainder of the uterus after **parturition** (childbirth). The **three regions of the decidua** are named according to their relation to the implantation site (see Fig. 7-1):

- The **decidua basalis** is the part of the decidua deep to the **conceptus** (embryo/fetus and membranes), which forms the *maternal part of the placenta.*
- The **decidua capsularis** is the superficial part of the decidua overlying the conceptus.
- The **decidua parietalis** represents the remaining parts of the decidua.

In response to increasing progesterone levels in maternal blood, the connective tissue cells of the decidua enlarge to form pale-staining **decidual cells.** These cells enlarge as glycogen and lipid accumulate in their **cytoplasm.**

The cellular and vascular changes occurring in the endometrium as the blastocyst implants constitute the **decidual reaction.** Many decidual cells degenerate near the **chorionic sac** in the region of the **syncytiotrophoblast** (syncytial outer layer of trophoblast), and, together with maternal blood and uterine secretions, they provide a rich source of nutrition for the embryo/fetus. It has also been suggested that these cells protect the maternal tissue against uncontrolled invasion by syncytiotrophoblast, and they may be involved in hormone production. *Decidual regions, clearly recognizable during ultrasonography, are important in diagnosing early pregnancy* (see Chapter 3, Fig. 3-7).

## Development of Placenta

Early development is characterized by rapid proliferation of trophoblast and development of the chorionic sac and chorionic villi (see Chapters 3 and 4). *Homeobox genes (HLX and DLX3) expressed in the trophoblast and its blood vessels regulate placental development.* By the end of the third week, the anatomical arrangements necessary for physiologic exchanges between the mother and embryo/fetus are established. A complex **vascular network** is established in the placenta by the end of the fourth week, which facilitates maternal–embryonic exchanges of gases, nutrients, and metabolic waste products.

**Chorionic villi** cover the entire chorionic sac until the beginning of the eighth week (Figs. 7-2 and 7-3, and see

Fig. 7-1C). As the chorionic sac grows, the villi associated with the decidua capsularis become compressed, so that the blood supply to them is reduced; hence, they soon degenerate (see Figs. 7-1D and 7-3B). This produces a relatively avascular bare area, the **smooth chorion** (chorion laeve). As the villi disappear, those associated with the decidua basalis rapidly increase, branch profusely, and enlarge. This forms the bushy area of the chorionic sac, the **villous chorion** (chorion frondosum).

---

### ULTRASONOGRAPHY OF CHORIONIC SAC

The size of the chorionic sac is useful in determining the gestational age of the embryo/fetus in patients with uncertain menstrual histories. Growth of the chorionic sac is extremely rapid between weeks 5 and 10. Modern ultrasound machines, especially instruments equipped with endovaginal transducers, enable ultrasonographers to view the chorionic sac when it has a median sac diameter of 2 to 3 mm (see Chapter 3, Fig. 3-7). Chorionic sacs with this diameter indicate that the gestational age is 31 to 32 days, which is approximately 18 days after fertilization.

---

The uterus, chorionic sac, and placenta enlarge as the embryo/fetus grows. Growth in the size and thickness of the placenta continues rapidly until the fetus is approximately 18 weeks old. The fully developed placenta covers 15% to 30% of the decidua of the endometrium of the uterus and weighs approximately one sixth as much as the fetus.

The placenta has two parts (Fig. 7-4, and see Fig. 7-1E and F):

- The **fetal part** is formed by the **villous chorion.** The chorionic villi that arise from the chorion project into the **intervillous space** containing maternal blood (see Fig. 7-1D).
- The **maternal part** is formed by the **decidua basalis,** the part of the decidua related to the fetal component of the placenta (see Fig. 7-1C to F). By the end of the fourth month, the decidua basalis is almost entirely replaced by the fetal part of the placenta.

The fetal part is attached to the maternal part of the placenta by the **cytotrophoblastic shell,** the external layer of trophoblastic cells on the maternal surface of the placenta (Fig. 7-5). The chorionic villi attach firmly to the decidua basalis through the cytotrophoblastic shell, which anchors the chorionic sac to the decidua basalis. **Endometrial arteries and veins** pass freely through gaps in the cytotrophoblastic shell and enter the intervillous space.

The shape of the placenta is determined by the persistent area of chorionic villi (see Fig. 7-1F). Usually this is a circular area, giving the placenta a **discoid shape** (shaped like a disc). As the chorionic villi invade the decidua

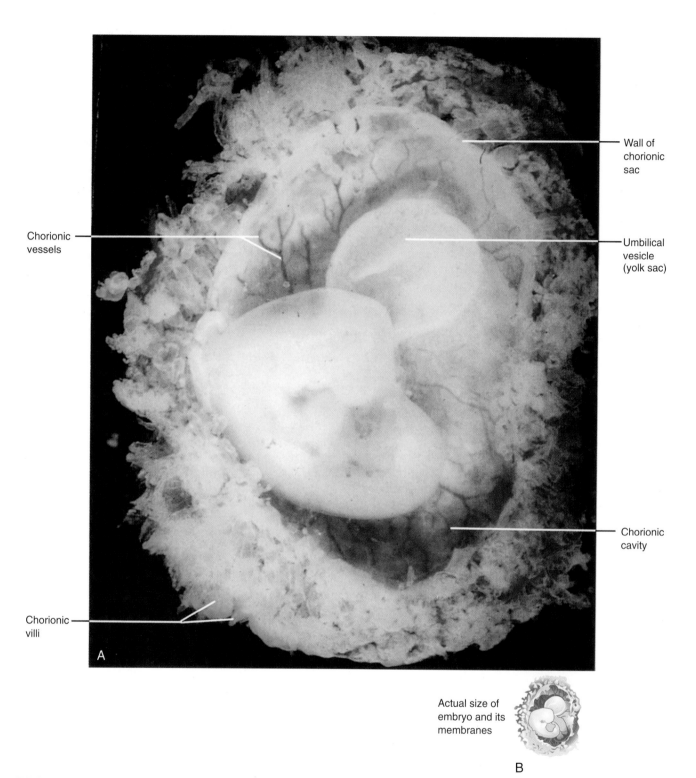

Chorionic vessels

Chorionic villi

Wall of chorionic sac

Umbilical vesicle (yolk sac)

Chorionic cavity

A

Actual size of embryo and its membranes

B

**FIGURE 7–2** A, Lateral view of a spontaneously aborted embryo at Carnegie stage 14, approximately 32 days. The chorionic and amniotic sacs have been opened to show the embryo. Note the large size of the umbilical vesicle. B, The sketch shows the actual size of the embryo and its membranes. (*A, From Moore KL, Persaud TVN, Shiota K: Color atlas of clinical embryology, ed 2, Philadelphia, 2000, Saunders.*)

Smooth chorion    Villous chorion

**FIGURE 7–3** Spontaneously aborted human chorionic sacs. **A,** At 21 days. The sac is covered with chorionic villi (×4). **B,** At 8 weeks. Some of the chorionic villi have degenerated, causing the smooth chorion to form. *(From Potter EL, Craig JM: Pathology of the fetus and the infant, ed 3. Copyright 1975 by Year Book Medical Publishers, Chicago.)*

basalis, decidual tissue is eroded to enlarge the **intervillous space** (see Fig. 7-4). This erosion produces several wedge-shaped areas of decidua, the **placental septa**, which project toward the **chorionic plate**, the part of the chorionic wall related to the placenta (Fig. 7-5). The septa divide the fetal part of the placenta into irregular convex areas, or **cotyledons**. Each cotyledon consists of two or more **stem villi** and many **branch villi** (Fig. 7-6A, and see Fig. 7-5). By the end of the fourth month, the decidua basalis is almost entirely replaced by cotyledons (see Fig. 7-11). *Expression of kinase genes (*MAP2K1 *and* MAP2K2*) and the transcription factor Gcm1 (glial cells missing-1) in trophoblast stem cells regulate the branching process of the stem villi to form the vascular network in the placenta.*

The **decidua capsularis**, the layer of decidua overlying the **chorionic sac**, forms a capsule over the external surface of the sac (see Fig. 7-1A to D). As the conceptus (embryo and membranes) enlarges, the decidua capsularis bulges into the uterine cavity and becomes greatly attenuated. Eventually the decidua capsularis contacts and fuses with the decidua parietalis on the opposite wall, thereby slowly obliterating the uterine cavity (see Fig. 7-1E and F). By 22 to 24 weeks, the reduced blood supply to the decidua capsularis causes it to degenerate and disappear.

After the disappearance of the decidua capsularis, the smooth part of the **chorionic sac** (smooth chorion) fuses with the decidua parietalis (see Fig. 7-1F). This fusion can be separated and usually occurs when blood escapes from the intervillous space (see Fig. 7-4). The collection of blood (**hematoma**) pushes the chorionic membrane away from the decidua parietalis, thereby reestablishing the potential space of the uterine cavity.

The **intervillous space of the placenta**, which by 8 to 10 weeks contains maternal blood, is derived from the **lacunae** (small spaces) that developed in the syncytiotrophoblast during the second week of development (see Chapter 3, Fig. 3-2A and B). This large blood-filled space results from the coalescence and enlargement of the **lacunar networks**. The intervillous space is divided into compartments by placental septa; however, there is free communication between the compartments because the septa do not reach the **chorionic plate** (see Fig. 7-5).

Maternal blood enters the intervillous space from the **spiral endometrial arteries** in the decidua basalis (see Figs. 7-4 and 7-5). The spiral arteries (corkscrew-like vessels) pass through gaps in the cytotrophoblastic shell and discharge blood into the intervillous space. This large space is drained by **endometrial veins**, which also penetrate the cytotrophoblastic shell. These veins are found over the entire surface of the decidua basalis.

The **numerous branch villi**, arising from **stem villi**, are continuously showered with maternal blood that circulates through the **intervillous space** (see Figs. 7-4 and 7-5). The blood in this space carries oxygen and nutritional materials that are necessary for fetal growth and development. The maternal blood also contains fetal waste, carbon dioxide, salts, and products of protein metabolism.

The amniotic sac enlarges faster than the chorionic sac. As a result, the amnion and smooth chorion fuse to form the **amniochorionic membrane** (see Figs. 7-4 and 7-5). This composite membrane fuses with the decidua capsularis and, after disappearance of the latter, adheres to the decidua parietalis (see Figs. 7-1F, 7-4, and 7-5). It is the amniochorionic membrane that ruptures during labor. *Preterm membrane rupture (i.e., at less than 37 weeks' gestation) is the most common event leading to premature labor.* Membrane rupture allows amniotic fluid to escape through the vagina.

## Placental Circulation

The branch chorionic villi of the placenta provide a large surface area where materials may be exchanged across the very thin **placental membrane** interposed between the fetal and maternal circulations (see Figs. 7-5 to 7-6). It is through the branch villi, which arise from stem villi, that the main exchange of material between the mother and fetus takes place. Fetal and maternal circulations

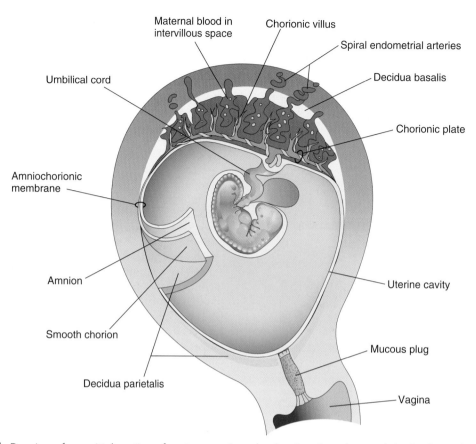

**FIGURE 7–4** Drawing of a sagittal section of a uterus at 4 weeks showing the relation of the fetal membranes to each other and the decidua and embryo. The amnion and smooth chorion have been cut and reflected to show their relationship to each other and the decidua parietalis.

are separated by the placental membrane consisting of extrafetal tissues (Fig. 7-7, and see Fig. 7-6B and C).

## Fetal Placental Circulation

Poorly oxygenated blood passes through the **umbilical arteries** to the placenta. At the site of attachment of the umbilical cord to the placenta, the arteries divide into several radially disposed **chorionic arteries** that branch freely in the **chorionic plate** before entering the chorionic villi (see Figs. 7-5 and 7-6). The blood vessels form an extensive **arteriocapillary–venous system** within the chorionic villi (see Fig. 7-6A), which brings the fetal blood extremely close to the maternal blood (see Fig. 7-7). This system provides a large surface area for the exchange of metabolic and gaseous products between the maternal and fetal bloodstreams.

*Normally, there is no intermingling of fetal and maternal blood;* however, very small amounts of fetal blood may enter the maternal circulation when minute defects develop in the placental membrane (see Fig. 7-6B and C). The **well-oxygenated fetal blood** in the fetal capillaries passes into thin-walled veins that follow the chorionic arteries to the site of attachment of the umbilical cord. They converge here to form the **umbilical vein** (see Figs. 7-5 and 7-7). This large vessel carries oxygen-rich blood to the fetus.

## Maternal Placental Circulation

The maternal blood in the intervillous space is temporarily outside the maternal circulatory system. It enters the intervillous space through 80 to 100 spiral endometrial arteries in the decidua basalis. These arteries discharge into the intervillous space through gaps in the cytotrophoblastic shell (see Fig. 7-5). The blood flow from the spiral arteries is pulsatile.

The entering blood is at a considerably higher pressure than that in the intervillous space, and therefore blood spurts toward the **chorionic plate**, which forms the "roof" of the intervillous space. As pressure dissipates, the blood flows slowly over the branch villi, allowing an exchange of metabolic and gaseous products with the fetal blood. The blood eventually returns through the **endometrial veins** to the maternal circulation.

*The welfare of the embryo/fetus depends more on the adequate bathing of the branch villi with maternal blood than any other factor.* Reductions of uteroplacental circulation result in **fetal hypoxia** and **intrauterine growth restriction (IUGR)**. Severe reductions of circulation may result in embryo/fetal death. The intervillous space of the mature placenta contains approximately 150 ml of blood, which is replenished three or four times per minute.

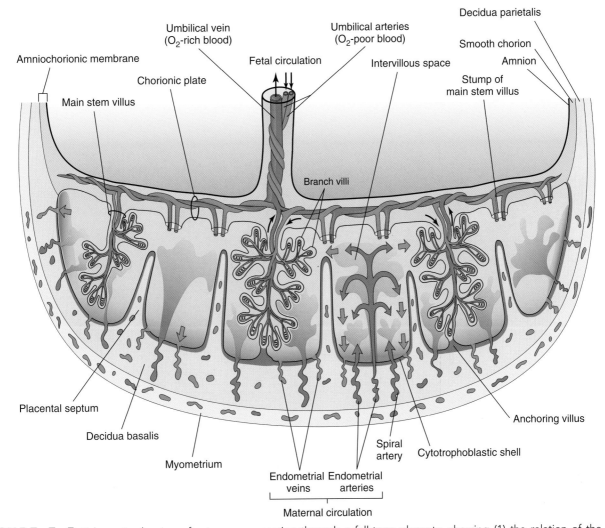

**FIGURE 7–5** Schematic drawing of a transverse section through a full-term placenta, showing (1) the relation of the villous chorion (fetal part of placenta) to the decidua basalis (maternal part of placenta), (2) the fetal placental circulation, and (3) the maternal placental circulation. Maternal blood flows into the intervillous spaces in spurts from the spiral arteries. Note that the umbilical arteries carry poorly oxygenated fetal blood (shown in *blue*) to the placenta and that the umbilical vein carries oxygenated blood (shown in *red*) to the fetus. Note that the cotyledons are separated from each other by placental septa, projections of the decidua basalis. Each cotyledon consists of two or more main stem villi and many branch villi. In this drawing, only one stem villus is shown in each cotyledon, but the stumps of those that have been removed are indicated.

## Placental Membrane

The **placental membrane** is a composite structure that consists of extrafetal tissues separating the maternal and fetal blood. Until approximately 20 weeks, the placental membrane consists of four layers (see Figs. 7-6 and 7-7): **syncytiotrophoblast, cytotrophoblast, connective tissue of the villi,** and **endothelium of fetal capillaries.** After the 20th week, cellular changes occur in the branch villi that result in the cytotrophoblast, in many of the villi, becoming attenuated.

Eventually cytotrophoblastic cells disappear over large areas of the villi, leaving only thin patches of syncytiotrophoblast. As a result, the placental membrane consists of three layers in most places (see Fig. 7-6C). In some areas, the placental membrane becomes markedly thinned and attenuated. At these sites, the syncytiotrophoblast comes into direct contact with the endothelium of the

fetal capillaries to form a **vasculosyncytial placental membrane.**

Sometimes the placental membrane is called the **placental barrier;** this is an inappropriate term because there are only a few substances, endogenous or exogenous, that are unable to pass through the membrane in detectable amounts. The placental membrane acts as a barrier only when a molecule is of a certain size, configuration, and charge, such as that of **heparin** (a compound occurring in the liver and lungs that inhibits blood coagulation). Some metabolites, toxins, and hormones, although present in the maternal circulation, do not pass through the placental membrane in sufficient concentrations to affect the embryo/fetus. Most drugs and other substances in the maternal blood plasma pass through the placental membrane and enter the fetal blood plasma (see Fig. 7-7). The **syncytiotrophoblast** free surface has many microvilli that increase the surface area for exchange between the

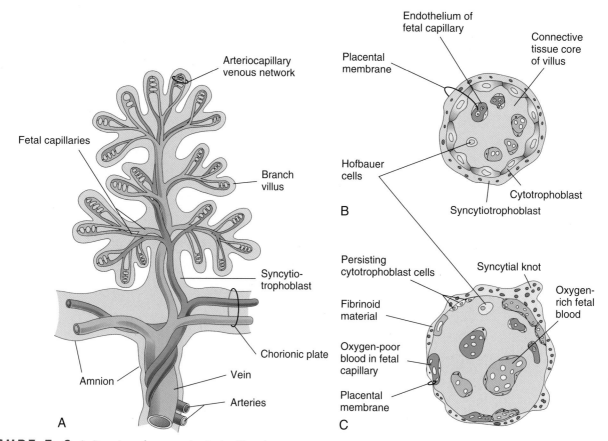

**FIGURE 7–6** A, Drawing of a stem chorionic villus showing its arteriocapillary–venous system. The arteries carry poorly oxygenated fetal blood and waste products from the fetus, whereas the vein carries oxygenated blood and nutrients to the fetus. B and C, Drawings of sections through a branch villus at 10 weeks and full term, respectively. The placental membrane, composed of extrafetal tissues, separates the maternal blood in the intervillous space from the fetal blood in the capillaries in the villi. Note that the placental membrane is very thin at full term. Hofbauer cells are thought to be phagocytic cells.

maternal and fetal circulations. As pregnancy advances, the placental membrane becomes progressively thinner, so that blood in many fetal capillaries is extremely close to the maternal blood in the intervillous space (see Figs. 7-6C and 7-7).

During the third trimester, numerous nuclei in the syncytiotrophoblast aggregate to form multinucleated protrusions, **syncytial knots** (see Fig. 7-6C). These aggregations regularly break off and are carried from the intervillous space into the maternal circulation. Some knots lodge in capillaries of the maternal lungs, where they are rapidly destroyed by local enzyme action. Toward the end of pregnancy, eosinophilic **fibrinoid material** thickens on the surfaces of villi (see Fig. 7-6C), which appears to reduce placental transfer.

## Functions of Placenta

*The placenta has several main functions:*

- **Metabolism** (e.g., synthesis of glycogen)
- **Transport** of gases and nutrients
- **Endocrine secretion** (e.g., human chorionic gonadotropin [hCG])

- **Protection**
- **Excretion** (fetal waste products)

These comprehensive activities are essential for maintaining pregnancy and promoting normal fetal development.

### Placental Metabolism

The placenta, particularly during early pregnancy, synthesizes glycogen, cholesterol, and fatty acids, which serve as sources of nutrients and energy for the embryo/fetus. Many of its metabolic activities are undoubtedly critical for its other two major placental activities (transport and endocrine secretion).

### Placental Transfer

The transport of substances in both directions between the fetal and maternal blood is facilitated by the great surface area of the placental membrane. Almost all materials are transported across this membrane by one of the following four main transport mechanisms: simple diffusion, facilitated diffusion, active transport, and pinocytosis.

**Passive transport by simple diffusion** is usually characteristic of substances moving from areas of higher to

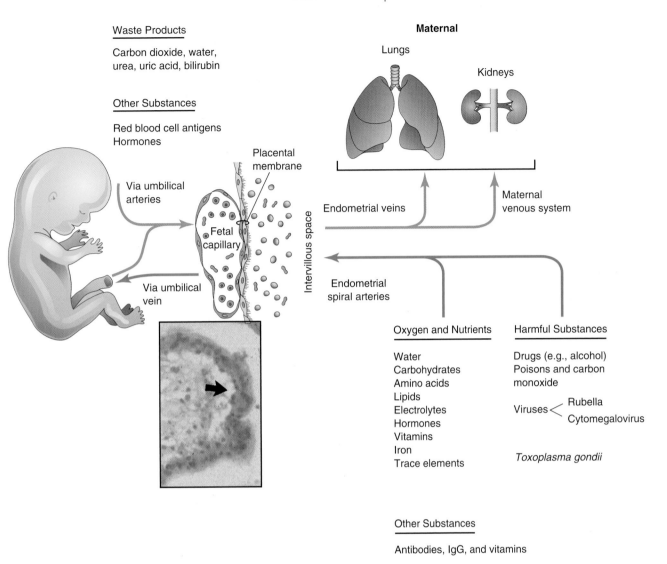

**Waste Products**

Carbon dioxide, water, urea, uric acid, bilirubin

**Other Substances**

Red blood cell antigens
Hormones

Via umbilical arteries

Via umbilical vein

Placental membrane

Fetal capillary

Intervillous space

**Maternal**

Lungs

Kidneys

Endometrial veins

Maternal venous system

Endometrial spiral arteries

**Oxygen and Nutrients**

Water
Carbohydrates
Amino acids
Lipids
Electrolytes
Hormones
Vitamins
Iron
Trace elements

**Harmful Substances**

Drugs (e.g., alcohol)
Poisons and carbon monoxide

Viruses < Rubella
Cytomegalovirus

*Toxoplasma gondii*

**Other Substances**

Antibodies, IgG, and vitamins

**Nontransferable Substances**

Bacteria, heparin, IgS, and IgM

**FIGURE 7–7** Diagrammatic illustration of transfer across the placental membrane. The extrafetal tissues, across which transport of substances between the mother and fetus occurs, collectively constitute the placental membrane. *Inset,* Light micrograph of chorionic villus showing a fetal capillary and placental membrane *(arrow)*.

lower concentration until equilibrium is established. In **facilitated diffusion**, there is transport through electrical gradients. Facilitated diffusion requires a transporter but no energy. Such systems may involve carrier molecules that temporarily combine with the substances to be transported. **Active transport** is the passage of ions or molecules across a cell membrane. **Pinocytosis** is a form of **endocytosis** (brings molecules and other substances into cells) in which the material being engulfed is a small amount of extracellular fluid. This method of transport is usually reserved for large molecules. Some proteins are transferred very slowly through the placenta by pinocytosis.

## Transfer of Gases

Oxygen, carbon dioxide, and carbon monoxide cross the placental membrane by **simple diffusion**. Interruption of oxygen transport for several minutes endangers the survival of the embryo/fetus. *The placental membrane approaches the efficiency of the lungs for gas exchange.* The quantity of oxygen reaching the fetus is primarily flow limited rather than diffusion limited; hence, **fetal hypoxia** (decreased levels of oxygen) results primarily from factors that diminish either the uterine blood flow or the embryo/fetal blood flow. **Maternal respiratory failure** (e.g., from pneumonia) will also reduce oxygen transport to the embryo/fetus.

## OTHER PLACENTAL TRANSPORT MECHANISMS

There are three other methods of transfer across the placental membrane. In the *first method of transport*, fetal red blood cells pass into the maternal circulation, particularly during **parturition** (childbirth), through microscopic breaks in the placental membrane. *Labeled maternal red blood cells have also been found in the fetal circulation.* Consequently, red blood cells may pass in either direction through very small defects in the placental membrane.

In the *second method of transport*, cells cross the placental membrane under their own power, for example, maternal leukocytes (white blood cells), which are involved in counteracting foreign substances and disease, and cells of *Treponema pallidum*, the organism that causes syphilis.

In the *third method of transport*, some bacteria and protozoa such as *Toxoplasma gondii* infect the placenta by creating lesions and then cross the placental membrane through the defects that are thus created.

## Nutritional Substances

Nutrients constitute the bulk of substances transferred from the mother to the embryo/fetus. *Water is rapidly exchanged by simple diffusion* and in increasing amounts as pregnancy advances. **Glucose** produced by the mother and the placenta is quickly transferred to the embryo/fetus by facilitated (active) diffusion mediated primarily by glucose transporter 1 (GLUT-1), an insulin-independent glucose carrier. Maternal cholesterol, triglycerides, and phospholipids are transferred. Although there is transport of free fatty acids (FFA), the amount transferred appears to be relatively small, with long-chain polyunsaturated fatty acids being the FFA transported in highest amounts.

**Amino acids** are actively transported across the placental membrane and are essential for fetal growth. For most amino acids, the plasma concentrations in the embryo/fetus are higher than in the mother. **Vitamins** cross the placental membrane and are essential for normal development. Water-soluble vitamins cross the placental membrane more quickly than fat-soluble vitamins.

## Hormones

Protein hormones (e.g., insulin or pituitary hormone) do not reach the embryo/fetus in significant amounts, except thyroxine and triiodothyronine by a slow transfer. Unconjugated steroid hormones cross the placental membrane rather freely. Testosterone and certain synthetic progestins cross the placental membrane and may cause masculinization of female fetuses (see Chapter 20, Fig. 20-41).

## Electrolytes

**Electrolytes** are freely exchanged across the placental membrane in significant quantities, each type at its own rate. When a mother receives intravenous fluids with electrolytes, they also pass to the embryo/fetus and affect the status of water and electrolytes.

## Maternal Antibodies and Proteins

The embryo/fetus produces only small amounts of antibodies because of its **immature immune system**. Some passive immunity is conferred on the fetus by the placental transfer of maternal antibodies. IgG gamma globulins are readily transported to the fetus by transcytosis. *Maternal antibodies confer fetal immunity to some diseases such as diphtheria, smallpox, and measles*; however, no immunity is acquired to **pertussis** (whooping cough) or **varicella** (chickenpox). A maternal protein, **transferrin**, crosses the placental membrane and carries iron to the embryo/fetus. The placental surface contains special receptors for this protein.

## HEMOLYTIC DISEASE OF THE NEONATE

Small amounts of fetal blood may pass to the maternal blood through microscopic breaks in the placental membrane. If the fetus is Rh positive and the mother Rh negative, the fetal blood cells may stimulate the formation of anti-Rh antibodies by the immune system of the mother. These antibodies pass to the fetal blood and cause hemolysis (destruction) of the fetal Rh-positive blood cells and jaundice and anemia in the fetus.

Some fetuses with hemolytic disease of the neonate, or **fetal erythroblastosis**, fail to make a satisfactory intrauterine adjustment. They may die unless delivered early or given intrauterine, intraperitoneal, or intravenous transfusions of packed Rh-negative blood cells until after birth. Hemolytic disease of the neonate due to Rh incompatibility is relatively uncommon now because **Rh(D) immunoglobulin** given to the mother usually prevents development of this disease in the fetus. Fetal anemia and consequent hyperbilirubinemia due to blood group incompatibility may still occur, though they are due to differences in other minor blood group antigens such as the Kell or Duffy group.

## Waste Products

Urea (formed in the liver) and uric acid pass through the placental membrane by simple diffusion. Conjugated bilirubin (which is fat soluble) is easily transported by the placenta for rapid clearance.

## Drugs and Drug Metabolites

*Drugs taken by the mother can affect the embryo/fetus directly or indirectly* by interfering with maternal or placental metabolism. The amount of drug or metabolite reaching the placenta is controlled by the maternal blood level and blood flow through the placenta. Most drugs and drug metabolites cross the placenta by simple diffusion, the exception being those with a structural similarity to amino acids, such as methyldopa and some antimetabolites.

*Some drugs cause major birth defects.* Fetal drug addiction may occur after maternal use of drugs such as heroin, and 55% to 90% of neonates of these mothers experience neonatal abstinence syndrome (withdrawal). The developmental outcomes of human in utero exposure to opioids are complex to evaluate, but animal studies have demonstrated that consequences may include somatic changes (including adrenal function), short-term spatial memory impairment, and alteration to the endogenous opiate system that may enhance addiction risk.

Most drugs used for the management of labor readily cross the placental membrane. Depending on the dose and timing in relation to parturition (childbirth), these drugs may cause respiratory depression of the neonate. All sedatives and analgesics affect the fetus to some degree. **Neuromuscular blocking agents** given to the mother during operative obstetrics cross the placenta in only small amounts. **Inhaled anesthetics** can also cross the placental membrane and affect fetal breathing if given during parturition.

### Infectious Agents

Cytomegalovirus, rubella virus, coxsackieviruses, and viruses associated with variola, varicella, measles, herpes, and poliomyelitis may pass through the placental membrane and cause **fetal infection**. In some cases, such as the **rubella virus infection**, severe birth defects such as **cataracts** may be produced. **Microorganisms** such as *Treponema pallidum*, which causes **syphilis**, and *Toxoplasma gondii*, which causes **toxoplasmosis**, produce destructive changes in the brain and eyes. These microscopic organisms cross the placental membrane, often causing severe **birth defects** and/or death of the embryo/fetus.

## Placental Endocrine Synthesis and Secretion

Using precursors derived from the fetus and/or the mother, the syncytiotrophoblast of the placenta synthesizes protein and steroid hormones. *The protein hormones synthesized by the placenta are*:

- Human chorionic gonadotropin (hCG)
- Human chorionic somatomammotropin (human placental lactogen)
- Human chorionic thyrotropin
- Human chorionic corticotropin

The glycoprotein **hCG**, similar to luteinizing hormone, is first secreted by the syncytiotrophoblast during the second week; hCG maintains the corpus luteum, preventing the onset of menstrual periods. The concentration of hCG in the maternal blood and urine increases to a maximum by the eighth week and then declines.

The **steroid hormones** synthesized by the placenta are **progesterone** and **estrogens**. Progesterone can be found in the placenta at all stages of gestation, indicating that progesterone is essential for the maintenance of pregnancy. The placenta forms progesterone from maternal cholesterol or pregnenolone. *The ovaries of a pregnant woman can be removed after the first trimester* without causing abortion because the placenta takes over the production of progesterone from the corpus luteum. Estrogens are also produced in large quantities by the syncytiotrophoblast.

## The Placenta as an Allograft*

The placenta can be regarded as an **allograft** (a graft transplanted between genetically nonidentical individuals) with respect to the mother. The fetal part of the placenta is a derivative of the conceptus, which inherits both paternal and maternal genes. What protects the placenta from rejection by the mother's immune system? This question remains a major biologic enigma in nature. The syncytiotrophoblast of the chorionic villi, although exposed to maternal immune cells within the blood sinusoids, lacks major histocompatibility (MHC) antigens and thus does not evoke rejection responses. However, extravillous trophoblast (EVT) cells, which invade the uterine decidua and its vasculature (spiral arteries), express class I MHC antigens. These antigens include HLA-G, which, being nonpolymorphic (class Ib), is poorly recognizable by T lymphocytes as an alloantigen, as well as HLA-C, which, being polymorphic (class Ia), is recognizable by T cells. In addition to averting T cells, EVT cells must also shield themselves from potential attack by natural killer (NK) lymphocytes and from injury inflicted by activation of complement.

Multiple mechanisms appear to be in place to guard the placenta:

- Expression of HLA-G is restricted to a few tissues, including placental EVT cells. Its strategic location in the placenta is believed to provide a dual immunoprotective role: evasion of T-cell recognition owing to its nonpolymorphic nature, and recognition by the "killer-inhibitory receptors" on NK cells, thus turning off their killer function. The inadequacy of this hypothesis is suggested by several observations: (1) healthy individuals showing biallelic loss of HLA-G1 have been identified, indicating that HLA-G is not essential for fetoplacental survival; (2) human EVT cells were found to be vulnerable to NK cell–mediated killing; and (3) the hypothesis does not explain why HLA-C, a polymorphic antigen, also expressed by EVT cells, does not evoke a rejection response in situ. Because both HLA-G and HLA-C were shown to have the unique ability to resist human cytomegalovirus-mediated MHC class I degradation, it is speculated that a selective location of these two antigens at the fetomaternal interface may help to withstand viral assault.
- Immunoprotection is provided locally by certain immunosuppressor molecules, such as prostaglandin $E_2$, transforming growth factor (TGF)-β and interleukin-10. Prostaglandin $E_2$ derived from the decidua was shown to block activation of maternal T cells as well as NK cells in situ. Indeed, the immunoregulatory function of decidual cells is consistent with

*The authors are grateful to Dr. Peeyush Lala, Professor Emeritus, Department of Anatomy and Cell Biology, Faculty of Medicine, Western University, London, Ontario, Canada, for preparing these sections: "The Placenta as an Allograft" and "The Placenta as an Invasive Tumor-like Structure."

their genealogy. It was shown that uterine endometrial stromal cells, which differentiate into decidual cells during pregnancy, are derived from progenitor (stem) cells that migrate from hemopoietic organs such as the fetal liver and bone marrow during ontogeny.

- Transient tolerance of the maternal T-cell repertoire to fetal MHC antigens may serve as a backup mechanism for placental immunoprotection. A similar B-cell tolerance has also been reported.
- A trafficking of activated maternal leukocytes into the placenta or fetus is prevented by deletion of these cells triggered by apoptosis-inducing ligands present on the trophoblast.
- Based on genetic manipulation in mice, it was shown that the presence of complement regulatory proteins (Crry in the mouse, membrane cofactor protein or CD46 in the human), which can block activation of the third component of complement (C3) in the complement cascade, protects the placenta from complement-mediated destruction, which may happen otherwise because of residual C3 activation remaining after defending against pathogens. Crry gene knockout mice died in utero because of complement-mediated placental damage, which could be averted by additional knockout of the C3 gene.
- Experiments in mice revealed that the presence of the enzyme indoleamine 2,3-deoxygenase in trophoblastic cells was critical for immunoprotection of the allogeneic conceptus. It suppresses T-cell–driven local inflammatory responses, including complement activation. Treatment of pregnant mice with an indoleamine 2,3-deoxygenase inhibitor, 1-methyltryptophan, caused selective death of allogeneic (but not syngeneic) conceptuses because of massive deposition of complement and hemorrhagic necrosis at the placental sites.

## The Placenta as an Invasive Tumor-like Structure

The placenta in many species, including humans, is a highly invasive **tumor-like structure** that invades the uterus to tap into its blood supply to establish an adequate exchange of key molecules between the mother and embryo/fetus. What protects the uterus from placental overinvasion? Following the development of chorionic villi, the invasive function of the placenta is provided by the subset of cytotrophoblastic cells (EVT cells), which are produced by proliferation and differentiation of stem cells located in the cytotrophoblastic layer of certain chorionic villi, the **anchoring villi** (see Fig. 7-5). They break out of the villous confines and migrate as cell columns to invade the decidua, where they reorganize as distinct subsets: a nearly continuous cell layer (**cytotrophoblastic shell**) separating the decidua from maternal blood sinusoids; cells dispersed within the decidua (interstitial trophoblast); multinucleate placental-bed giant cells produced by EVT cell fusion; and endovascular trophoblast, which invades and remodels the uteroplacental (spiral) arteries within the endometrium and a part of the myometrium. Optimal arterial remodeling (loss of tunica media and replacement of endothelium by the EVT cells)

allows steady placental perfusion with maternal blood unhindered by the presence of vasoactive molecules. Inadequate EVT cell invasion leading to poor placental perfusion underlies the pathogenesis of **preeclampsia** (a major hypertensive disorder associated with pregnancy in the mother) and certain forms of IUGR of the fetus, whereas excessive invasion is a hallmark of **gestational trophoblastic neoplasias** and **choriocarcinomas**.

Trophoblastic stem cells have been successfully propagated from the murine (mouse) placenta but not from the human placenta. However, normal human EVT cells have been successfully propagated from first-trimester human placentas. Using these cells for functional assays in vitro, it was shown that molecular mechanisms responsible for their invasiveness are identical to those of cancer cells, whereas their proliferation, migration, and invasiveness are stringently regulated in situ by a variety of locally produced molecules: growth factors, growth factor–binding proteins, proteoglycans, and components of the extracellular matrix. Numerous growth factors, such as epidermal growth factor, TGF-α, amphiregulin, colony-stimulating factor 1, vascular endothelial growth factor, and placental growth factor, were shown to stimulate EVT cell proliferation without affecting migration or invasiveness, whereas insulin-like growth factor II and an insulin-like, growth factor–binding protein, IGFBP-1, were shown to stimulate EVT cell migration and invasiveness without affecting proliferation. TGF-β, primarily produced by the decidua, was shown to provide the key control of EVT cell proliferation, migration, and invasiveness, whereas trophoblastic cancer (choriocarcinoma) cells were shown to be resistant to the inhibitory signals of TGF-β. *Thus, it appears that the decidua plays a dual role in uteroplacental homeostasis by providing immunoprotection of the placenta and also protection of the uterus from placental overinvasion.*

## PREECLAMPSIA

Preeclampsia (high blood pressure) is a serious disorder that may occur during pregnancy, usually after the 20th week of gestation. **Maternal hypertension**, **proteinuria** (abnormal quantities of protein in the urine), and **edema** (excess of watery fluid) are essential features of this condition. Preeclampsia can lead to **eclampsia** (one or more convulsions), resulting in miscarriage and maternal death. The cause of preeclampsia is uncertain, but recent studies have implicated the **renin–angiotensin system** in the development of high blood pressure and edema. In eclampsia, extensive placental infarcts are present that reduce the uteroplacental circulation. This may lead to fetal malnutrition, fetal growth restriction, miscarriage, or fetal death.

## Uterine Growth during Pregnancy

The uterus of a nonpregnant woman is in the pelvis (Fig. 7-8A). To accommodate the growing conceptus (embryo

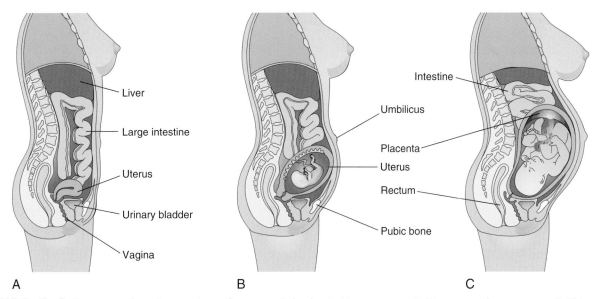

**FIGURE 7–8** Drawings of median sections of a woman's body. **A,** Not pregnant. **B,** Twenty weeks pregnant. **C,** Thirty weeks pregnant. Note that as the conceptus enlarges, the uterus increases in size to accommodate the rapidly growing fetus. By 20 weeks, the uterus and fetus reach the level of the umbilicus, and by 30 weeks, they reach the epigastric region. The mother's abdominal viscera are displaced and compressed, and the skin and muscles of her anterior abdominal wall are stretched.

and membranes), the uterus increases in size. It also increases in weight, and its walls become thinner (see Fig. 7-8B and C). During the first trimester, the uterus moves out of the pelvis, and by 20 weeks, it reaches the level of the umbilicus. By 28 to 30 weeks, the uterus reaches the epigastric region, the area between the xiphoid process of the sternum and the umbilicus. The increase in size of the uterus largely results from **hypertrophy** (enlargement) of preexisting smooth muscular fibers and partly from the development of new fibers.

## PARTURITION

**Parturition** is the process during which the fetus, placenta, and fetal membranes are expelled from the mother's reproductive tract (Fig. 7-9A to E). **Labor** is a sequence of involuntary **uterine contractions**, which result in dilation of the uterine cervix and expulsion of the fetus and placenta from the uterus (see Fig. 7-9F to H). The factors that trigger labor are not completely understood; however, several hormones are related to the initiation of contractions.

The **fetal hypothalamus** secretes **corticotropin-releasing hormone**, which stimulates the anterior **hypophysis** (pituitary) to produce **adrenocorticotropin**. This hormone causes the secretion of **cortisol** from the suprarenal (adrenal) cortex, which is involved in the synthesis of **estrogens** that are formed by the ovaries, placenta, testes, and, possibly, adrenal cortex.

**Peristaltic contractions** of uterine smooth muscle are elicited by **oxytocin**, a hormone released by the neurohypophysis of the pituitary gland. This hormone is administered clinically when it is necessary to induce labor. Oxytocin also stimulates release of **prostaglandins** (promoters of uterine contractions) from the decidua,

increasing myometrial contractility by sensitizing the myometrial cells to oxytocin.

**Estrogens** (sex hormones) also increase myometrial contractile activity and stimulate the release of oxytocin and prostaglandins. From studies carried out in sheep and nonhuman primates, it seems that the duration of pregnancy and process of birth are under the direct control of the fetus.

## Stages of Labor

Labor is a continuous process; however, for clinical purposes, it is usually divided into three stages:

- **Dilation** begins with progressive dilation of the cervix (see Fig. 7-9A and B) and ends when the cervix is completely dilated. During this **first stage**, regular painful contractions of the uterus occur less than 10 minutes apart. The average duration of the first stage is approximately 12 hours for first pregnancies (**primigravida**) and approximately 7 hours for women who have had a baby previously (**multigravida**).
- **Expulsion**, the **first stage of labor**, begins when the cervix is completely dilated and ends with delivery of the fetus (Fig. 7-10, and see Fig. 7-9C to E). During the **second stage of labor**, the fetus descends through the cervix and vagina. When the fetus is outside the mother, it is called a **neonate**. The average duration of the second stage is 50 minutes for primigravidas and 20 minutes for multigravidas.
- The **placental stage** begins as soon as the **fetus** is born and ends with the expulsion of the placenta and membranes. The duration of this **third stage of labor** is 15 minutes in approximately 90% of pregnancies. A **retained placenta** is one that is not expelled within 60 minutes of delivery.

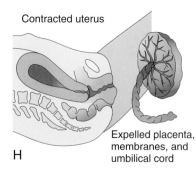

**FIGURE 7–9** Drawings illustrating parturition (childbirth). A and B, The cervix is dilating during the first stage of labor. C to E, The fetus is passing through the cervix and vagina during the second stage of labor. F and G, As the uterus contracts during the third stage of labor, the placenta folds and pulls away from the uterine wall. Separation of the placenta results in bleeding and formation of a large hematoma (mass of blood). Pressure on the abdomen facilitates placental separation. H, The placenta is expelled and the uterus contracts.

**FIGURE 7-10** Delivery of the fetus's head during the second stage of labor. **A,** The crown of the fetal head distends the mother's perineum. **B,** The perineum slips over the head and face. **C,** The head is delivered; subsequently, the body of the fetus is expelled. *(From Greenhill JB, Friedman EA:* Biological principles and modern practice of obstetrics, *Philadelphia, 1974, Saunders.)*

Retraction of the uterus reduces the area of placental attachment (Fig. 7-9*G*). A **hematoma** (localized mass of extravasated blood) soon forms deep to the placenta and separates it from the uterine wall. The placenta and fetal membranes are expelled through the vaginal canal. The placenta separates through the spongy layer of the decidua basalis. After delivery of the fetus, the uterus continues to contract (see Fig. 7-9*H*). The **myometrial contractions** of the uterus constrict the spiral arteries that supplied blood to the intervillous space (see Fig. 7-5). These contractions prevent excessive uterine bleeding.

## Placenta and Fetal Membranes after Birth

The **placenta** usually has a discoid shape, with a diameter of 15 to 20 cm and a thickness of 2 to 3 cm (Fig. 7-11). It weighs 500 to 600 g, which is approximately one sixth the weight of the average fetus. The margins of the placenta are continuous with the ruptured amniotic and chorionic sacs (see Fig 7-11*C*).

When chorionic villi persist on the entire surface of the chorionic sac (an uncommon occurrence), a thin layer of placenta attaches to a large area of the uterus. This type of placenta is a **membranous placenta** (placenta membranacea). When villi persist elsewhere, several variations in placental shape occur: **accessory placenta** (Fig. 7-12), **bidiscoid placenta**, and **horseshoe placenta**. Although there are variations in the size and shape of the placenta, most of them are of little physiologic or clinical significance.

## Maternal Surface of Placenta

The characteristic cobblestone appearance of the maternal surface is produced by slightly bulging villous areas, or **cotyledons,** which are separated by grooves that were formerly occupied by placental septa (see Figs. 7-5 and

### GESTATIONAL CHORIOCARCINOMA

Abnormal proliferation of the trophoblast results in **gestational trophoblastic disease,** a spectrum of lesions including highly malignant tumors. The cells invade the decidua basalis, penetrate its blood vessels and lymphatics, and may metastasize (spread) to the maternal lungs, bone marrow, liver, and other organs. *Gestational choriocarcinomas are highly sensitive to chemotherapy, and cures are usually achieved.*

7-11*A*). The surface of the cotyledons is covered by thin, grayish shreds of decidua basalis that separated from the uterine wall when the placenta was extruded. Most of the decidua is temporarily retained in the uterus and is shed with the uterine bleeding after delivery of the fetus.

Examination of the placenta prenatally by ultrasonography or magnetic resonance imaging (Fig. 7-13), or postnatally by gross and microscopic study, may provide clinical information about the causes of IUGR, placental dysfunction, fetal distress and death, and neonatal illness. Placental studies can also determine whether the expelled placenta is complete. Retention of a cotyledon, **accessory placenta,** in the uterus may cause severe uterine hemorrhage (see Fig. 7-12).

## Fetal Surface of Placenta

The umbilical cord usually attaches to the fetal surface of the placenta, and its epithelium is continuous with the amnion adhering to the fetal surface (see Figs. 7-5 and 7-11*B*). The fetal surface of a freshly delivered placenta is smooth and shiny because it is covered by the amnion. The chorionic vessels radiating to and from the umbilical

Umbilical cord

Smooth chorion

Cotyledon

Groove

A

Umbilical cord

Umbilical vessels radiating to form chorionic vessels

Amnion (transparent)

Chorionic vessels (under amnion)

B

**FIGURE 7–11** Placentas and fetal membranes after birth, approximately one third actual size. **A**, Maternal surface showing cotyledons and grooves around them. Each cotyledon consists of a number of main stem villi with their many branch villi. The grooves were occupied by the placental septa when the maternal and fetal parts of the placenta were together (see Fig. 7-5). **B**, Fetal surface showing blood vessels running in the chorionic plate deep to the amnion and converging to form the umbilical vessels at the attachment of the umbilical cord.

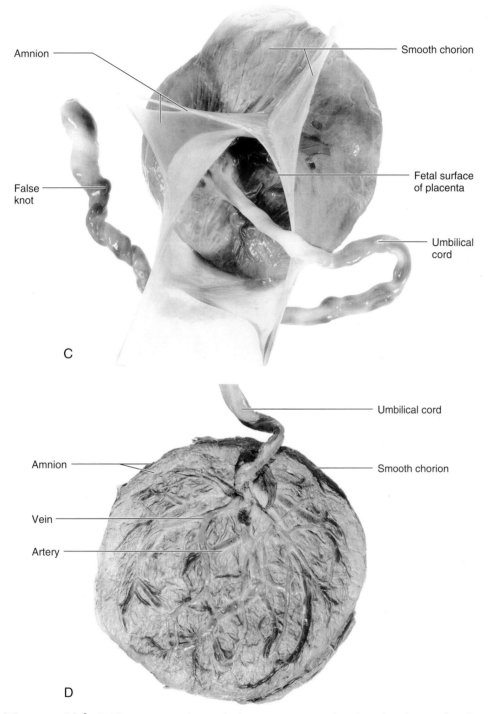

FIGURE 7–11, cont'd  C, The amnion and smooth chorion are arranged to show that they are fused and continuous with the margins of the placenta. D, Placenta with a marginal attachment of the cord. *(From Moore KL, Persaud TVN, Shiota K: Color atlas of clinical embryology, ed 2, Philadelphia, 2000, Saunders.)*

Umbilical
cord

Accessory
placenta

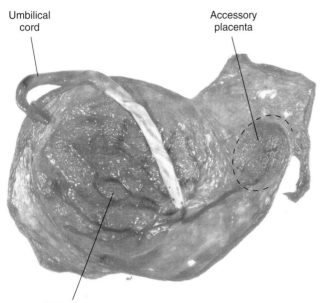

Main placenta

**FIGURE 7–12** A full-term placenta and an accessory placenta. The accessory placenta developed from a patch of chorionic villi that persisted a short distance from the main placenta.

cord are clearly visible through the transparent amnion. The umbilical vessels branch on the fetal surface to form **chorionic vessels**, which enter the chorionic villi and form the **arteriocapillary–venous system** (see Fig. 7-6A).

## PLACENTAL ABNORMALITIES

Abnormal adherence of chorionic villi to the myometrium is called **placenta accreta** (Fig. 7-14). When chorionic villi penetrate the full thickness of the **myometrium** (muscular wall of the uterus) to or through the perimetrium (peritoneal covering), the abnormality is called **placenta percreta**. *Third-trimester bleeding is the common presenting sign of these placental abnormalities.* Most women with placenta accreta have normal pregnancies and labors. After birth, the placenta fails to separate from the uterine wall, and attempts to remove it may cause hemorrhage that is difficult to control.

When the blastocyst implants close to or overlying the internal os of the uterus, the abnormality is called **placenta previa** (see Fig. 7-14). Late pregnancy bleeding may result from this placental abnormality. The fetus has to be delivered by cesarean section when the placenta completely obstructs the internal uterine os. Ultrasound scanning of the placenta is invaluable for clinical diagnosis of placental abnormalities.

## Umbilical Cord

The attachment of the umbilical cord to the placenta is usually near the center of the fetal surface (see Fig. 7-11B), but it may attach at any point (e.g., insertion of the cord near the placental margin produces a **battledore placenta**) (see Fig. 7-11D). The attachment of the cord to the fetal membranes is termed a **velamentous insertion of the cord** (Fig. 7-15).

**Doppler ultrasonography** may be used for prenatal diagnosis of the position and structural abnormalities of the umbilical cord and its vessels, as well as blood flow. The cord is usually 1 to 2 cm in diameter and 30 to 90 cm in length (average, 55 cm). Excessively long or short cords are uncommon. *Long cords have a tendency to prolapse and/or to coil around the fetus* (see Fig. 7-19B). Prompt recognition of prolapse of the cord is important because the cord may be compressed between the presenting body part of the fetus and the mother's bony pelvis, causing fetal hypoxia or anoxia. If the deficiency of oxygen persists for more than 5 minutes, the neonate's brain may be damaged. A very short cord may cause premature separation of the placenta from the wall of the uterus during delivery.

The umbilical cord usually has two arteries and one large vein, which are surrounded by mucoid connective tissue (**Wharton jelly**). Because the umbilical vessels are longer than the cord, twisting and bending of the vessels are common. They frequently form loops, producing **false knots** that are of no significance; however, in approximately 1% of pregnancies, **true knots** form in the cord,

**FIGURE 7–13** Sagittal magnetic resonance image of the pelvis of a pregnant woman. The vertebral column and pelvis of the mother are visible, as are the fetal brain, limbs, and placenta (*P*).

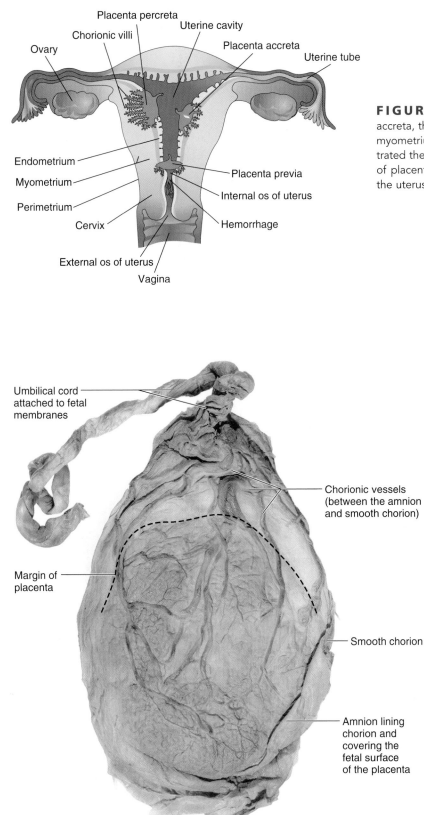

**FIGURE 7–14** Placental abnormalities. In placenta accreta, there is abnormal adherence of the placenta to the myometrium. In placenta percreta, the placenta has penetrated the full thickness of the myometrium. In this example of placenta previa, the placenta overlies the internal os of the uterus and blocks the cervical canal.

**FIGURE 7–15** A placenta with a velamentous insertion of the umbilical cord. The cord is attached to the membranes, not to the placenta. The umbilical vessels leave the cord and run between the amnion and chorion before spreading over the placenta. The vessels are easily torn in this location, especially when they cross over the inferior uterine segment; the latter condition is called vasa previa. If the vessels rupture before birth, the fetus loses blood and could be near exsanguination when born. *(From Moore KL, Persaud TVN, Shiota K: Color atlas of clinical embryology, ed 2, Philadelphia, 2000, Saunders.)*

**FIGURE 7–16** Photograph of an umbilical cord showing a true knot. Such a knot will cause severe anoxia (decreased oxygen in fetal tissues and organs).

**FIGURE 7–17** Doppler velocimetry of the umbilical cord. The arterial waveform *(top)* illustrates pulsatile forward flow, with high peaks and low velocities during diastole. This combination suggests high resistance in the placenta to placental blood flow. Because this index changes over gestation, it is important to know that the pregnancy was 18 weeks' gestation. For this period, the flow pattern is normal. The nonpulsatile flow in the opposite, negative direction represents venous return from the placenta. Both waveforms are normal for this gestational age.

which may tighten and cause fetal death resulting from anoxia (Fig. 7-16). In most cases, the knots form during labor as a result of the fetus passing through a loop in the cord. Simple looping of the cord around the fetus (e.g., around the ankle) occasionally occurs (see Fig. 7-19*B*). If the coil is tight, then blood circulation to the ankle is affected. In approximately one fifth of deliveries, the cord is loosely looped around the neck without increased fetal risk.

## UMBILICAL ARTERY DOPPLER VELOCIMETRY

As gestation and trophoblastic invasion of the decidua basalis progress, there is a corresponding increase in the diastolic flow velocity in the umbilical arteries. Doppler velocimetry of the uteroplacental and fetoplacental circulation is used to investigate complications of pregnancy, such as IUGR and fetal distress resulting from fetal hypoxia and asphyxia (Fig. 7-17). For example, there is a statistically significant association between IUGR and abnormally increased resistance in an umbilical artery.

## ABSENCE OF UMBILICAL ARTERY

In approximately 1 in 100 neonates, only one umbilical artery is present (Fig. 7-18), a condition that may be associated with chromosomal and fetal abnormalities. Absence of an umbilical artery is accompanied by a 15% to 20% incidence of cardiovascular defects in the fetus. Absence of an artery results from either agenesis or degeneration of one of the two umbilical arteries. A single umbilical artery and the defects associated with it can be detected before birth by ultrasonography.

Amnion
Mucous connective tissue
Umbilical artery
Umbilical vein

**FIGURE 7–18** Transverse section of an umbilical cord. Observe that the cord is covered by epithelium derived from the enveloping amnion. It has a core of mucous connective tissue (Wharton jelly). Observe also that the cord has one vein and only one umbilical artery instead of the normal two arteries.

## Amnion and Amniotic Fluid

The thin but tough **amnion** forms a fluid-filled, membranous **amniotic sac** that surrounds the embryo and later the fetus. The sac contains **amniotic fluid** (Figs. 7-19 and 7-20). As the amnion enlarges, it gradually obliterates the chorionic cavity and forms the epithelial covering of the umbilical cord (see Figs. 7-18 and 7-20*C* and *D*).

### Amniotic Fluid

**Amniotic fluid** plays a major role in fetal growth and embryo/fetal development. Initially, some amniotic fluid is secreted by cells of the amnion. Most fluid is derived from maternal tissue and interstitial fluid by diffusion across the amniochorionic membrane from the decidua parietalis (see Fig. 7-5). Later there is diffusion of fluid

**FIGURE 7–19** A, A 12-week fetus in its amniotic sac. The fetus and its membranes aborted spontaneously. It was removed from its chorionic sac with its amniotic sac intact. Actual size. B, Note that the umbilical cord is looped around the left ankle of the fetus. Coiling of the cord around parts of the fetus affects development when the coils are so tight that the circulation to the parts is affected.

through the chorionic plate from blood in the intervillous space of the placenta.

Before **keratinization** (formation of keratin) of the skin occurs, a major pathway for passage of water and solutes in tissue fluid from the fetus to the amniotic cavity is through the skin; thus, amniotic fluid is similar to fetal tissue fluid. Fluid is also secreted by the fetal respiratory and gastrointestinal tracts and enters the amniotic cavity. The daily rate of contribution of fluid to the amniotic cavity from the respiratory tract is 300 to 400 ml.

Beginning in the 11th week, *the fetus contributes to the amniotic fluid by excreting urine into the amniotic cavity.* By late pregnancy, approximately 500 ml of urine is added daily. The volume of amniotic fluid normally increases slowly, reaching approximately 30 ml at 10 weeks, 350 ml at 20 weeks, and 700 to 1000 ml by 37 weeks.

### Circulation of Amniotic Fluid

The water content of amniotic fluid changes every 3 hours. Large amounts of water pass through the **amniochorionic membrane** (see Fig. 7-5) into the maternal tissue fluid and enter the uterine capillaries. An exchange of fluid with fetal blood also occurs through the umbilical cord and where the amnion adheres to the chorionic plate on the fetal surface of the placenta (see Figs. 7-5 and 7-11B); thus, amniotic fluid is in balance with the fetal circulation.

Amniotic fluid is swallowed by the fetus and absorbed by the fetus's respiratory and digestive tracts. It has been estimated that during the final stages of pregnancy, the fetus swallows up to 400 ml of amniotic fluid per day. The fluid passes into the fetal bloodstream, and the waste products in it cross the placental membrane and enter the maternal blood in the intervillous space. Excess water in the fetal blood is excreted by the fetal kidneys and returned to the amniotic sac through the fetal urinary tract.

### Composition of Amniotic Fluid

Amniotic fluid is an aqueous solution in which undissolved material (e.g., desquamated fetal epithelial cells) is suspended. Amniotic fluid contains approximately equal portions of organic compounds and inorganic salts. Half of the organic constituents are protein; the other half consists of carbohydrates, fats, enzymes, hormones, and pigments. As pregnancy advances, the composition of the amniotic fluid changes.

Because fetal urine enters the amniotic fluid, studies of fetal enzyme systems, amino acids, hormones, and other substances can be conducted on fluid removed by amniocentesis (see Fig. 6-13A). Studies of cells in the amniotic fluid permit diagnosis of chromosomal abnormalities such as trisomy 21 (Down syndrome). High levels of alpha fetoprotein usually indicate the presence of a severe neural tube defect. Low levels of alpha fetoprotein may indicate chromosomal aberrations such as trisomy 21.

### Significance of Amniotic Fluid

The embryo, suspended in amniotic fluid by the umbilical cord, floats freely. Amniotic fluid has critical functions in the normal development of the fetus:

- Permits symmetric external growth of the embryo/fetus
- Acts as a barrier to infection

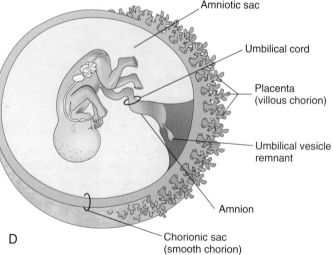

**FIGURE 7–20** Illustrations showing how the amnion enlarges, obliterates the chorionic cavity, and envelops the umbilical cord. Observe that part of the umbilical vesicle is incorporated into the embryo as the primordial gut. Formation of the fetal part of the placenta and degeneration of chorionic villi are also shown. **A,** At 3 weeks. **B,** At 4 weeks. **C,** At 10 weeks. **D,** At 20 weeks.

## DISORDERS OF AMNIOTIC FLUID VOLUME

A condition in which a low volume of amniotic fluid is present for a given gestational age, **oligohydramnios**, results in many cases from placental insufficiency with diminished placental blood flow. Preterm rupture of the amniochorionic membrane occurs in approximately 10% of pregnancies and is the most common cause of oligohydramnios.

When there is **renal agenesis** (failure of kidney formation), the absence of fetal urine contribution to the amniotic fluid is the main cause of oligohydramnios. A similar decrease in fluid occurs when there is obstructive uropathy (urinary tract obstruction). Complications of oligohydramnios include fetal birth defects (pulmonary hypoplasia and facial and limb defects) that are caused by fetal compression by the uterine wall. In extreme cases, as in renal agenesis, **Potter sequence** results from lethal pulmonary hypoplasia due to severe oligohydramnios. Compression of the umbilical cord is also a potential complication of severe oligohydramnios.

Most cases (60%) of **polyhydramnios**, or a large volume of amniotic fluid for a given gestational age, are idiopathic (or of unknown cause), 20% are caused by maternal factors, and 20% are fetal in origin. Polyhydramnios may be associated with severe defects of the central nervous system, such as **meroencephaly**. When there are other defects, such as **esophageal atresia** (blockage), amniotic fluid accumulates because it is unable to pass to the fetal stomach and intestines for absorption.

Ultrasonography has become the technique of choice for diagnosing oligohydramnios and polyhydramnios. Premature rupture of the amniochorionic membrane is the most common event leading to premature labor and delivery and the most common complication resulting in oligohydramnios. Loss of amniotic fluid removes the major protection that the fetus has against infection.

- Permits normal fetal lung development
- Prevents adherence of the amnion to the embryo/fetus
- Cushions the embryo/fetus against injuries by distributing impacts the mother receives
- Helps control the embryo/fetus's body temperature by maintaining a relatively constant temperature
- Enables the fetus to move freely, thereby aiding muscular development (e.g., by movements of the limbs)
- Assists in maintaining homeostasis of fluid and electrolytes

## AMNIOTIC BAND SYNDROME

Amniotic band syndrome (ABS), or **amniotic band disruption complex**, may result in a variety of fetal birth defects (Fig. 7-21). The incidence of ABS is approximately 1 in every 1200 live births. The defects caused by ABS vary from simple digital constriction to major scalp, craniofacial, and visceral defects. Prenatal ultrasound diagnosis of ABS is possible. **There appears to be two possible causes of these defects**: exogenous causes, which **result** from delamination of the amnion due to rupturing or tearing, causing an encircling amniotic band (see Figs. 7-19 and 7-21), and endogenous causes, which result from vascular disruption.

## UMBILICAL VESICLE

The umbilical vesicle can be observed with ultrasound early in the fifth week. Early development of the umbilical vesicle was described in Chapters 3 and 5. At 32 days, the umbilical vesicle is large (see Figs. 7-1C and 7-2). By 10 weeks, the umbilical vesicle has shrunk to a pear-shaped remnant approximately 5 mm in diameter (see Fig. 7-20) and is connected to the midgut by a narrow **omphaloenteric duct** (yolk stalk). By 20 weeks, the umbilical vesicle is very small (see Fig. 7-20D); thereafter, it is

Chorion

Fibrous bands of disrupted amnion

Fetal surface of placenta

Umbilical cord

**FIGURE 7–21** A fetus with amniotic band syndrome showing amniotic bands constricting the left arm.

usually not visible. The presence of the amniotic sac and umbilical vesicle enables early recognition and measurement of the embryo. The umbilical vesicle is recognizable in ultrasound examinations until the end of the first trimester.

## Significance of Umbilical Vesicle

The umbilical vesicle is essential for several reasons:

- It has a role in the **transfer of nutrients** to the embryo during the second and third weeks when the uteroplacental circulation is being established.
- **Blood cell development** first occurs in the well-vascularized extraembryonic mesoderm covering the wall of the umbilical vesicle beginning in the third week (see Chapter 4) and continues to form there until hemopoietic activity begins in the liver during the sixth week.
- During the fourth week, the endoderm of the umbilical vesicle is incorporated into the embryo as the primordial gut (see Chapter 5, Fig. 5-1C$_2$). Its endoderm, derived from epiblast, gives rise to the epithelium of the trachea, bronchi, lungs, and alimentary canal.
- **Primordial germ cells** appear in the endodermal lining of the wall of the umbilical vesicle in the third week and subsequently migrate to the developing gonads (see Chapter 12, Fig. 12-31). The cells differentiate into spermatogonia in males and oogonia in females.

## Fate of Umbilical Vesicle

At 10 weeks, the small vesicle lies in the chorionic cavity between the amniotic and chorionic sacs (see Fig. 7-20C). It atrophies as pregnancy advances, eventually becoming very small (Fig. 7-20D). In very unusual cases, the umbilical vesicle persists throughout pregnancy and appears under the amnion as a small structure on the fetal surface of the placenta near the attachment of the umbilical cord. Persistence of the umbilical vesicle is of no significance. The **omphaloenteric duct** usually detaches from the midgut loop by the end of the sixth week. In approximately 2% of adults, the proximal intra-abdominal part of the omphaloenteric duct persists as an **ileal diverticulum** (Meckel diverticulum; see Chapter 11, Fig. 11-21).

## ▶ ALLANTOIS

5  Early development of the allantois is described in Chapter 4. In the third week, it appears as a sausage-like diverticulum from the caudal wall of the umbilical vesicle that extends into the connecting stalk (Fig. 7-22A). During the second month, the extraembryonic part of the allantois degenerates (see Fig. 7-22B). Although the allantois is not functional in human embryos, it is important for three reasons:

- Blood cell formation occurs in its wall during the third to fifth weeks.
- Its blood vessels persist as the umbilical vein and arteries.

- The intraembryonic part of the allantois passes from the umbilicus to the urinary bladder, with which it is continuous. As the bladder enlarges, the allantois involutes to form a thick tube, the **urachus**. After birth, the urachus becomes a fibrous cord, the **median umbilical ligament**, which extends from the apex of the urinary bladder to the umbilicus (see Fig. 7-22D).

### ALLANTOIC CYSTS

A cystic mass in the umbilical cord may represent the remains of the extraembryonic part of the allantois (Fig. 7-23). These cysts usually resolve, but they may be associated with an **omphalocele**, the congenital herniation of viscera into the proximal part of the umbilical cord (see Chapter 11, Fig. 11-23).

## MULTIPLE PREGNANCIES

The risks of chromosomal anomalies and fetal morbidity and mortality are higher in multiple gestations than in single pregnancies. As the number of fetuses increases, the risks are progressively greater. In most countries, multiple births are more common now because of greater access to fertility therapies, including induction of ovulation that occurs when exogenous gonadotropins are administered to women with ovulatory failure and to those being treated for infertility by assisted reproductive technologies. In North America, twins normally occur approximately once in every 85 pregnancies, triplets approximately once in $90^2$ pregnancies, quadruplets once in $90^3$ pregnancies, and quintuplets approximately once in every $90^4$ pregnancies.

## Twins and Fetal Membranes

Twins that originate from two zygotes are dizygotic (DZ) twins, or fraternal twins (Fig. 7-24), whereas twins that originate from one zygote are monozygotic (MZ) twins, or identical twins (Fig. 7-25). The fetal membranes and placentas vary according to the origin of the twins (Table 7-1). In the case of MZ twins, the type of placenta and membranes formed depends on when the twinning process occurs. Approximately two thirds of twins are DZ. The frequency of DZ twinning shows marked racial differences, but the incidence of MZ twinning is approximately the same in all populations. In addition, the rate of MZ twinning shows little variation with the mother's age, whereas the rate of DZ twinning increases with maternal age.

The study of twins is important in human genetics because it is useful for comparing the effects of genes and the environment on development. If an abnormal condition does not show a simple genetic pattern, comparison of its incidence in MZ and DZ twins may reveal that heredity is involved. The tendency for DZ, but not MZ, twins to repeat in families is evidence of hereditary

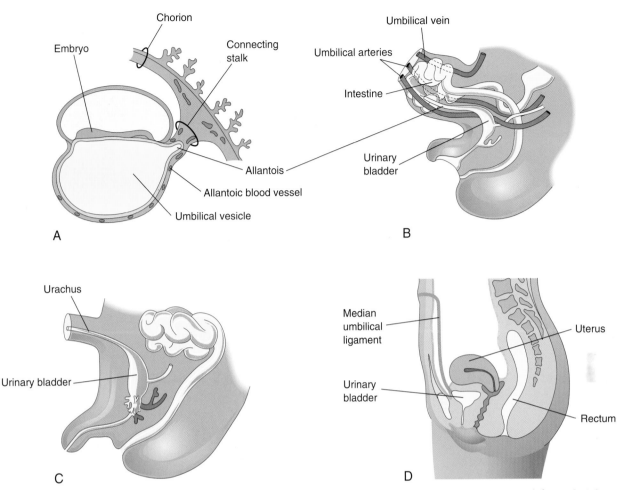

**FIGURE 7–22** Illustrations of development and usual fate of the allantois. **A,** A 3-week embryo. **B,** A 9-week fetus. **C,** A 3-month male fetus. **D,** Adult female. The nonfunctional allantois forms the urachus in the fetus and the median umbilical ligament in the adult.

**FIGURE 7–23** Sonogram of the umbilical cord of a 7-week embryo exhibiting an allantoic cyst *(at calipers)*.

influence. Studies in a Mormon population showed that the genotype of the mother affects the frequency of DZ twins but the genotype of the father has no effect. It has also been observed that if the firstborns are twins, a repetition of twinning or some other form of multiple birth is approximately five times more likely to occur with the next pregnancy than in the general population.

## Dizygotic Twins

Because they result from the fertilization of two oocytes, DZ twins develop from two zygotes and may be of the same sex or different sexes (see Fig. 7-24). For the same reason, they are no more alike genetically than brothers or sisters born at different times. The only thing they have in common is that they were in their mother's uterus at the same time. DZ twins always have two amnions and two chorions, but the chorions and placentas may be fused. *DZ twinning shows a hereditary tendency.* Recurrence in families is approximately three times that of the general population. The incidence of DZ twinning shows considerable racial variation, being approximately 1 in 500 in Asians, 1 in 125 in whites, and as high as 1 in 20 in some African populations.

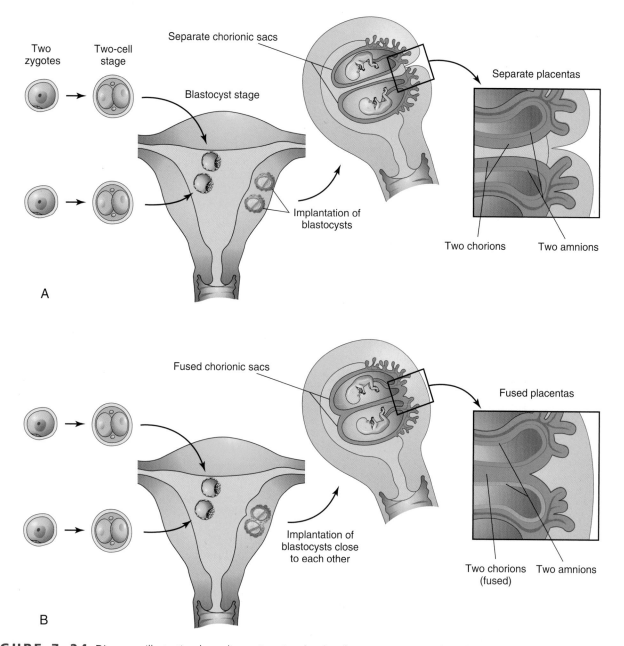

**FIGURE 7–24** Diagrams illustrating how dizygotic twins develop from two zygotes. The relationships of the fetal membranes and placentas are shown for instances in which the blastocysts implant separately (**A**) and the blastocysts implant close together (**B**). In both cases, there are two amnions and two chorions. The placentas are usually fused when they implant close together.

## ANASTOMOSIS OF PLACENTAL BLOOD VESSELS

Anastomoses between blood vessels of fused placentas of DZ twins may result in erythrocyte **mosaicism**. The members of these DZ twins have red blood cells of two different blood groups because red cells were exchanged between the circulations of the twins. In cases in which one fetus is a male and the other is a female, masculinization of the female fetus does not occur.

## Monozygotic Twins

Because they result from the fertilization of one oocyte and develop from one zygote (see Fig. 7-25), MZ twins are of the same sex, genetically identical, and very similar in physical appearance. Physical differences between MZ twins are caused by many factors (see the box titled Establishing the Zygosity of Twins) (Fig. 7-26). MZ twinning usually begins in the blastocyst stage, approximately at the end of the first week, and results from division of the embryoblast into two embryonic primordia. Subsequently, two embryos, each in its own amniotic sac, develop within the same chorionic sac and share a

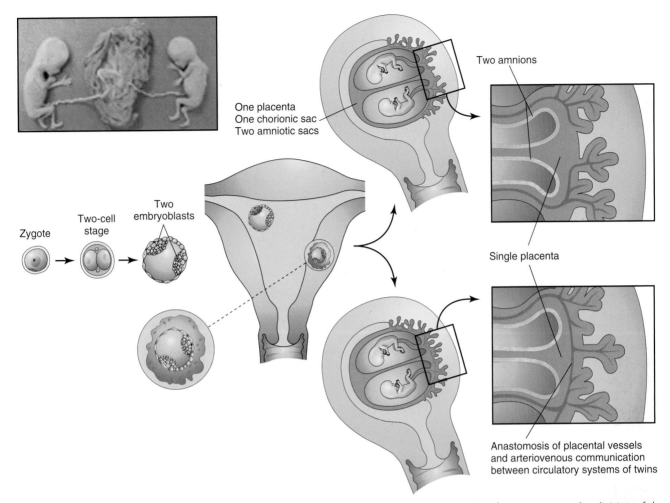

**FIGURE 7–25** Diagrams illustrating how approximately 65% of monozygotic twins develop from one zygote by division of the embryoblast of the blastocyst. These twins always have separate amnions, a single chorionic sac, and a common placenta. If there is anastomosis of the placental vessels, one twin may receive most of the nutrition from the placenta. *Inset,* Monozygotic twins, 17 weeks' gestation.

| Table 7–1 | Frequency of Types of Placentas and Fetal Membranes in Monozygotic (MZ) and Dizygotic (DZ) Twins | | | |
|---|---|---|---|---|
| | **SINGLE CHORION** | | **TWO CHORIONS** | |
| **ZYGOSITY** | **Single Amnion** | **Two Amnions** | **Fused Placentas*** | **Two Placentas** |
| MZ | Very rare | 65% | 25% | 10% |
| DZ | — | — | 40% | 60% |

Data from Thompson MW, McInnes RR, Willard HF: *Thompson and Thompson genetics in medicine*, ed 5, Philadelphia, 1991, Saunders.
*Results from secondary fusion after implantation.

common placenta, that is, a monochorionic–diamniotic twin placenta.

Uncommonly, early separation of embryonic blastomeres (e.g., during the two-cell to eight-cell stages) results in MZ twins with two amnions, two chorions, and two placentas that may or may not be fused (Fig. 7-27). In such cases, it is impossible to determine from the membranes alone whether the twins are MZ or DZ.

## Other Types of Multiple Births

**Triplets** may be derived from:

- One zygote and be identical
- Two zygotes and consist of identical twins and a singleton
- Three zygotes and be of the same sex or of different sexes

**FIGURE 7–26** A, Three-dimensional ultrasound scan of 6-week monochorionic–diamniotic discordant twins. The normal twin *(right)* is seen surrounded by the amniotic membrane and adjacent to the umbilical vesicle. The arms and legs can also be seen. The smaller fetus is also visible *(above left)*. B, Monozygotic–monochorionic–diamniotic twins showing a wide discrepancy in size resulting from an uncompensated arteriovenous anastomosis of placental vessels. Blood was shunted from the smaller twin to the larger one, producing the twin transfusion syndrome.

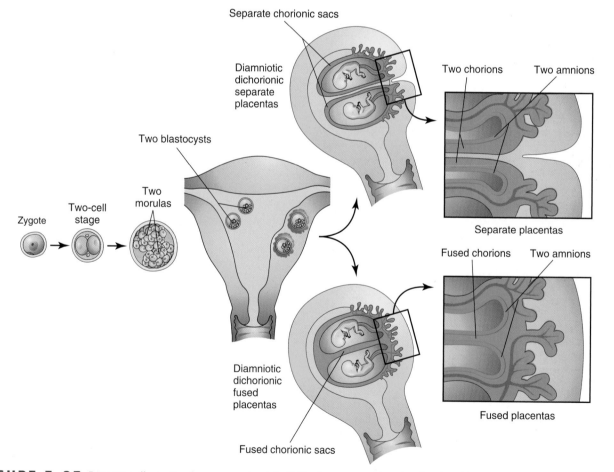

**FIGURE 7–27** Diagrams illustrating how approximately 35% of monozygotic twins develop from one zygote. Separation of the blastomeres may occur anywhere from the two-cell stage to the morula stage, producing two identical blastocysts. Each embryo subsequently develops its own amniotic and chorionic sacs. The placentas may be separate or fused. In 25% of cases, there is a single placenta resulting from secondary fusion, and in 10% of cases, there are two placentas. In the latter cases, examination of the placenta would suggest that the twins were dizygotic twins. This explains why some monozygotic twins are wrongly stated to be dizygotic twins at birth.

## TWIN TRANSFUSION SYNDROME

**Twin transfusion syndrome** occurs in as many as 10% to 15% of monochorionic–diamniotic MZ twins. There is shunting of arterial blood from one twin through **arteriovenous anastomoses** into the venous circulation of the other twin. The donor twin is small, pale, and anemic (see Fig. 7-26), whereas the recipient twin is large and has **polycythemia**, an increase above the normal in the number of red blood cells. The placenta shows similar abnormalities; the part of the placenta supplying the anemic twin is pale, whereas the part supplying the polycythemic twin is dark red. In lethal cases, death results from anemia in the donor twin and congestive heart failure in the recipient twin. Fetoscopic laser coagulation of placental vascular anastomoses is the established method of treatment of twin transfusion syndrome.

## ESTABLISHING THE ZYGOSITY OF TWINS

Establishing the zygosity of twins is important for clinical care as well as in tissue and organ transplantation (e.g., bone marrow transplantations). The determination of twin zygosity is now done by molecular diagnosis because any two people who are not MZ twins are virtually certain to show differences in some of the large number of DNA markers that can be studied.

Late division of early embryonic cells, such as division of the embryonic disc during the second week, results in MZ twins that are in one amniotic sac and one chorionic sac (Fig. 7-28A). A monochorionic–monoamniotic twin placenta is associated with fetal mortality rates that are higher by up to 10%, with the cause being cord entanglement. This compromises the circulation of blood through the umbilical vessels, leading to the death of one or both fetuses. Sonography plays an important role in the diagnosis and management of twin pregnancies (Fig. 7-29, and see Fig. 7-26A). Ultrasound evaluation is necessary to identify various conditions that may complicate MZ twinning, such as IUGR, fetal distress, and premature labor.

*MZ twins may be discordant for a variety of birth defects and genetic disorders*, despite their origin from the same zygote. In addition to environmental differences and chance variation, the following have been implicated:

- Mechanisms of embryologic development, such as vascular abnormalities, that can lead to discordance for anomalies
- Postzygotic changes, such as somatic mutation leading to discordance for cancer, or somatic rearrangement of immunoglobulin or T-cell–receptor genes
- Chromosome aberrations originating in one blastocyst after the twinning event
- Uneven X chromosome inactivation between female MZ twins, with the result that one twin preferentially expresses the paternal X and the other the maternal X

## EARLY DEATH OF A TWIN

Because ultrasonographic studies are a common part of prenatal care, it is known that early death and resorption of one member of a twin pair is common. Awareness of this possibility must be considered when discrepancies occur between prenatal cytogenetic findings and the karyotype of an infant. Errors in prenatal cytogenetic diagnosis may arise if extraembryonic tissues (e.g., part of a chorionic villus) from the resorbed twin are examined.

## CONJOINED MONOZYGOTIC TWINS

If the embryonic disc does not divide completely or adjacent embryonic discs fuse, various types of conjoined MZ twins may form (Figs. 7-30, 7-31, and 7-32, and see Fig. 7-28B and C). The twin phenotype is named according to the regions that are attached, for instance, **thoracopagus** indicates that there is anterior union of the thoracic regions. It has been estimated that the incidence of conjoined twins is 1 in 50,000 to 100,000 births. In some cases, the twins are connected to each other by skin only or by cutaneous and other tissues (see Fig. 7-31). Some conjoined twins can be successfully separated by surgical procedures (see Fig. 7-30B); however, the anatomic relations in many conjoined twins do not permit surgical separation with sustained viability (see Fig. 7-32).

## SUPERFECUNDATION

**Superfecundation** is the fertilization of two or more oocytes at different times. In humans, the presence of two fetuses in the uterus caused by fertilization at different times (**superfetation**) is rare. DZ human twins with different fathers have been confirmed by genetic markers.

In the last case, the infants are no more similar than infants from three separate pregnancies. Similar combinations occur in quadruplets, quintuplets, sextuplets, and septuplets.

## SUMMARY OF PLACENTA AND FETAL MEMBRANES

- The placenta consists of two parts: a larger fetal part derived from the villous chorion and a smaller maternal part developed from the decidua basalis. The two parts are held together by stem chorionic villi that attach to the cytotrophoblastic shell surrounding the

**FIGURE 7–28** Diagrams illustrating how some monozygotic twins develop. This method of development is very uncommon. Division of the embryonic disc results in two embryos within one amniotic sac. **A,** Complete division of the embryonic disc gives rise to twins. Such twins rarely survive because their umbilical cords are often so entangled that interruption of the blood supply to the fetuses occurs. **B** and **C,** Incomplete division of the embryonic disc results in various types of conjoined twins.

**FIGURE 7-29** Serial ultrasound scans of a dichorionic pregnancy. **A,** At 3 weeks' gestation. **B,** At 7 weeks' gestation.

chorionic sac, which attaches the sac to the decidua basalis.

● The principal activities of the placenta are metabolism (synthesis of glycogen, cholesterol, and fatty acids), respiratory gas exchange (oxygen, carbon dioxide, and carbon monoxide), transfer of nutrients (vitamins, hormones, and antibodies), elimination of waste products, and endocrine secretion (e.g., of hCG) for maintenance of pregnancy.

● The fetal circulation is separated from the maternal circulation by a thin layer of extrafetal tissues, the placental membrane. This permeable membrane allows water, oxygen, nutritive substances, hormones, and noxious agents to pass from the mother to the embryo/fetus. Excretory products pass through the placental membrane from the fetus to the mother.

● The fetal membranes and placentas in multiple pregnancies vary considerably, depending on the derivation of the embryos and the time when division of embryonic cells occurs. The common type of twins is DZ twins, with two amnions, two chorions, and two placentas that may or may not be fused.

● MZ twins, the less common type, represent approximately one third of all twins; they are derived from one zygote. MZ twins commonly have one chorion, two amnions, and one placenta. Twins with one

**FIGURE 7-30** **A,** Newborn monozygotic conjoined twins showing union in the thoracic regions (thoracopagus). **B,** The twins approximately 4 years after separation. *(From deVries PA: Case history: the San Francisco twins. In Bergsma D, editor: Birth defects original article series: conjoined twins, New York, 1967, Alan R. Liss for the National Foundation–March of Dimes, pp 141–142, with permission of the copyright holder.)*

**FIGURE 7–31** Parasitic twins, anterior view. Note the normal tone and posture of the fully developed host twin with meconium staining, exstrophy of the bladder in both host and parasitic twins, exposed small bowel in parasitic twin, and fully formed right lower limb with normal tone and flexion in the parasitic twin.

**FIGURE 7–32** Dicephalic (two heads) conjoined twins, alizarin stained, showing bone *(red)* and cartilage *(blue)*. Note the two clavicles supporting the midline upper limb, fused thoracic cage, and parallel vertebral columns.

amnion, one chorion, and one placenta are always monozygotic, and their umbilical cords are often entangled. Other types of multiple births (e.g., triplets) may be derived from one or more zygotes.

● The umbilical vesicle and allantois are vestigial structures; however, their presence is essential to normal embryonic development. Both are early sites of blood formation and both are partly incorporated into the embryo. Primordial germ cells also originate in the wall of the umbilical vesicle.

● The amnion forms an amniotic sac for amniotic fluid and provides a covering for the umbilical cord. The amniotic fluid has three main functions: to provide a protective buffer for the embryo/fetus, to allow room for fetal movements, and to assist in the regulation of fetal body temperature.

## NEONATAL PERIOD

The neonatal period pertains to the first four weeks after birth. The **early neonatal period** is from birth to 7 days. The **neonate** (newborn) is not a "miniature adult," and an extremely preterm infant is not the same as a full-term infant. The **late neonatal period** is from 7 to 28 days. The umbilical cord typically falls off 7 to 8 days after birth. The head of a neonate is large in proportion to the rest of its body, but thereafter, the head grows more slowly than the trunk (torso). Usually a neonate loses about 10% of its birth weight 3 to 4 days after birth, owing to the loss of excess extracellular fluid and the discharge of **meconium**, the first greenish intestinal discharges from the rectum.

When someone touches a neonate's hand, the baby will usually grasp a finger. If someone holds a baby close to his or her chest, the baby will search (root) for the breast to find the nipple. Similarly, a gentle stroke on the baby's cheek makes the baby turn toward the touch with its mouth open. Neonates quickly develop basic visual capacity, but this improves dramatically over the next 12 months as they prefer to look at faces. In some cases, the eyes of a neonate are crossed (**strabismus**) because the eye muscles are not yet fully developed, but this typically corrects itself within a few months.

## CLINICALLY ORIENTED PROBLEMS

*CASE 7–1*

*A physician told a pregnant woman that she had polyhydramnios.*

* If you were asked to explain the meaning of this clinical condition, what would be your answer?
* What conditions are often associated with polyhydramnios?
* Explain why polyhydramnios occurs and how it is identified.

### CASE 7–2

*A patient with a twin (dizygotic) sister asked her physician whether twinning runs in families.*

* Is maternal age a factor?
* Is there a difference in incidence of monozygotic and dizygotic twinning?

### CASE 7–3

*A pathologist noted that an umbilical cord had only one umbilical artery.*

* How often does this anomaly occur?
* What kind of birth defects might be associated with this condition?

### CASE 7–4

*An ultrasound examination revealed a twin pregnancy with a single placenta. Chorionic villus sampling and chromosome analysis revealed that the twins were likely female. At birth, the twins were of different sexes.*

* How could this error have occurred?

### CASE 7–5

*An ultrasound examination of a pregnant woman during the second trimester revealed multiple amniotic bands associated with the fetus.*

* What produces these bands?
* What birth defects may result from them?
* What is the syndrome called?

Discussion of these problems appears in the Appendix at the back of the book.

## BIBLIOGRAPHY AND SUGGESTED READING

Abuhamad AZ: Doppler ultrasound in obstetrics. In Callen PW, editor: *Ultrasonography in obstetrics and gynecology*, ed 5, Philadelphia, 2008, Saunders.

Alexander GR, Wingate MS, Salihu H, et al: Fetal and neonatal mortality risks of multiple births, *Obstet Gynecol Clin North Am* 32:1, 2005.

Banks CL: Labour. In Magowan BA, Owen P, Thomson A, editors: *Clinical obstetrics and gynaecology*, ed 3, Philadelphia, 2014, Saunders.

Baschatt AA: Fetal growth restriction: from observation to intervention, *J Perinat Med* 38:239, 2010.

Benirschke K, Kaufmann P: *Pathology of the human placenta*, ed 4, New York, 2000, Springer-Verlag.

Brémond-Gignac D, Copin H, Lapillonne A, et al: Visual development in infants: physiological and pathological mechanisms, *Curr Opin Ophthalmol* 22(Clinical Update 1):S1, 2011.

Callen PW: The role of amniotic fluid volume in fetal health and disease. In Callen PW, editor: *Ultrasonography in obstetrics and gynecology*, ed 5, Philadelphia, 2008, Saunders.

Chauhan SP, Scardo JA, Hayes E, et al: Twins: prevalence, problems, and preterm births, *Am J Obstet Gynecol* 203:305, 2010.

Collins JH: Umbilical cord accidents: human studies, *Semin Perinatol* 26:79, 2002.

Cross JC: Formation of the placenta and extraembryonic membranes, *Ann N Y Acad Sci* 857:23, 1998.

Cunningham FG, Leveno KJ, Bloom SL, et al, editors: *Williams' obstetrics*, ed 24, New York, 2014, McGraw-Hill.

D'Antonio F, Bhide A: Ultrasound in placental disorders, *Best Pract Res Clin Obstet Gynaecol* 2014. doi:10.1016/j.bpobgyn.2014.01.001.

Egan JFX, Borgida AF: Ultrasound evaluation of multiple pregnancies. In Callen PW, editor: *Ultrasonography in obstetrics and gynecology*, ed 5, Philadelphia, 2008, Saunders.

Feldstein VA, Harris RD, Machin GA: Ultrasound evaluation of the placenta and umbilical cord. In Callen PW, editor: *Ultrasonography in obstetrics and gynecology*, ed 5, Philadelphia, 2008, Saunders.

Fodor A, Tímár J, Zelena D: Behavioral effects of perinatal opioid exposure, *Life Sci* 104:1, 2014.

Forbes K: IFPA Gabor Than Award lecture: molecular control of placental growth: the emerging role of microRNAs, *Placenta* 34(Suppl):S27–S33, 2013.

Gibson J: Multiple pregnancy. In Magowan BA, Owen P, Thomson A, editors: *Clinical obstetrics and gynaecology*, ed 3, Philadelphia, 2014, Saunders.

Jabrane-Ferrat N, Siewiera J: The up side of decidual natural killer cells: new developments in immunology of pregnancy, *Immunology* 141:490, 2014.

James JL, Whitley GS, Cartwright JE: Pre-eclampsia: fitting together the placental, immune and cardiovascular pieces, *J Pathol* 221:363, 2010.

Kazandi M: Conservative and surgical treatment of abnormal placentation: report of five cases and review of the literature, *Clin Exp Obstet Gynecol* 37:310, 2010.

Knöfler M, Pollheimer J: Human placental trophoblast invasion and differentiation: a particular focus on Wnt signaling, *Front Genet* 4:190, 2013.

Laing FC, Frates MC, Benson CB: Ultrasound evaluation during the first trimester. In Callen PW, editor: *Ultrasonography in obstetrics and gynecology*, ed 5, Philadelphia, 2008, Saunders.

Lala N, Girish GV, Cloutier-Bosworth A, et al: Mechanisms in decorin regulation of vascular endothelial growth factor-induced human trophoblast migration and acquisition of endothelial phenotype, *Biol Reprod* 87:59, 2012.

Lala PK, Chatterjee-Hasrouni S, Kearns M, et al: Immunobiology of the feto-maternal interface, *Immunol Rev* 75:87, 1983.

Lala PK, Kearns M, Colavincenzo V: Cells of the fetomaternal interface: their role in the maintenance of viviparous pregnancy, *Am J Anat* 170:501, 1984.

Lurain JR: Gestational trophoblastic disease I: epidemiology, pathology, clinical presentation and diagnosis of gestational trophoblastic disease, and management of hydatidiform mole, *Am J Obstet Gynecol* 203:531, 2010.

Masselli G, Gualdi G: MRI imaging of the placenta: what a radiologist should know, *Abdom Imaging J* 38:573, 2013.

Moore KL, Dalley AD, Agur AMR: *Clinically oriented anatomy*, ed 7, Baltimore, 2014, Williams and Wilkins.

Silasi M, Cohen B, Karumanchi SA, et al: Abnormal placentation, angiogenic factors, and the pathogenesis of preeclampsia, *Obstet Gynecol Clin North Am* 37:239, 2010.

Williams PJ, Mistry HD, Innes BA, et al: Expression of AT1R, AT2R and AT4R and their roles in extravillous trophoblast invasion in the human, *Placenta* 31:448, 2010.

# Body Cavities, Mesenteries, and Diaphragm

**E**arly in the fourth week of development, the **intraembryonic coelom** appears as a horseshoe-shaped cavity (Fig. 8-1A). The bend in the cavity at the cranial end of the embryo represents the future *pericardial cavity*, and its limbs (lateral extensions) indicate the future *pleural* and *peritoneal cavities*. The distal part of each limb of the intraembryonic coelom is continuous with the **extraembryonic coelom** at the lateral edges of the embryonic disc (see Fig. 8-1B). The intraembryonic coelom provides room for the organs to develop and move. For instance, it allows the normal herniation of the midgut into the umbilical cord (Fig. 8-2E; see Chapter 11, Fig. 11-14). During embryonic folding in the horizontal plane, the limbs of the coelom are brought together on the ventral aspect of the embryo (see Fig. 8-2C). The ventral mesentery degenerates in the region of the future peritoneal cavity (see Fig. 8-2F), resulting in a large embryonic **peritoneal cavity** extending from the heart to the pelvic region.

## EMBRYONIC BODY CAVITY

The intraembryonic coelom becomes the embryonic body cavity, which is divided into three well-defined cavities during the fourth week (Fig. 8-3; see Figs. 8-1A and 8-2):

- A pericardial cavity
- Two pericardioperitoneal canals
- A peritoneal cavity

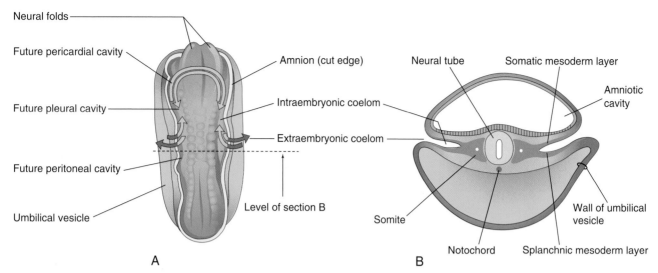

**FIGURE 8–1** A, Drawing of a dorsal view of a 22-day embryo shows the outline of the horseshoe-shaped intraembryonic coelom. The amnion has been removed, and the coelom is shown as if the embryo were translucent. The continuity of the coelom and the communication of its right and left limbs with the extraembryonic coelom are indicated by arrows. B, Transverse section through the embryo at the level shown in A.

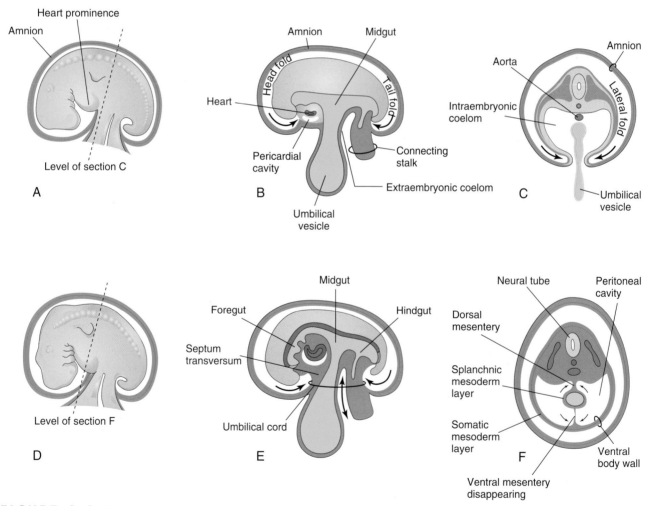

**FIGURE 8–2** Illustrations of embryonic folding and its effects on the intraembryonic coelom and other structures. A, Lateral view of an embryo (approximately 26 days). B, Schematic sagittal section of the same embryo shows the head and tail folds. C, Transverse section at the level shown in A indicates how fusion of the lateral folds gives the embryo a cylindrical form. D, Lateral view of an embryo (at approximately 28 days). E, Schematic sagittal section of the same embryo shows the reduced communication between the intraembryonic and extraembryonic coeloms (*double-headed arrow*). F, Transverse section at the level shown in D illustrates formation of the ventral body wall and disappearance of the ventral mesentery. The *arrows* indicate the junction of the somatic and splanchnic layers of mesoderm. The somatic mesoderm will form the parietal peritoneum lining the abdominal wall, and the splanchnic mesoderm will form the visceral peritoneum covering the organs (e.g., the stomach).

**FIGURE 8−3** Illustrations of the mesenteries and body cavities at the beginning of the fifth week of development. **A,** Schematic sagittal section. Notice that the dorsal mesentery serves as a pathway for the arteries supplying the developing midgut. Nerves and lymphatics also pass between the layers of this mesentery. **B to E,** Transverse sections through the embryo at the levels indicated in **A.** The ventral mesentery disappears, except in the region of the terminal esophagus, stomach, and first part of the duodenum. Notice that the right and left parts of the peritoneal cavity separate in **C** but are continuous in **E.**

These cavities have a parietal wall, lined by mesothelium (future parietal layer of peritoneum), that is derived from somatic mesoderm and a visceral wall, also covered by mesothelium (future visceral layer of peritoneum), that is derived from splanchnic mesoderm (see Fig. 8-3E). The **peritoneal cavity** is connected with the extraembryonic coelom at the umbilicus (Fig. 8-4A and D). The cavity loses its connection with the extraembryonic coelom during the 11th week of gestation as the intestines return to the abdomen from the umbilical cord (see Chapter 11, Fig. 11-13C).

During formation of the head fold, the **heart** and **pericardial cavity** are relocated ventrally, anterior to the foregut (see Fig. 8-2B). As a result, the pericardial cavity opens into **pericardioperitoneal canals**, which pass dorsal to the foregut (see Fig. 8-4B and D). After embryonic folding, the caudal part of the foregut, midgut, and hindgut are suspended in the peritoneal cavity from the dorsal abdominal wall by the **dorsal mesentery** (see Figs. 8-2F and 8-3B, D, and E).

## Mesenteries

A **mesentery** is a double layer of peritoneum that begins as an extension of the visceral peritoneum covering an organ. The mesentery connects the organ to the body wall and conveys vessels and nerves to it. Transiently, the **dorsal and ventral mesenteries** divide the peritoneal cavity into right and left halves (see Fig. 8-3C). The ventral mesentery soon disappears (see Fig. 8-3E), except where it is attached to the caudal part of the foregut (primordium of stomach and proximal part of duodenum). The peritoneal cavity then becomes a continuous space (see Fig. 8-4D). The arteries supplying the primordial gut—celiac arterial trunk (foregut), superior mesenteric artery (midgut), and inferior mesenteric artery (hindgut)—pass between the layers of the dorsal mesentery (see Fig. 8-3C).

## Division of Embryonic Body Cavity

Each pericardioperitoneal canal lies lateral to the proximal part of the foregut (future esophagus) and dorsal to

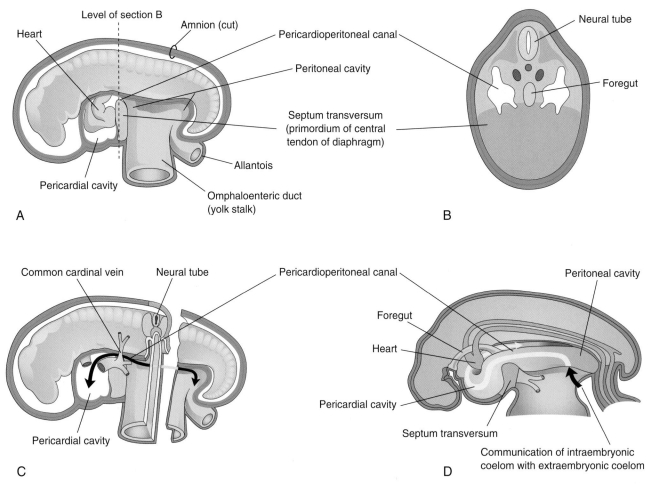

**FIGURE 8–4** Schematic drawings of an embryo (at approximately 24 days). **A**, The lateral wall of the pericardial cavity has been removed to show the primordial heart. **B**, Transverse section of the embryo illustrates the relationship of the pericardioperitoneal canals to the septum transversum (primordium of central tendon of diaphragm) and the foregut. **C**, Lateral view of the embryo with heart removed. The embryo has also been sectioned transversely to show the continuity of the intraembryonic and extraembryonic coeloms (*arrow*). **D**, Sketch shows the pericardioperitoneal canals arising from the dorsal wall of the pericardial cavity and passing on each side of the foregut to join the peritoneal cavity. The *arrow* shows the communication of the extraembryonic coelom with the intraembryonic coelom and the continuity of the intraembryonic coelom at this stage.

**FIGURE 8–5** Drawings of transverse sections through embryos cranial to the septum transversum illustrate successive stages in the separation of the pleural cavities from the pericardial cavity. Growth and development of the lungs, expansion of the pleural cavities, and formation of fibrous pericardium are also shown. **A,** At 5 weeks. The arrows indicate the communications between the pericardioperitoneal canals and the pericardial cavity. **B,** At 6 weeks. The *arrows* indicate development of the pleural cavities as they expand into the body wall. **C,** At 7 weeks. Expansion of the pleural cavities ventrally around the heart is shown. The pleuropericardial membranes are now fused in the median plane and with the mesoderm ventral to the esophagus. **D,** At 8 weeks. Continued expansion of the lungs and pleural cavities and formation of the fibrous pericardium and thoracic wall are illustrated.

the **septum transversum**—a plate of mesodermal tissue that occupies the space between the thoracic cavity and the omphaloenteric duct (see Fig. 8-4A and B).

*The septum transversum is the primordium of the central tendon of the diaphragm.* Partitions form in each pericardioperitoneal canal separating the pericardial cavity from the pleural cavities and the pleural cavities from the peritoneal cavity. Because of the growth of the **bronchial buds** (primordia of bronchi and lungs) into the **pericardioperitoneal canals**, a pair of membranous ridges is produced in the lateral wall of each canal (Fig. 8-5A and B):

- The cranial ridges—*pleuropericardial folds*—are located superior to the developing lungs.
- The caudal ridges—*pleuroperitoneal folds*—are located inferior to the lungs.

### Pleuropericardial Membranes

As the pleuropericardial folds enlarge, they form partitions that separate the pericardial cavity from the

## CONGENITAL PERICARDIAL DEFECT

Defective formation and/or fusion of the pleuropericardial membranes separating the pericardial and pleural cavities is uncommon. This anomaly results in a congenital defect of the pericardium, usually asymptomatic and on the left side. Consequently, the pericardial cavity communicates with the pleural cavity. In very unusual cases, a part of the left atrium of the heart herniates into the pleural cavity at each heartbeat.

pleural cavities. These partitions—the **pleuropericardial membranes**—contain the common cardinal veins (see Figs. 8-4C and 8-5A), which drain the venous system into the sinus venosus of the heart. Initially, the **bronchial buds** are small relative to the heart and pericardial cavity (see Fig. 8-5A). They soon grow laterally from the caudal end of the trachea into the **pericardioperitoneal canals** (future pleural canals). As the primordial pleural cavities expand ventrally around the heart, they extend into the body wall, splitting the mesenchyme into

- An outer layer that becomes the thoracic wall
- An inner layer that becomes the fibrous pericardium, the outer layer of the pericardial sac enclosing the heart (see Fig. 8-5C and D)

The pleuropericardial membranes project into the cranial ends of the pericardioperitoneal canals (see Fig. 8-5B). With subsequent growth of the common cardinal veins, positional displacement of the heart, and expansion of the pleural cavities, the membranes become mesentery-like folds extending from the lateral thoracic wall. By the seventh week, the membranes fuse with the mesenchyme ventral to the esophagus, separating the pericardial cavity from the pleural cavities (see Fig. 8-5C). This **primordial mediastinum** consists of a mass of mesenchyme that extends from the sternum to the vertebral column, separating the developing lungs (see Fig. 8-5D). The right pleuropericardial opening closes slightly earlier than the left one and produces a larger pleuropericardial membrane.

### Pleuroperitoneal Membranes

As the pleuroperitoneal folds enlarge, they project into the pericardioperitoneal canals. Gradually the folds become membranous, forming the **pleuroperitoneal membranes** (Fig. 8-6 and Fig. 8-7). Eventually, these membranes separate the pleural cavities from the peritoneal cavity. The pleuroperitoneal membranes are produced as the developing lungs and pleural cavities expand and invade the body wall. They are attached dorsolaterally to the abdominal wall, and initially their crescentic free edges project into the caudal ends of the **pericardioperitoneal canals**.

During the sixth week of gestation, the pleuroperitoneal membranes extend ventromedially until their free edges fuse with the dorsal mesentery of the esophagus and septum transversum (see Fig. 8-7C). This separates the pleural cavities from the peritoneal cavity. Closure of the pleuroperitoneal openings is completed by the migration of **myoblasts** (primordial muscle cells) into the pleuroperitoneal membranes (see Fig. 8-7E). The pleuroperitoneal opening on the right side closes slightly before the left one. The reason for this is uncertain, but it may be related to the relatively large size of the right lobe of the liver at this stage of development.

### ▶ DEVELOPMENT OF DIAPHRAGM

6   The diaphragm is a dome-shaped, musculotendinous partition that separates the thoracic and abdominal cavities. It is a composite structure that develops from four embryonic components (see Fig. 8-7):

- Septum transversum
- Pleuroperitoneal membranes
- Dorsal mesentery of esophagus
- Muscular ingrowth from lateral body walls

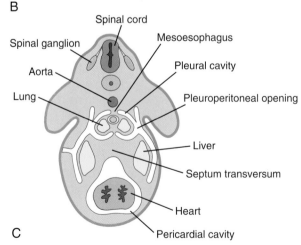

**FIGURE 8–6** A, The primordial body cavities are viewed from the left side after removal of the lateral body wall. B, Photograph of a 5-week-old embryo shows the developing septum transversum (*arrow*), heart tube (*H*), and liver (*L*). C, Transverse section through an embryo at the level shown in A.

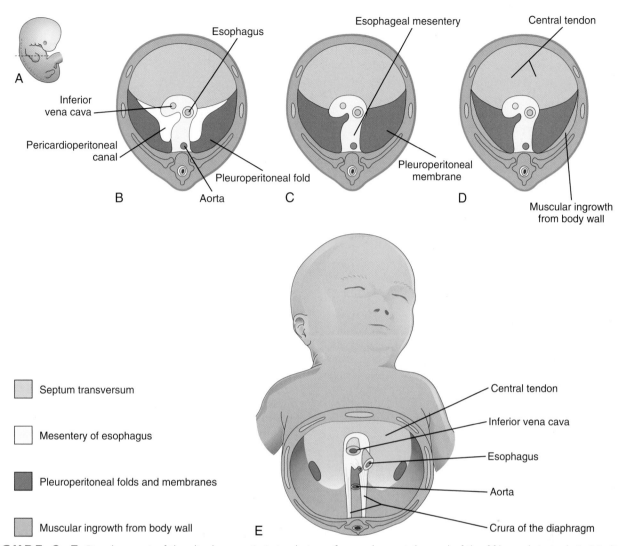

**FIGURE 8–7** Development of the diaphragm. **A,** Lateral view of an embryo at the end of the fifth week (actual size) indicates the level of sections B to D. **B,** Transverse section shows the unfused pleuroperitoneal membranes. **C,** Similar section at the end of the sixth week after fusion of the pleuroperitoneal membranes with the other two diaphragmatic components. **D,** Transverse section of a 12-week fetus after ingrowth of the fourth diaphragmatic component from the body wall. **E,** Inferior view of the diaphragm of a neonate indicates the embryologic origin of its components.

*Several candidate genes on the long arm of chromosome 15 (15q) play a critical role in the development of the diaphragm.*

## Septum Transversum

The transverse septum grows dorsally from the ventro-lateral body wall and forms a semicircular shelf that separates the heart from the liver (see Fig. 8-6A). This septum, which is composed of mesodermal tissue, forms the **central tendon of diaphragm** (see Fig. 8-7D and E). After the head folds ventrally during the fourth week, the septum forms a thick, incomplete connective tissue partition between the pericardial and abdominal cavities (see Fig. 8-4). The septum does not completely separate the thoracic and abdominal cavities.

During early development, a large part of the liver is embedded in the septum transversum. There are large openings, the **pericardioperitoneal canals**, along the sides of the esophagus (see Fig. 8-7B). The septum expands and fuses with the dorsal mesentery of the esophagus and pleuroperitoneal membranes (see Fig. 8-7C).

## Pleuroperitoneal Membranes

The pleuroperitoneal membranes fuse with the dorsal mesentery of the esophagus and the septum transversum (see Fig. 8-7C). This completes the partition between the thoracic and abdominal cavities and forms the **primordial diaphragm**. Although the pleuroperitoneal membranes form large portions of the early fetal diaphragm, they represent relatively small portions of the neonate's diaphragm (see Fig. 8-7E).

## Dorsal Mesentery of Esophagus

The septum transversum and pleuroperitoneal membranes fuse with the dorsal mesentery of the esophagus.

This mesentery constitutes the median portion of the diaphragm. The **crura of the diaphragm**, a leg-like pair of diverging muscle bundles that cross in the median plane anterior to the aorta (see Fig. 8-7E), develop from myoblasts that grow into the dorsal mesentery of the esophagus.

## Muscular Ingrowth from Lateral Body Walls

During the 9th to 12th weeks, the lungs and pleural cavities enlarge, burrowing into the lateral body walls (see Fig. 8-5). During this process, the body-wall tissue is split into two layers:

- An external layer that becomes part of the definitive abdominal wall
- An internal layer that contributes to peripheral parts of the diaphragm, external to the parts derived from the pleuroperitoneal membranes (see Fig. 8-7D and E)

Further extension of the developing **pleural cavities** into the lateral body walls forms the **costodiaphragmatic recesses** (Fig. 8-8A and B), establishing the characteristic dome-shaped configuration of the diaphragm. After birth, the costodiaphragmatic recesses become alternately smaller and larger as the lungs move in and out during inspiration and expiration.

## Positional Changes and Innervation of Diaphragm

During the fourth week of gestation, the septum transversum, before relocation of the heart, lies opposite the third to fifth cervical somites. During the fifth week, myoblasts from the somites migrate into the developing diaphragm, bringing their nerve fibers with them. Consequently, the **phrenic nerves** that supply motor innervation to the diaphragm arise from the ventral primary rami of the third, fourth, and fifth cervical spinal nerves (see Fig. 8-5A and C). The three twigs on each side join to form a phrenic nerve. The phrenic nerves also supply sensory fibers to the superior and inferior surfaces of the right and left domes of the diaphragm.

Rapid growth of the dorsal part of the embryo's body results in an apparent descent of the diaphragm. By the

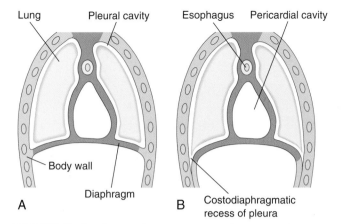

Lung    Pleural cavity          Esophagus    Pericardial cavity

Body wall

Diaphragm

A

Costodiaphragmatic recess of pleura

B

**FIGURE 8–8** A and B, Extensions of the pleural cavities into the body walls form peripheral parts of the diaphragm and costodiaphragmatic recesses and establish the characteristic dome-shaped configuration of the diaphragm. Notice that body-wall tissue is added peripherally to the diaphragm as the lungs and pleural cavities enlarge.

sixth week, the diaphragm is at the level of the thoracic somites. The **phrenic nerves** now have a descending course. As the diaphragm appears relatively farther caudally in the body, the nerves are correspondingly lengthened. By the beginning of the eighth week, the dorsal part of the diaphragm lies at the level of the first lumbar vertebra. Because of the cervical origin of the phrenic nerves, they are approximately 30 cm long in adults.

The phrenic nerves in the embryo enter the diaphragm by passing through the pleuropericardial membranes. This explains why the phrenic nerves subsequently lie on the fibrous pericardium, the adult derivative of the pleuropericardial membranes (see Fig. 8-5C and D).

As the four parts of the diaphragm fuse (see Fig. 8-7), mesenchyme in the septum transversum extends into the other three parts. It forms myoblasts that differentiate into the skeletal muscle of the diaphragm. The costal border receives sensory fibers from the lower intercostal nerves because of the origin of the peripheral part of the diaphragm from the lateral body walls (see Fig. 8-7D and E).

## POSTEROLATERAL DEFECT OF DIAPHRAGM

The only relatively common birth defect of the diaphragm is a posterolateral defect (Fig. 8-9A and B and Fig. 8-10), which occurs in about 1 in 2200 neonates. It is associated with **congenital diaphragmatic hernia (CDH)**, which leads to herniation of abdominal contents into the thoracic cavity.

Life-threatening breathing difficulties may be associated with CDH because of inhibition of development and inflation of the lungs (Fig. 8-11). Moreover, fetal lung maturation may be delayed. **Polyhydramnios** (excess amniotic fluid)

may also be present. *CDH is the most common cause of pulmonary hypoplasia. The candidate gene region for CDH has been reported to be a chromosome 15q26 gene mutation that includes zinc finger formation (GATA6).*

CDH, usually unilateral, results from defective formation and/or fusion of the pleuroperitoneal membranes with the other three parts of the diaphragm (see Fig. 8-7). This results in a large opening in the posterolateral region of the diaphragm. As a result, the peritoneal and pleural cavities are continuous with one another along the posterior body

## POSTEROLATERAL DEFECT OF DIAPHRAGM—cont'd

wall. This birth defect (sometimes referred to as the *foramen of Bochdalek*) occurs on the left side in 85% to 90% of cases. The preponderance of left-sided defects may be related to the earlier closure of the right pleuroperitoneal opening. Prenatal diagnosis of CDH depends on ultrasound examination and magnetic resonance imaging of abdominal organs in the thorax.

The pleuroperitoneal membranes normally fuse with the other three diaphragmatic components by the end of the sixth week of gestation (see Fig. 8-7*C*). If a pleuroperitoneal canal is still open when the intestines return to the abdomen from the physiologic hernia of the umbilical cord in the 10th week, some of the intestines and other viscera may pass into the thorax. The presence of abdominal viscera in the thorax pushes the lungs and heart anteriorly and compresses the lungs. Often, the stomach, spleen, and most of the intestines herniate (see Fig. 8-11). Mortality in cases of CDH results not because there is a defect in the diaphragm or that abdominal viscera are in the chest but because the lungs are hypoplastic due to compression during development.

The severity of pulmonary developmental abnormalities depends on when and to what extent the abdominal viscera herniate into the thorax (i.e., the timing and degree of compression of the fetal lungs). The effect on the ipsilateral (same-side) lung is greater, but the contralateral lung also shows morphologic changes. If the abdominal viscera are in the thoracic cavity at birth, the initiation of respiration is likely to be impaired. The intestines dilate, and this compromises the functioning of the heart and lungs. Because the abdominal organs are most often in the left side of the thorax, the heart and mediastinum are usually displaced to the right.

The lungs in infants with CDH are often hypoplastic. The growth retardation of the lungs results from the lack of room for them to develop normally. Further complicating the neonatal course is the associated pulmonary hypertension resulting from decreased vascular cross-sectional area. Hypoxia may also trigger pulmonary vasoconstriction, which in some cases may be reversible with inhaled nitric oxide, a potent pulmonary vasodilator. The lungs often become aerated and achieve their normal size after reduction (repositioning) of the herniated viscera and repair of the defect in the diaphragm. Prenatal detection of CDH occurs in about 50% of cases. Most infants with CDH now survive because of improvements in ventilator care.

## EVENTRATION OF DIAPHRAGM

In eventration of the diaphragm, an uncommon condition, half of the diaphragm has defective musculature and balloons into the thoracic cavity as an aponeurotic (membranous) sheet, forming a **diaphragmatic pouch** (see Fig. 8-9*C* and *D*). The abdominal viscera are displaced superiorly into the pocket-like outpouching of the diaphragm. This defect results mainly from failure of muscular tissue from the body wall to extend into the pleuroperitoneal membrane on the affected side.

Eventration of the diaphragm is not a true diaphragmatic herniation; it is a superior displacement of viscera into a sac-like part of the diaphragm. However, the clinical manifestations of diaphragmatic eventration may simulate CDH.

## GASTROSCHISIS AND CONGENITAL EPIGASTRIC HERNIA

Gastroschisis is a congenital fissure in the anterior abdominal wall that occurs in approximately 1 in 3000 live births. Usually, there is protrusion of viscera. The site of the abdominal defect is to the right of the umbilical cord rather than truly in the midline. This defect differs from an umbilical hernia (see Chapter 11) in that the bowel is uncovered and floating in the amniotic fluid. Although it is not a true covering, an inflammatory peel may form secondary to exposure of the bowel to amniotic fluid. If this is present, the bowel at birth appears to be covered in a membrane, and the individual loops are not easily discernible. This defect is usually detected prenatally with routine ultrasound examination.

Congenital epigastric hernia, on the other hand, is found in the midline as a bulging of the abdominal wall located between the xiphoid process and the umbilicus. The bowel is not exposed to the amniotic fluid because it remains covered by skin and subcutaneous tissues.

Gastroschisis and epigastric hernias result from failure of the lateral body folds to fuse completely when the anterior abdominal wall forms during the fourth week of gestation (see Fig. 8-2*C* and *F*).

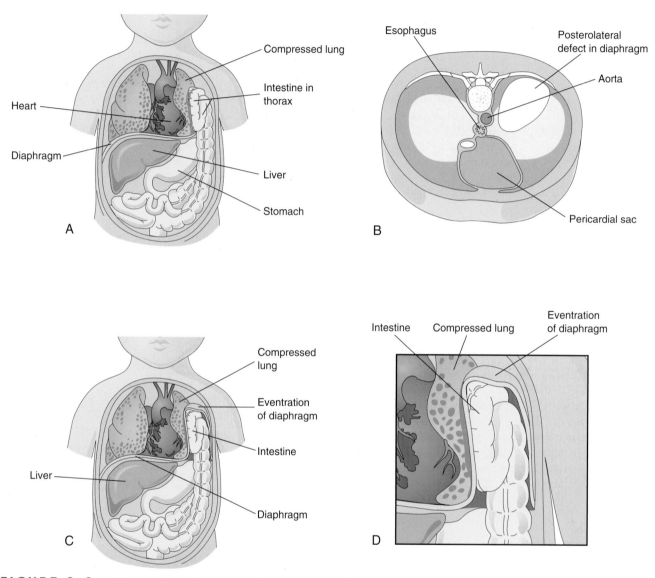

**FIGURE 8-9** A, Diagram shows herniation of the intestine into the thorax through a posterolateral defect in the left side of the diaphragm. Notice that the left lung is compressed and hypoplastic. B, Drawing of a diaphragm with a large posterolateral defect on the left side due to abnormal formation and/or abnormal fusion of the pleuroperitoneal membrane on the left side with the meso-esophagus and septum transversum. C and D, Eventration of the diaphragm resulting from defective muscular development of the diaphragm. The abdominal viscera are displaced in the thorax within a pouch of diaphragmatic tissue.

## CONGENITAL HIATAL HERNIA

Herniation of part of the fetal stomach may occur through an excessively large **esophageal hiatus**—the opening in the diaphragm through which the esophagus and the vagus nerves pass. A **hiatal hernia** is usually acquired during adult life; a congenitally enlarged esophageal hiatus may be the predisposing factor in some cases.

## RETROSTERNAL (PARASTERNAL) HERNIA

Herniations may occur through the **sternocostal hiatus** (also called foramen of Morgagni)—the opening for the superior epigastric vessels in the retrosternal area. However, they are uncommon. This hiatus is located between the sternal and costal parts of the diaphragm. Herniation of intestine into the pericardial sac may occur, or, conversely, part of the heart may descend into the peritoneal cavity in the epigastric region. Large defects are commonly associated with body-wall defects in the umbilical region. Radiologists and pathologists often observe fatty herniations through the sternocostal hiatus; however, they are usually of no clinical significance.

## ACCESSORY DIAPHRAGM

More than 30 cases of this rare anomaly known as accessory diaphragm have been reported. It is most often on the right side and associated with lung hypoplasia and other respiratory complications. An accessory diaphragm can be diagnosed by magnetic resonance imaging or computed tomography. It is treated by surgical excision.

## SUMMARY OF DEVELOPMENT OF BODY CAVITIES, MESENTERIES, AND DIAPHRAGM

- The **intraembryonic coelom** begins to develop near the end of the third week. By the fourth week, it is a horseshoe-shaped cavity in the cardiogenic and lateral mesoderm. The bend in the cavity represents the future pericardial cavity, and its lateral extensions represent the future pleural and peritoneal cavities.
- During folding of the embryonic disc in the fourth week (see Chapter 5, Fig. 5-1*B*), lateral parts of the intraembryonic coelom move together on the ventral aspect of the embryo. When the caudal part of the ventral mesentery disappears, the right and left parts of the intraembryonic coelom merge to form the **peritoneal cavity**.

**FIGURE 8–10** Coronal magnetic resonance image of a fetus with right-sided congenital diaphragmatic hernia. Notice the liver (*L*) and loops of small intestine (*arrowheads*) in the thoracic cavity. Ascites is present (*asterisks*), with accumulation of serous fluid in the peritoneal cavity and extending into the thoracic cavity. *Arrows* indicate abnormal skin thickening.

- As peritoneal parts of the intraembryonic coelom come together, the splanchnic layer of mesoderm encloses the primordial gut and suspends it from the dorsal body wall by a double-layered peritoneal membrane, the **dorsal mesentery**.
- The parts of the parietal layer of mesoderm lining the peritoneal, pleural, and pericardial cavities become the parietal peritoneum, parietal pleura, and serous pericardium, respectively.
- By the seventh week, the embryonic pericardial cavity communicates with the peritoneal cavity through paired **pericardioperitoneal canals**. During the fifth and sixth weeks, folds (later to become membranes) form near the cranial and caudal ends of the canals.
- Fusion of the cranial pleuropericardial membranes with mesoderm ventral to the esophagus separates the **pericardial cavity** from the **pleural cavities**. Fusion of the caudal pleuroperitoneal membranes during formation of the diaphragm separates the pleural cavities from the peritoneal cavity.
- The diaphragm develops from the septum transversum, mesentery of the esophagus, pleuroperitoneal folds and membranes, and muscular outgrowth from the body wall.
- The diaphragm divides the body cavity into thoracic and peritoneal cavities.
- A birth defect (opening) in the pleuroperitoneal membrane on the left side becomes a CDH.

**FIGURE 8–11** Diaphragmatic hernia on the left side of a female fetus (19 to 20 weeks) with herniation of liver (**A**), stomach, and bowel (**B**), underneath the liver into left thoracic cavity. Notice the pulmonary hypoplasia visible after liver removal. **C,** Diaphragmatic hernia (posterolateral defect). Chest radiograph of a neonate shows herniation of intestinal loops (*I*) into the left side of the thorax. Notice that the heart (*H*) is displaced to the right side and that the stomach (*S*) is on the left side of the upper abdominal cavity.

# CLINICALLY ORIENTED PROBLEMS

## CASE 8–1

*A neonate had severe respiratory distress. The abdomen was unusually flat, and intestinal peristaltic movements were heard over the left side of the thorax.*

* What birth defect do you think this is?
* Explain the basis of the signs described.
* How would the diagnosis likely be established?

## CASE 8–2

*An ultrasound scan of an infant's thorax revealed intestine in the pericardial sac.*

* What birth defect could result in herniation of intestine into the pericardial cavity?
* What is the embryologic basis of this defect?

## CASE 8–3

*CDH was diagnosed prenatally during an ultrasound examination.*

* How common is a posterolateral defect of the diaphragm?
* How do you think a neonate in whom this diagnosis is suspected should be positioned?
* Why would this positional treatment be given?
* Briefly describe surgical repair of a CDH.

## CASE 8–4

*A baby was born with a hernia in the median plane, between the xiphoid process and the umbilicus.*

* What is this type of hernia called?
* Is it common?
* What is the embryologic basis of this birth defect?

Discussion of these problems appears in the Appendix at the back of the book.

## BIBLIOGRAPHY AND SUGGESTED READING

Badillo A, Gingalewski C: Congenital diaphragmatic hernia: treatment and outcome, *Semin Perinatol* 38:92, 2014.

Clugston RD, Greer JJ: Diaphragmatic development and congenital diaphragmatic hernia, *Semin Pediatr Surg* 16:94, 2007.

Groth SS, Andrade RS: Diaphragmatic eventration, *Thorac Surg Clin* 19:511, 2009.

Hayashi S, Fukuzawa Y, Rodríguez-Vázquez JF, et al: Pleuroperitoneal canal closure and the fetal adrenal gland, *Anat Rec* 294:633, 2011.

Hedrick HL: Management of prenatally diagnosed congenital diaphragmatic hernia, *Semin Pediatr Surg* 22:37, 2013.

Mayer S, Metzger R, Kluth D: The embryology of the diaphragm, *Semin Pediatr Surg* 20:161, 2011.

Merrell AJ, Kardon G: Development of the diaphragm—a skeletal muscle essential for mammalian respiration, *FEBS J* 280:4026, 2013.

Moore KL, Dalley AF, Agur AMR: *Clinically oriented anatomy*, ed 7, Baltimore, 2014, Williams & Wilkins.

Wells LJ: Development of the human diaphragm and pleural sacs, *Contrib Embryol* 35:107, 1954.

Yu L, Bennett JT, Wynn J, et al: Whole exome sequencing identifies de novo mutations in GATA6 associated with congenital diaphragmatic hernia, *J Med Genet* 51:197, 2014.

# Pharyngeal Apparatus, Face, and Neck

T he **pharyngeal apparatus** consists of pharyngeal arches, pouches, grooves, and membranes (Fig. 9-1). These early embryonic structures contribute to the formation of the face and neck.

## PHARYNGEAL ARCHES

The pharyngeal arches begin to develop early in the fourth week as **neural crest cells** migrate into the future head and neck regions (see Chapter 5, Fig. 5-5). *Sonic hedgehog signaling plays an important role in the formation of the first pharyngeal arches.* The first pair of arches, the **primordial jaws**, appears as surface elevations lateral to the developing pharynx (see Fig. 9-1A and B). Other arches soon appear as ridges on each side of the future head and neck regions (see Fig. 9-1C and D). By the end of the fourth week, four pairs of arches are visible externally (see Fig. 9-1D). The fifth and sixth arches are rudimentary and are not visible on the surface of the embryo.

The pharyngeal arches are separated by pharyngeal grooves (clefts). Like the arches, the grooves are numbered in a craniocaudal sequence (see Fig. 9-1D). The **first arch** separates into the maxillary and mandibular prominences (Fig. 9-2; see Fig. 9-1E). The **maxillary**

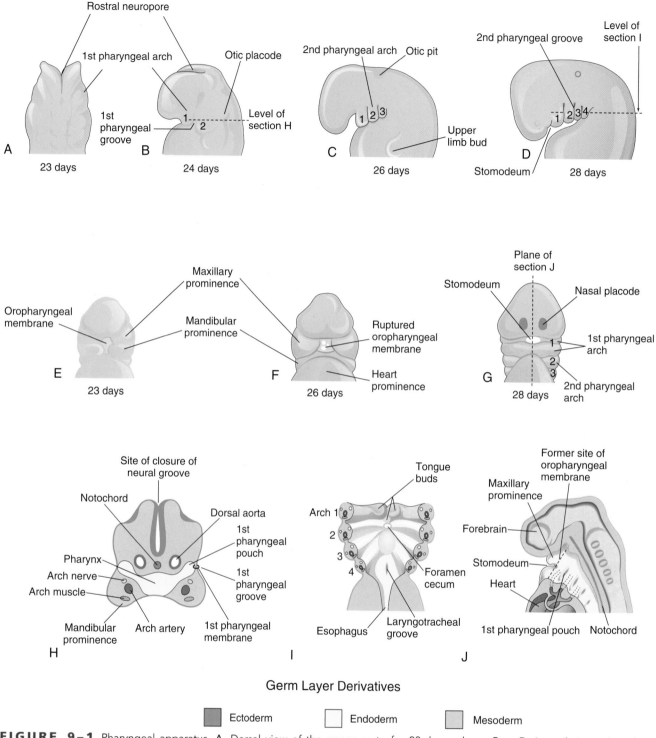

Germ Layer Derivatives

☐ Ectoderm   ☐ Endoderm   ☐ Mesoderm

**FIGURE 9–1** Pharyngeal apparatus. **A,** Dorsal view of the upper part of a 23-day embryo. **B** to **D,** Lateral views show later development of the pharyngeal arches. **E** to **G,** Ventral or facial views show the relationship of the first arch to the stomodeum. **H,** Horizontal section through the cranial region of an embryo. **I,** Similar section shows the arch components and floor of the primordial pharynx. **J,** Sagittal section of the cranial region of an embryo shows the openings of the pouches in the lateral wall of the primordial pharynx.

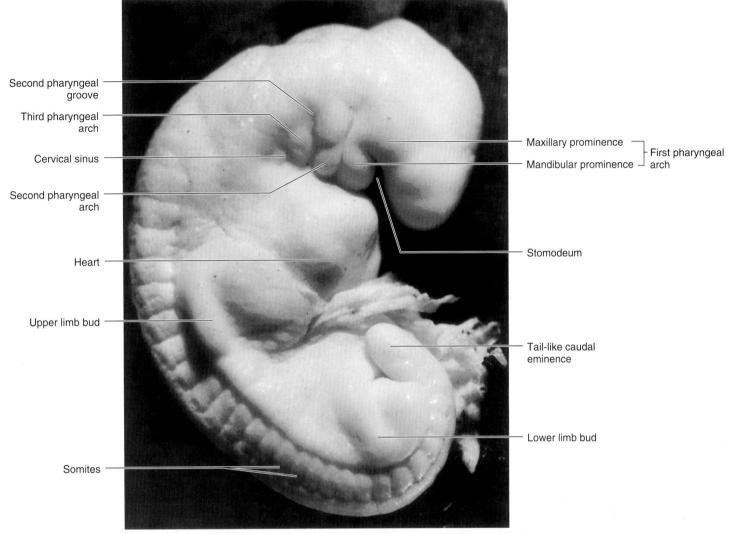

Second pharyngeal groove

Third pharyngeal arch

Cervical sinus

Second pharyngeal arch

Heart

Upper limb bud

Somites

Maxillary prominence ⎫ First pharyngeal
Mandibular prominence ⎭ arch

Stomodeum

Tail-like caudal eminence

Lower limb bud

**FIGURE 9–2** Photograph of a stage 13, 4.5-week human embryo.

**prominence** forms the maxilla, zygomatic bone, and a portion of the vomer bone. The **mandibular prominence** forms the mandible and squamous temporal bone. Along with the third arch, the **second arch** (hyoid arch) contributes to the formation of the hyoid bone.

The arches support the lateral walls of the **primordial pharynx**, which is derived from the cranial part of the foregut. The **stomodeum** (primordial mouth) initially appears as a slight depression of the surface ectoderm (see Fig. 9-1D and G). It is separated from the cavity of the primordial pharynx by a bilaminar membrane, the **oropharyngeal membrane**, which is composed of ectoderm externally and endoderm internally (see Fig. 9-1E and F). This membrane ruptures at approximately 26 days, bringing the pharynx and foregut in communication with the amniotic cavity. The ectodermal lining of the first arch forms the oral epithelium.

## Pharyngeal Arch Components

Each arch consists of a core of **mesenchyme** (embryonic connective tissue) and is covered externally by ectoderm

and internally by endoderm (see Fig. 9-1H and I). Originally, the mesenchyme is derived during the third week from mesoderm. During the fourth week, most of the mesenchyme is derived from **neural crest cells** that migrate into the arches. Migration of neural crest cells into the arches and their differentiation into mesenchyme produce the **maxillary** and **mandibular prominences** (see Fig. 9-2) in addition to all connective tissue, including the dermis (layer of skin) and smooth muscle.

Coincident with immigration of neural crest cells, **myogenic mesoderm** from paraxial regions moves into each arch, forming a central core of **muscle primordium**. Endothelial cells in the arches are derived from the lateral mesoderm and invasive **angioblasts** (cells that differentiate into blood vessel endothelium) that move into the arches. The **pharyngeal endoderm** plays an essential role in regulating the development of the arches.

A typical pharyngeal arch contains several structures:

● An **artery** arises from the **truncus arteriosus** of the primordial heart (Fig. 9-3B) and passes around the primordial pharynx to enter the dorsal aorta.
● A **cartilaginous rod** forms the skeleton of the arch.

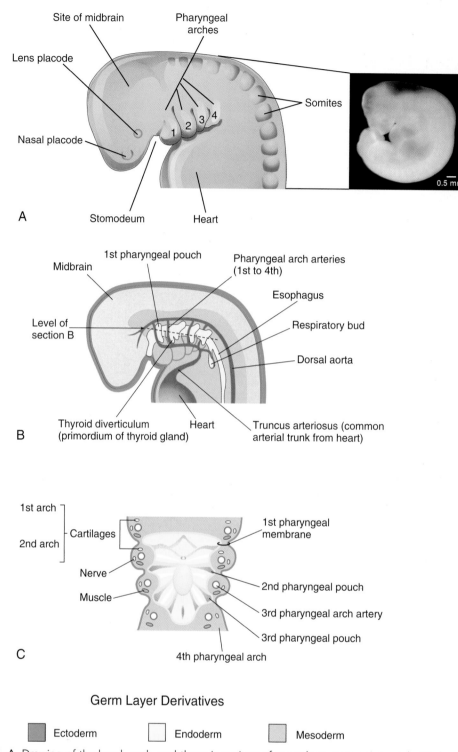

Germ Layer Derivatives

| Ectoderm | Endoderm | Mesoderm |

**FIGURE 9–3** A, Drawing of the head, neck, and thoracic regions of an embryo at approximately 28 days' gestation shows the pharyngeal apparatus. *Inset,* Photograph of an embryo of approximately the same age as shown in A. B, Schematic drawing shows the pouches and arch arteries. C, Horizontal section through the embryo shows the floor of the primordial pharynx and the germ layer of origin of the arch components.

- A **muscular component** differentiates into muscles in the head and neck.
- **Sensory and motor nerves** supply the mucosa (tissue lining) and muscles derived from each arch. The nerves that grow into the arches are derived from neuroectoderm of the primordial brain.

### Fate of Pharyngeal Arches

The arches contribute extensively to the formation of the face, nasal cavities, mouth, larynx, pharynx, and neck (see Figs. 9-3 and 9-25). During the fifth week, the second arch enlarges and overgrows the third and fourth arches, forming an ectodermal depression, the **cervical sinus** (see

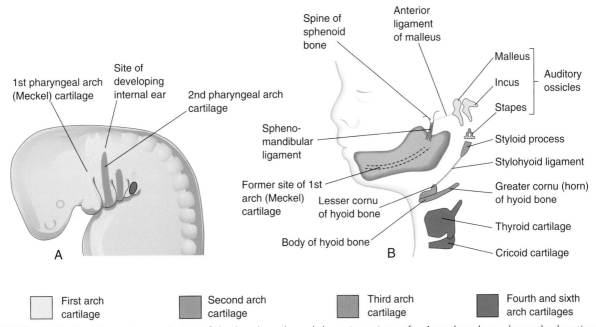

**FIGURE 9–4** **A,** Schematic lateral view of the head, neck, and thoracic regions of a 4-week embryo shows the location of the cartilages in the pharyngeal arches. **B,** Similar view of a 24-week fetus shows the derivatives of the arch cartilages. The mandible is formed by intramembranous ossification of mesenchymal tissue surrounding the first arch cartilage. The cartilage acts as a template for development of the mandible but does not contribute directly to its formation. Occasionally, ossification of the second arch cartilage may extend from the styloid process along the stylohyoid ligament. When this occurs, it may cause pain in the region of the palatine tonsil.

Figs. 9-2 and 9-7). By the end of the seventh week, the second to fourth grooves and cervical sinus have disappeared, giving the neck a smooth contour.

## Derivatives of Pharyngeal Arch Cartilages

The dorsal end of the **first arch cartilage** (Meckel cartilage) is closely related to the developing ear. Early in development, small nodules break away from the proximal part of the cartilage and form two of the middle ear bones, the **malleus** and **incus** (Fig. 9-4 and Table 9-1). The middle part of the cartilage regresses, but its *perichondrium* (connective tissue membrane around cartilage) forms the *anterior ligament of malleus* and *sphenomandibular ligament.*

Ventral parts of the first arch cartilages form the horseshoe-shaped primordium of the mandible, and by keeping pace with its growth, they guide its early **morphogenesis.** Each half of the mandible forms lateral to and in close association with its cartilage. The cartilage disappears as the mandible develops around it by **intramembranous ossification** (see Fig. 9-4*B*). *Multiple signaling pathways involving expression of homeobox genes (BMP, PRRX1, and PRRX2), and fibroblast growth factors regulate the morphogenesis of the mandible.*

An independent cartilage, the **anlage** (primordium) near the dorsal end of the **second arch cartilage** (Reichert cartilage), participates in ear development. It contributes to the formation of the **stapes of the middle ear** and the **styloid process of the temporal bone** (see Fig. 9-4*B*). The cartilage between the styloid process and hyoid bone regresses; its *perichondrium* (connective tissue membrane) forms the **stylohyoid ligament.** The ventral end of

the second arch cartilage ossifies to form the **lesser cornu** (lesser horn) (see Fig. 9-4*B*).

The **third arch cartilage**, located in the ventral part of the arch, ossifies to form the **greater cornu** of the hyoid bone. The **body of the hyoid bone** is formed by the hypobranchial eminence (see Fig. 9-23).

The **fourth and sixth arch cartilages** fuse to form the **laryngeal cartilages** (see Fig. 9-4*B* and Table 9-1), except for the epiglottis. The cartilage of the epiglottis develops from mesenchyme in the **hypopharyngeal eminence** (see Fig. 9-23*A*), a prominence in the floor of the embryonic pharynx that is derived from the third and fourth arches. The **fifth arch**, if present, is rudimentary and has no derivatives.

## Derivatives of Pharyngeal Arch Muscles

The muscular components of the arches derived from unsegmented *paraxial mesoderm* and **prechordal plate** form various muscles in the head and neck. The musculature of the first arch forms the **muscles of mastication** and other muscles (Fig. 9-5; see Table 9-1). The musculature of the second arch forms the **stapedius**, stylohyoid, posterior belly of digastric, auricular, and **muscles of facial expression.** The musculature of the third arch forms the **stylopharyngeus.** The musculature of the fourth arch forms the **cricothyroid, levator veli palatini,** and **constrictors of pharynx.** The musculature of the sixth arch forms the intrinsic muscles of the larynx.

## Derivatives of Pharyngeal Arch Nerves

Each arch is supplied by its own **cranial nerve** (CN). The special visceral efferent (branchial) components of these

## Table 9–1    Structures Derived from Pharyngeal Arch Components

| ARCHES* | CRANIAL NERVES | MUSCLES | SKELETAL STRUCTURES | LIGAMENTS |
|---|---|---|---|---|
| First (mandibular) | Trigeminal (CN V)[†] | Muscles of mastication[‡]<br>Mylohyoid and anterior belly of digastric<br>Tensor tympani<br>Tensor veli palatini | Malleus<br>Incus | Anterior ligament of malleus<br>Sphenomandibular ligament |
| Second (hyoid) | Facial (CN VII) | Muscles of facial expression[§]<br>Stapedius<br>Stylohyoid<br>Posterior belly of digastric | Stapes<br>Styloid process<br>Lesser cornu of hyoid bone | Stylohyoid ligament |
| Third | Glossopharyngeal (CN IX) | Stylopharyngeus | Greater cornu of hyoid bone | |
| Fourth and sixth[¶] | Superior laryngeal branch of vagus (CN X)<br>Recurrent laryngeal branch of vagus (CN X) | Cricothyroid<br>Levator veli palatini<br>Constrictors of pharynx<br>Intrinsic muscles of larynx<br>Striated muscles of esophagus | Thyroid cartilage<br>Cricoid cartilage<br>Arytenoid cartilage<br>Corniculate cartilage<br>Cuneiform cartilage | |

*The derivatives of the pharyngeal arch arteries are described in Fig. 13-38 in Chapter 13.
†The ophthalmic division of the fifth cranial nerve (CN V) does not supply any pharyngeal arch components.
‡Temporalis, masseter, medial, and lateral pterygoids.
§Buccinator, auricularis, frontalis, platysma, orbicularis oris, and orbicularis oculi.
¶The fifth pharyngeal arch is often absent. When present, it is rudimentary and usually has no recognizable cartilage bar. The cartilaginous components of the fourth and sixth arches fuse to form the cartilages of the larynx.

**FIGURE 9–5**  A, Lateral view of the head, neck, and thoracic regions of a 4-week embryo shows the muscles derived from the pharyngeal arches. The *arrow* shows the pathway taken by myoblasts from the occipital myotomes to form the tongue musculature. B, Sketch of the dissected head and neck regions of a 20-week fetus shows the muscles derived from the arches. Parts of the platysma and sternocleidomastoid muscles have been removed to show the deeper muscles. The myoblasts from the second arch migrate from the neck to the head, where they give rise to the muscles of facial expression. These muscles are supplied by the facial nerve (cranial nerve VII), which is the nerve of the second arch.

nerves supply muscles derived from the arches (Fig. 9-6, see Table 9-1). Because mesenchyme from the arches contributes to the dermis and mucous membranes of the head and neck, these areas are supplied with special visceral afferent nerves.

The **facial skin** is supplied by the **trigeminal nerve** (CN V); however, only its caudal two branches (maxillary and mandibular) supply derivatives of the first arch (see Fig. 9-6B). CN V is the principal sensory nerve of the head and neck and is the motor nerve for the muscles of mastication (see Table 9-1). Its sensory branches innervate the face, teeth, and mucous membranes of nasal cavities, palate, mouth, and tongue (see Fig. 9-6C).

The **facial nerve** (CN VII), **glossopharyngeal nerve** (CN IX), and **vagus nerve** (CN X) supply the second, third, and fourth to sixth (caudal) arches, respectively. The fourth arch is supplied by the superior laryngeal branch of CN X and by its recurrent laryngeal branch. The nerves of the second to sixth arches have little cutaneous distribution (see Fig. 9-6C), but they innervate the mucous membranes of the tongue, pharynx, and larynx.

## PHARYNGEAL POUCHES

The **primordial pharynx**, which is derived from the foregut, widens cranially as it joins the **stomodeum** (see Figs. 9-3A and B and 9-4B) and narrows as it joins the esophagus. The endoderm of the pharynx lines the internal aspects of the arches and the **pharyngeal pouches** (see Figs. 9-1H to J and 9-3B and C). The pouches develop in a craniocaudal sequence between the arches. The first pair of pouches, for example, lies between the first and second arches. Four pairs of pouches are well defined; the fifth pair (if present) is rudimentary. The endoderm of the pouches contacts the ectoderm of the pharyngeal grooves, and they form the double-layered **pharyngeal membranes** that separate the pouches from the grooves (see Figs. 9-1H and 9-3C). *Formation of the arches and pouches requires TBX2 gene expression in these tissues.*

### Derivatives of Pharyngeal Pouches

The endodermal epithelial lining of the pouches forms important organs in the head and neck.

#### First Pharyngeal Pouch

The first pouch expands into an elongated **tubotympanic recess** (Fig. 9-7B). The expanded distal part of this recess contacts the first groove, where it later contributes to the formation of the **tympanic membrane** (eardrum). The cavity of the tubotympanic recess becomes the **tympanic cavity** and **mastoid antrum**. The connection of the tubotympanic recess with the pharynx gradually elongates to form the **pharyngotympanic tube** (auditory tube).

#### Second Pharyngeal Pouch

Although the second pouch is largely obliterated as the palatine tonsil develops, part of the cavity of this pouch remains as the **tonsillar sinus** (fossa), the depression between the **palatoglossal** and **palatopharyngeal arches** (Fig. 9-8; see Fig. 9-7C). The endoderm of the

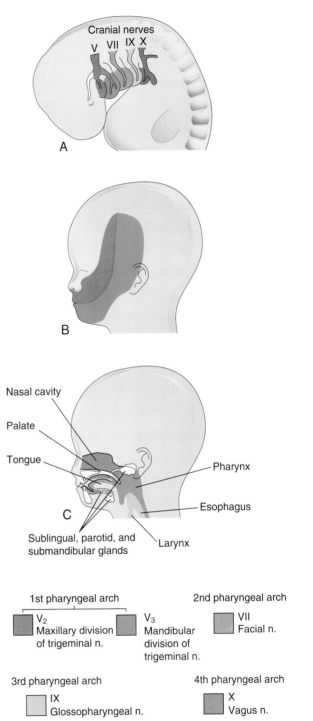

**FIGURE 9–6** A, Lateral view of the head, neck, and thoracic regions of a 4-week embryo shows the cranial nerves supplying the pharyngeal arches. B, Sketch of the head and neck regions of a 20-week fetus shows the superficial distribution of the two caudal branches of the first arch nerve (cranial nerve V). C, Sagittal section of the fetal head and neck shows the deep distribution of sensory fibers of the nerves to the teeth and mucosa of the tongue, pharynx, nasal cavity, palate, and larynx.

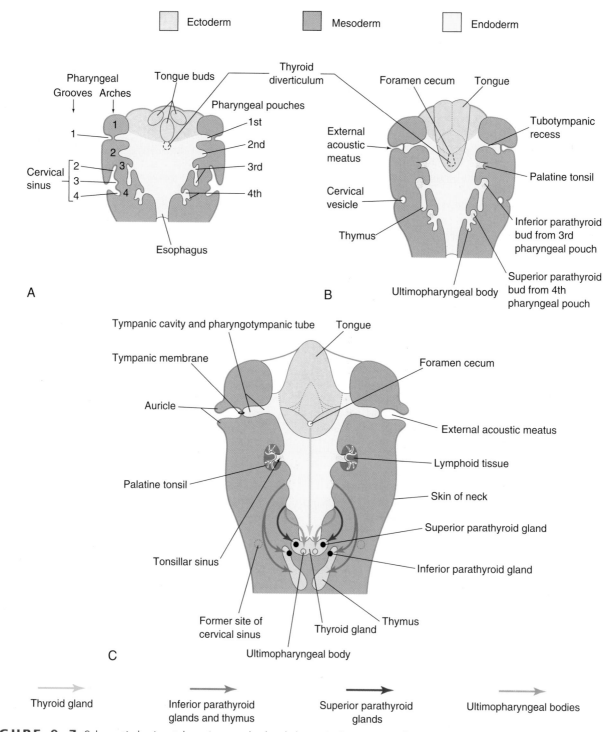

## Germ Layer Derivatives

**FIGURE 9–7** Schematic horizontal sections at the level shown in Figure 9-5A illustrate the adult derivatives of the pharyngeal pouches. **A,** At 5 weeks, the second arch grows over the third and fourth arches, burying the second to fourth grooves in the cervical sinus. **B,** Development at 6 weeks. **C,** At 7 weeks, the developing thymus, parathyroid, and thyroid glands migrate into the neck (*arrows*).

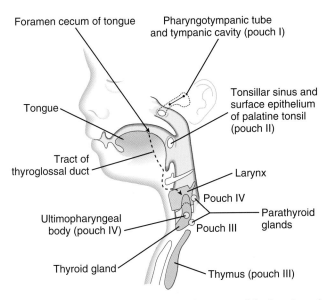

**FIGURE 9-8** Schematic sagittal section of the head, neck, and upper thoracic regions of a 20-week fetus shows the adult derivatives of the pharyngeal pouches and the descent of the thyroid gland into the neck (*broken line*).

second pouch proliferates and grows into the underlying mesenchyme. The central parts of these buds break down, forming **tonsillar crypts** (pit-like depressions). The pouch endoderm forms the surface epithelium and lining of the tonsillar crypts. At approximately 20 weeks, the mesenchyme around the crypts differentiates into **lymphoid tissue**, which soon organizes into the **lymphatic nodules** of the palatine tonsil (see Fig. 9-7C). Initial lymphoid cell infiltration occurs at approximately the seventh month, with germinal centers forming in the neonatal period and active germinal centers within the first year of life.

### Third Pharyngeal Pouch

The third pouch expands and forms a solid, dorsal, bulbar part and a hollow, elongated, ventral part (see Fig. 9-7B). Its connection with the pharynx is reduced to a narrow duct that soon degenerates. By the sixth week, the epithelium of each *dorsal bulbar part of the pouch* begins to differentiate into an **inferior parathyroid gland**. The epithelium of the elongated *ventral parts of the pouch* proliferates, obliterating their cavities. These parts come together in the median plane to form the **thymus**, which is a primary lymphoid organ (see Fig. 9-7C). The bilobed structure of this lymphatic organ remains throughout life, discretely encapsulated.

Each lobe has its own blood supply, lymphatic drainage, and nerve supply. The developing **thymus** and **inferior parathyroid glands** lose their connections with the pharynx when the brain and associated structures expand rostrally, and the pharynx and cardiac structures expand caudally. The derivatives of pouches two to four become displaced caudally. Later, the **parathyroid glands** separate from the thymus and lie on the dorsal surface of the thyroid gland (see Figs. 9-7C and 9-8). *The fibroblast growth factor signaling pathways, acting through*

*fibroblast growth factor receptor substrate 2 (FRS2), are involved in the development of the thymus and parathyroid glands.*

### Histogenesis of Thymus

The thymus is a primary lymphoid organ that develops from epithelial cells derived from endoderm of the third pair of pouches and from mesenchyme into which epithelial tubes grow. The tubes soon become solid cords that proliferate and form side branches. Each side branch becomes the core of a lobule of the thymus. Some cells of the epithelial cords become arranged around a central point, forming small groups of cells called **thymic corpuscles** (Hassall corpuscles). Other cells of the epithelial cords spread apart, but they retain connections with each other to form an epithelial reticulum. The mesenchyme between the epithelial cords forms thin, incomplete septa between the lobules.

**Lymphocytes** soon appear and fill the interstices between the epithelial cells. The lymphocytes are derived from **hematopoietic stem cells**. The thymic primordium is surrounded by a thin layer of mesenchyme that is essential for its development. **Neural crest cells** also contribute to thymic organogenesis.

Growth and development of the thymus are not complete at birth. It is a relatively large organ during the perinatal period and may extend through the superior thoracic aperture at the root of the neck. As puberty is reached, the thymus begins to diminish in relative size as it undergoes involution. By adulthood, it is often scarcely recognizable because of fat infiltrating the cortex of the gland; however, it is still functional and important for the maintenance of health. In addition to secreting thymic hormones, the thymus primes **thymocytes** (T-cell precursors) before releasing them to the periphery.

### Fourth Pharyngeal Pouch

The fourth pouch expands into dorsal bulbar and elongated ventral parts (see Figs. 9-7 and 9-8). Its connection with the pharynx is reduced to a narrow duct that soon degenerates. By the sixth week, each dorsal part develops into a **superior parathyroid gland**, which lies on the dorsal surface of the thyroid gland. Because the parathyroid glands derived from the third pouches accompany the thymus, they are in a more inferior position than the parathyroid glands derived from the fourth pouches (see Fig. 9-8).

### Histogenesis of Parathyroid and Thyroid Glands

The epithelium of the dorsal parts of the third and fourth pouches proliferates during the fifth week and forms small nodules on the dorsal aspect of each pouch. Vascular mesenchyme soon grows into these nodules, forming a capillary network. The *chief* or *principal cells* differentiate during the embryonic period and are thought to become functionally active in regulating fetal calcium metabolism. The **oxyphil cells** of the parathyroid gland differentiate 5 to 7 years after birth.

The elongated ventral part of each fourth pouch develops into an **ultimopharyngeal body**, which fuses with the thyroid gland (see Fig. 9-8). Its cells disseminate within the thyroid and form **parafollicular cells**. These cells are also called C cells, indicating that they produce **calcitonin**, a hormone that lowers blood calcium levels. C cells differentiate from **neural crest cells** that migrate from the arches into the fourth pair of pouches. *The basic helix-loop-helix (bHLH) transcription factor MASH1 regulates C-cell differentiation.*

## ▶ PHARYNGEAL GROOVES

7  The head and neck regions of the embryo exhibit four grooves (branchial clefts) on each side during the fourth and fifth weeks (see Figs. 9-1B to D and 9-2). These grooves separate the arches externally. Only one pair of grooves contributes to postnatal structures; the first pair persists as the **external acoustic meatus** (ear canals) (see Fig. 9-7C). The other grooves lie in a slit-like depression (**cervical sinus**) and are normally obliterated along with the sinus as the neck develops (see Fig. 9-4A, D, and F). Birth defects of the second groove are relatively common.

## ▶ PHARYNGEAL MEMBRANES

7  The pharyngeal membranes appear in the floors of the pharyngeal grooves (see Figs. 9-1H and 9-3C). These membranes form where the epithelia of the grooves and pouches approach each other. The endoderm of the pouches and ectoderm of the grooves are soon infiltrated and separated by mesenchyme. Only one pair of membranes contributes to the formation of adult structures; the first membrane and the intervening layer of mesenchyme become the **tympanic membrane** (see Fig. 9-7C).

### CERVICAL (BRANCHIAL) SINUSES

**External cervical sinuses** are uncommon, and most result from failure of the second groove and cervical sinus to obliterate (Figs. 9-9D and 9-10A and B). The sinus typically opens along the anterior border of the sternocleidomastoid muscle in the inferior third of the neck. Anomalies of the other pharyngeal grooves occur in approximately 5% of neonates. External sinuses are commonly detected during infancy because of the discharge of mucus from them (see Fig. 9-10A). The **external cervical sinuses** are bilateral in approximately 10% of affected neonates and are commonly associated with auricular sinuses.

**Internal cervical sinuses** open into the tonsillar sinus or near the palatopharyngeal arch (see Fig. 9-9D and F). These sinuses are rare. Most result from persistence of the proximal part of the second pouch. This pouch usually disappears as the palatine tonsil develops; its normal remnant is the tonsillar sinus.

### CERVICAL (BRANCHIAL) FISTULA

A cervical fistula is an abnormal canal that typically opens internally into the **tonsillar sinus** and externally in the side of the neck. The canal results from persistence of parts of the second groove and second pouch (see Figs. 9-9E and F and 9-10B). The fistula ascends from its opening in the neck through the subcutaneous tissue and platysma muscle to reach the **carotid sheath**. The fistula then passes between the internal and external carotid arteries and opens into the tonsillar sinus.

### PIRIFORM SINUS FISTULA

The piriform sinus fistula is thought to result from persistence of remnants of the **ultimopharyngeal body** along its path to the thyroid gland (see Figs. 9-7C and 9-8).

### CERVICAL (BRANCHIAL) CYSTS

Remnants of parts of the cervical sinus and/or the second groove may persist and form a spherical or elongated cyst (see Fig. 9-9F). Although they may be associated with cervical sinuses and drain through them, the cysts often lie free in the neck just inferior to the angle of the mandible. However, they can develop anywhere along the anterior border of the sternocleidomastoid muscle. **Cervical cysts** do not usually become apparent until late childhood or early adulthood, when they produce a slowly enlarging, painless swelling in the neck (Fig. 9-11). The cyst enlarges because of the accumulation of fluid and cellular debris derived from desquamation of their epithelial linings (Fig. 9-12).

### CERVICAL (BRANCHIAL) VESTIGES

The pharyngeal cartilages normally disappear, except for parts that form ligaments or bones. However, in unusual cases, cartilaginous or bony remnants of pharyngeal arch cartilages appear under the skin in the side of the neck (Fig. 9-13). They are usually found anterior to the inferior third of the sternocleidomastoid muscle (see Fig. 9-9F).

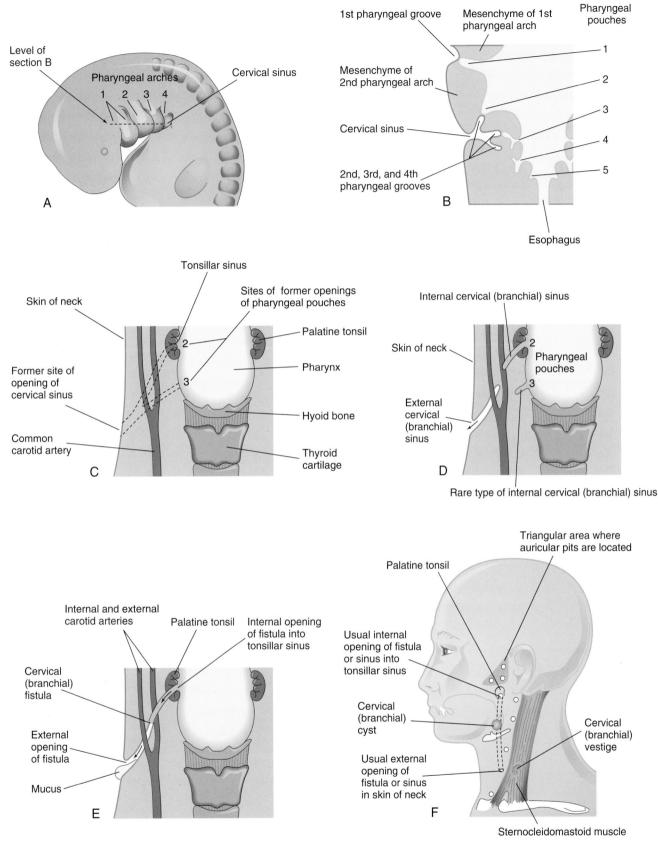

**FIGURE 9–9** *A,* Lateral view of the head, neck, and thoracic regions of a 5-week embryo shows the cervical sinus that is normally present at this stage. *B,* Horizontal section of the embryo at the level shown in *A* illustrates the relationship between the cervical sinus and the pharyngeal arches and pouches. *C,* Diagrammatic sketch of the adult pharyngeal and neck regions shows the former sites of openings of the cervical sinus and pharyngeal pouches. The *broken lines* indicate possible tracts of cervical fistulas. *D,* Similar sketch shows the embryologic basis of various cervical sinus types. *E,* Drawing shows a cervical fistula that resulted from persistence of parts of the second groove and second pouch. *F,* Sketch shows possible sites of cervical cysts, the openings of cervical sinuses and fistulas, and a branchial vestige (see Fig. 9-13).

**FIGURE 9–10** A, A catheter is inserted into the external opening of a cervical sinus in a child's neck. The catheter allows definition of the length of the tract, which facilitates surgical excision. B, After injection of contrast material, the fistulogram shows the course of a complete cervical fistula through the neck.

**FIGURE 9–11** The swelling in a boy's neck was produced by a cervical cyst. These large cysts often lie free in the neck just inferior to the angle of the mandible, but they may develop anywhere along the anterior border of the sternocleidomastoid muscle, as in this case.

**FIGURE 9–12** Computed tomography of the neck region of a 24-year-old woman with a 2-month history of a lump in the neck shows a low-density cervical cyst (C) that is anterior to the sternocleidomastoid muscle (S). Notice the external carotid artery (arrow) and external jugular vein (dotted arrow).

**FIGURE 9–13** A cartilaginous branchial vestige *(arrow)* in a child's neck (see Fig. 9-9F). *(From Raffensperger JG: Swenson's pediatric surgery, ed 5, New York, 1990, Appleton-Century-Crofts.)*

## FIRST PHARYNGEAL ARCH SYNDROME

Abnormal development of the components of the first arch results in various birth defects of the eyes, ears, mandible, and palate, which together constitute the first arch syndrome (Fig. 9-14). This birth defect is thought to result from insufficient migration of neural crest cells into the first arch during the fourth week. There are two main manifestations of the first arch syndrome:

**Treacher Collins syndrome** (mandibulofacial dysostosis) is an autosomal dominant disorder characterized by **malar hypoplasia** (underdevelopment of zygomatic bones of the face) with down-slanting **palpebral fissures**, defects of the lower eyelids, deformed external ears, and sometimes defects of the middle and internal ears.

*The Treacher Collins–Franceschetti syndrome 1 gene (TCOF1) is responsible for the production of a protein called treacle. Treacle is involved in the biogenesis of ribosomal RNA that contributes to the development of bones and cartilage of the face. Mutation in the TCOF1 gene is associated with Treacher Collins syndrome.*

**Pierre Robin sequence** typically occurs de novo in most patients and is associated with **hypoplasia** (underdevelopment) of the mandible, cleft palate, and defects of the eyes and ears. Rarely, it is inherited in an autosomal dominant pattern. In the Robin morphogenetic complex, the initiating defect is a small mandible (**micrognathia**), which results in posterior displacement of the tongue and obstruction to full closure of the palatal processes, resulting in a **bilateral cleft palate** (see Figs. 9-39 and 9-40).

**FIGURE 9–14** This infant has first arch syndrome, a pattern of birth defects that results from insufficient migration of neural crest cells into the first pharyngeal arch. Notice the deformed auricle of the external ear, preauricular appendage, defect in the cheek between the auricle and mouth, hypoplasia (underdevelopment) of the mandible, and macrostomia (large mouth).

## DIGEORGE SYNDROME

Infants with DiGeorge syndrome are born without a thymus and parathyroid glands and have defects in the cardiac outflow tracts. In some cases, ectopic glandular tissue has been found (Fig. 9-15). The disease is characterized by *congenital hypoparathyroidism*, increased susceptibility to infections (from immune deficiency, specifically defective T-cell function), birth defects of the mouth (shortened philtrum of upper lip), low-set and notched ears, nasal clefts, thyroid hypoplasia, and cardiac abnormalities (defects of the aortic arch and heart). Features of this syndrome vary widely, but most infants have some of the classic characteristics previously described. Only 1.5% of infants have the complete form of T-cell deficiency, and approximately 30% have only a partial deficiency.

DiGeorge syndrome occurs because the third and fourth pharyngeal pouches fail to differentiate into the thymus and parathyroid glands. This is the result of a breakdown in signaling between pharyngeal endoderm and adjacent neural crest cells. The facial abnormalities result primarily from abnormal development of the first arch components because neural crest cells are disrupted, and the cardiac anomalies arise in the sites normally occupied by neural crest cells. *Most cases of DiGeorge syndrome have a microdeletion in the q11.2 region of chromosome 22 (inactivating the TBX1, HIRA, and UFDIL genes) and have neural crest cell defects.*

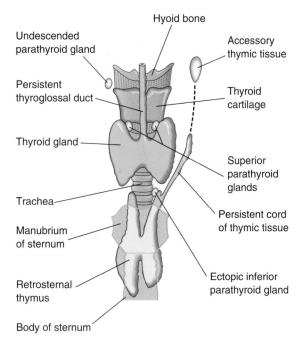

**FIGURE 9–15** Anterior view of the thyroid gland, thymus, and parathyroid glands illustrates various birth defects that may occur.

## ACCESSORY THYMIC TISSUE

An isolated mass of thymic tissue may persist in the neck and often lies close to an inferior parathyroid gland (see Fig. 9-15). This tissue breaks free from the developing thymus as it shifts caudally in the neck.

## ECTOPIC PARATHYROID GLANDS

Ectopic parathyroid glands may be found anywhere near or within the thyroid gland or thymus. The superior glands are more constant in position than the inferior ones. Occasionally, an inferior parathyroid gland remains near the bifurcation of the common carotid artery. In other cases, it may be in the thorax.

## ABNORMAL NUMBER OF PARATHYROID GLANDS

Uncommonly, there are more than four parathyroid glands. **Supernumerary parathyroid glands** probably result from division of the primordia of the original glands. Absence of a gland results from failure of one of the primordia to differentiate or from atrophy of a gland early in development.

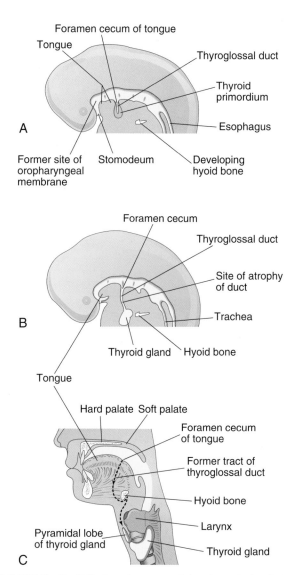

**FIGURE 9–16** Development of the thyroid gland. **A** and **B**, Schematic sagittal sections of the head and neck regions of embryos at 5 and 6 weeks, respectively, illustrate successive stages in the development of the gland. **C**, Similar section of an adult head and neck shows the path taken by the gland during its embryonic descent (indicated by the former tract of the thyroglossal duct).

## DEVELOPMENT OF THYROID GLAND

The thyroid gland is the first endocrine gland to develop in the embryo. Under the influence of fibroblast growth factor signaling pathways, it begins to form approximately 24 days after fertilization from a median endodermal thickening in the floor of the primordial pharynx. This thickening soon forms a small outpouching, the **thyroid primordium** (Fig. 9-16A).

As the embryo and tongue grow, the developing thyroid gland descends in the neck, passing ventral to the developing hyoid bone and laryngeal cartilages. For a short time, the gland is connected to the tongue by a narrow tube, the **thyroglossal duct** (see Fig. 9-16A and B). At

Persistent thyroglossal duct

Pyramidal lobe

Isthmus of thyroid gland

**FIGURE 9–17** The anterior surface of a dissected adult thyroid gland shows persistence of the thyroglossal duct. Notice the pyramidal lobe ascending from the superior border of the isthmus of the gland. It represents a persistent portion of the inferior end of the thyroglossal duct that has formed thyroid tissue.

first, the thyroid primordium is hollow, but it soon becomes a solid mass of cells. It divides into right and left lobes that are connected by the **isthmus of thyroid gland** (Fig. 9-17), which lies anterior to the developing second and third tracheal rings.

At 7 weeks, the thyroid gland has assumed its definitive shape and is usually located in its final site in the neck (see Fig. 9-16C). By this time, the **thyroglossal duct** has normally degenerated and disappeared. The proximal opening of the duct persists as a small pit in the dorsum (posterosuperior surface) of the tongue, the **foramen cecum** (see Fig. 9-16D). A **pyramidal lobe** of the thyroid gland extends superiorly from the isthmus in approximately 50% of people (see Fig. 9-17). This lobe may be attached to the hyoid bone by fibrous tissue or smooth muscle, or both.

## Histogenesis of Thyroid Gland

The thyroid primordium consists of a solid mass of endodermal cells. This cellular aggregation later breaks up into a network of epithelial cords as it is invaded by the surrounding vascular mesenchyme. By the 10th week, the cords have divided into small cellular groups. A lumen soon forms in each cell cluster, and the cells become arranged in a single layer around **thyroid follicles**. During

the 11th week, colloid (semifluid material in follicles) begins to appear; thereafter, iodine concentration and synthesis of thyroid hormones can be demonstrated. By 20 weeks, the levels of fetal **thyroid-stimulating hormone** and **thyroxine** begin to increase, reaching adult levels at 35 weeks.

## CONGENITAL HYPOTHYROIDISM

Congenital hypothyroidism is *the most common metabolic disorder in neonates.* It is a **heterogeneous disorder** for which several candidate genes, including those for the thyroid-stimulating hormone receptor and thyroid transcription factors (*TTF1, TTF2,* and *PAX8*), have been identified. Congenital hypothyroidism may result in neurodevelopmental disorders and infertility if untreated. An increased incidence of renal and urinary tract defects has been reported in infants with **congenital hypothyroidism**.

## THYROGLOSSAL DUCT CYSTS AND SINUSES

Cysts may form anywhere along the course of the **thyroglossal duct** (Fig. 9-18). The duct typically atrophies and disappears, but a remnant of it may persist and form a cyst in the tongue or in the anterior part of the neck, usually just inferior to the hyoid bone (Fig. 9-19). Most cysts are observed by the age of 5 years. Unless the lesions become infected, most of them are asymptomatic. The swelling produced by a **thyroglossal duct cyst** usually develops as a painless, progressively enlarging, movable mass (Fig. 9-20; see Figs. 9-18 and 9-19A and B). The cyst may contain some thyroid tissue. If infection of a cyst occurs, a perforation of the skin may develop, forming a **thyroglossal duct sinus** that usually opens in the median plane of the neck anterior to the laryngeal cartilages.

## ECTOPIC THYROID GLAND

An **ectopic thyroid gland** is an uncommon birth defect, and it is usually located along the course of the thyroglossal duct (see Fig. 9-16C). **Lingual thyroid glandular tissue** is the most common of ectopic thyroid tissues. **Intralingual thyroid masses** are found in up to 10% of autopsies, although they are clinically relevant in only 1 of 4000 persons with thyroid disease.

Incomplete movement of the thyroid gland results in a **sublingual thyroid gland** that appears high in the neck at

or just inferior to the hyoid bone (Figs. 9-21 and 9-22). In 70% of cases, an ectopic sublingual thyroid gland is the only thyroid tissue present. *It is clinically important to differentiate an ectopic thyroid gland from a thyroglossal duct cyst or accessory thyroid tissue to prevent inadvertent surgical removal of the thyroid gland.* Failure to do so may leave the person permanently dependent on thyroid medication. Ultrasound is commonly used to investigate an ectopic sublingual thyroid gland.

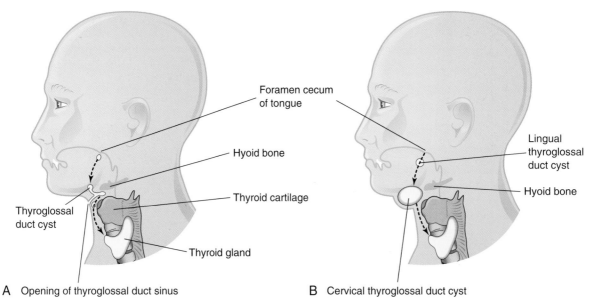

**FIGURE 9–18** A, Sketch of the head and neck shows possible locations of thyroglossal duct cysts and a duct sinus. The *broken line* indicates the course taken by the duct during descent of the developing thyroid gland from the foramen cecum to its final position in the anterior part of the neck. B, Similar sketch illustrates lingual and cervical thyroglossal duct cysts. Most cysts are located inferior to the hyoid bone.

**FIGURE 9–19** A, Large thyroglossal duct cyst *(arrow)* in a male patient. B, Computed tomogram of a thyroglossal duct cyst in a child shows that it is located in the neck anterior to the thyroid cartilage.

Epiglottis

Thyroglossal duct cyst

Thyroid cartilage

**FIGURE 9–20** Computed tomography at the level of the thyrohyoid membrane and base of the epiglottis (**A**) and at the level of the calcified thyroid cartilage (**B**). The thyroglossal duct cyst extends cranially to the margin of the hyoid bone.

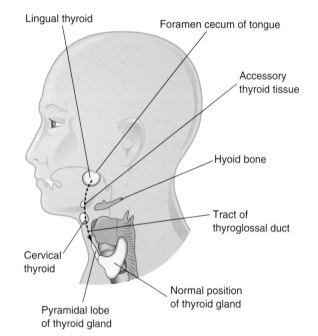

Lingual thyroid

Foramen cecum of tongue

Accessory thyroid tissue

Hyoid bone

Tract of thyroglossal duct

Cervical thyroid

Normal position of thyroid gland

Pyramidal lobe of thyroid gland

**FIGURE 9–21** Sketch of the head and neck shows the usual sites of ectopic thyroid tissue. The *broken line* indicates the path followed by the thyroid gland during its descent and the former tract of the thyroglossal duct.

**FIGURE 9–22** A, Sublingual thyroid mass in a 5-year-old girl. B, Technetium-99m pertechnetate scan (scintigram) shows a sublingual thyroid gland (*asterisk*) without evidence of functioning thyroid tissue in the anterior part of the neck. (*From Leung AK, Wong AL, Robson WL: Ectopic thyroid gland simulating a thyroglossal duct cyst, Can J Surg 38:87, 1995.*)

## AGENESIS OF THYROID GLAND

Absence of a thyroid gland or one of its lobes is a rare anomaly. In **thyroid hemiagenesis** (unilateral failure of formation), the left lobe is more commonly absent. Mutations in the receptor for thyroid-stimulating hormone are probably involved in some cases.

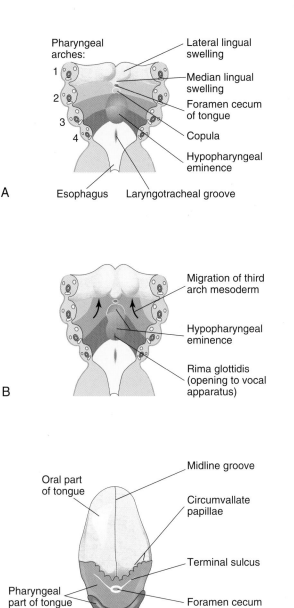

A

B

C

### Pharyngeal Arch Derivatives of Tongue

☐ 1st pharyngeal arch (CN V—mandibular division)

☐ 2nd pharyngeal arch (CN VII—chorda tympani)

☐ 3rd pharyngeal arch (CN IX—glossopharyngeal)

☐ 4th pharyngeal arch (CN X—vagus)

**FIGURE 9–23** A and B, Schematic horizontal sections through the pharynx at the level shown in Figure 9-5A illustrate successive stages in the development of the tongue during the fourth and fifth weeks. C, Drawing of the adult tongue shows the pharyngeal arch derivation of the nerve supply of its mucosa. *CN,* Cranial nerve.

## DEVELOPMENT OF TONGUE

8 Near the end of the fourth week, a median triangular elevation appears in the floor of the **primordial pharynx** just rostral to the foramen cecum (Fig. 9-23A). This **median lingual swelling** (tongue bud) is the first indication of tongue development. Soon, two oval, **lateral lingual swellings** (distal tongue buds) develop on each side of the median lingual swelling. The three swellings result from the proliferation of mesenchyme in ventromedial parts of the first pair of pharyngeal arches. The lateral lingual swellings rapidly increase in size, merge with each other, and overgrow the median lingual swelling.

The merged lateral lingual swellings form the anterior two thirds of the tongue (**oral part**) (see Fig. 9-23C). The fusion site of the swellings is indicated by the **midline groove** and internally by the fibrous **lingual septum**. The median lingual swelling does not form a recognizable part of the adult tongue. Formation of the posterior third of the tongue (pharyngeal part) is indicated in the fetus by two elevations that develop caudal to the **foramen cecum** (see Fig. 9-23A). The **copula** forms by fusion of the ventromedial parts of the second pair of pharyngeal arches. The **hypopharyngeal eminence** develops caudal to the copula from mesenchyme in the ventromedial parts of the third and fourth pairs of pharyngeal arches.

As the tongue develops, the copula is gradually overgrown by the hypopharyngeal eminence and disappears (see Fig. 9-23B and C). As a result, the posterior third of the tongue develops from the rostral part of the hypopharyngeal eminence. The line of fusion of the anterior and posterior parts of the tongue is roughly indicated by a V-shaped groove, the **terminal sulcus** (see Fig. 9-23C). Cranial neural crest cells migrate into the developing tongue and give rise to its connective tissue and vasculature.

Most of the tongue muscles are derived from **myoblasts** (primordial muscle cells) that migrate from the second to fifth occipital myotomes (see Fig. 9-5A). The **hypoglossal nerve** (CN XII) accompanies the myoblasts (myogenic precursors) during their migration and innervates the tongue muscles as they develop. The anterior and posterior parts of the tongue are located within the oral cavity at birth; the posterior third of the tongue descends into the **oropharynx** (oral part of the pharynx) by 4 years of age. *The molecular mechanisms involved in the development of the tongue include myogenic regulatory factors and paired box genes PAX3 and PAX7.*

## Lingual Papillae and Taste Buds

**Lingual papillae** appear toward the end of the eighth week. The *vallate and foliate papillae* appear first and lie close to terminal branches of the glossopharyngeal nerve (CN IX). The *fungiform papillae* appear later near terminations of the chorda tympani branch of the facial nerve (CN VII). The long and numerous papillae are called **filiform papillae** because of their thread-like shape. They develop during the early fetal period (10–11 weeks). They contain afferent nerve endings that are sensitive to touch.

**Taste buds** (cell nests in the papillae) develop during weeks 11 to 13 by inductive interaction between the epithelial cells of the tongue and invading gustatory (relating to taste) nerve cells from the chorda tympani, glossopharyngeal, and vagus nerves. Most taste buds form on the dorsal surface of the tongue, and some develop on the palatoglossal (palate and tongue) arches, palate, posterior surface of the epiglottis, and posterior wall of the oropharynx. **Fetal facial responses** can be induced by bitter-tasting substances at 26 to 28 weeks, indicating that reflex pathways between taste buds and facial muscles are established.

## Nerve Supply of Tongue

The development of the tongue explains its nerve supply (see Fig. 9-23). The sensory supply to the mucosa of almost two thirds of the tongue is from the lingual branch of the mandibular division of the **trigeminal nerve** (CN V), the nerve of the first pharyngeal arch. This arch forms the median and lateral lingual swellings. Although the **facial nerve** (CN VII) is the nerve of the second pharyngeal arch, its **chorda tympani branch** supplies the taste buds in the anterior two thirds of the tongue except for the vallate papillae. Because the second arch component, the **copula** (narrow part connecting two structures), is overgrown by the third arch, CN VII does not supply the tongue mucosa, except for the taste buds in the anterior part of the tongue. The **vallate papillae** in the anterior part of the tongue are innervated by the **glossopharyngeal nerve** (CN IX) of the third arch (see Fig. 9-23C). The usual explanation is that the mucosa of the posterior third of the tongue is pulled slightly anteriorly as the tongue develops.

The posterior third of the tongue is innervated mainly by the **glossopharyngeal nerve** (CN IX) of the third arch. The superior laryngeal branch of the **vagus nerve** (CN X) of the fourth arch supplies a small area of the tongue anterior to the epiglottis (see Fig. 9-23C). All muscles of the tongue are supplied by the **hypoglossal nerve** (CN XII), except for the palatoglossus, which is supplied from the pharyngeal plexus by fibers arising from the **vagus nerve** (CN X).

### CONGENITAL ANOMALIES OF TONGUE

Abnormalities of the tongue are uncommon, except for fissuring (forming a cleft) of the tongue and **hypertrophy** of the lingual papillae, which are characteristics of infants with Down syndrome (see Chapter 20, Fig. 20-6*D*).

### CONGENITAL LINGUAL CYSTS AND FISTULAS

Cysts (sacs containing fluid or semisolid material) in the tongue may be derived from remnants of the thyroglossal duct (see Fig. 9-16). They may enlarge and produce symptoms of pharyngeal discomfort or **dysphagia** (difficulty in swallowing), or both. Fistulas are also derived from persistent lingual parts of the thyroglossal duct. They open through the **foramen cecum** into the oral cavity.

### ANKYLOGLOSSIA

The **lingual frenulum** normally connects the inferior surface of the tongue to the floor of the mouth. Sometimes, the frenulum is short and extends to the tip of the tongue (Fig. 9-24). This interferes with the tongue's free protrusion and may make breast-feeding difficult. **Ankyloglossia** (tongue-tie) occurs in approximately 1 of 300 North American neonates, but it usually has no permanent functional significance. A short frenulum usually stretches with time, making surgical correction of the defect unnecessary.

### MACROGLOSSIA

An excessively large tongue is uncommon. It is caused by generalized hypertrophy of the developing tongue, usually resulting from **lymphangioma** (lymph tumor) or muscular hypertrophy. Macroglossia is often seen in infants with Down or Beckwith-Wiedemann syndrome.

**FIGURE 9–24** Infant with ankyloglossia (tongue-tie). Notice the short frenulum of the tongue, a fold of mucous membrane extending from the floor of the mouth to the midline of the undersurface of the tongue. Ankyloglossia interferes with protrusion of the tongue, and it may make breast-feeding difficult.

---

### MICROGLOSSIA

An abnormally small tongue is rare. It is usually associated with **micrognathia** (underdeveloped mandible and chin recession) and limb defects **(Hanhart syndrome)**.

---

### BIFID OR CLEFT TONGUE (GLOSSOSCHISIS)

Incomplete fusion of the **lateral lingual swellings** (see Fig. 9-23A) results in a deep **midline groove** in the tongue (see Fig. 9-23A and C). This groove usually does not extend to the tip of the tongue. Glossoschisis is a very uncommon birth defect.

---

## DEVELOPMENT OF SALIVARY GLANDS

During the sixth and seventh weeks, the salivary glands, under the influence of the *Notch signaling pathway*, develop as highly branched structure by branching morphogenesis from solid epithelial buds of the primordial oral cavity (see Fig. 9-6C). The club-shaped ends of these buds grow into the underlying mesenchyme. The connective tissue in the glands is derived from neural crest cells. All parenchymal (secretory) tissue arises by proliferation of the oral epithelium.

The **parotid glands** are the first to develop and appear early in the sixth week (see Fig. 9-6C). They develop from buds that arise from the oral ectodermal lining near the angles of the stomodeum. Elongation of the jaws causes lengthening of the **parotid duct**, with the gland remaining close to its site of origin. Later the buds canalize (develop lumina) and become ducts by approximately 10 weeks. The rounded ends of the cords differentiate into **acini** (grape-shaped structures). Secretory activity begins at 18 weeks. The capsule and connective tissue of the glands develop from the surrounding mesenchyme.

The **submandibular glands** appear late in the sixth week. They develop from endodermal buds in the floor of the stomodeum. Solid cellular processes grow posteriorly, lateral to the developing tongue. Later, they branch and differentiate. Acini begin to form at 12 weeks and secretory activity begins at 16 weeks. Growth of the glands continues after birth with the formation of mucous acini. Lateral to the developing tongue, a linear groove forms that soon closes to form the **submandibular duct**.

The **sublingual glands** appear during the eighth week, approximately 2 weeks later than the other glands (see Fig. 9-6C). They develop from multiple endodermal epithelial buds that branch and canalize to form 10 to 12 ducts that open independently into the floor of the mouth.

## DEVELOPMENT OF FACE

The **facial primordia** appear early in the fourth week around the **stomodeum** (primordium of the mouth) (Fig. 9-25A and B). Facial development depends on the inductive influence of the forebrain (through sonic hedgehog morphogenic gradients), frontonasal ectodermal zone, and developing eye. **Five facial primordia** appear as prominences around the stomodeum (see Fig. 9-25A):

- A frontonasal prominence
- Paired maxillary prominences
- Paired mandibular prominences

The maxillary and mandibular prominences are derivatives of the first pair of pharyngeal arches. The prominences are produced mainly by the expansion of **neural crest populations** that originate from the mesencephalic and rostral rhombencephalic neural folds during the fourth week. These cells are the major source of connective tissue components, including cartilage, bone, and ligaments in the facial and oral regions.

The **frontonasal prominence** surrounds the ventrolateral part of the forebrain, which gives rise to the **optic vesicles** that form the eyes (see Fig. 9-25C). The frontal part of the frontonasal prominence forms the forehead; the nasal part forms the rostral boundary of the stomodeum and nose. The **maxillary prominences** form the lateral boundaries of the **stomodeum**, and **mandibular prominences** constitute the caudal boundary of the stomodeum (Fig. 9-26). The facial prominences are **active centers of growth** in the underlying mesenchyme. This embryonic connective tissue is continuous from one prominence to the other.

Facial development occurs mainly between the fourth and eighth weeks (see Fig. 9-25A to G). By the end of the embryonic period, the face has an unquestionably human appearance. Facial proportions develop during the fetal period (see Fig. 9-25H and I). The lower jaw and lower lip are the first parts of the face to form. They result from merging of the medial ends of the mandibular prominences in the median plane. The common chin dimple results from incomplete fusion of the prominences.

By the end of the fourth week, bilateral oval thickenings of the surface ectoderm (**nasal placodes**, the primordia of the *nasal epithelium*) have developed on the inferolateral parts of the **frontonasal prominence** (Fig. 9-27 and Fig. 9-28A and B).These placodes are initially convex, but they are later stretched to produce a flat depression in each **placode**. Mesenchyme in the margins of the placodes proliferates, producing horseshoe-shaped elevations, the **medial and lateral nasal prominences**. As a result, the nasal placodes lie in depressions, the **nasal pits** (see Fig. 9-28C and D). These pits are the primordia of the anterior **nares** (nostrils) and **nasal cavities** (see Fig. 9-28E), and the lateral nasal prominences form the alae (sides) of the nose.

Proliferation of mesenchyme in the **maxillary prominences** makes them enlarge and grow medially toward each other and the **nasal prominences** (see Figs. 9-25D to G, 9-26, and 9-27). This proliferation-driven expansion results in movement of the **medial nasal prominences** toward the median plane and each other; a process

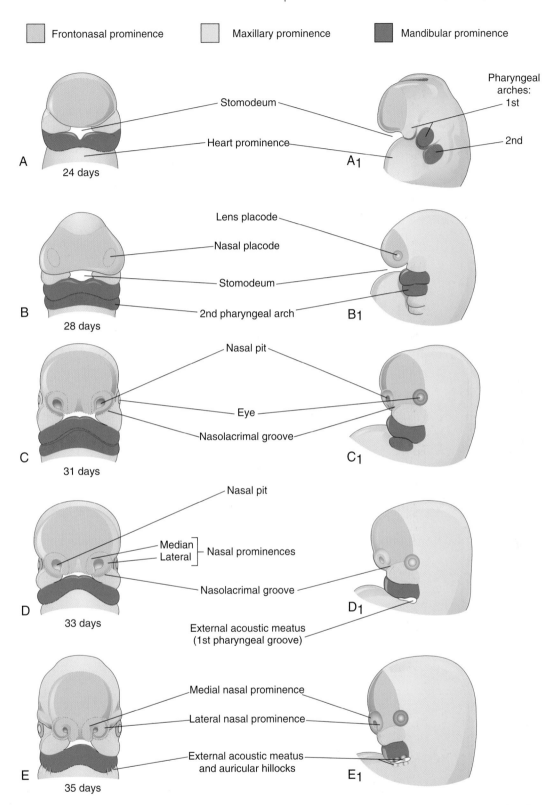

Frontonasal prominence    Maxillary prominence    Mandibular prominence

**A** 24 days

Stomodeum

Heart prominence

**A₁**

Pharyngeal arches:
1st
2nd

**B** 28 days

Lens placode

Nasal placode

Stomodeum

2nd pharyngeal arch

**B₁**

**C** 31 days

Nasal pit

Eye

Nasolacrimal groove

**C₁**

**D** 33 days

Nasal pit

Median
Lateral
Nasal prominences

Nasolacrimal groove

**D₁**

External acoustic meatus
(1st pharyngeal groove)

**E** 35 days

Medial nasal prominence

Lateral nasal prominence

External acoustic meatus
and auricular hillocks

**E₁**

**FIGURE 9-25** A through I, Diagrams show frontal and lateral views illustrating progressive stages in the development of the face.
*Continued*

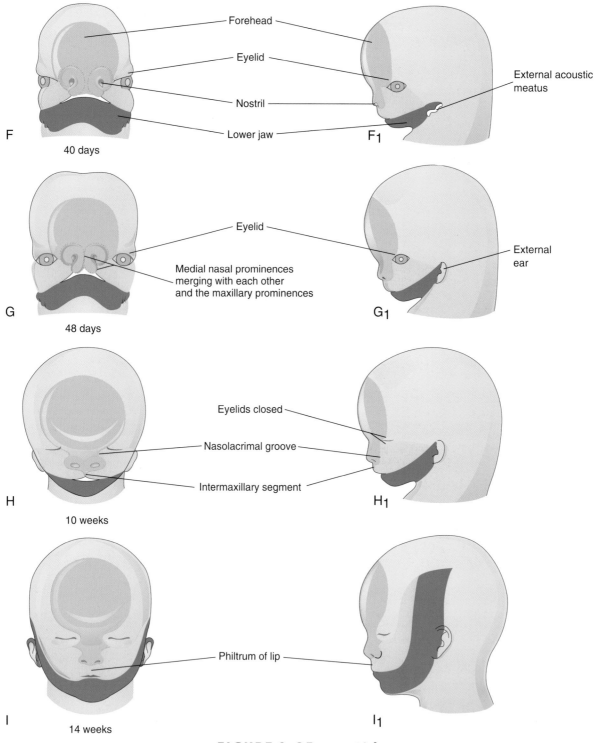

F — 40 days — Forehead, Eyelid, Nostril, Lower jaw

F₁ — External acoustic meatus

G — 48 days — Eyelid, Medial nasal prominences merging with each other and the maxillary prominences

G₁ — External ear

H — 10 weeks — Eyelids closed, Nasolacrimal groove, Intermaxillary segment

H₁

I — 14 weeks — Philtrum of lip

I₁

**FIGURE 9–25, cont'd**

Eye

Maxillary prominence

Entrance to stomodeum

Mandibular prominence

2nd pharyngeal arch

3rd pharyngeal arch

4th pharyngeal arch

Entrance to intraembryonic coelom

Frontonasal prominence

Umbilical vein

Spinal cord

**FIGURE 9-26** Scanning electron micrograph shows the ventral view of a Carnegie stage 14 embryo (30 to 32 days).

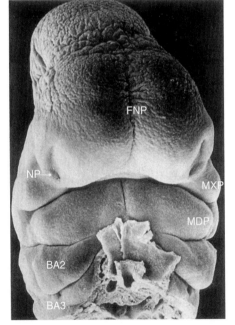

FNP

NP

MXP

MDP

BA2

BA3

**FIGURE 9-27** Scanning electron micrograph shows the ventral view of a Carnegie stage 15 embryo of approximately 33 days with a crown–rump length of 8 mm. Notice the prominent frontonasal process *(FNP)* surrounding the telencephalon (forebrain) and the nasal pits *(NP)* located in the ventrolateral regions of the FNP. Medial and lateral nasal prominences surround these pits. The maxillary prominences *(MXP)* form the lateral boundaries of the stomodeum. The fusing mandibular prominences *(MDP)* are located just caudal to the stomodeum. The second pharyngeal arch *(BA2)* shows overhanging margins (opercula), and the third arch *(BA3)* is also clearly visible. *(From Hinrichsen K: The early development of morphology and patterns of the face in the human embryo, Adv Anat Embryol Cell Biol 98:1, 1985.)*

regulated by platelet-derived growth factor receptor α-polypeptide (PDGFRA) signaling. Each **lateral nasal prominence** is separated from the maxillary prominence by a cleft, the **nasolacrimal groove** (see Figs. 9-25C and D).

By the end of the fifth week, the **primordia of the auricles** (external part of ears) have begun to develop (Fig. 9-29; see Fig. 9-25E). **Six auricular hillocks** (three mesenchymal swellings on each side) form around the first pharyngeal groove, the primordia of the auricle, and the **external acoustic meatus**, respectively. Initially, the external ears are located in the neck region (Fig. 9-30); however, as the mandible develops, they become located on the side of the head at the level of the eyes (see Fig. 9-25H).

By the end of the sixth week, each **maxillary prominence** has begun to merge with the **lateral nasal prominence** along the line of the nasolacrimal groove (Figs. 9-31 and 9-32). This establishes continuity between the side of the nose, which is formed by the lateral nasal prominence, and the cheek region formed by the maxillary prominence.

The **nasolacrimal duct** develops from a rod-like thickening of ectoderm in the floor of the **nasolacrimal groove**. This thickening forms a solid epithelial cord that separates from the ectoderm and sinks into the mesenchyme. Later, as a result of apoptosis (programmed cell death), the epithelial cord canalizes to form a duct. The superior end of the duct expands to form the **lacrimal sac**. By the late fetal period, the **nasolacrimal duct** drains into the inferior meatus in the lateral wall of the nasal cavity. The duct becomes completely patent after birth.

Between the 7th and 10th weeks, the **medial nasal prominences** merge with the maxillary and **lateral nasal prominences** (see Fig. 9-25G and H). Merging the prominences requires disintegration of their contacting surface epithelia, which results in intermingling of the

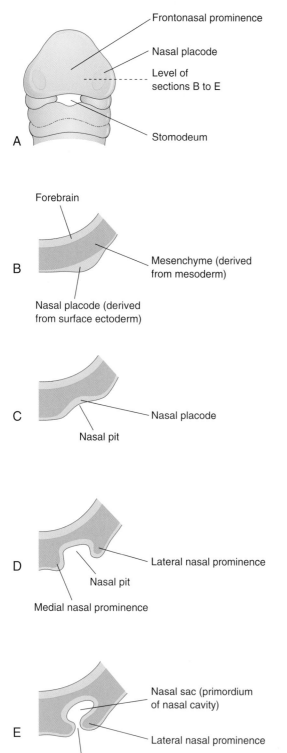

**FIGURE 9–28** Progressive stages in the development of a nasal sac (primordial nasal cavity). **A,** Ventral view of an embryo of approximately 28 days. **B** to **E,** Transverse sections through the left side of the developing nasal sac.

**FIGURE 9–29** Scanning electron micrograph shows the oblique view of the craniofacial region of a stage 16 embryo of approximately 41 days with a crown–rump length of 10.8 mm. The maxillary prominence *(MXP)* appears puffed up laterally and wedged between the lateral *(LNP)* and medial *(MNP)* nasal prominences surrounding the nasal pit *(NP)*. The auricular hillocks *(AH)* are present on both sides of the pharyngeal groove between the first and second arches, which will form the external acoustic meatus *(EAM)*. *MDP,* Mandibular prominence; *ST,* stomodeum. *(From Hinrichsen K: The early development of morphology and patterns of the face in the human embryo,* Adv Anat Embryol Cell Biol *98:1, 1985.)*

underlying mesenchymal cells. Merging the medial nasal and maxillary prominences results in continuity of the upper jaw and lip and separation of the nasal pits from the stomodeum.

As the medial nasal prominences merge, they form an **intermaxillary segment** (see Figs. 9-25H and 9-32E and F). This segment forms the middle part (philtrum) of the upper lip, the premaxillary part of the maxilla and its associated gingiva (gum), and the primary palate.

Clinical and embryologic studies indicate that the upper lip is formed entirely from the maxillary prominences. The lower parts of the medial nasal prominences appear to have become deeply positioned and covered by medial extensions of the maxillary prominences to form the **philtrum** (see Fig. 9-25H and I). In addition to connective tissue and muscular derivatives, various bones are derived from mesenchyme in the facial prominences.

Until the end of the sixth week, the primordial jaws are composed of masses of mesenchymal tissue. The lips and gingivae begin to develop when a linear thickening of the ectoderm, the **labiogingival lamina**, grows into the underlying mesenchyme (see Fig. 9-36B). Gradually, most of the lamina degenerates, leaving a **labiogingival groove**

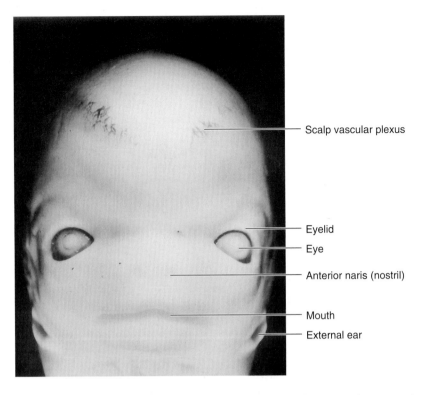

- Scalp vascular plexus
- Eyelid
- Eye
- Anterior naris (nostril)
- Mouth
- External ear

**FIGURE 9–30** Ventral view of the face of a stage 22 embryo at approximately 54 days. The eyes are widely separated, and the ears are low set at this stage. *(From Nishimura H, Semba R, Tanimura T, Tanaka O: Prenatal development of the human with special reference to craniofacial structures: an atlas. Bethesda, MD, 1977, U.S. Department of Health, Education, and Welfare, National Institutes of Health.)*

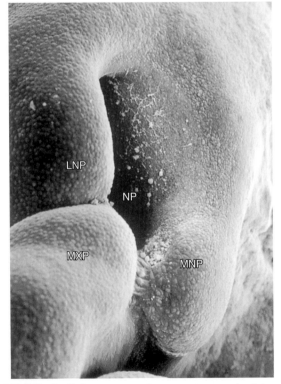

**FIGURE 9–31** Scanning electron micrograph of the right nasal region of a stage 17 embryo of approximately 41 days with a crown–rump length of 10.8 mm shows the maxillary prominence *(MXP)* fusing with the medial nasal prominence *(MNP)*. Epithelial bridges can be seen between these prominences. The furrow representing the nasolacrimal groove lies between the MXP and the lateral nasal prominence *(LNP)*. Notice the large nasal pit *(NP)*. *(From Hinrichsen K: The early development of morphology and patterns of the face in the human embryo, Adv Anat Embryol Cell Biol 98:1, 1985.)*

between the lips and gingivae (see Fig. 9-36H). A small area of the labiogingival lamina persists in the median plane to form the frenulum of the upper lip, which attaches the lip to the gum.

Further development of the face occurs slowly during the fetal period and results mainly from changes in the proportion and relative positions of the facial components. During the early fetal period, the nose is flat, and the mandible is underdeveloped (see Fig. 9-25H). At 14 weeks, the nose and mandible have their characteristic form as facial development is completed (see Fig. 9-25I).

As the brain enlarges, the **cranial cavity** (space occupied by the brain) expands bilaterally. This causes the orbits (bony cavities containing the eyeballs), which were oriented laterally, to assume a forward-facing orientation. The opening of the **external acoustic meatus** (auditory canal) appears to elevate, but it remains stationary; elongation of the lower jaw creates the false impression. The small appearance of the face prenatally results from the rudimentary upper and lower jaws, unerupted deciduous teethe (primary dentition), and small nasal cavities and maxillary sinuses.

Facial development requires all of the following components:

- The **frontal nasal prominence** forms the forehead and dorsum and apex of the nose (see Fig. 9-25F).
- The **lateral nasal prominences** form the alae (sides) of the nose.
- The **medial nasal prominences** form the nasal septum, ethmoid bone, and **cribriform plate** (openings for passage of olfactory nerves).
- The **maxillary prominences** form the upper cheek regions and lip.
- The **mandibular prominences** form the chin, lower lip, and cheek regions.

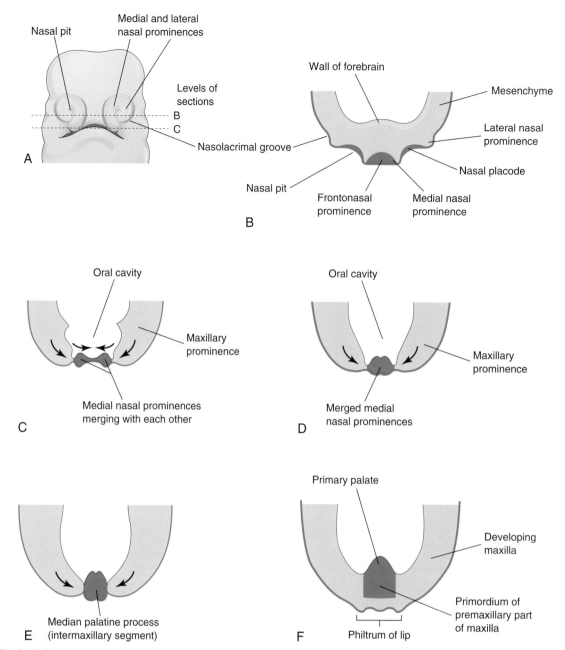

**FIGURE 9–32** Early development of the maxilla, palate, and upper lip. **A,** Diagram of a facial view of a 5-week embryo. **B** and **C,** Sketches of horizontal sections at the levels shown in **A**. The *arrows* indicate subsequent growth of the maxillary and medial nasal prominences toward the median plane and merging of the prominences with each other. **D** to **F,** Similar sections of older embryos illustrate merging of the medial nasal prominences with each other and the maxillary prominences to form the upper lip. Studies suggest that the upper lip is formed entirely from the maxillary prominences.

## ATRESIA OF THE NASOLACRIMAL DUCT

Part of the nasolacrimal duct occasionally fails to canalize, resulting in **congenital atresia** (lack of an opening) of the nasolacrimal duct. Obstruction of this duct with clinical symptoms occurs in approximately 6% of neonates.

## CONGENITAL AURICULAR SINUSES AND CYSTS

Small auricular sinuses and cysts are usually located in a triangular area of skin anterior to the auricle of the external ear (see Fig. 9-9F); however, they may occur in other sites around the auricle or in the lobule (earlobe). Although some sinuses and cysts are remnants of the first pharyngeal groove, others represent ectodermal folds sequestered during formation of the auricle from six **auricular hillocks** (nodular masses of mesenchyme from the first and second arches that coalesce to form the auricle). The sinuses and cysts are classified as minor defects that have no serious medical consequences.

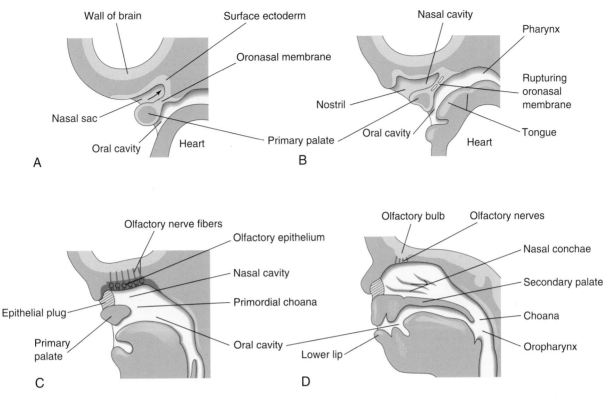

**FIGURE 9–33** Sagittal sections of the head show development of the nasal cavities. The nasal septum has been removed. **A,** Development at 5 weeks. **B,** At 6 weeks, the oronasal membrane breaks down. **C,** At 7 weeks, the nasal cavity communicates with the oral cavity and the olfactory epithelium develops. **D,** At 12 weeks, the palate and lateral wall of the nasal cavity develop.

## DEVELOPMENT OF NASAL CAVITIES

As the face develops, the **nasal placodes** become depressed, forming **nasal pits** (see Figs. 9-27, 9-28, and 9-31). Proliferation of the surrounding mesenchyme forms the medial and lateral **nasal prominences**, which results in deepening of the nasal pits and formation of **primordial nasal sacs.** Each sac grows dorsally and ventral to the developing forebrain. At first, the sacs are separated from the oral cavity by the **oronasal membrane** (Fig. 9-33*A*). This membrane ruptures by the end of the sixth week, bringing the nasal and oral cavities into communication (see Fig. 9-33*B* and *C*). Temporary epithelial plugs are formed in the nasal cavities from proliferation of the cells lining them. By the middle of the 16th week, the nasal plugs disappear.

The regions of continuity between the nasal and oral cavities are the **primordial choanae** (openings from the nasal cavity into the nasal pharynx). After the **secondary palate** develops, the choanae are located at the junction of the nasal cavity and pharynx (see Figs. 9-33*D* and 9-36). While these changes are occurring, the superior, middle, and inferior **nasal conchae** develop as elevations of the lateral walls of the nasal cavities (see Fig. 9-33*D*). Concurrently, the ectodermal epithelium in the roof of each nasal cavity becomes specialized to form the **olfactory epithelium** (see Fig. 9-33*C*). Some epithelial cells differentiate into **olfactory receptor cells** (neurons). The neuronal axons constitute the **olfactory nerves**, which grow into the **olfactory bulbs** of brain (see Fig. 9-33*C* and *D*).

Most of the upper lip, maxilla, and secondary palate forms from the **maxillary prominences** (see Fig. 9-25*H*). These prominences merge laterally with the **mandibular prominences.** The primordial lips and cheeks are invaded by mesenchyme from the second pair of pharyngeal arches, which differentiates into the facial muscles (see Fig. 9-5 and Table 9-1). The muscles of facial expression are supplied by the **facial nerve** (CN VII), the nerve of the second arch. The mesenchyme in the first pair of arches differentiates into the muscles of mastication (chewing) and a few others, all of which are innervated by the **trigeminal nerves** (CN V), which supply the first pair of arches.

### Paranasal Sinuses

Some paranasal sinuses, such as **maxillary sinuses,** begin to develop during late fetal life; the remaining sinuses develop after birth. They form from diverticula (outgrowths) of the walls of the nasal cavities and become pneumatic (air-filled) extensions of the nasal cavities in the adjacent bones, such as the maxillary sinuses in the maxillae, and the **frontal sinuses** in the frontal bones. The original openings of the diverticula persist as the orifices of the adult sinuses.

### Vomeronasal Organ

The first appearance of the **vomeronasal primordia** is in the form of bilateral epithelial thickenings on the nasal septum. Further invagination of the primordia and breaking away from the nasal septal epithelium forms a tubular **vomeronasal organ** (VNO) between days 37 and 43

Olfactory epithelium

Nasal septum

Nasal cavity

Vomeronasal nerve

Vomeronasal organ

Paraseptal cartilage

Tongue

Lateral palatine process

Oral cavity

**FIGURE 9–34** Photomicrograph of a frontal section through the developing oral cavity and nasal regions of a 22-mm human embryo of approximately 54 days shows the bilateral, tubular vomeronasal organ.

(Fig. 9-34). This chemosensory structure, which ends blindly posteriorly, reaches its greatest development between 12 and 14 weeks. Later, the receptor population is gradually replaced with patchy ciliated cells. The VNO is consistently present in the form of a bilateral duct-like structure on the nasal septum, superior to the paraseptal cartilage (see Fig. 9-34). The tubular human VNO with its minute anterior opening is a true homolog of the VNO in other mammals, reptiles, and amphibians used as an auxiliary olfactory sense organ typically to detect pheromones.

## POSTNATAL DEVELOPMENT OF PARANASAL SINUSES

Most of paranasal sinuses are rudimentary or absent in neonates. The **maxillary sinuses** are small at birth. They grow slowly until puberty and are not fully developed until all the permanent teeth have erupted in early adulthood.

No **frontal or sphenoidal sinuses** are present at birth. The **ethmoidal cells (sinuses)** are small before the age of 2 years, and they do not begin to grow rapidly until 6 to 8 years of age. At approximately 2 years of age, the two most anterior ethmoidal cells grow into the frontal bone, forming a **frontal sinus** on each side. Usually, the frontal sinuses are visible in radiographs by the seventh year.

The two most posterior ethmoidal cells grow into the sphenoid bone at approximately 2 years of age, forming two **sphenoidal sinuses**. Growth of the paranasal sinuses is important in altering the size and shape of the face during infancy and childhood and in adding resonance to the voice during adolescence.

## DEVELOPMENT OF PALATE

The palate develops from two primordia, the primary and secondary palates. **Palatogenesis** (regulated morphogenetic process) begins in the sixth week, but it is not completed until the 12th week. *Molecular pathways, including WNT and PRICKLE1, are involved in this process.* The critical period of palatogenesis is from the end of the sixth week until the beginning of the ninth week. The palate develops in two stages: primary and secondary.

### Primary Palate

Early in the sixth week, the primary palate (**median process**) begins to develop (see Figs. 9-32F and 9-33). Formed by merging the **medial nasal prominences**, this segment is initially a wedge-shaped mass of mesenchyme between the internal surfaces of the **maxillary prominences** of the developing maxillae. The primary palate forms the anterior and midline aspect of the maxilla, the **premaxillary part of the maxilla** (Fig. 9-35B). It represents only a small part of the adult **hard palate** (anterior to the incisive fossa).

### Secondary Palate

The secondary palate (definitive palate) is the primordium of the hard and soft parts of the palate (see Figs. 9-33D and 9-35). The palate begins to develop early in the sixth week from two mesenchymal projections that extend from the internal aspects of the **maxillary prominences**. These **lateral palatine processes** (palatal shelves) initially project inferomedially on each side of the tongue (Figs. 9-36B and 9-37A and B). As the jaws elongate, they pull the tongue away from its root, and it is brought lower in the mouth.

During the seventh and eighth weeks, the **lateral palatine processes** assume a horizontal position above the tongue (see Figs. 9-36E to H and 9-37C). This change in orientation occurs by a flowing process facilitated in part by the release of hyaluronic acid by the mesenchyme of the palatine processes.

Bone gradually develops in the primary palate, forming the **premaxillary part of maxilla**, which lodges the incisor teeth (see Fig. 9-35B). Concurrently, bone extends from the maxillae and palatine bones into the lateral palatine processes to form the **hard palate** (see Fig. 9-36E and G). The posterior parts of these processes do not ossify. They extend posteriorly beyond the nasal septum and fuse to form the **soft palate**, including its soft conical projection, the **uvula** (see Fig. 9-36D, F, and H). The palatine raphe indicates the line of fusion of the palatine processes (see Fig. 9-36H).

A small **nasopalatine canal** persists in the median plane of the palate between the anterior part of the maxilla and the palatine processes of the maxillae. This canal is represented in the adult hard palate by the **incisive fossa** (see Fig. 9-35B), which is the common opening for the small right and left incisive canals. An irregular suture runs on each side from the fossa to the alveolar process of the maxilla between the lateral incisor and canine teeth on

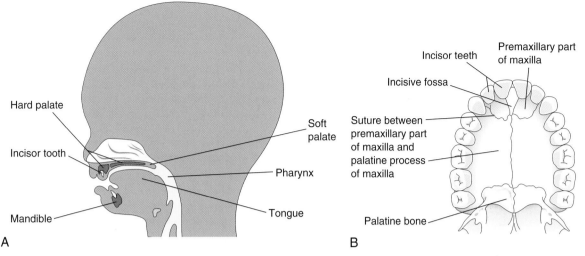

**FIGURE 9–35** A, Sagittal section of the head of a 20-week fetus shows the location of the palate. **B**, Bony palate and alveolar arch of a young adult. The suture between the premaxillary part of the maxilla and the fused palatine processes of the maxillae is usually visible in the cranium (skulls) of a young adult. Most dried crania are from older adults, and the suture is not visible.

each side (see Fig. 9-35B). It is visible in the anterior region of the palates of young persons. This suture indicates where the embryonic primary and secondary palates fused.

The **nasal septum** develops as a down growth from internal parts of the merged medial nasal prominences (see Figs. 9-36 and 9-37). The fusion between the nasal septum and palatine processes begins anteriorly during the ninth week, and it is completed posteriorly by the 12th week superior to the primordium of the hard palate (see Fig. 9-36D to H).

*Text continued on p. 191*

## CLEFT LIP AND CLEFT PALATE

Clefts of the upper lip and palate are common craniofacial birth defects. A 2014 report from the U.S. Department of Health and Human Services indicated that approximately 7000 neonates have orofacial clefts each year in the United States. The defects are usually classified according to developmental criteria, with the incisive fossa used as a reference landmark (see Fig. 9-35B). These clefts are especially conspicuous because they result in an abnormal facial appearance and defective speech. There are **two major groups of cleft lip and cleft palat**e (Figs. 9-38, 9-39, and 9-40):

- **Anterior cleft defects** include cleft lip with or without a cleft of the alveolar part of the maxilla. In a complete anterior cleft defect, the cleft extends through the upper lip and alveolar part of the maxilla to the incisive fossa, separating the anterior and posterior parts of the palate (see Fig. 9-39E and F). Anterior cleft defects result from a deficiency of mesenchyme in the maxillary prominences and the median palatine process (see Fig. 9-32E).
- **Posterior cleft defects** include clefts of the secondary palate that extend through the soft and hard regions of the palate to the incisive fossa, separating the anterior and posterior parts of the palate (see

Fig. 9-39G and H). Posterior cleft defects result from defective development of the secondary palate and growth distortions of the lateral palatine processes that prevent their fusion. Other factors such as the width of the stomodeum, mobility of the lateral **palatine processes** (palatal shelves), and altered focal degeneration sites of the palatal epithelium may contribute to these birth defects.

A cleft lip with or without a cleft palate occurs approximately once in 1000 births, but the frequency varies widely among ethnic groups. Between 60% and 80% of affected neonates are male. The clefts vary from incomplete cleft lip to those that extend into the nose and through the alveolar part of the maxilla (see Figs. 9-38 and 9-40A and B). Cleft lip may be unilateral or bilateral.

A **unilateral cleft lip** (see Figs. 9-38, 9-39E and F, and 9-40A) results from failure of the **maxillary prominence** on the affected side to unite with the merged **medial nasal prominences**. Failure of the mesenchymal masses to merge and mesenchyme to proliferate and smooth the overlying epithelium results in *a persistent labia groove* (Fig. 9-41D). The epithelium in the labial groove becomes stretched, and the tissue in the floor of the groove breaks down, resulting in a lip that is divided into medial and lateral parts (see

*Continued*

## CLEFT LIP AND CLEFT PALATE—cont'd

Fig. 9-41*G* and *H*). A bridge of tissue, called the *Simonart band*, sometimes joins the parts of the incomplete unilateral cleft lip.

A **bilateral cleft lip** results from failure of the mesenchymal masses in both maxillary prominences to meet and unite with the merged medial nasal prominences (Fig. 9-42*C* and *D*; see Fig. 9-40*B*). The epithelium in both labial grooves becomes stretched and breaks down (see Fig. 9-41*H*). In bilateral cases, the defects may be dissimilar, with various degrees of defect on each side. When there is a complete **bilateral cleft of lip and alveolar part of the maxilla**, the median palatal process hangs free and projects anteriorly (see Fig. 9-40*B*). These defects are especially deforming because of the loss of continuity of the **orbicularis oris muscle** (see Fig. 9-5*B*), which closes the mouth and purses the lips.

A **median cleft lip** is a rare defect that results from a mesenchymal deficiency. This defect causes partial or complete failure of the medial nasal prominences to merge and form the median palatal process. A median cleft lip is a characteristic feature of the **Mohr syndrome**, which is transmitted as an autosomal recessive trait. A median cleft of the lower lip is also rare and results from failure of the mesenchymal masses in the mandibular prominences to merge completely and smooth the embryonic cleft between them (see Fig. 9-25*A*).

A **cleft palate** with or without a cleft lip occurs approximately once in 2500 births, and it is more common in girls than in boys. The cleft may involve only the uvula (a **cleft uvula** has a fishtail appearance; see Fig. 9-39*B*), or the cleft may extend through the soft and hard regions of the palate (see Figs. 9-39*C* and *D* and 9-42). In severe cases associated with a cleft lip, the cleft in the palate extends through the alveolar part of the maxilla and lips on both sides (see Figs. 9-39*G* and *H* and 9-40*B*).

A **complete cleft palate** is the maximum degree of clefting of any particular type. For example, a complete cleft of the posterior palate is a defect in which the cleft extends through the soft palate and anteriorly to the incisive fossa.

The landmark for distinguishing anterior from posterior cleft defects is the incisive fossa. Unilateral and bilateral clefts of the palate are classified in three groups:

- *Clefts of the anterior palate* (clefts anterior to the incisive fossa) result from failure of mesenchymal masses in the lateral palatal processes to meet and fuse with the mesenchyme in the primary palate (see Fig. 9-39*E* and *F*).
- *Clefts of the posterior palate* (clefts posterior to the incisive fossa) result from failure of mesenchymal masses in the lateral palatine processes to meet and fuse with each other and the nasal septum (see Fig. 9-39*C* and *D*).
- *Clefts of the secondary parts of the palate* (clefts of the anterior and posterior palates) result from failure of the mesenchymal masses in the lateral palatine processes to meet and fuse with mesenchyme in the primary palate, with each other, and the nasal septum (see Fig. 9-39*G* and *H*).

Most clefts of the upper lip and palate result from multiple genetic and nongenetic factors (**multifactorial inheritance**; see Chapter 20, Fig. 20-1), with each causing a minor developmental disturbance. Several studies show that the interferon regulatory factor 6 gene (*IRF6*) is involved in the formation of isolated clefts.

Some clefts of the lip and/or palate appear as part of syndromes determined by single mutant genes. Other clefts are parts of chromosomal syndromes, especially **trisomy 13** (see Chapter 20, Fig. 20-8). A few cases of cleft lip and/or palate appear to have been caused by **teratogenic agents** (e.g., anticonvulsant drugs). Studies of twins indicate that genetic factors are more important in cases of cleft lip with or without a cleft palate than in cleft palate alone.

A sibling of a child with a cleft palate has an elevated risk of cleft palate but has no increased risk of cleft lip. A cleft of the lip and alveolar process of the maxilla that continues through the palate is usually transmitted through a male sex-linked gene. When neither parent is affected, the recurrence risk in subsequent siblings is approximately 4%.

## OTHER FACIAL DEFECTS

**Congenital microstomia** (small mouth) results from excessive merging of the mesenchymal masses in the maxillary and mandibular prominences of the first pharyngeal arch. In severe cases, the defect may be associated with underdevelopment (hypoplasia) of the mandible. A **single nostril** results when only one nasal placode forms. A **bifid nose** results when the medial nasal prominences do not merge completely; the nostrils are widely separated and the nasal bridge is bifid. In mild forms, there is a groove in the tip of the nose.

At the beginning of the second trimester (see Fig. 9-25), features of the fetal face can be identified sonographically. Using this imaging technique (Fig. 9-43), facial defects such as a cleft lip are readily recognizable.

**FIGURE 9–36** A, Drawings of sagittal section of the embryonic head at the end of the sixth week shows the median palatal process. B, D, F, and H, Sections of the roof of the mouth from the 6th to 12th week show development of the palate. The *broken lines* in D and F indicate sites of fusion of the palatine processes. The *arrows* indicate medial and posterior growth of the lateral palatine processes. C, E, and G, Frontal sections of the head show fusion of the lateral palatine processes with each other, the nasal septum, and separation of the nasal and oral cavities.

**FIGURE 9–38** An infant with a unilateral cleft lip and cleft palate. Clefts of the lip, with or without a cleft palate, occur in approximately 1 in 1000 births, and most affected infants are male.

**FIGURE 9–37** Frontal sections of embryonic heads show development of the lateral palatal processes (P), nasal septum (NS), and tongue (T) during the eighth week. **A,** Section of an embryo with a crown–rump length (CRL) of 24 mm shows early development of the palatine processes. **B,** Section of an embryo with a CRL of 27 mm shows the palate just before palatine process elevation. **C,** In an embryo with a CRL of 29 mm (near the end of the eighth week), the palatine processes are elevated and fused. (From Sandham A: Embryonic facial vertical dimension and its relationship to palatal shelf elevation, Early Hum Dev 12:241, 1985.)

## FACIAL CLEFTS

Various types of facial clefts occur, but all are rare. Severe clefts are usually associated with gross defects of the head. **Oblique facial clefts** are often bilateral and extend from the upper lip to the medial margin of the **orbit** (bony cavity containing the eyeball). When this occurs, the nasolacrimal ducts are open grooves (persistent nasolacrimal grooves) (Fig. 9-44). Oblique facial clefts associated with cleft lip result from failure of the mesenchymal masses in the maxillary prominences to merge with the lateral and medial nasal prominences. **Lateral or transverse facial clefts** run from the mouth toward the ear. **Bilateral clefts** result in a very large mouth (**macrostomia**). In severe cases, the clefts in the cheeks extend almost to the ears.

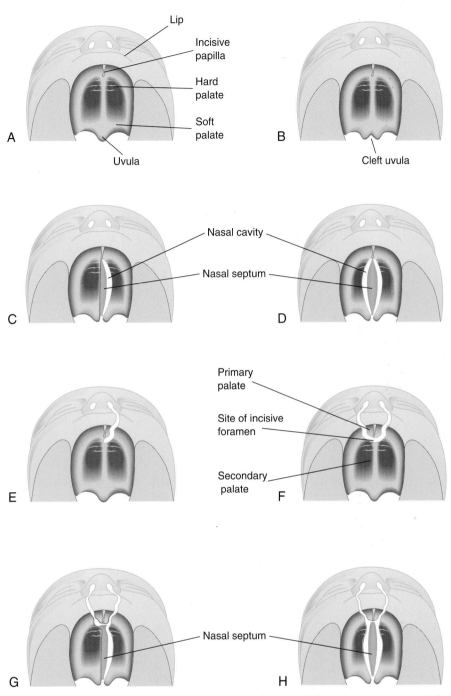

**FIGURE 9–39** Types of cleft lip and palate. A, Normal lip and palate. B, Cleft uvula. C, Unilateral cleft of the secondary (posterior) palate. D, Bilateral cleft of the posterior part of the palate. E, Complete unilateral cleft of the lip and alveolar process of the maxilla with a unilateral cleft of the primary (anterior) palate. F, Complete bilateral cleft of the lip and alveolar processes of the maxillae with bilateral cleft of the anterior part of the palate. G, Complete bilateral cleft of the lip and alveolar processes of the maxillae with bilateral cleft of the anterior part of the palate and unilateral cleft of the posterior part of the palate. H, Complete bilateral cleft of the lip and alveolar processes of the maxillae with complete bilateral cleft of the anterior and posterior palate.

**FIGURE 9–40** Birth defects of the lip and palate. **A,** Infant with a left unilateral cleft lip and cleft palate. **B,** Infant with a bilateral cleft lip and cleft palate.

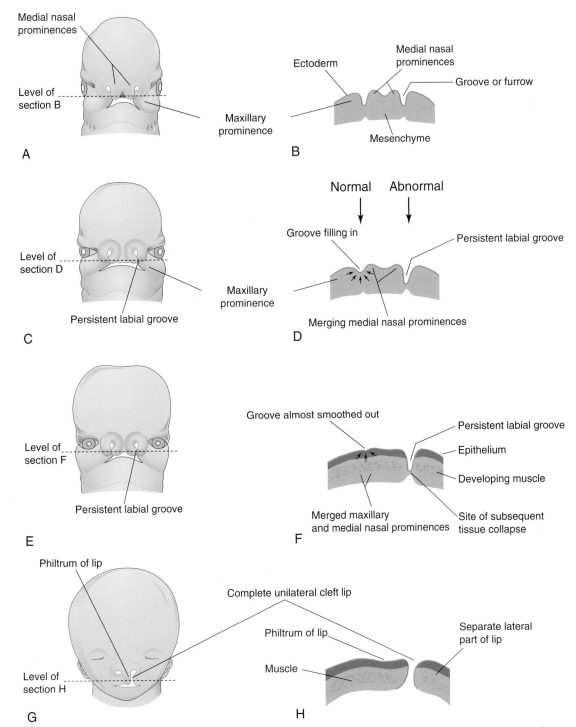

**FIGURE 9–41** Embryologic basis of complete unilateral cleft lip. **A,** Drawing of a 5-week embryo. **B,** Horizontal section through the head shows the grooves between the maxillary prominences and merging medial nasal prominences. **C,** Drawing of a 6-week embryo shows a persistent labial groove on the left side. **D,** Horizontal section through the head shows the groove gradually filling in on the right side after proliferation of mesenchyme *(arrows)*. **E,** Drawing of a 7-week embryo. **F,** Horizontal section through the head shows that the epithelium on the right has almost been pushed out of the groove between the maxillary and medial nasal prominences. **G,** Drawing of a 10-week fetus with a complete unilateral cleft lip. **H,** Horizontal section through the head after stretching of the epithelium and breakdown of the tissues in the floor of the persistent labial groove on the left side shows formation of a complete unilateral cleft lip.

**FIGURE 9–42** Birth defects of the lip and palate. **A**, Male neonate with a unilateral complete cleft lip and cleft palate. **B**, Intraoral photograph (taken with a mirror) shows a left unilateral complete cleft of the primary and secondary parts of the palate. **C**, Female neonate with a bilateral complete cleft lip and cleft palate. **D**, Intraoral photograph shows a bilateral complete cleft palate. Notice the maxillary protrusion and natal tooth (present at birth) in the gingival apex in each lesser segment.

**FIGURE 9–43** **A**, Three-dimensional ultrasound surface rendering of a fetus with a unilateral cleft lip. **B**, Coronal sonogram shows a fetal mouth with a cleft lip extending into the left nostril *(plus sign)*. **C**, Coronal sonogram shows a fetus with a bilateral cleft lip *(arrows)*, lower lip *(L)*, and chin *(C)*. **D**, Sagittal magnetic resonance image of a fetus shows the absence of the middle part of the hard palate. Notice the fluid above the tongue *(t)* without intervening palate.

**FIGURE 9–44** Photographs of a child with an oblique facial cleft. Notice the persistent nasolacrimal cleft. **A,** Before surgical correction. **B,** After surgical correction.

## SUMMARY OF PHARYNGEAL APPARATUS, FACE, AND NECK

- The **primordial pharynx** is bounded laterally by **pharyngeal arches.** Each arch consists of a core of mesenchyme covered externally by ectoderm and internally by endoderm. The original mesenchyme of each arch is derived from mesoderm. Later, **neural crest cells** migrate into the arches and are the major source of the connective tissue components, including cartilage, bone, and ligaments in the oral and facial regions. Each arch contains an artery, cartilage rod, nerve, and a muscular component.

- **Externally, the pharyngeal arches** are separated by pharyngeal grooves. Internally, the arches are separated by evaginations of the pharynx (**pharyngeal pouches**). Where the ectoderm of a groove contacts the endoderm of a pouch, **pharyngeal membranes** are formed. The adult derivatives of the various pharyngeal arch components are summarized in Table 9-1, and the derivatives of the pouches are illustrated in Figure 9-7.

- The **pharyngeal grooves** disappear except for the first pair, which persists as the external acoustic meatus. The **pharyngeal membranes** also disappear, except for the first pair, which becomes the tympanic membranes. The **first pharyngeal pouch** forms the tympanic cavity, mastoid antrum, and pharyngotympanic tube. The **second pharyngeal pouch** is associated with the development of the palatine tonsil.

- The **thymus** is derived from the **third pair of pharyngeal pouches,** and the **parathyroid glands** are formed from the **third and fourth pairs of pouches.**

- The **thyroid gland** develops from a down growth from the floor of the *primordial pharynx* in the region where the tongue develops. The parafollicular cells (C cells) in the thyroid gland are derived from the **ultimopharyngeal bodies,** which are derived mainly from the fourth pair of pharyngeal pouches.

- Cervical cysts, sinuses, and fistulas may develop from parts of the second pharyngeal groove, the **cervical sinus,** or the second pharyngeal pouch that fail to obliterate.

- An **ectopic thyroid gland** results when the gland fails to descend completely from its site of origin in the tongue. The **thyroglossal duct** may persist, or remnants of it may form **thyroglossal duct cysts** and ectopic thyroid tissue masses. Infected cysts may perforate the skin and form thyroglossal duct sinuses that open anteriorly in the median plane of the neck.

- **Cleft of the upper lip** is a common birth defect. Although frequently associated with cleft palate, cleft lip and cleft palate are etiologically distinct defects that involve different developmental processes occurring at different times. *Cleft of the upper lip results from failure of mesenchymal masses in the medial nasal and maxillary prominences to merge, whereas cleft palate results from failure of mesenchymal masses in the palatal processes to meet and fuse.* Most cases of cleft lip, with or without cleft palate, are caused by a combination of genetic and environmental factors (**multifactorial inheritance;** see Chapter 20).

## CLINICALLY ORIENTED PROBLEMS

### CASE 9–1

*The mother of a 2-year-old boy consulted her pediatrician about an intermittent discharge of mucoid material from a small opening in the side of the boy's neck. There was also extensive redness and swelling in the inferior third of his neck just anterior to the sternocleidomastoid muscle.*

* What is the most likely diagnosis?
* What is the probable embryologic basis of this intermittent mucoid discharge?
* Discuss the cause of this birth defect.

## CASE 9–2

*During a subtotal thyroidectomy, the surgeon located only one inferior parathyroid gland.*

* Where might the other one be located?
* What is the embryologic basis for the ectopic location of this gland?

## CASE 9–3

*A young woman consulted her physician about a swelling in the anterior part of her neck, just inferior to the hyoid bone.*

* What kind of a cyst is this?
* Are they always in the median plane?
* Discuss the embryologic basis of these cysts.
* What other condition may be confused with the swelling?

## CASE 9–4

*A male neonate has a unilateral cleft lip extending into his nose and through the alveolar process of his maxilla.*

* Are the terms *harelip* and *cleft lip* synonymous?
* What is the embryologic basis of this birth defect?
* Neither parent had a cleft lip or cleft palate. Are genetic factors likely involved?
* Are these defects more common in males?
* What is the chance that the next child will have a cleft lip?

## CASE 9–5

*A mother with epilepsy who was treated with an anticonvulsant drug during pregnancy gave birth to a child with a cleft lip and palate.*

* Is there evidence indicating that these drugs increase the incidence of these birth defects?
* Discuss the causes of these two birth defects.

Discussion of these problems appears in the Appendix at the back of the book.

## BIBLIOGRAPHY AND SUGGESTED READING

Abbott BD: The etiology of cleft palate: a 50-year search for mechanistic and molecular understanding, *Birth Defects Res B Dev Reprod Toxicol* 89:266, 2010.

Arnold JS, Werling U, Braunstein EM, et al: Inactivation of Tbx1 in the pharyngeal endoderm results in 22q11DS malformations, *Development* 133:977, 2006.

Bajaj Y, Ifeacho S, Tweedie D, et al: Branchial anomalies in children, *Int J Pediatr Otorhinolaryngol* 75:1020, 2011.

Berkovitz BKB, Holland GR, Moxham B: *Oral anatomy, histology, and embryology*, ed 4, Edinburgh, 2009, Mosby.

Bothe I, Tenin G, Oseni A, et al: Dynamic control of head mesoderm patterning, *Development* 138:2807, 2011.

Edmunds J, Fulbrook P, Miles S: My baby has tongue-tie: what does this mean?, *J Hum Lact* 30:244, 2014.

Edmunds J, Miles SC, Fulbrook P: Tongue-tie and breastfeeding: a review of the literature, *Breastfeed Rev* 19:19, 2011.

Gartner LP, Hiatt JL: *Color textbook of histology*, ed 3, Philadelphia, 2007, Saunders.

Gitton Y, Heude E, Vieux-Rochas M, et al: Evolving maps in craniofacial development, *Semin Cell Develop Biol* 21:301, 2010.

Greene RM, Pisano MM: Palate morphogenesis: current understanding and future directions, *Birth Defects Res C* 90:133, 2010.

Gross E, Sichel JY: Congenital neck lesions, *Surg Clin North Am* 86:383, 2006.

Hennekam R, Allanson J, Krantz I: *Gorlin's syndromes of the head and neck*, ed 5, New York, 2010, Oxford University Press.

Hinrichsen K: The early development of morphology and patterns of the face in the human embryo, *Adv Anat Embryol Cell Biol* 98:1, 1985.

Hong P, Lago D, Seargeant J, et al: Defining ankyloglossia: a case series of anterior and posterior tongue ties, *Int J Pediatr Otorhinolaryngol* 74:1003, 2010.

Jirásel JE: *An atlas of human prenatal developmental mechanics. anatomy and staging*, London, 2004, Taylor & Francis.

Jones KL, Jones MC, Campo MD: *Smith's recognizable patterns of human malformation: Smith's recognizable patterns of human malformation*, ed 7, Philadelphia, 2013, Saunders.

Kurosaka H, Iulianella A, Williams T, et al: Disrupting hedgehog and WNT signaling interactions promotes cleft lip pathogenesis, *J Clin Invest* 124:2014, 1660.

Lale SM, Lele MS, Anderson VM: The thymus in infancy and childhood, *Chest Surg Clin North Am* 11:233, 2001.

Minoux M, Rijii FM: Molecular mechanisms of cranial neural crest cell migration and patterning in craniofacial development, *Development* 137:2605, 2010.

Moore KL, Dalley AD, Agur AMR: *Clinically oriented anatomy*, ed 7, Baltimore, 2014, Lippincott Williams & Wilkins.

Mueller DT, Callanan VP: Congenital malformations of the oral cavity, *Otolaryngol Clin North Am* 40:141, 2007.

Nishimura Y: Embryological study of nasal cavity development in human embryos with reference to congenital nostril atresia, *Acta Anat* 147:140, 1993.

Noden DM: Cell movements and control of patterned tissue assembly during craniofacial development, *J Craniofac Genet Dev Biol* 11: 192, 1991.

Noden DM: Vertebrate craniofacial development: novel approaches and new dilemmas, *Curr Opin Genet Dev* 2:576, 1992.

Noden DM, Francis-West P: The differentiation and morphogenesis of craniofacial muscles, *Dev Dyn* 235:1194, 2006.

Noden DM, Trainor PA: Relations and interactions between cranial mesoderm and neural crest populations, *J Anat* 207:575, 2005.

Ozolek JA: Selective pathologies of the head and neck in children—a developmental perspective, *Adv Anat Pathol* 16:332, 2009.

Passos-Bueno MR, Ornelas CC, Fanganiello RD: Syndromes of the first and second pharyngeal arches: a review, *Am J Med Genet A* 149A:1853, 2009.

Pilu G, Segata M, Perola A: Fetal craniofacial and neck anomalies. In Callen PW, editor: *Ultrasonography in obstetrics and gynecology*, ed 5, Philadelphia, 2008, Saunders.

Rice DPC: Craniofacial anomalies: from development to molecular pathogenesis, *Curr Mol Med* 5:699, 2009.

Rodriguez-Vázquez JF: Development of the stapes and associated structures in human embryos, *J Anat* 207:165, 2005.

Sperber GH, Sperber SM, Guttmann GD: *Craniofacial embryogenetics and development*, ed 2, Beijing, 2010, People's Medical Publishing House/PMPH-Global.

Thi Thu HN, Haw Tien SF, Loh SL: Tbx2a is required for specification of endodermal pouches during development of the pharyngeal arches, *PLoS One* 10:e77171, 2013.

Thompson H, Ohazama A, Sharpe PT, et al: The origin of the stapes and relationship to the otic capsule and oval window, *Dev Dyn* 241:1396, 2012.

Tovar JA: The neural crest in pediatric surgery, *J Pediatr Surg* 42:915, 2007.

Yatzey KE: Di George syndrome, Tbx1, and retinoic acid signaling come full circle, *Circ Res* 106:630, 2010.

# Respiratory System

**T**he lower respiratory organs (larynx, trachea, bronchi, and lungs) begin to form during the fourth week of development.

## RESPIRATORY PRIMORDIUM

The respiratory system starts as a median outgrowth, the **laryngotracheal groove**, which appears in the floor of the caudal end of the anterior foregut (primordial pharynx) (Fig. 10-1*B* and *C*; see also Fig. 10-4*A*). This primordium of the **tracheobronchial tree** develops caudal to the fourth pair of pharyngeal pouches. The endodermal lining of the laryngotracheal groove forms the pulmonary epithelium and glands of the larynx, trachea, and bronchi. The connective tissue, cartilage, and smooth muscle in these structures develop from splanchnic mesoderm surrounding the foregut (see Fig. 10-5*A*).

By the end of the fourth week, the laryngotracheal groove has evaginated (protruded) to form a pouch-like **laryngotracheal diverticulum** (lung bud), which is located ventral to the caudal part of the foregut (Fig. 10-2*A*, and see also Fig. 10-1*B*). As this diverticulum elongates, it is invested with **splanchnic mesenchyme**. Its distal end enlarges to form a globular **respiratory bud** that denotes the single bud from which the respiratory tree originates (see Fig. 10-2*B*).

The **laryngotracheal diverticulum** soon separates from the primordial pharynx; however, it maintains communication with it through the **primordial laryngeal inlet** (see Fig. 10-2*C*). Longitudinal **tracheoesophageal folds** develop in the diverticulum, approach each other, and fuse to form a partition, the **tracheoesophageal septum,** at the end of the fifth week (see Fig. 10-2*D* and *E*). This septum divides the cranial portion of the foregut into a ventral part, the **laryngotracheal tube** (the primordium of the larynx, trachea, bronchi, and lungs), and a dorsal part (the primordium of the oropharynx and esophagus; see Fig. 10-2*F*). The

**A**    Lateral view

The pharyngeal arches are indicated.

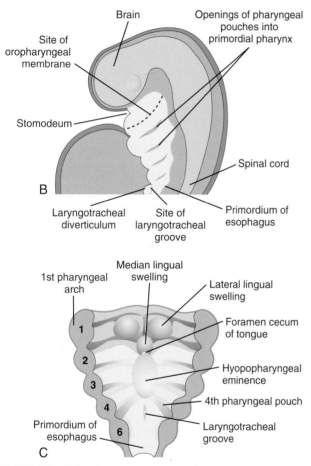

**FIGURE 10–1** *A,* Lateral view of a 4-week embryo illustrating the relationship of the pharyngeal apparatus to the developing respiratory system. *B,* Sagittal section of the cranial half of the embryo. *C,* Horizontal section of the embryo illustrating the floor of the primordial pharynx and the location of the laryngotracheal groove.

opening of the laryngotracheal tube into the pharynx becomes the **primordial laryngeal inlet** (see Figs. 10-2*C* and 10-4*B* to *D*). *The separation of the single foregut tube into the trachea and esophagus results from a complex and coordinated process of multiple signaling pathways and transcription factors* (Fig. 10-3).

# DEVELOPMENT OF LARYNX

The epithelial lining of the larynx develops from the endoderm of the cranial end of the **laryngotracheal tube.** The cartilages of the larynx develop from the fourth and sixth pairs of pharyngeal arches (see Fig. 10-1*A* and *C*). The **laryngeal cartilages** develop from mesenchyme that is derived from **neural crest cells.** The mesenchyme at the cranial end of the laryngotracheal tube proliferates rapidly, producing paired **arytenoid swellings** (Fig. 10-4*B*). The swellings grow toward the tongue, converting the slit-like aperture, the **primordial glottis**, into a T-shaped **laryngeal inlet** and reducing the developing laryngeal lumen to a narrow slit (see Fig. 10-4*C*).

The laryngeal epithelium proliferates rapidly, resulting in temporary occlusion of the laryngeal lumen. Recanalization normally occurs by the 10th week (see Fig. 10-4*D*); laryngeal ventricles form during this recanalization process. These recesses are bounded by folds of mucous membrane that become the **vocal folds** (cords) and **vestibular folds.**

The **epiglottis** develops from the caudal part of the **hypopharyngeal eminence,** a prominence produced by proliferation of mesenchyme in the ventral ends of the third and fourth pharyngeal arches (see Fig. 10-4*B* to *D*). The rostral part of this eminence forms the posterior third or pharyngeal part of the tongue (see Fig. 10-4*C* and *D*).

Because the **laryngeal muscles** develop from myoblasts in the fourth and sixth pairs of pharyngeal arches, they are innervated by the laryngeal branches of the **vagus nerves** (cranial nerve X) that supply these arches (see Chapter 9, Table 9-1). The larynx is found in a high position in the neck of the neonate; this positioning allows the epiglottis to come into contact with the soft palate. This provides an almost separate respiratory and digestive tract, facilitating nursing, but also means that neonates almost obligatorily breathe through their noses. Structural descent of the larynx occurs over the first 2 years of life.

## LARYNGEAL ATRESIA

Laryngeal atresia (obstruction), a rare birth defect, results from failure of recanalization of the larynx, which produces obstruction of the upper fetal airway, or **congenital high airway obstruction syndrome (CHAOS syndrome)**. Distal to the region of atresia or stenosis (narrowing), the airways become dilated and the lungs are enlarged and filled with fluid. The diaphragm is either flattened or inverted, and there is **fetal ascites** (accumulation of serous fluid in the peritoneal cavity) and/or **hydrops** (accumulation of fluid in the intracellular spaces, causing severe edema).

Incomplete atresia, or laryngeal web, is a defect in which the connective tissue between the vocal folds is covered with a mucous membrane; this causes airway obstruction and a hoarse cry in the neonate. This defect results from incomplete recanalization of the larynx during the 10th week. Treatment is by endoscopic dilation of the laryngeal web.

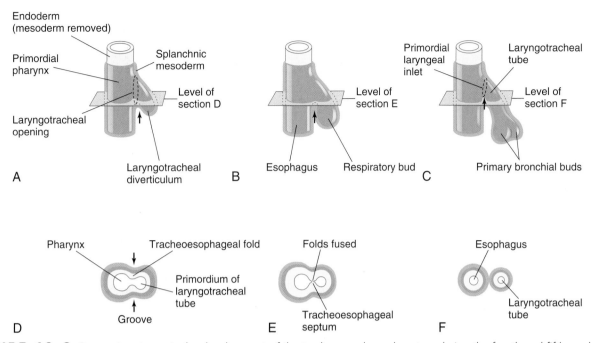

**FIGURE 10-2** Successive stages in the development of the tracheoesophageal septum during the fourth and fifth weeks. **A** to **C**, Lateral views of the caudal part of the primordial pharynx showing the laryngotracheal diverticulum and partitioning of the foregut into the esophagus and laryngotracheal tube. **D** to **F**, Transverse sections illustrating formation of the tracheoesophageal septum and showing how it separates the foregut into the laryngotracheal tube and esophagus. The *arrows* indicate cellular changes resulting from growth.

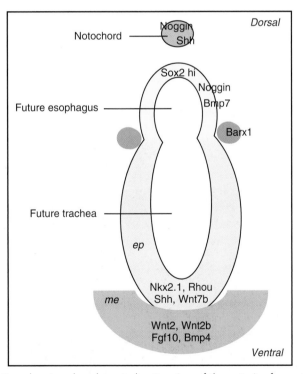

**FIGURE 10-3** Schematic section showing dorsal–ventral patterning of the anterior foregut (mouse). The unseparated anterior foregut tube shows high levels of Sox2, Noggin, and Bmp7 in the dorsal epithelium that will give rise to the esophagus. The ventral epithelium, which will contribute to the trachea, highly expresses transcription factor Nkx2.1 and signaling molecules Shh and Wnt7b, along with Rhou. Homeobox gene Barx1 is expressed at the demarcation between the dorsal and ventral foregut separation. The ventral mesenchyme factors Wnt2, Wnt2b, Fgf10, and Bmp4 support gene expression in the epithelium. Defects in the Shh, Wnt, or Bmp pathway or mutations of Sox2, Nkx2.1, or Rhou can result in abnormal foregut development, leading to esophageal atresia with or without tracheoesophageal fistula.

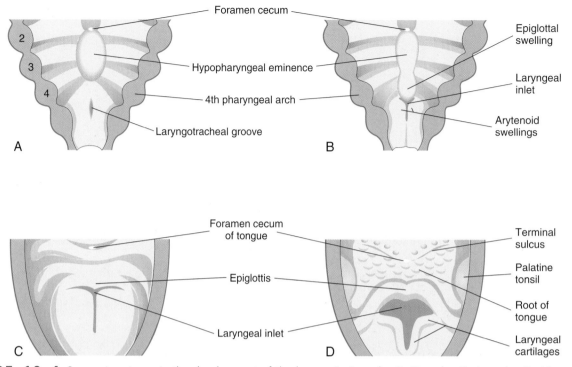

**FIGURE 10–4** Successive stages in the development of the larynx. **A,** 4 weeks. **B,** 5 weeks. **C,** 6 weeks. **D,** 10 weeks. The epithelium lining the larynx is of endodermal origin. The cartilages and muscles of the larynx arise from mesenchyme in the fourth and sixth pairs of pharyngeal arches. Note that the laryngeal inlet changes in shape from a slit-like opening to a T-shaped inlet as the mesenchyme surrounding the developing larynx proliferates.

## DEVELOPMENT OF TRACHEA

During its separation from the foregut, the **laryngotracheal diverticulum** forms the trachea and two lateral outpouchings, the **primary bronchial buds** (see Figs. 10-2C, 10-8A, and 10-9). The endodermal lining of the laryngotracheal tube distal to the larynx differentiates into the epithelium and glands of the trachea and the pulmonary epithelium. The cartilage, connective tissue, and muscles of the trachea are derived from the splanchnic mesenchyme surrounding the laryngotracheal tube (Fig. 10-5).

### TRACHEOESOPHAGEAL FISTULA

A **fistula** (abnormal passage) between the trachea and esophagus occurs once in 3000 to 4500 infants. (Figs. 10-6 and 10-7); most affected infants are males. In more than 85% of cases, the **tracheoesophageal fistula** (TEF) is associated with esophageal **atresia**. A TEF results from incomplete division of the cranial part of the foregut into respiratory and esophageal parts during the fourth week. Incomplete fusion of the tracheoesophageal folds results in a defective tracheoesophageal septum and a TEF between the trachea and esophagus.

*TEF is the most common birth defect of the lower respiratory tract.* Four main varieties of TEF may develop (see Fig. 10-6). The usual defect is for the superior part of the esophagus to end blindly (**esophageal atresia**) and for the inferior part to join the trachea near its bifurcation (see Figs. 10-6A and 10-7). Other varieties of this defect are illustrated in Figure 10-6B to D.

Infants with the common type of TEF and esophageal atresia cannot swallow, so they frequently drool saliva and immediately regurgitate milk when fed. Gastric and intestinal contents may also reflux from the stomach through the fistula into the trachea and lungs. This refluxed acid, and in some cases bile, can cause **pneumonitis** (inflammation of the lungs), leading to respiratory compromise. **Polyhydramnios** is often associated with esophageal atresia. The excess amniotic fluid develops because fluid cannot enter the stomach and intestines for absorption and subsequent transfer through the placenta to the mother's blood for disposal.

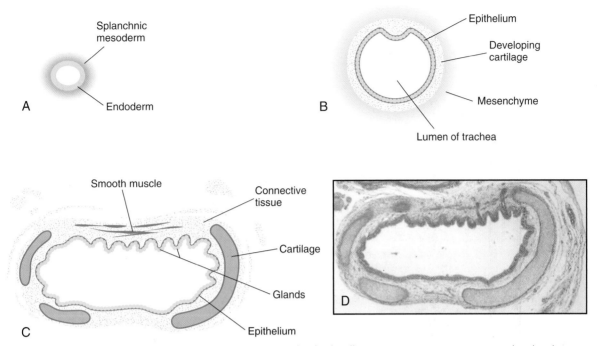

**FIGURE 10–5** Transverse sections through the laryngotracheal tube illustrating progressive stages in the development of the trachea. **A,** 4 weeks. **B,** 10 weeks. **C,** 12 weeks (drawing of micrograph in **D**). Note that endoderm of the tube gives rise to the epithelium and glands of the trachea and that mesenchyme surrounding the tube forms the connective tissue, muscle, and cartilage. **D,** Photomicrograph of a transverse section of the developing trachea at 12 weeks. (*D, From Moore KL, Persaud TVN, Shiota K: Color atlas of clinical embryology, ed 2, Philadelphia, 2000, Saunders.*)

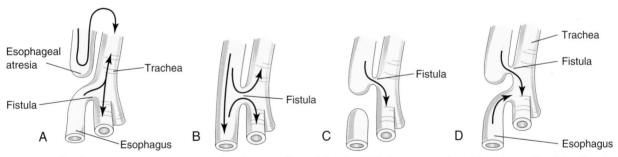

**FIGURE 10–6** The four main varieties of tracheoesophageal fistula (TEF) shown in order of frequency. Possible directions of the flow of the contents are indicated by *arrows*. Esophageal atresia, as illustrated in **A,** is associated with TEF in more than 85% of cases. **B,** Fistula between the trachea and esophagus. **C,** Air cannot enter the distal esophagus and stomach. **D,** Air can enter the distal esophagus and stomach, and the esophageal and gastric contents may enter the trachea and lungs.

## LARYNGOTRACHEOESOPHAGEAL CLEFT

Uncommonly, the larynx and upper trachea may fail to separate completely from the esophagus. This results in a persistent connection of variable lengths between these normally separated structures, or **laryngotracheoesophageal cleft.** Symptoms of this birth defect are similar to those of TEF because of aspiration of fluid and/or food into the lungs. **Aphonia** (inability to speak) is a distinguishing feature.

## TRACHEAL STENOSIS AND ATRESIA

**Stenosis** (narrowing) and **atresia** of the trachea are uncommon birth defects, which are usually associated with one of the varieties of TEF. Stenoses and atresias probably result from unequal partitioning of the foregut into the esophagus and trachea (see Fig. 10-6). Sometimes there is a web of tissue obstructing airflow (**incomplete tracheal atresia**). Atresia or **agenesis** (absence) of the trachea is uniformly fatal.

**FIGURE 10–7 A,** Tracheoesophageal fistula (TEF) in a 17-week male fetus. The upper esophageal segment ends blindly (*pointer*). **B,** Contrast radiograph of a neonate with TEF. Note the communication (*arrow*) between the esophagus (*E*) and trachea (*T*). **C,** Radiograph of esophageal atresia and tracheoesophageal fistula. The blind proximal esophageal sac is clearly visible. Note the air present in the distal gastrointestinal tract, indicating the presence of the tracheoesophageal fistula. An umbilical venous catheter can also been seen. (*A, From Kalousek DK, Fitch N, Paradice B:* Pathology of the human embryo and previable fetus, *New York, 1990, Springer-Verlag.*)

**FIGURE 10–8** Illustrations of the growth of the developing lungs into the splanchnic mesenchyme adjacent to the medial walls of the pericardioperitoneal canals (primordial pleural cavities). Development of the layers of the pleura is also shown. **A,** 5 weeks. **B,** 6 weeks.

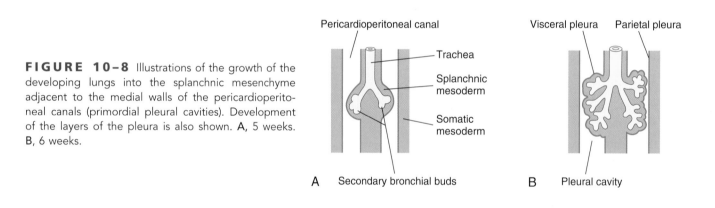

## TRACHEAL DIVERTICULUM (TRACHEAL BRONCHUS)

**Tracheal diverticulum,** or **bronchus,** consists of a blind, bronchus-like projection from the trachea. The outgrowth may terminate in normal-appearing lung tissue, forming a tracheal lobe of the lung. This diverticulum may cause recurrent infection and respiratory distress in infants.

## DEVELOPMENT OF BRONCHI AND LUNGS

A **respiratory bud (lung bud)** develops at the caudal end of the **laryngotracheal diverticulum** during the fourth week (see Fig. 10-2A and B). The bud soon divides into two outpouchings, the **primary bronchial buds** (Figs. 10-8A and 10-9, and see Fig. 10-2C). These buds grow laterally into the **pericardioperitoneal canals,** the primordia of the pleural cavities (see Fig. 10-8B). **Secondary** and **tertiary bronchial buds** soon develop.

Together with the surrounding splanchnic mesenchyme, the bronchial buds differentiate into bronchi and their ramifications in the lungs. Early in the fifth week, the connection of each bronchial bud with the trachea enlarges to form the primordia of the **main bronchi** (see Fig. 10-9).

The embryonic right main bronchus is slightly larger than the left one and is oriented more vertically. This relationship persists in the adult; consequently, a foreign body is more likely to enter the right main bronchus than the left one.

The main bronchi subdivide into **secondary bronchi** that form **lobar, segmental,** and **intrasegmental** branches (see Fig. 10-9). On the right, the superior lobar bronchus will supply the upper (superior) lobe of the lung, whereas the inferior bronchus subdivides into two bronchi, one to the middle lobe of the right lung and the other to the lower (inferior) lobe. On the left, the two secondary bronchi supply the upper and lower lobes of the lung. Each **lobar bronchus** undergoes progressive branching.

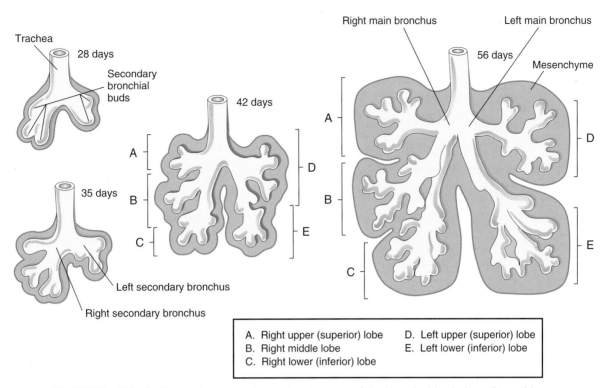

**FIGURE 10–9** Successive stages in the development of the bronchial buds, bronchi, and lungs.

The **segmental bronchi**, 10 in the right lung and 8 or 9 in the left lung, begin to form by the seventh week. As this occurs, the surrounding mesenchyme also divides. The segmental bronchi, with the surrounding mass of mesenchyme, form the primordia of the **bronchopulmonary segments**. By 24 weeks, approximately 17 orders of branches have formed and **respiratory bronchioles** have developed (Fig. 10-10*B*). An additional seven orders of airways develop after birth.

As the bronchi develop, cartilaginous plates develop from the surrounding splanchnic mesenchyme. The bronchial smooth muscle and connective tissue and the pulmonary connective tissue and capillaries are also derived from this mesenchyme. As the lungs develop, they acquire a layer of **visceral pleura** from the splanchnic mesenchyme (see Fig. 10-8). With expansion, the lungs and pleural cavities grow caudally into the mesenchyme of the body wall and soon lie close to the heart. The thoracic body wall becomes lined by a layer of **parietal pleura** derived from the somatic mesoderm (see Fig. 10-8*B*). The space between the parietal and visceral pleura is the **pleural cavity**.

## Maturation of Lungs

Maturation of the lungs is divided into four histologic stages: the **pseudoglandular**, **canalicular**, **terminal sac**, and **alveolar stages**.

### Pseudoglandular Stage (5 to 17 Weeks)

From a histologic standpoint, the developing lungs somewhat resemble exocrine glands during the **pseudoglandular stage** (Fig. 10-11A, and see Fig. 10-10*A*). By 16 weeks, all major elements of the lung have formed, except those involved with gas exchange. Respiration is not possible; therefore *fetuses born during this period are unable to survive*.

### Canalicular Stage (16 to 25 Weeks)

The **canalicular stage** overlaps the pseudoglandular stage because cranial segments of the lungs mature faster than caudal ones. During the canalicular stage, the lumina of bronchi and **terminal bronchioles** become larger and the lung tissue becomes highly vascular (see Figs. 10-10*B* and 10-11*B*). By 24 weeks, each terminal bronchiole has formed two or more **respiratory bronchioles**, each of which divides into three to six passages, the **primordial alveolar ducts**.

Respiration is possible at the end of the canalicular stage (26 weeks) because some thin-walled **terminal sacs** (primordial alveoli) have developed at the ends of the respiratory bronchioles and *lung tissue is well vascularized*. Although a fetus born toward the end of this period may survive if given intensive care, this premature neonate may die because its respiratory and other systems are still relatively immature.

### Terminal Sac Stage (24 Weeks to Late Fetal Period)

During the **terminal sac stage**, many more terminal sacs (primordial alveoli) develop (see Figs. 10-10*C* and 10-11*D*) and their *epithelium becomes very thin*. Capillaries begin to bulge into these sacs. The intimate contact between epithelial and endothelial cells establishes a

**FIGURE 10–10** Diagrammatic sketches of histologic sections illustrating the stages of lung development. **A** and **B**, Early stages of lung development. **C** and **D**, Note that the alveolocapillary membrane is thin and that some capillaries bulge into the terminal sacs and alveoli.

**blood–air barrier**, which permits adequate gas exchange for survival of the fetus if it is born prematurely.

At 26 weeks, the terminal sacs are lined mainly by squamous epithelial cells of endodermal origin, **type I pneumocytes**, across which gas exchange occurs. The capillary network proliferates rapidly in the mesenchyme around the developing alveoli, and there is concurrent active development of lymphatic capillaries. Scattered among the squamous epithelial cells are rounded secretory epithelial cells, **type II pneumocytes**, *which secrete pulmonary surfactant*, a complex mixture of phospholipids and proteins.

**Surfactant** forms as a monomolecular film over the internal walls of the **alveolar sacs** and counteracts surface tension forces at the air–alveolar interface. This facilitates expansion of the terminal sacs by preventing **atelectasis** (collapse of sacs during exhalation). The maturation of type II pneumocytes and surfactant production varies widely in fetuses of different gestational ages. The production of surfactant increases during the terminal stages of pregnancy, particularly during the last 2 weeks.

*Surfactant production begins at 20 to 22 weeks*, but surfactant is present in only small amounts in premature infants; it does not reach adequate levels until the late fetal period. By 26 to 28 weeks, the fetus usually weighs approximately 1000 g and sufficient alveolar sacs and surfactant are present to permit survival of a prematurely born infant. Before this, the lungs are usually incapable of providing adequate gas exchange, partly because the alveolar surface area is insufficient and the vascularity underdeveloped.

It is not the presence of thin terminal sacs or a primordial alveolar epithelium so much as the development of an adequate pulmonary vasculature and **surfactant** that is critical to the survival and neurodevelopmental outcome of premature infants.

Fetuses born at 24 to 26 weeks after fertilization may survive if given intensive care; however, they may suffer from **respiratory distress** because of surfactant deficiency. Survival of these infants has improved with the use of antenatal corticosteroids (steroids produced by the adrenal cortex), which induces surfactant production, and also with postnatal surfactant replacement therapy.

**FIGURE 10–11** Photomicrographs of sections of developing embryonic and fetal lungs. **A,** Pseudoglandular stage, 8 weeks. Note the "glandular" appearance of the lung. **B,** Canalicular stage, 16 weeks. The lumina of the bronchi and terminal bronchioles are enlarging. **C,** Canalicular stage, 18 weeks. **D,** Terminal sac stage, 24 weeks. Observe the thin-walled terminal sacs (primordial alveoli) that have developed at the ends of the respiratory bronchioles. Also observe that the numbers of capillaries have increased and that some of them are closely associated with the developing alveoli. *(From Moore KL, Persaud TVN, Shiota K: Color atlas of clinical embryology, ed 2, Philadelphia, 2000, Saunders.)*

## Alveolar Stage (Late Fetal Period to 8 Years)

Exactly when the terminal sac stage ends and the **alveolar stage** begins depends on the definition of the term **alveolus.** Terminal sacs analogous to alveoli are present at 32 weeks. The epithelial lining of the sacs attenuates to a thin squamous epithelial layer. The **type I pneumocytes** become so thin that the adjacent capillaries bulge into the alveolar sacs (see Figs. 10-10*D* and 10-11*D*). By the late fetal period (38 weeks), the lungs are capable of respiration because the **alveolocapillary membrane** (pulmonary diffusion barrier or respiratory membrane) is sufficiently thin to allow gas exchange. Although the lungs do not begin to perform this vital function until birth, they are well developed so that they are capable of functioning as soon as the baby is born.

At the beginning of the alveolar stage (32 weeks), each respiratory bronchiole terminates in a cluster of thin-walled **alveolar sacs,** separated from one another by loose connective tissue. These sacs represent future **alveolar ducts** (see Figs. 10-10*D* and 10-11*D*). The transition from dependence on the placenta for gas exchange to autonomous gas exchange requires the following adaptive changes in the lungs:

- Production of surfactant in the alveolar sacs
- Transformation of the lungs from secretory organs into organs capable of gas exchange
- Establishment of parallel pulmonary and systemic circulations

*Approximately 95% of mature alveoli develop postnatally.* Before birth, the primordial alveoli appear as small bulges on the walls of **respiratory bronchioles** and **alveolar sacs,** terminal dilations of alveolar ducts (see Fig. 10-10*D*). After birth, the primordial alveoli enlarge as the lungs expand, but the greatest increase in size of the lungs results from an increase in the number of **respiratory bronchioles** and **primordial alveoli** rather than from an increase in the size of the alveoli (see Fig. 10-11*B* and *D*).

Alveolar development is largely completed by 3 years of age, but new alveoli are added until approximately 8 years of age. Unlike mature alveoli, *immature alveoli have the potential for forming additional primordial alveoli.* As these alveoli increase in size, they become mature alveoli. The major mechanism for increasing the number of alveoli is the formation of secondary connective tissue septa that subdivide existing primordial alveoli. Initially, the septa are relatively thick, but they are soon transformed into mature thin septa that are capable of gas exchange.

**Lung development** during the first few months after birth is characterized by an exponential *increase in the surface area of the air–blood barrier* through the multiplication of alveoli and capillaries. Approximately 150 million primordial alveoli, one half of the adult number, are present in the lungs of a full-term neonate. On chest radiographs, therefore, the lungs of neonates are denser than adult lungs. Between the third and eighth years, the adult complement of 300 million alveoli is achieved.

*Molecular studies indicate that lung development is controlled by a cascade of signaling pathways that are regulated by the temporal and sequential expression of highly conserved genes. The commitment and differentiation of endodermal foregut cells to form respiratory-type epithelial cells are associated with expression of several transcription factors, including thyroid transcription factor 1, hepatocyte nuclear factor 3β, and GATA-6, as well as other Zinc-finger family members, retinoic acid receptors, and homeobox (Hox) domain-containing genes. Hox genes specify the anteroposterior axis in the embryo. Fibroblast growth factor 10 and other signals from splanchnic mesenchyme probably induce the outgrowth of the respiratory buds.*

*Branching of the buds (branching morphogenesis, or production) and its proliferation depend on epithelial (endodermal foregut)–mesenchymal (mesoderm) interactions. The Wnt signaling pathway plays an essential role in the inductive interactions between epithelium and mesenchyme. Recent studies suggest that the transcription factor SOX17 and Wnt7b signaling from the epithelium regulates mesenchymal proliferation and blood vessel formation in the lung. The patterning morphogen sonic hedgehog (Shh-Gli) modulates the expression of fibroblast growth factor 10, which controls the branching of the bronchial buds. Also, the morphogen retinoic acid regulates Hox a5, b5, and c4, which are expressed in the developing lung.*

**Fetal breathing movements (FBMs),** which can be detected by real-time ultrasonography, occur before birth, exerting sufficient force to cause aspiration of some amniotic fluid into the lungs. *FBMs occur intermittently (approximately 30% of them during rapid eye movement sleep) and are essential for normal lung development* (Fig. 10-12). The pattern of FBMs is widely used in the

**FIGURE 10–12** Fetal breathing movements (*FBMs*) seem to play a role in lung growth through their effects on lung cell cycle kinetics by regulating the expression of growth factors, such as platelet-derived growth factors (*PDGFs*) and insulin-like growth factors (*IGFs*), and establishing the gradient of thyroid transcription factor 1 (*TTF-1*) expression at the last stage of lung organogenesis (i.e., late mediators). It is also suggested that FBMs influence the expression of other unknown growth factors (i.e., early mediators) that are responsible for changes in cell cycle kinetics at earlier stages of lung development. FBMs appear to also be required for the accomplishment of the morphologic differentiation of type I and II pneumocytes. (*From Inanlou MR, Baguma-Nibasheka M, Kablar B: The role of fetal breathing–like movements in lung organogenesis, Histol Histopathol 20:1261, 2005.*)

monitoring of labor and as a predictor of fetal outcome in a preterm delivery. By birth, the fetus has had the advantage of several months of breathing exercise. FBMs, which increase as the time of delivery approaches, probably condition the respiratory muscles. In addition, these movements stimulate lung development, possibly by creating a pressure gradient between the lungs and the amniotic fluid.

*At birth, the lungs are approximately half filled with fluid derived from the amniotic cavity, lungs, and tracheal glands.* Aeration of the lungs at birth is not so much the inflation of empty collapsed organs but rather the rapid replacement of intra-alveolar fluid by air.

*The fluid in the lungs is cleared at birth by three routes:*

- Through the mouth and nose by pressure on the fetal thorax during vaginal delivery
- Into the pulmonary capillaries, arteries, and veins
- Into the lymphatics

In the near-term fetus, the pulmonary lymphatic vessels are relatively larger and more numerous than in the adult. Lymph flow is rapid during the first few hours after birth and then diminishes. Three factors are important for normal lung development: adequate thoracic space for lung growth, FBMs, and adequate amniotic fluid volume (Fig. 10-13).

## OLIGOHYDRAMNIOS AND LUNG DEVELOPMENT

When **oligohydramnios** (insufficient amount of amniotic fluid) is severe and chronic because of amniotic fluid leakage or decreased production, lung development is retarded, and severe **pulmonary hypoplasia** may result from restriction of the fetal thorax. The risk of pulmonary hypoplasia increases significantly with oligohydramnios prior to 26 weeks. It has also been shown that oligohydramnios results in decreased hydraulic pressure on the lungs, which affects stretch receptors, which in turn affect $Ca^+$ regulation and lung growth.

## LUNGS OF NEONATES

Fresh healthy lungs of neonates always contain some air; consequently, pulmonary tissue removed from them will float in water. A diseased lung, partly filled with fluid, may not float. Of medicolegal significance is the fact that the lungs of a stillborn infant are firm and sink when placed in water because they contain fluid, not air.

## RESPIRATORY DISTRESS SYNDROME

Respiratory distress syndrome (RDS) affects approximately 2% of neonates; those born prematurely are most susceptible. These infants develop rapid, labored breathing shortly after birth. RDS is also known as **hyaline membrane disease**. An estimated 30% of all neonatal diseases result from RDS or its complications.

*Surfactant deficiency is a major cause of RDS.* The lungs are underinflated and the alveoli contain a fluid with a high protein content that resembles a glassy, or hyaline, membrane. This membrane is thought to be derived from a combination of substances in the circulation and from the injured pulmonary epithelium. It has been suggested that prolonged intrauterine **asphyxia** (impaired or absent exchange of oxygen and carbon dioxide) may produce irreversible changes in the **type II alveolar cells**, making them incapable of producing surfactant. Other factors such as sepsis, aspiration, and pneumonia may inactivate surfactant, leading to an absence of deficiency of surfactant in premature and full-term infants.

All growth factors and hormones controlling surfactant production have not been identified, but corticosteroids and thyroxine, which are involved in fetal lung maturation, are potent stimulators of surfactant production. Maternal glucocorticoid treatment during pregnancy accelerates fetal lung development and surfactant production. This finding has led to the routine clinical use of corticosteroids (betamethasone) for the prevention of RDS in preterm labor. In addition, administration of exogenous surfactant (**surfactant replacement therapy**) reduces the severity of RDS and the chance of neonatal mortality.

## LOBE OF AZYGOS VEIN

A **lobe of the azygos vein** appears in the right lung in *approximately* 1% of people. It develops when the apical bronchus grows superiorly, medial to the arch of the azygos vein, instead of lateral to it. As a result, the vein lies at the bottom of a fissure in the superior (upper) lobe, which produces a linear marking on a radiograph of the lungs.

## CONGENITAL LUNG CYSTS

Cysts (filled with fluid or air) are thought to be formed by the dilation of terminal bronchi. They probably result from a disturbance in bronchial development during late fetal life. If several cysts are present, the lungs have a honeycomb appearance on radiographs. These lung cysts are usually located at the periphery of the lung (see Fig. 10-13).

**FIGURE 10–13** Congenital lung cysts. **A,** Chest radiograph (posteroanterior) of an infant showing a large left-sided congenital cystic adenomatoid malformation *(arrow).* The heart *(asterisk)* has shifted to the right. Note the chest tube on the left side, which was placed on the initial diagnosis of a pneumothorax (air in pleural cavity). **B,** Axial computed tomography image of the thorax in an infant with a large right-sided congenital bronchogenic cyst *(asterisk).*

## AGENESIS OF LUNGS

Absence of the lungs results from failure of the respiratory bud to develop. **Agenesis** of one lung is more common than bilateral agenesis, but both conditions are rare. Unilateral pulmonary agenesis is compatible with life. The heart and other mediastinal structures are shifted to the affected side, and the existing lung is hyperexpanded.

## ACCESSORY LUNG

A small **accessory lung (pulmonary sequestration)** is uncommon. It is almost always located at the base of the left lung and nonfunctional. It does not communicate with the tracheobronchial tree, and its blood supply is usually systemic. Larger masses should be removed because they have a tendency for overcirculation from their systemic arterial blood supply.

## LUNG HYPOPLASIA

In infants with **congenital diaphragmatic hernia** (see Chapter 8, Figs. 8-9A and B and 8-10), the lung is unable to develop normally because it is compressed by the abnormally positioned abdominal viscera. **Lung hypoplasia** is characterized by a markedly reduced lung volume and hypertrophy of smooth muscle in the pulmonary arteries. The pulmonary hypertension leads to decreased blood flow through the pulmonary vascular system as the blood continues to shunt through the ductus arteriosus.

Approximately 25% of infants with congenital diaphragmatic hernia die of pulmonary insufficiency, despite optimal postnatal care, because their lungs are too hypoplastic for air exchange and there is too much resistance for pulmonary blood flow to support extrauterine life.

## SUMMARY OF RESPIRATORY SYSTEM

- By the fourth week, a **laryngotracheal diverticulum** develops from the floor of the primordial pharynx.
- The laryngotracheal diverticulum becomes separated from the foregut by **tracheoesophageal folds** that fuse to form a tracheoesophageal septum. This septum results in the formation of the esophagus and laryngotracheal tube (see Fig. 10-2C and E).
- The endoderm of the laryngotracheal tube gives rise to the epithelium of the lower respiratory organs and tracheobronchial glands. The splanchnic mesenchyme surrounding the laryngotracheal tube forms the connective tissue, cartilage, muscle, and blood and lymphatic vessels of these organs.
- Pharyngeal arch mesenchyme contributes to formation of the epiglottis and connective tissue of the larynx. The laryngeal muscles are derived from mesenchyme in the caudal pharyngeal arches. The laryngeal cartilages are derived from neural crest cells.
- The distal end of the laryngotracheal diverticulum forms a **respiratory bud** that divides into two **bronchial**

**buds.** Each bronchial bud soon enlarges to form a **main bronchus**, and then the main bronchus subdivides to form lobar, segmental, and subsegmental branches (see Figs. 10-2C and 10-9).

- **Each tertiary bronchial bud** (segmental bronchial bud), with its surrounding mesenchyme, is the primordium of a **bronchopulmonary segment**. Branching continues until *approximately* 17 orders of branches have formed. Additional airways are formed after birth, until *approximately* 24 orders of branches are present.
- Lung development is divided into four stages: the **pseudoglandular** (6–16 weeks), **canalicular** (16–26 weeks), **terminal sac** (26 weeks to birth), and **alveolar** (32 weeks to approximately 8 years of age) **stages**.
- By 20 to 22 weeks, **type II pneumocytes** begin to secrete pulmonary **surfactant**. Deficiency of surfactant results in **RDS** or **hyaline membrane disease**.
- A **TEF**, which results from faulty partitioning of the foregut into the esophagus and trachea, is usually associated with esophageal atresia.

# CLINICALLY ORIENTED PROBLEMS

### CASE 10–1

*Choking and continuous coughing were observed in a male neonate. There was an excessive amount of secreted mucus and saliva in his mouth. He also experienced considerable difficulty in breathing. The pediatrician was unable to pass a catheter through the esophagus into the stomach.*

- ※ What birth defect would be suspected?
- ※ Discuss the embryologic basis of these defects.
- ※ What kind of an examination or testing do you think would be used to confirm the tentative diagnosis?

### CASE 10–2

*A premature infant developed rapid, shallow respiration shortly after birth. A diagnosis of RDS was made.*

- ※ How do you think the infant might attempt to overcome his or her inadequate exchange of oxygen and carbon dioxide?
- ※ What usually causes RDS?
- ※ What treatment is currently used clinically to prevent RDS?
- ※ A deficiency of what substance is associated with RDS?

### CASE 10–3

*The parents of a neonate were told that their son had a fistula between his trachea and esophagus.*

- ※ What is the most common type of TEF?
- ※ What is its embryologic basis?
- ※ What defect of the alimentary (digestive) tract is frequently associated with this abnormality?

### CASE 10–4

*A neonate with esophageal atresia experienced respiratory distress with cyanosis shortly after birth. Radiographs demonstrated air in the infant's stomach.*

- ※ How did the air enter the stomach?
- ※ What other problem might result in an infant with this fairly common type of birth defect?

Discussion of these problems appears in the Appendix at the back of the book.

## BIBLIOGRAPHY AND SUGGESTED READING

Abel R, Bush A, Chitty RS, et al: Congenital lung disease. In Chernick V, Boat T, Wilmott R, et al, editors: *Kendig's disorders of the respiratory tract in children*, ed 7, Philadelphia, 2006, Saunders.

Brunner HG, van Bokhoven H: Genetic players in esophageal atresia and tracheoesophageal fistula, *Curr Opin Genet Dev* 15:341, 2005.

Domyan ET, Sun X: Patterning and plasticity in development of the respiratory lineage, *Dev Dyn* 240:477, 2011.

Herriges M, Morrisey EE: Lung development: orchestrating the generation and regeneration of a complex organ, *Development* 141:502, 2014.

Holinger LD: Congenital anomalies of the larynx; congenital anomalies of the trachea and bronchi. In Behrman RE, Kliegman Jenson HB, editors: *Nelson textbook of pediatrics*, ed 17, Philadelphia, 2004, Saunders.

Ioannides AS, Massa V, Ferraro E, et al: Foregut separation and tracheoesophageal malformations: the role of tracheal outgrowth, dorsoventral patterning and programmed cell death, *Dev Dyn* 237:351, 2010.

Jobe AH: Lung development and maturation. In Martin RJ, Fanaroff AA, Walsh MC, editors: *Fanaroff and Martin's neonatal-perinatal medicine: diseases of the fetus and infant*, ed 8, Philadelphia, 2006, Mosby.

Kays DW: Congenital diaphragmatic hernia and neonatal lung lesions, *Surg Clin North Am* 86:329, 2006.

Laitman JT, Reidenberg JS: The evolution and development of human swallowing, *Otolaryngol Clin North Am* 46:923, 2013.

Lange AW, Haitchi HM, LeCras TD, et al: Sox17 is required for normal pulmonary vascular morphogenesis, *Dev Biol* 387:109, 2014.

Moore KL, Dalley AF, Agur AMR: *Clinically oriented anatomy*, ed 7, Baltimore, 2014, Williams & Wilkins.

Morrisey EE, Cardoso WV, Lane RH, et al: Molecular determinants of lung development, *Ann Am Thorac Soc* 10:S12–S16, 2013.

Morrisey EE, Hogan BL: Preparing for the first breath: genetic and cellular mechanisms in lung development, *Dev Cell* 18:8, 2010.

O'Rahilly R, Boyden E: The timing and sequence of events in the development of the human respiratory system during the embryonic period proper, *Z Anat Entwicklungsgesch* 141:237, 1973.

Rawlins EL: The building blocks of mammalian lung development, *Dev Dyn* 240:463, 2011.

Shanks A, Gross G, Shim T, et al: Administration of steroids after 34 weeks of gestation enhances fetal lung maturity profiles, *Am J Obstet Gynecol* 203:47, 2010.

Shi W, Chen F, Cardoso WV: Mechanisms of lung development, *Proc Am Thorac Soc* 6:558, 2009.

Sluiter I, van de Ven CP, Wijnen RM, et al: Congenital diaphragmatic hernia, *Semin Fetal Neonatal Med* 16(3):139, 2011.

Turell DC: Advances with surfactant, *Emerg Med Clin North Am* 26:921, 2008.

Turner BS, Bradshaw W, Brandon D: Neonatal lung remodeling, *J Perinat Neonat Nurs* 19:362, 2006.

Warburton D, El-Hashash A, Carraro G, et al: Lung organogenesis, *Curr Top Dev Biol* 90:73, 2010.

Wells LJ, Boyden EA: The development of the bronchopulmonary segments in human embryos of horizons XVII and XIX, *Am J Anat* 95:163, 1954.

Whitsett JA: The molecular era of surfactant biology, *Neonatology* 105:337, 2014.

Wladimiroff JW, Cohen-Overbeek TE, Laudy JAM: Ultrasound evaluation of the fetal thorax. In Callen PW, editor: *Ultrasonography in obstetrics and gynecology*, ed 5, Philadelphia, 2008, Saunders.

# Alimentary System

**T**he **alimentary system** (digestive system) is the digestive tract from the mouth to the anus, with all its associated glands and organs. The **primordial gut** forms during the fourth week as the head, caudal eminence (tail), and lateral folds incorporate the dorsal part of the umbilical vesicle (yolk sac) (see Chapter 5, Fig. 5-1). The primordial gut is initially closed at its cranial end by the **oropharyngeal membrane** (see Chapter 9, Fig. 9-1E) and at its caudal end by the **cloacal membrane** (Fig. 11-1B). The endoderm of the primordial gut forms most of the gut, epithelium, and glands. *Mesenchymal factors, FoxF proteins, control proliferation of the endodermal epithelium that secretes sonic hedgehog (Shh).* The epithelium of the cranial and caudal ends of the alimentary tract is derived from ectoderm of the **stomodeum and anal pit (proctodeum)** (see Fig. 11-1A and B).

*Fibroblast growth factors (FGFs) are involved in early anteroposterior axial patterning, and it appears that FGF-4 signals from the adjacent ectoderm and mesoderm induce the endoderm. Other secreted factors, such as activins, members of the transforming growth factor-β superfamily, contribute to the formation of the endoderm.* The endoderm specifies temporal and positional information, which is essential for the development of the gut. The muscular, connective tissue, and other layers of the wall of the alimentary tract are derived from the splanchnic mesenchyme surrounding the primordial gut.

For descriptive purposes, the primordial gut is divided into three parts: foregut, midgut, and hindgut. *Molecular studies indicate that* Hox *and ParaHox genes, as well as Shh, BMP, and Wnt signals, regulate the regional differentiation of the primordial gut to form its three parts.*

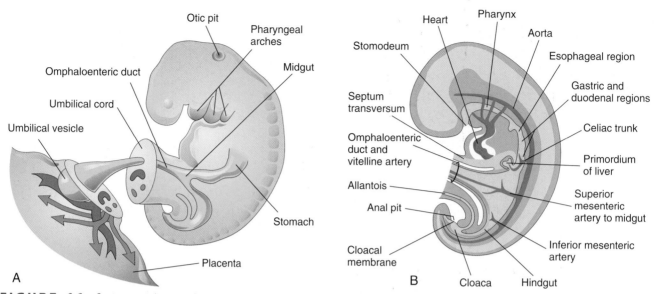

**FIGURE 11–1** *A,* Lateral view of a 4-week embryo showing the relationship of the primordial gut to the omphaloenteric duct. *B,* Drawing of median section of the embryo showing the early alimentary system and its blood supply.

## FOREGUT

The derivatives of the foregut are the:

- Primordial pharynx and its derivatives
- Lower respiratory system
- Esophagus and stomach
- Duodenum, distal to the opening of the bile duct
- Liver, biliary apparatus (hepatic ducts, gallbladder, and bile duct), and pancreas

These foregut derivatives, other than the pharynx, lower respiratory tract, and most of the esophagus, are supplied by the **celiac trunk**, the artery of the foregut (see Fig. 11-1*B*).

## ▶ Development of Esophagus

10

The **esophagus** develops from the foregut immediately caudal to the pharynx (see Fig. 11-1*B*). The partitioning of the trachea from the esophagus by the **tracheoesophageal septum** is described in Chapter 10, Figure 10-2*E*. Initially, the esophagus is short, but it elongates rapidly, mainly because of the growth and relocation of the heart and lungs.

The esophagus reaches its final relative length by the seventh week. Its epithelium and glands are derived from endoderm that proliferates and, partly or completely, obliterates the lumen of the esophagus. However, recanalization of the esophagus normally occurs by the end of the eighth week. The **striated muscle** forming the muscularis externa (external muscle) of the superior third of the esophagus is derived from mesenchyme in the fourth and sixth pharyngeal arches. The **smooth muscle**, mainly in the inferior third of the esophagus, develops from the surrounding splanchnic mesenchyme.

Recent studies indicate transdifferentiation of smooth muscle cells in the superior part of the esophagus to striated muscle, which is dependent on myogenic regulatory factors. Both types of muscle are innervated by branches

of the vagus nerves (cranial nerve X), which supply the caudal pharyngeal arches (see Chapter 9, Table 9-1).

### ESOPHAGEAL ATRESIA

Blockage (atresia) of the esophageal lumen occurs with an incidence of 1 in 3000 to 4500 neonates. Approximately one third of affected infants are born prematurely. This defect is associated with **tracheoesophageal fistula** in more than 90% of cases (see Chapter 10, Fig. 10-6). **Esophageal atresia** results from deviation of the tracheoesophageal septum in a posterior direction (see Chapter 10, Fig. 10-7) and incomplete separation of the esophagus from the laryngotracheal tube. Isolated atresia (5% to 7% of cases) results from failure of recanalization of the esophagus during the eighth week of development.

A fetus with esophageal atresia is unable to swallow amniotic fluid; consequently, the fluid cannot pass to the intestine for absorption and transfer through the placenta to the maternal blood for disposal. This results in **polyhydramnios**, the accumulation of an excessive amount of amniotic fluid. Neonates with esophageal atresia usually appear healthy initially. Excessive drooling may be noted soon after birth, and the diagnosis of esophageal atresia should be considered if the baby rejects oral feeding with immediate regurgitation and coughing.

Inability to pass a catheter through the esophagus into the stomach strongly suggests esophageal atresia. A radiographic examination demonstrates the defect by imaging the nasogastric tube arrested in the proximal esophageal pouch. In neonates weighing more than 2 kg and without associated cardiac anomalies, the survival rate now approaches 100% with surgical repair. As the birth weight decreases and cardiovascular anomalies become more severe, the survival rate decreases to as low as 1%.

Narrowing of the lumen of the esophagus (**stenosis**) can occur anywhere along the esophagus, but it usually occurs in its distal third, either as a web or a long segment with a thread-like lumen. Stenosis results from incomplete recanalization of the esophagus during the eighth week, or from a failure of esophageal blood vessels to develop in the affected area.

## Development of Stomach

Initially the distal part of the foregut is a tubular structure (see Fig. 11-1*B*). During the fourth week, a slight dilation indicates the site of the primordial stomach. The dilation first appears as a fusiform enlargement of the caudal (distal) part of the foregut and is initially oriented in the median plane (see Figs. 11-1 and 11-2*B*). The primordial stomach soon enlarges and broadens ventrodorsally. During the next 2 weeks, the dorsal border of the stomach grows faster than its ventral border; this demarcates the developing **greater curvature of the stomach** (see Fig. 11-2*D*).

### Rotation of Stomach

Enlargement of the mesentery and adjacent organs, as well as growth of the stomach walls, contributes to the rotation of the stomach. As the stomach enlarges and acquires its final shape, it slowly rotates 90 degrees in a clockwise direction (viewed from the cranial end) around its longitudinal axis. The effects of rotation on the stomach are (Figs. 11-2 and 11-3):

- The ventral border (lesser curvature) moves to the right, and the dorsal border (greater curvature) moves to the left (see Fig. 11-2*C* and *F*).
- The original left side becomes the ventral surface, and the original right side becomes the dorsal surface.
- Before rotation, the cranial and caudal ends of the stomach are in the median plane (see Fig. 11-2*B*). During rotation and growth of the stomach, its cranial region moves to the left and slightly inferiorly and its caudal region moves to the right and superiorly.
- After rotation, the stomach assumes its final position, with its long axis almost transverse to the long axis of the body (see Fig. 11-2*E*). The rotation and growth of the stomach explain why the **left vagus nerve** supplies the anterior wall of the adult stomach and the **right vagus nerve** innervates its posterior wall.

### Mesenteries of Stomach

The stomach is suspended from the dorsal wall of the abdominal cavity by a dorsal mesentery, the **primordial dorsal mesogastrium** (see Figs. 11-2*B* and *C* and 11-3*A*). This mesentery, originally in the median plane, is carried to the left during rotation of the stomach and formation of the **omental bursa** or lesser sac of the peritoneum (see

Fig. 11-3*A* to *E*). The mesentery also contains the spleen and celiac artery. The **primordial ventral mesogastrium** attaches to the stomach; it also attaches the duodenum to the liver and ventral abdominal wall (see Figs. 11-2*C* and 11-3*A* and *B*).

## Omental Bursa

Isolated clefts develop in the mesenchyme, forming the thick **dorsal mesogastrium** (see Fig. 11-3*A* and *B*). The clefts soon coalesce to form a single cavity, the **omental bursa** or lesser peritoneal sac (see Fig. 11-3*C* and *D*). Rotation of the stomach pulls the mesogastrium to the left, thereby enlarging the bursa, a large recess in the peritoneal cavity. The bursa expands transversely and cranially and soon lies between the stomach and posterior abdominal wall. The pouch-like bursa facilitates movements of the stomach (see Fig. 11-3*H*).

The superior part of the omental bursa is cut off as the diaphragm develops, forming a closed space, the **infracardiac bursa**. If the space persists, it usually lies medial to the base of the right lung. The inferior region of the superior part of the bursa persists as the **superior recess of the omental bursa** (see Fig. 11-3*C*).

As the stomach enlarges, the omental bursa expands and acquires an **inferior recess of the omental bursa** between the layers of the elongated dorsal mesogastrium, the **greater omentum** (see Fig. 11-3*J*). This membrane overhangs the developing intestines. The inferior recess disappears as the layers of the greater omentum fuse (see Fig. 11-15*F*). The omental bursa communicates with the peritoneal cavity through an opening, the **omental foramen** (see Figs. 11-2*D* and *F* and 11-3*C* and *F*).

Anomalies of the stomach are uncommon, except for **hypertrophic pyloric stenosis**. This defect affects one in every 150 males and one in every 750 females. In infants there is a marked **muscular thickening of the pylorus**, the distal sphincteric region of the stomach (Fig. 11-4*A* and *B*). The circular muscles and, to a lesser degree, the longitudinal muscles in the pyloric region are hypertrophied (increased in bulk). This results in severe stenosis of the pyloric canal and obstruction of the passage of food. As a result, the stomach becomes markedly distended (see Fig. 11-4*C*) and the infant expels the stomach's contents with considerable force (projectile vomiting).

Surgical relief of the pyloric obstruction by **pyloromyotomy**, in which a longitudinal incision is made through the anterior wall of the pyloric canal, is the usual treatment. The cause of congenital pyloric stenosis is unknown, but the high rate of concordance in monozygotic twins suggests genetic factors may be involved.

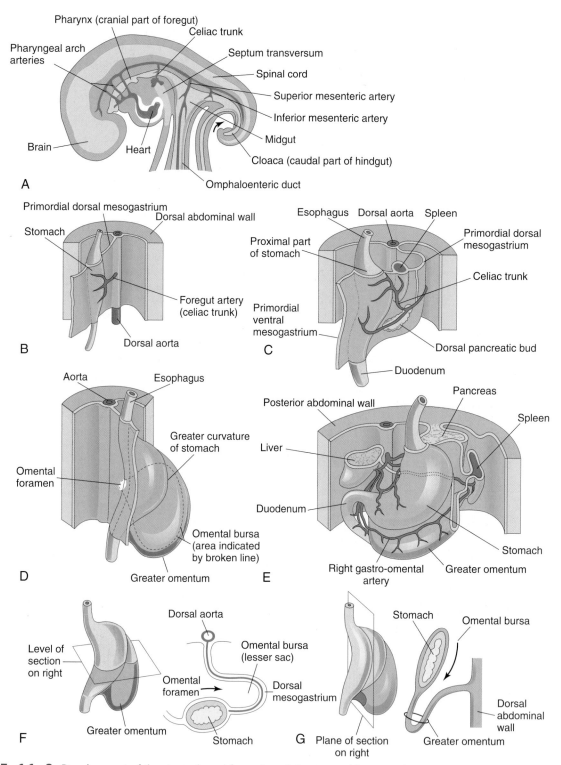

**FIGURE 11–2** Development of the stomach and formation of the omental bursa and greater omentum. **A,** Median section of the abdomen of a 28-day embryo. **B,** Anterolateral view of the embryo shown in **A. C,** Embryo of approximately 35 days. **D,** Embryo of approximately 40 days. **E,** Embryo of approximately 48 days. **F,** Lateral view of the stomach and greater omentum of an embryo of approximately 52 days. **G,** Sagittal section showing the omental bursa and greater omentum. The *arrow* in **F** and **G** indicates the site of the omental foramen.

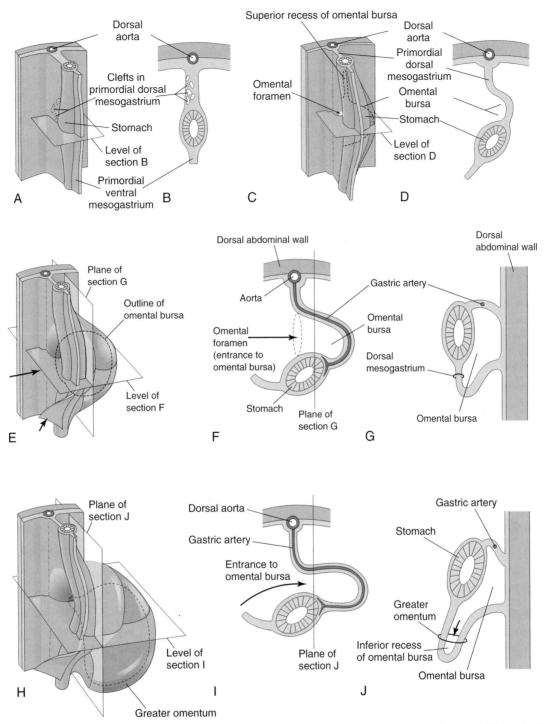

**FIGURE 11–3** Development of stomach and mesenteries and formation of omental bursa. **A**, Embryo of 5 weeks. **B**, Transverse section showing clefts in the dorsal mesogastrium. **C**, Later stage after coalescence of the clefts to form the omental bursa. **D**, Transverse section showing the initial appearance of the omental bursa. **E**, The dorsal mesentery has elongated and the omental bursa has enlarged. **F** and **G**, Transverse and sagittal sections, respectively, showing elongation of the dorsal mesogastrium and expansion of the omental bursa. **H**, Embryo of 6 weeks showing the greater omentum and expansion of the omental bursa. **I** and **J**, Transverse and sagittal sections, respectively, showing the inferior recess of the omental bursa and the omental foramen. The *arrows* in **E**, **F**, and **I** indicate the site of the omental foramen. In **J**, the *arrow* indicates the inferior recess of the omental bursa.

**FIGURE 11-4** A, Transverse abdominal sonogram demonstrating a pyloric muscle wall thickness of greater than 4 mm (*distance between crosses*). B, Horizontal image demonstrating a pyloric channel length greater than 14 mm in an infant with hypertrophic pyloric stenosis. C, Contrast radiograph of the stomach in a 1-month-old male infant with pyloric stenosis. Note the narrowed pyloric end (*arrow*) and the distended fundus (F) of the stomach, filled with contrast material. (*A and B, From Wyllie R: Pyloric stenosis and other congenital anomalies of the stomach. In Behrman RE, Kliegman RM, Arvin AM, editors: Nelson textbook of pediatrics, ed 15, Philadelphia, 1996, Saunders.*)

## Development of Duodenum

Early in the fourth week, the duodenum begins to develop from the caudal part of the foregut, cranial part of the midgut, and splanchnic mesenchyme associated with these parts of the primordial gut (Fig. 11-5A). The junction of the two parts of the duodenum is just distal to the origin of the bile duct (see Fig. 11-5D). The developing duodenum grows rapidly, forming a C-shaped loop that projects ventrally (see Fig. 11-5B to D).

As the stomach rotates, the duodenal loop rotates to the right and is pressed against the posterior wall of the abdominal cavity, or in a retroperitoneal position (external to the peritoneum). Because of its derivation from the foregut and midgut, the duodenum is supplied by branches of the celiac trunk and superior mesenteric arteries that supply these parts of the primordial gut (see Fig. 11-1).

During the fifth and sixth weeks, the lumen of the duodenum becomes progressively smaller and is temporarily obliterated because of proliferation of its epithelial cells. Normally, **vacuolation** (formation of vacuoles) occurs as the epithelial cells degenerate; as a result, the duodenum normally becomes recanalized by the end of the embryonic period (Fig. 11-6C and D). By this time, most of the ventral mesentery of the duodenum has disappeared.

### DUODENAL STENOSIS

Partial occlusion of the duodenal lumen, or **duodenal stenosis** (see Fig. 11-6A), usually results from incomplete recanalization of the duodenum, resulting from defective vacuolization (see Fig. 11-6E and $E_3$). Most stenoses involve the horizontal (third) and/or ascending (fourth) parts of the duodenum. Because of the stenosis, the stomach's contents (usually containing bile) are often vomited.

### DUODENAL ATRESIA

Complete occlusion of the duodenal lumen, or **duodenal atresia** (see Fig. 11-6B), is not common. During early duodenal development, the lumen is completely occluded by epithelial cells. If complete recanalization of the lumen fails to occur (see Fig. 11-6$D_3$), a short segment of the duodenum is occluded (see Fig. 11-6$F_3$). The blockage usually occurs at the junction of the bile duct and pancreatic duct, or **hepatopancreatic ampulla**, a dilated area within the major duodenal papilla that receives the bile duct and main pancreatic duct; occasionally, the blockage involves the horizontal (third) part of the duodenum. Investigation of families with **familial duodenal atresia** suggests an autosomal recessive inheritance pattern.

In neonates with duodenal atresia, vomiting begins a few hours after birth. The vomitus almost always contains bile; often there is distention of the epigastrium, the upper

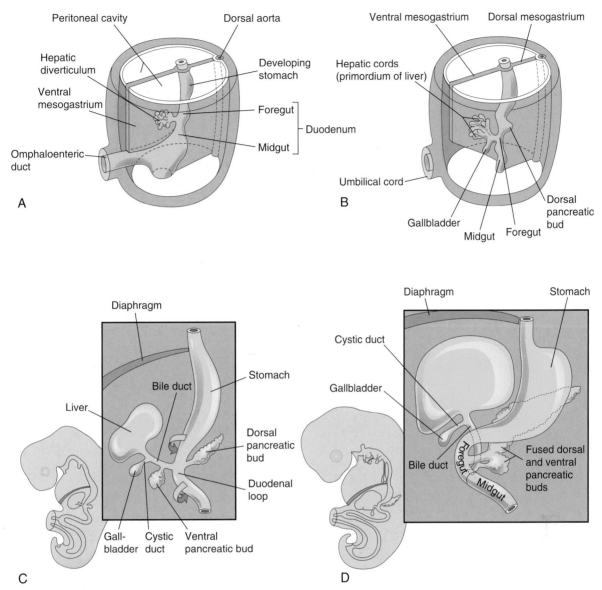

**FIGURE 11–5** Progressive stages in the development of the duodenum, liver, pancreas, and extrahepatic biliary apparatus. **A,** Embryo of 4 weeks. **B** and **C,** Embryo of 5 weeks. **D,** Embryo of 6 weeks. During embryologic development, the dorsal and ventral pancreatic buds eventually fuse, forming the pancreas. Note that the entrance of the bile duct into the duodenum gradually shifts from its initial position to a posterior one. This explains why the bile duct in adults passes posterior to the duodenum and the head of the pancreas.

## DUODENAL ATRESIA—cont'd

central area of the abdomen, resulting from an overfilled stomach and superior part of the duodenum. The atresia is associated with bilious emesis (vomiting of bile) because the blockage occurs distal to the opening of the bile duct. The atresia may occur as an isolated birth defect, but other defects are often associated with it, such as annular pancreas (see Fig. 11-11C), cardiovascular defects, anorectal defects, and malrotation of the gut (see Fig. 11-20). The presence of nonbilious emesis does not exclude duodenal atresia as a diagnosis, because some infants will have

obstruction proximal to the ampula. Importantly, approximately one third of affected infants have Down syndrome and an additional 20% are premature.

Polyhydramnios (an **excess of amniotic fluid**) also occurs because duodenal atresia prevents normal intestinal absorption of swallowed amniotic fluid. The diagnosis of duodenal atresia is suggested by the presence of a "double-bubble" sign on plain radiographs and ultrasound scans (Fig. 11-7). This appearance is caused by a distended, gas-filled stomach and the proximal duodenum.

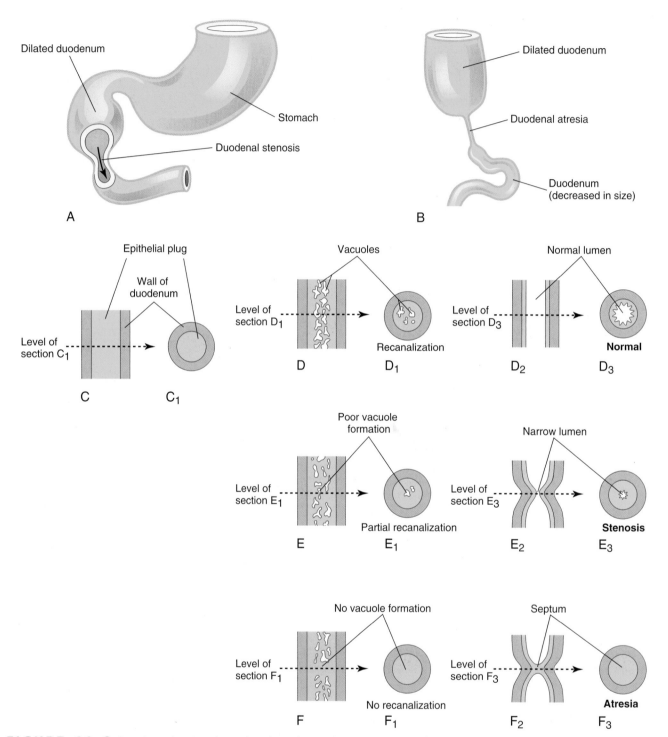

**FIGURE 11-6** Drawings showing the embryologic basis of common types of congenital intestinal obstruction. **A,** Duodenal stenosis. **B,** Duodenal atresia. **C** to **F,** Diagrammatic longitudinal and transverse sections of the duodenum showing (1) normal recanalization (D to $D_3$), (2) stenosis (E to $E_3$), and atresia (F to $F_3$).

**FIGURE 11–7** Ultrasound scans of a fetus of 33 weeks showing duodenal atresia. **A,** An oblique scan showing the dilated, fluid-filled stomach *(St)* entering the proximal duodenum *(D)*, which is also enlarged because of atresia (blockage) distal to it. **B,** Transverse scan illustrating the characteristic "double-bubble" appearance of the stomach and duodenum when there is duodenal atresia.

## Development of Liver and Biliary Apparatus

The liver, gallbladder, and biliary duct system arise as a ventral outgrowth, the **hepatic diverticulum**, from the distal part of the foregut early in the fourth week (Fig. 11-8A, and see also Fig. 11-5A). *The Wnt/β–catenin signaling pathway plays a key role in this process, which includes the proliferation and differentiation of the hepatic progenitor cells to form hepatocytes. It has been suggested that both the hepatic diverticulum and the ventral bud of the pancreas develop from two cell populations in the embryonic endoderm. At sufficient levels, FGFs secreted by the developing heart interact with the bipotential cells and induce formation of the hepatic diverticulum.*

The diverticulum extends into the **septum transversum,** a mass of splanchnic mesoderm separating the pericardial and peritoneal cavities. The septum forms the ventral mesogastrium in this region. The hepatic diverticulum enlarges rapidly and divides into two parts as it grows between the layers of the **ventral mesogastrium,** or mesentery of the dilated portion of the foregut and the future stomach (see Fig. 11-5A).

The larger cranial part of the **hepatic diverticulum** is the primordium of the liver (see Figs. 11-8A and C and 11-10A and B); the smaller caudal part becomes the primordium of the gallbladder. The proliferating endodermal cells form interlacing cords of hepatocytes and give rise to the epithelial lining of the intrahepatic part of the biliary apparatus. The **hepatic cords** anastomose around endothelium-lined spaces, the primordia of the **hepatic sinusoids.** *Vascular endothelial growth factor Flk-1 signaling appears to be important for the early morphogenesis of the hepatic sinusoids (primitive vascular system).* The fibrous and hematopoietic tissue and Kupffer cells of the liver are derived from mesenchyme in the septum transversum.

The liver grows rapidly from the 5th to 10th weeks and fills a large part of the upper abdominal cavity (see Fig. 11-8C and D). The quantity of oxygenated blood flowing from the umbilical vein into the liver determines the development and functional segmentation of the liver. Initially, the right and left lobes are approximately the same size, but the right lobe soon becomes larger.

**Hematopoiesis** (formation and development of various types of blood cells) begins in the liver during the sixth week, giving the liver a bright reddish appearance. By the ninth week, the liver accounts for approximately 10% of the total weight of the fetus. **Bile formation** by hepatic cells begins during the 12th week.

The small caudal part of the hepatic diverticulum becomes the **gallbladder,** and the stalk of the diverticulum forms the **cystic duct** (see Fig. 11-5C). Initially, the **extrahepatic biliary apparatus** is occluded with epithelial cells, but it is later canalized because of vacuolation resulting from degeneration of these cells.

The stalk of the diverticulum connecting the hepatic and cystic ducts to the duodenum becomes the **bile duct.** Initially, this duct attaches to the ventral aspect of the duodenal loop; however, as the duodenum grows and rotates, the entrance of the bile duct is carried to the dorsal aspect of the duodenum (see Fig. 11-5C and D). The bile entering the duodenum through the bile duct after the 13th week gives the **meconium** (intestinal discharges of the fetus) a dark green color.

### Ventral Mesentery

The **ventral mesentery,** a thin, double-layered membrane (see Fig. 11-8C and D), gives rise to:

- The **lesser omentum,** passing from the liver to the lesser curvature of the stomach (**hepatogastric ligament**) and from the liver to the duodenum (**hepatoduodenal ligament**)
- The **falciform ligament,** extending from the liver to the ventral abdominal wall

The **umbilical vein** passes in the free border of the **falciform ligament** on its way from the umbilical cord to the liver. The ventral mesentery, derived from the mesogastrium, also forms the visceral peritoneum of the liver. The liver is covered by peritoneum, except for the **bare area,** which is in direct contact with the diaphragm (Fig. 11-9).

**FIGURE 11–8** *A,* Median section of a 4-week embryo. *B,* Transverse section of the embryo showing expansion of the peritoneal cavity *(arrows)*. *C,* Sagittal section of a 5-week embryo. *D,* Transverse section of the embryo after formation of the dorsal and ventral mesenteries.

## ANOMALIES OF LIVER

Minor variations of liver lobulation are common; however, birth defects of the liver are rare. Variations of the hepatic ducts, bile duct, and cystic duct are common and clinically significant. **Accessory hepatic ducts** are present in approximately 5% of the population, and awareness of their possible presence is of importance in surgery (e.g., liver transplantation). The accessory ducts are narrow channels running from the right lobe of the liver into the anterior surface of the body of the gallbladder. In some cases, the **cystic duct** opens into an accessory hepatic duct rather than into the common hepatic duct.

## EXTRAHEPATIC BILIARY ATRESIA

This is the most serious defect of the extrahepatic biliary system, and it occurs in 1 in 5000 to 20,000 live births. The most common form of extrahepatic biliary atresia (present in 85% of cases) is **obliteration of the bile ducts** at or superior to the **porta hepatis**, a deep transverse fissure on the visceral surface of the liver.

Previous speculations that there is a failure of the bile ducts to canalize may not be true. Biliary atresia (absence of a normal opening) of the major bile ducts could result from a failure of the remodeling process at the hepatic hilum or from infections or immunologic reactions during late fetal development.

Jaundice occurs soon after birth, the stools are acholic (clay colored), and the urine appears dark colored. Biliary atresia can be palliated surgically in most patients, but in more than 70% of those treated, the disease continues to progress.

Agenesis of the gallbladder occurs rarely and is usually associated with absence of the cystic duct.

**FIGURE 11-9** Median section of caudal half of an embryo at the end of the fifth week, showing the liver and associated ligaments. The *arrow* indicates the communication of the peritoneal cavity with the extraembryonic coelom.

## Development of Pancreas

The pancreas develops between the layers of the mesentery from dorsal and ventral **pancreatic buds** of endodermal cells, which arise from the caudal part of the foregut (Fig. 11-10*A* and *B*, and see also Fig. 11-9). Most of the pancreas is derived from the larger **dorsal pancreatic bud**, which appears first and develops at a slight distance cranial to the ventral bud.

The smaller **ventral pancreatic bud** develops near the entry of the bile duct into the duodenum and grows between the layers of the ventral mesentery. As the duodenum rotates to the right and becomes C shaped, the bud is carried dorsally with the bile duct (see Fig. 11-10*C* to *G*). It soon lies posterior to the dorsal pancreatic bud and later fuses with it. The ventral pancreatic bud forms the **uncinate process** and part of the **head of the pancreas**.

As the stomach, duodenum, and ventral mesentery rotate, the pancreas comes to lie along the dorsal abdominal wall (in a retroperitoneal position). As the pancreatic buds fuse, their ducts anastomose, or open into one another (see Fig. 11-10*C*). The **pancreatic duct** forms from the duct of the ventral bud and the distal part of the duct of the dorsal bud (see Fig. 11-10*G*). The proximal part of the duct of the dorsal bud often persists as an **accessory pancreatic duct** that opens into the **minor duodenal papilla**, located approximately 2 cm cranial to the main duct (see Fig. 11-10*G*). The two ducts often communicate with each other. In approximately 9% of people, the pancreatic ducts fail to fuse, resulting in two ducts.

*Molecular studies show that the ventral pancreas develops from a bipotential cell population in the ventral region of the duodenum where the transcription factor*

*PDX1 is expressed. A default mechanism involving FGF-2, which is secreted by the developing heart, appears to play a role. Formation of the dorsal pancreatic bud depends on the notochord secreting activin and FGF-2, which block the expression of Shh in the associated endoderm.*

### Histogenesis of Pancreas

The **parenchyma** (basic cellular tissue) of the pancreas is derived from the endoderm of the pancreatic buds, which forms a network of tubules. Early in the fetal period, **pancreatic acini** (secretory portions of an acinous gland) begin to develop from cell clusters around the ends of these tubules (**primordial pancreatic ducts**). The **pancreatic islets** develop from groups of cells that separate from the tubules and lie between the acini.

*Recent studies show that the chemokine, stromal-cell derived factor 1 (SDF-1), expressed in the mesenchyme, controls the formation and branching of the tubules.* Expression of transcription factor neurogenin-3 is required for differentiation of pancreatic islet endocrine cells.

**Insulin secretion** begins during the early fetal period (at 10 weeks). The cells containing glucagon and somatostatin develop before differentiation of the **beta cells that secrete insulin.** Glucagon has been detected in fetal plasma at 15 weeks.

The connective tissue sheath and interlobular septa of the pancreas develop from the surrounding splanchnic mesenchyme. When there is **maternal diabetes mellitus**, the beta cells that secrete insulin in the fetal pancreas are chronically exposed to high levels of glucose. As a result, these cells undergo hypertrophy to increase the rate of insulin secretion.

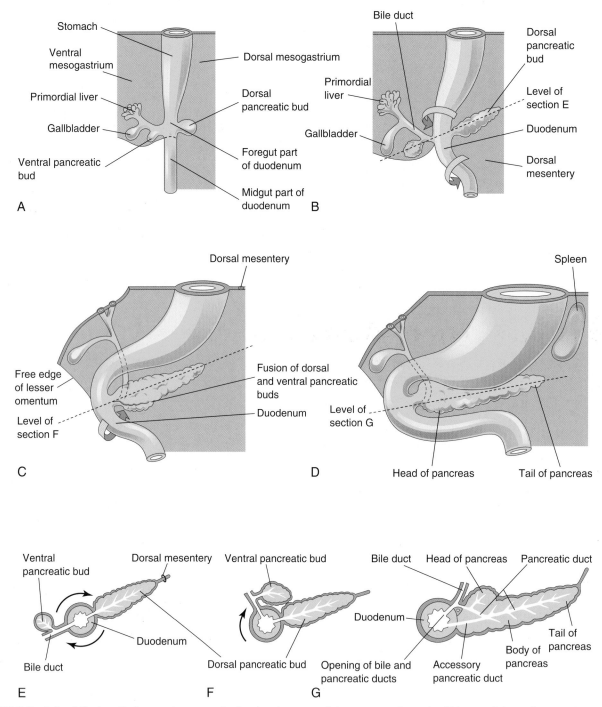

**FIGURE 11–10** A to D, Successive stages in the development of the pancreas from the fifth to eighth weeks. E to G, Diagrammatic transverse sections through the duodenum and developing pancreas. Growth and rotation (arrows) of the duodenum bring the ventral pancreatic bud toward the dorsal bud, and the two buds subsequently fuse.

## ECTOPIC PANCREAS

Ectopic pancreas (ectopic pancreatic tissue) is located separate from the pancreas. Locations for the tissue are the mucosa of the stomach, the proximal duodenum, the jejunum, the pyloric antrum, and the ileal diverticulum (of Meckel). This defect is usually asymptomatic and is discovered incidentally (e.g., by computed tomography scanning); however, it may present with gastrointestinal symptoms, obstruction, bleeding, or even cancer.

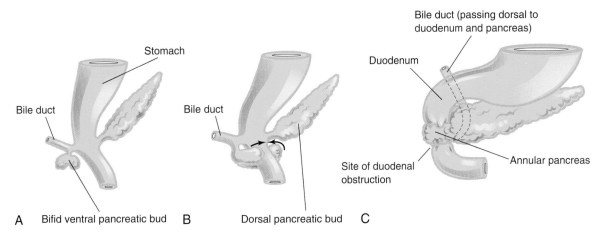

**FIGURE 11–11** A and B show the probable basis of an annular pancreas. C, An annular pancreas encircling the duodenum. This birth defect produces complete obstruction (atresia) or partial obstruction (stenosis) of the duodenum.

## ANNULAR PANCREAS

Although an **annular pancreas** is rare, the defect warrants description because it may cause duodenal obstruction (Fig. 11-11C). The ring-like, annular part of the pancreas consists of a thin, flat band of pancreatic tissue surrounding the descending or second part of the duodenum. An annular pancreas may cause obstruction of the duodenum. Infants present with symptoms of complete or partial bowel obstruction.

Blockage of the duodenum develops if inflammation (**pancreatitis**) develops in the annular pancreas. The defect may be associated with Down syndrome, intestinal malrotation, and cardiac defects. Females are affected more frequently than males. An annular pancreas probably results from the growth of a bifid ventral pancreatic bud around the duodenum (see Fig. 11-11A to C). The parts of the bifid ventral bud then fuse with the dorsal bud, forming a pancreatic ring. Surgical intervention may be required for management of this condition.

### Development of Spleen

**10** The **spleen** is derived from a mass of mesenchymal cells located between the layers of the **dorsal mesogastrium** (Fig. 11-12A and B). The spleen, a vascular lymphatic organ, begins to develop during the fifth week, but it does not acquire its characteristic shape until early in the fetal period.

*Gene-targeting experiments show that capsulin, a basic helix–loop transcription factor, and homeobox genes NKx2-5, Hox11, and Bapx1 regulate the development of the spleen.*

The fetal spleen is lobulated, but the lobules normally disappear before birth. The notches in the superior border of the adult spleen are remnants of the grooves that separated the fetal lobules. As the stomach rotates, the left surface of the mesogastrium fuses with the peritoneum over the left kidney. This fusion explains why the **splenorenal ligament** has a dorsal attachment and why the adult **splenic artery**, the largest branch of the **celiac trunk**, follows a tortuous course posterior to the omental bursa and anterior to the left kidney (see Fig. 11-12C).

The mesenchymal cells in the splenic primordium differentiate to form the capsule, connective tissue framework, and parenchyma of the spleen. The spleen functions as a **hematopoietic center** until late fetal life; however, it retains its potential for blood cell formation even in adult life.

## ACCESSORY SPLEENS

One or more small splenic masses (~1 cm in diameter) of fully functional splenic tissue may exist in addition to the main body of the spleen, in one of the peritoneal folds, commonly near the hilum of the spleen, in the tail of the pancreas, or within the gastrosplenic ligament (see Fig. 11-10D). In **polysplenia**, multiple small accessory spleens are present in an infant *without* a main body of the spleen. Although the multiple spleens are functional tissue, the infant's immune function may still be compromised, resulting in an increased susceptibility to infection. An accessory spleen occurs in approximately 10% of people.

## MIDGUT

The derivatives of the midgut are the:

- Small intestine, including the duodenum distal to the opening of the bile duct
- Cecum, appendix, ascending colon, and right one half to two thirds of the transverse colon

These derivatives are supplied by the **superior mesenteric artery** (see Figs. 11-1 and 11-9).

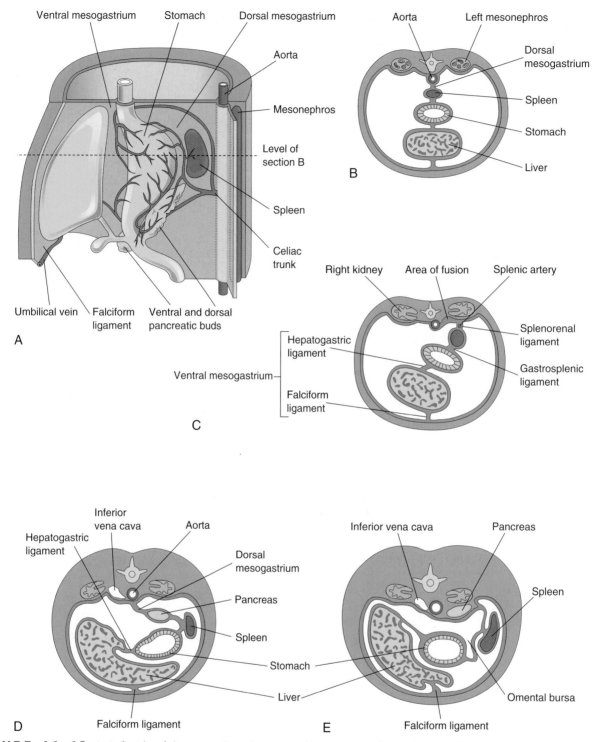

**FIGURE 11–12** A, Left side of the stomach and associated structures at the end of the fifth week. Note that the pancreas, spleen, and celiac trunk are between the layers of the dorsal mesogastrium. B, Transverse section of the liver, stomach, and spleen at the level shown in A, illustrating the relationship of these structures to the dorsal and ventral mesenteries. C, Transverse section of a fetus showing fusion of the dorsal mesogastrium with the peritoneum on the posterior abdominal wall. D and E, Similar sections showing movement of the liver to the right and rotation of the stomach. Observe the fusion of the dorsal mesogastrium with the dorsal abdominal wall. As a result, the pancreas becomes situated in a retroperitoneal position.

## Herniation of Midgut Loop

As the midgut elongates, it forms a ventral U-shaped loop of intestine, the **midgut loop**, that projects into the remains of the **extraembryonic coelom** in the proximal part of the umbilical cord (Fig. 11-13A). The loop is a **physiologic umbilical herniation**, which occurs at the beginning of the sixth week (Fig. 11-14A, and see also Fig. 11-13A and B). The loop communicates with the **umbilical vesicle** (yolk sac) through the narrow **omphaloenteric duct** until the 10th week.

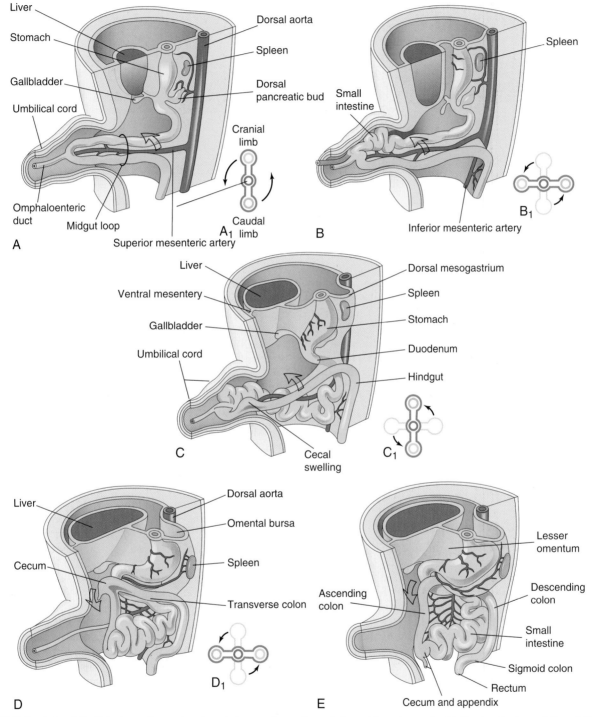

**FIGURE 11-13** Drawings illustrating herniation and rotation of the midgut loop. **A,** At the beginning of the sixth week. **A₁,** Transverse section through the midgut loop, illustrating the initial relationship of the limbs of the loop to the superior mesenteric artery. Note that the midgut loop is in the proximal part of the umbilical cord. **B,** Later stage showing the beginning of midgut rotation. **B₁,** Illustration of the 90-degree counterclockwise rotation that carries the cranial limb of the midgut to the right. **C,** At approximately 10 weeks, showing the intestine returning to the abdomen. **C₁,** Illustration of a further rotation of 90 degrees. **D,** At approximately 11 weeks, showing the location of the viscera after retraction of the intestine. **D₁,** Illustration of a further 90-degree rotation of the viscera, for a total of 270 degrees. **E,** Later in the fetal period, showing the cecum rotating to its normal position in the lower right quadrant of the abdomen.

A

B

- Umbilical vein
- Umbilical artery
- Allantois
- Umbilical artery
- Intestine
- Amnion covering umbilical cord

**FIGURE 11–14** A, Physiologic hernia in a fetus of approximately 58 days (attached to its placenta). Note the herniated intestine *(arrow)* in the proximal part of the umbilical cord. B, Schematic drawing showing the structures in the distal part of the umbilical cord.

The herniation occurs because there is not enough room in the abdominal cavity for the rapidly growing midgut. The shortage of space is caused mainly by the relatively massive liver and kidneys. The midgut loop has a cranial (proximal) limb and a caudal (distal) limb and is suspended from the dorsal abdominal wall by an elongated mesentery, the **dorsal mesogastrium** (see Fig. 11-13A).

The **omphaloenteric duct** is attached to the apex of the midgut loop where the two limbs join (see Fig. 11-13A). The cranial limb grows rapidly and forms **small intestinal loops** (see Fig. 11-13B), but the caudal limb undergoes very little change except for development of the **cecal swelling** (diverticulum), the primordium of the cecum and appendix (see Fig. 11-13C).

## Rotation of Midgut Loop

While it is in the umbilical cord, the midgut loop rotates 90 degrees counterclockwise around the axis of the **superior mesenteric artery** (see Fig. 11-13B and C). This brings the **cranial limb** (small intestine) of the loop to the right and the **caudal limb** (large intestine) to the left. During rotation, the cranial limb elongates and forms **intestinal loops** (e.g., the primordia of the jejunum and ileum).

## Retraction of Intestinal Loops

During the 10th week, the intestines return to the abdomen; this is the **reduction of the midgut hernia** (see Fig. 11-13C and D). It is not known what causes the intestine to return; however, the enlargement of the abdominal cavity and relative decrease in the size of the liver and kidneys are important factors. The small intestine (formed from the cranial limb) returns first,

passing posterior to the superior mesenteric artery, and occupies the central part of the abdomen.

As the large intestine returns, it undergoes a further 180-degree counterclockwise rotation (see Fig. 11-13$C_1$ and $D_1$). The descending colon and sigmoid colon move to the right side of the abdomen. The ascending colon becomes recognizable with the elongation of the posterior abdominal wall (see Fig. 11-13E).

### Fixation of Intestines

Rotation of the stomach and duodenum causes the duodenum and pancreas to fall to the right. The enlarged colon presses the duodenum and pancreas against the posterior abdominal wall. As a result, most of the **duodenal mesentery** is absorbed (Fig. 11-15C, D, and F). Consequently, the duodenum, except for the first part (derived from the foregut), has no mesentery and lies retroperitoneally (external or posterior to the peritoneum). Similarly, the head of the pancreas becomes retroperitoneal.

The attachment of the dorsal mesentery to the posterior abdominal wall is greatly modified after the intestines return to the abdominal cavity. At first, the dorsal mesentery is in the median plane. As the intestines enlarge, lengthen, and assume their final positions, their mesenteries are pressed against the posterior abdominal wall. The mesentery of the ascending colon fuses with the parietal peritoneum on this wall and disappears; consequently, the ascending colon also becomes retroperitoneal (see Fig. 11-15B and E).

Other derivatives of the midgut loop (e.g., jejunum and ileum) retain their mesenteries. The mesentery is at first attached to the median plane of the posterior abdominal wall (see Fig. 11-13B and C). After the mesentery of the ascending colon disappears, the fan-shaped mesentery of the small intestine acquires a new line of attachment that

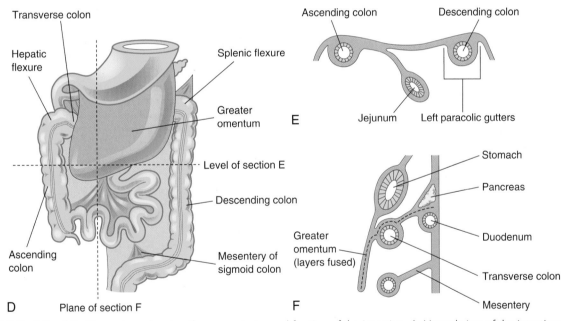

**FIGURE 11–15** Illustrations showing the mesenteries and fixation of the intestine. A, Ventral view of the intestines before fixation. B, Transverse section at the level shown in A. The *arrows* indicate areas of subsequent fusion. C, Sagittal section at the plane shown in A, illustrating the greater omentum overhanging the transverse colon. The *arrows* indicate areas of subsequent fusion. D, Ventral view of the intestine after fixation. E, Transverse section at the level shown in D after disappearance of the mesentery of the ascending colon and descending colon. F, Sagittal section at the plane shown in D, illustrating fusion of the greater omentum with the mesentery of the transverse colon and fusion of the layers of the greater omentum.

passes from the duodenojejunal junction inferolaterally to the ileocecal junction.

## Cecum and Appendix

The primordium of the cecum and appendix, the **cecal swelling**, appears in the sixth week as an elevation on the antimesenteric border of the caudal limb of the midgut loop (Fig. 11-16*A* to *C*, and see also Fig. 11-13*C* and *E*). The apex of the cecal swelling does not grow as rapidly as the rest of it; therefore, the **appendix** is initially a small pouch or sac opening from the cecum (see Fig. 11-16*B*). The appendix increases rapidly in length, so that at birth it is a relatively long tube arising from

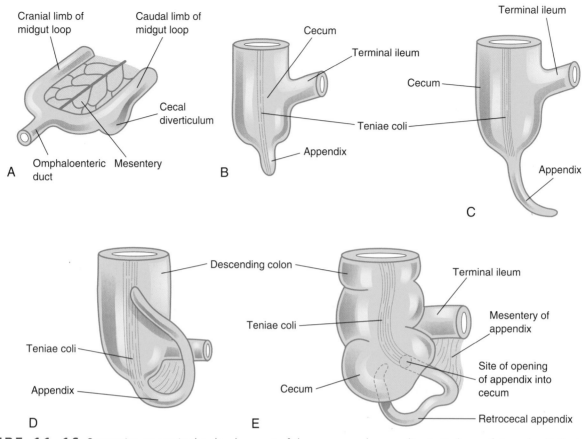

**FIGURE 11–16** Successive stages in the development of the cecum and appendix. **A**, Embryo of 6 weeks. **B**, Embryo of 8 weeks. **C**, Fetus of 12 weeks. **D**, Fetus at birth. Note that the appendix is relatively long and is continuous with the apex of the cecum. **E**, Child. Note that the opening of the appendix lies on the medial side of the cecum. In approximately 64% of people, the appendix is located posterior to the cecum (retrocecal). The teniae coli is a thickened band of longitudinal muscle in the wall of the colon.

the distal end of the cecum (see Fig. 11-16*D* and *E*). After birth, the wall of the cecum grows unequally, with the result that the appendix comes to enter its medial side.

There are variations of the position of the appendix. As the ascending colon elongates, the appendix may pass posterior to the cecum (**retrocecal appendix**) or colon (**retrocolic appendix**). It may also descend over the brim of the pelvis (**pelvic appendix**). In approximately 64% of people, the appendix is located **retrocecally** (see Fig. 11-16*E*).

*Text continued on p. 233*

## CONGENITAL OMPHALOCELE

**Congenital omphalocele** is a birth defect in which herniation of abdominal contents into the proximal part of the umbilical cord persists (Figs. 11-17 and 11-18). Herniation of the intestine into the cord occurs in approximately 1 in 5000 births, and herniation of the liver and intestine occurs in approximately 1 in 10,000 births. Up to 50% of cases are associated with chromosomal abnormalities. The abdominal cavity is proportionately small when there is an omphalocele because the impetus for it to grow is absent.

Surgical repair of omphaloceles is required. Minor omphaloceles may be treated with primary closure. A staged reduction is often planned if the visceral–abdominal disproportion is large. Infants with very large omphaloceles can also suffer from pulmonary and thoracic hypoplasia (underdevelopment).

The covering of the hernia sac is the peritoneum and the amnion. Omphalocele results from impaired growth of mesodermal (muscle) and ectodermal (skin) components of the abdominal wall. Because the formation of the abdominal compartment occurs during gastrulation, a critical failure of growth at this time is often associated with other birth defects of the cardiovascular and urogenital systems.

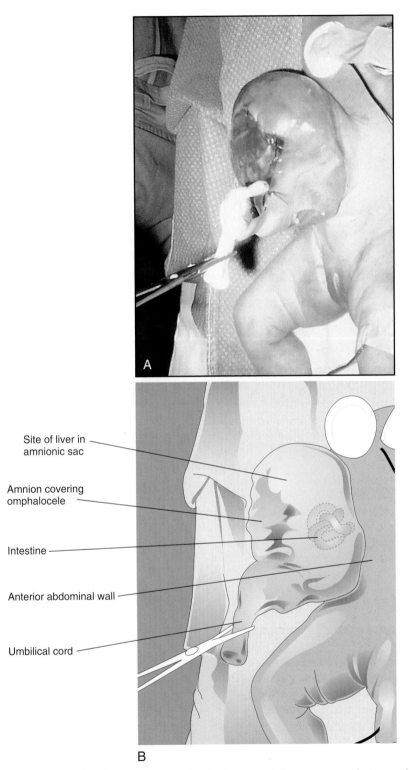

Site of liver in
amnionic sac

Amnion covering
omphalocele

Intestine

Anterior abdominal wall

Umbilical cord

**FIGURE 11–17** A, A neonate with a large omphalocele. B, Drawing of the neonate with an omphalocele resulting from a median defect of the abdominal muscles, fascia, and skin near the umbilicus. This defect resulted in the herniation of intra-abdominal structures (liver and intestine) into the proximal end of the umbilical cord. The omphalocele is covered by a membrane composed of peritoneum and amnion.

**FIGURE 11-18** Sonogram of the abdomen of a fetus showing a large omphalocele. Note that the liver (L) is protruding (herniating) from the abdomen (asterisk). Also observe the stomach (S).

## UMBILICAL HERNIA

When the intestines return to the abdominal cavity during the 10th week and then later herniate again through an imperfectly closed umbilicus, an umbilical hernia forms. This common type of hernia is different from an omphalocele. In an umbilical hernia, the protruding mass (usually the greater omentum and part of the small intestine) is covered by subcutaneous tissue and skin.

Usually the hernia does not reach its maximum size until the end of the neonatal period (28 days). It usually ranges in diameter from 1 to 5 cm. The defect through which the hernia occurs is in the linea alba (fibrous band in the median line of the anterior abdominal wall between the rectus muscles). The hernia protrudes during crying, straining, or coughing and can be easily reduced through the fibrous ring at the umbilicus. Surgery is not usually performed, unless the hernia persists to the age of 3 to 5 years.

## GASTROSCHISIS

Gastroschisis, a birth defect of the abdominal wall (prevalence 1 in 2000), (Fig. 11-19) results from a defect lateral to the median plane of the anterior abdominal wall. The linear defect permits extrusion of the abdominal viscera without involving the umbilical cord. The viscera protrude into the amniotic cavity and are bathed by amniotic fluid. The term *gastroschisis*, which literally means a "split or open stomach," is a misnomer because it is the anterior abdominal wall that is split, not the stomach.

This defect usually occurs on the right side lateral to the umbilicus; it is more common in males than females. The exact cause of gastroschisis is uncertain, but various suggestions have been proposed, such as ischemic injury to the anterior abdominal wall; absence of the right omphalomesenteric artery; rupture of the abdominal wall; weakness of the wall caused by abnormal involution of the right umbilical vein; and perhaps rupture of an omphalocele (herniation of viscera into the base of the umbilical cord) before the sides of the anterior abdominal wall have closed.

## ANOMALIES OF MIDGUT

Birth defects of the intestine are common; most of them are defects of gut rotation, or **malrotation of the gut**, which result from incomplete rotation and/or fixation of the intestine. **Nonrotation of the midgut** occurs when the intestine does not rotate as it reenters the abdomen. As a result, the caudal limb of the midgut loop returns to the abdomen first, the small intestine lies on the right side of the abdomen, and the entire large intestine is on the left side (Fig. 11-20A). The usual 270-degree counterclockwise rotation is not completed, and the cecum and appendix lie just inferior to the pylorus of the stomach, a condition known as **subhepatic cecum and appendix** (see Fig. 11-20D). The cecum is fixed to the posterolateral abdominal wall by peritoneal bands that pass over the duodenum (see Fig. 11-20B). The peritoneal bands and the volvulus (twisting) of the intestine cause **intestinal atresia** (duodenal obstruction).

This type of malrotation results from failure of the midgut loop to complete the final 90 degrees of rotation (see Fig. 11-13D). Only two parts of the intestine are attached to the posterior abdominal wall, the duodenum and proximal colon. This improperly positioned and incompletely fixed intestine may lead to a twisting of the midgut, or **midgut volvulus** (see Fig. 11-20F). The small intestine hangs by a narrow stalk that contains the superior mesenteric artery and vein.

When midgut volvulus occurs, the superior mesenteric artery may be obstructed, resulting in infarction and **gangrene** of the intestine supplied by it (see Fig. 11-20A and B). Infants with intestinal malrotation are prone to volvulus and present with **bilious emesis** (vomiting bile). A contrast x-ray study can determine the presence of rotational abnormalities.

**FIGURE 11-19** **A,** Photograph of a neonate with viscera protruding from an anterior abdominal wall birth defect (gastroschisis). The defect was 2 to 4 cm long and involved all layers of the abdominal wall. **B,** Photograph of the infant after the viscera were returned to the abdomen and the defect was surgically closed. **C** (sagittal) and **D** (axial) sonograms of a fetus at 18 weeks with gastroschisis. Loops of intestine (*arrow*) can be seen in the amniotic fluid anterior to the fetus (*F*).

## REVERSED ROTATION

In rare cases, the midgut loop rotates in a clockwise rather than a counterclockwise direction (see Fig. 11-20C). As a result, the duodenum lies anterior to the superior mesenteric artery rather than posterior to it and the transverse colon lies posterior instead of anterior to it. In these infants, the transverse colon may be obstructed by pressure from the superior mesenteric artery. In more unusual cases, the small intestine lies on the left side of the abdomen and the large intestine lies on the right side with the cecum in the center. This unusual situation results from malrotation of the midgut followed by failure of fixation of the intestines.

A

B

C

D

E

F

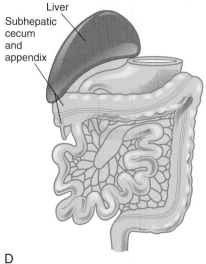

G

**FIGURE 11–20** Birth defects of midgut rotation. **A,** Nonrotation. **B,** Mixed rotation and volvulus (twisting); the *arrow* indicates the twisting of the intestine. **C,** Reversed rotation. **D,** Subhepatic (below liver) cecum and appendix. **E,** Internal hernia. **F,** Midgut volvulus. **G,** Computed tomography enterographic image of non-rotation in an adolescent patient with chronic abdominal pain. The large intestine is completely on the left side of the abdomen (stool-filled). The small intestine (fluid-filled) is seen on the right.

## SUBHEPATIC CECUM AND APPENDIX

If the cecum adheres to the inferior surface of the liver when it returns to the abdomen, it will be drawn superiorly as the liver diminishes in size; as a result, the cecum and appendix remain in their fetal positions (see Fig. 11-20D). **Subhepatic cecum and appendix** are more common in males and occur in approximately 6% of fetuses. A subhepatic cecum and "high-riding" appendix may be seen in adults. When this situation occurs, it may create a problem in the diagnosis of appendicitis and during surgical removal of the appendix (**appendectomy**).

## MOBILE CECUM

In approximately 10% of people, the cecum has an abnormal amount of freedom. In very unusual cases, it may herniate into the right inguinal canal. A **mobile cecum** results from incomplete fixation of the ascending colon (see Fig. 11-20F). This condition is clinically significant because of the possible variations in the position of the appendix and because twisting, or **volvulus**, of the cecum may occur (see Fig. 11-20B).

## INTERNAL HERNIA

In **internal hernia**, a rare birth defect, the small intestine passes into the mesentery of the midgut loop during the return of the intestine to the abdomen (see Fig. 11-20E). As a result, a hernia-like sac forms. This usually does not produce symptoms and is often detected only on postmortem examination.

## STENOSIS AND ATRESIA OF INTESTINE

Partial occlusion and complete occlusion (**atresia**) of the intestinal lumen account for approximately one third of cases of **intestinal obstruction** (see Fig. 11-6). The obstructive lesion occurs most often in the duodenum (25%) and ileum (50%). The length of the area affected varies. These birth defects result from failure of an adequate number of vacuoles to form during recanalization (**restoration of the lumen**) of the intestine. In some cases, a transverse septum or web forms, producing the blockage (see Fig. 11-6F$_2$).

Another possible cause of stenoses and atresias is interruption of the blood supply to a loop of fetal intestine resulting from a **fetal vascular accident** caused by impaired microcirculation associated with *fetal distress*, *drug exposure*, or a *volvulus*. The loss of blood supply leads to **necrosis** of the intestine and development of a fibrous cord connecting the proximal and distal ends of normal intestine. Malfixation of the gut most likely occurs during the 10th week; it predisposes the gut to volvulus, strangulation, and impairment of its blood supply.

## ILEAL DIVERTICULUM AND OMPHALOENTERIC REMNANTS

Outpouching of part of the ileum is a common defect of the alimentary tract (Figs. 11-21 and 11-22A). A **congenital ileal diverticulum (Meckel diverticulum)** occurs in 2% to 4% of people, and it is three to five times more prevalent in males than females. *An ileal diverticulum is of clinical significance* because it may become inflamed and cause symptoms that mimic appendicitis.

The wall of the diverticulum contains all layers of the ileum and may contain small patches of gastric and pancreatic tissues. This ectopic gastric mucosa often secretes acid, producing ulceration (ulcer) and bleeding (see Fig. 11-22A). An ileal diverticulum is the remnant of the proximal part of the omphaloenteric duct. It typically appears as a finger-like pouch approximately 3 to 6 cm long that arises from the antimesenteric border of the ileum (see Fig. 11-21), 40 to 50 cm from the ileocecal junction. An ileal diverticulum may be connected to the umbilicus by a fibrous cord. This may predispose the person to intestinal obstruction because the intestine may wrap around this cord or it may form an **omphaloenteric fistula** (Fig. 11-23; also see Fig. 11-22B and C). Similarly, cysts may form within a remnant of the duct and can be found within the abdominal cavity or the anterior abdominal wall (see Figs. 11-22D and 11-23); other possible remnants of the omphaloenteric duct are illustrated in Figure 11-22E and F.

**FIGURE 11–21** Photograph of a large ileal diverticulum (Meckel diverticulum). Only a small percentage of these diverticula produce symptoms. Ileal diverticula are some of the most common birth defects of the alimentary tract.

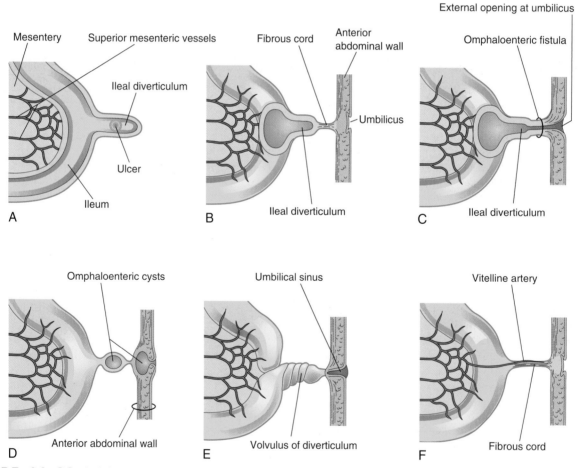

**FIGURE 11–22** Ileal diverticula and remnants of the omphaloenteric duct. A, Section of the ileum and a diverticulum with an ulcer. B, A diverticulum connected to the umbilicus by a fibrous remnant of the omphaloenteric duct. C, Omphaloenteric fistula resulting from persistence of the intra-abdominal part of the omphaloenteric duct. D, Omphaloenteric cysts at the umbilicus and in the fibrous remnant of the omphaloenteric duct. E, Volvulus (twisted) ileal diverticulum and an umbilical sinus resulting from the persistence of the omphaloenteric duct in the umbilicus. F, The omphaloenteric duct has persisted as a fibrous cord connecting the ileum with the umbilicus. A persistent vitelline artery extends along the fibrous cord to the umbilicus. This artery carried blood to the umbilical vesicle from the anterior wall of the embryo.

**FIGURE 11–23** A contrast-enhanced computed tomogram of the abdomen of a 6-year-old girl demonstrating a cyst within an omphaloenteric duct remnant, located just below the level of the umbilicus. A portion of the cyst wall contained ectopic gastric tissue with obvious glandular components. (*From Iwasaki M, Taira K, Kobayashi H, et al: Umbilical cyst containing ectopic gastric mucosa originating from an omphalomesenteric duct remnant, J Pediatr Surg 44:2399, 2009.*)

## DUPLICATION OF INTESTINE

Most intestinal duplications are cystic or tubular. **Cystic duplications** are more common than **tubular duplications** (Fig. 11-24A to D). Tubular duplications usually communicate with the intestinal lumen (see Fig. 11-24C). Almost all duplications are caused by failure of normal recanalization of the small intestine; as a result, two lumina form (see Fig. 11-24H and I). The duplicated segment lies on the mesenteric side of the intestine. The duplication often contains **ectopic gastric mucosa**, which may result in local peptic ulceration and gastrointestinal bleeding.

## HINDGUT

The derivatives of the hindgut are the:

- Left one third to one half of the transverse colon, the descending colon, the sigmoid colon, the rectum, and the superior part of the anal canal
- Epithelium of the urinary bladder and most of the urethra

All hindgut derivatives are supplied by the **inferior mesenteric artery**. The junction between the segment of transverse colon derived from the midgut and that originating from the hindgut is indicated by the change in blood supply from a branch of the superior mesenteric artery to a branch of the inferior mesenteric artery.

The descending colon becomes retroperitoneal as its mesentery fuses with the parietal peritoneum on the left posterior abdominal wall and then disappears (see Fig.

11-15B and E). The mesentery of the fetal sigmoid colon is retained, but it is smaller than in the embryo (see Fig. 11-15D).

## Cloaca

In early embryos, the cloaca is a chamber into which the hindgut and allantois empty. The expanded terminal part of the hindgut, the **cloaca**, is an endoderm-lined chamber that is in contact with the surface ectoderm at the **cloacal membrane** (Fig. 11-25A and B). This membrane is composed of endoderm of the cloaca and ectoderm of the anal pit (see Fig. 11-25D). The cloaca receives the **allantois** ventrally, which is a finger-like diverticulum (see Fig. 11-25A).

### Partitioning of the Cloaca

The cloaca is divided into dorsal and ventral parts by a wedge of mesenchyme, the **urorectal septum**, that develops in the angle between the allantois and hindgut. *Endodermal β-catenin signaling is required for the formation of the urorectal septum.* As the septum grows toward the cloacal membrane, it develops fork-like extensions that produce infoldings of the lateral walls of the cloaca (see Fig. 11-25B). These folds grow toward each other and fuse, forming a partition that divides the cloaca into three parts: the **rectum**, the cranial part of the anal canal, and the **urogenital sinus** (see Fig. 11-25D and E).

The cloaca plays a crucial role in anorectal development. New information indicates that the urorectal septum does not fuse with the cloacal membrane; therefore, an anal membrane does not exist. After the cloacal membrane ruptures by **apoptosis** (programmed cell death), the **anorectal lumen** is temporarily closed by an **epithelial plug** (which may have been misinterpreted as the anal membrane). Mesenchymal proliferations produce elevations of the surface ectoderm around the epithelial anal plug. Recanalization of the anorectal canal occurs by apoptotic cell death of the epithelial anal plug, which forms the **anal pit** (proctodeum) (see Fig. 11-25E).

## Anal Canal

The superior two thirds of the adult anal canal are derived from the **hindgut**; the inferior one third develops from the **anal pit** (Fig. 11-26). The junction of the epithelium derived from the ectoderm of the anal pit and endoderm of the hindgut is roughly indicated by the irregular **pectinate line**, located at the inferior limit of the anal valves. Approximately 2 cm superior to the anus is the **anocutaneous line** (white line). This is approximately where the composition of the anal epithelium changes from columnar to stratified squamous cells. At the anus, the epithelium is **keratinized** (made keratinous) and continuous with the skin around the anus. The other layers of the wall of the anal canal are derived from splanchnic mesenchyme. *The formation of the anal sphincter appears to be under Hox D genetic control.*

Because of its hindgut origin, the superior two thirds of the anal canal are mainly supplied by the **superior rectal artery**, the continuation of the inferior mesenteric artery (hindgut artery). The venous drainage of this

**FIGURE 11–24** A, Cystic duplication of the small intestine on the mesenteric side of the intestine; it receives branches from the arteries supplying the intestine. B, Longitudinal section of the duplication shown in A; its musculature is continuous with the intestinal wall. C, A short tubular duplication. D, A long duplication showing a partition consisting of the fused muscular walls. E, Transverse section of the intestine during the solid stage. F, Normal vacuole formation. G, Coalescence of the vacuoles and reformation of the lumen. H, Two groups of vacuoles have formed. I, Coalescence of vacuoles illustrated in H results in intestinal duplication.

superior part is mainly via the **superior rectal vein**, a tributary of the inferior mesenteric vein. The lymphatic drainage of the superior part is eventually to the **inferior mesenteric lymph nodes**. Its nerves are from the **autonomic nervous system**.

Because of its origin from the anal pit, the inferior one third of the anal canal is supplied mainly by the **inferior rectal arteries**, branches of the internal pudendal artery. The venous drainage is through the **inferior rectal vein**, a tributary of the internal pudendal vein that drains into the internal iliac vein. The **lymphatic drainage** of the inferior part of the anal canal is to the **superficial inguinal lymph nodes**. Its nerve supply is from the **inferior rectal nerve**; hence, it is sensitive to pain, temperature, touch, and pressure.

*The differences in blood supply, nerve supply, and venous and lymphatic drainage of the anal canal are important clinically*, as when one may be considering the **metastasis** (spread) of cancer cells. The characteristics of a **carcinoma** *(cancer arising in the epithelial tissue)* in the two parts is also different. *Tumors in the superior part are painless* and arise from columnar epithelium, whereas *tumors in the inferior part are painful* and arise from stratified squamous epithelium.

## SUMMARY OF ALIMENTARY SYSTEM

- The **primordial gut** forms from the dorsal part of the umbilical vesicle, which is incorporated into the embryo. The endoderm of the primordial gut gives rise to the epithelial lining of the alimentary tract, except for the cranial and caudal parts, which are derived from ectoderm of the stomodeum and cloacal membrane, respectively. The muscular and connective tissue components of the alimentary tract are derived from splanchnic mesenchyme surrounding the primordial gut.

- The **foregut** gives rise to the pharynx, lower respiratory system, esophagus, stomach, proximal part of the

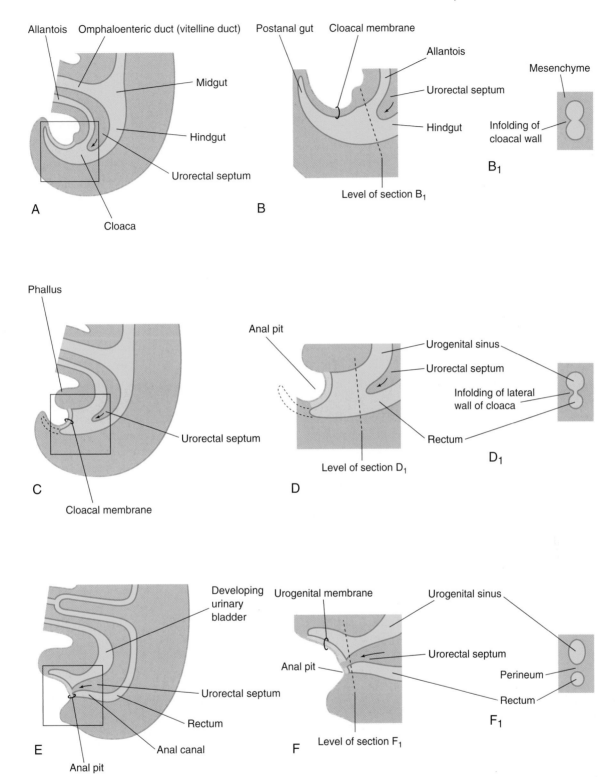

**FIGURE 11–25** Successive stages in the partitioning of the cloaca into the rectum and urogenital sinus by the urorectal septum. A, C, and E, Views from the left side at 4, 6, and 7 weeks, respectively. B, D, and F, Enlargements of the cloacal region. B₁ and D₁, Transverse sections of the cloaca at the levels shown in B and D. Note that the postanal portion (shown in B) degenerates and disappears as the rectum forms.

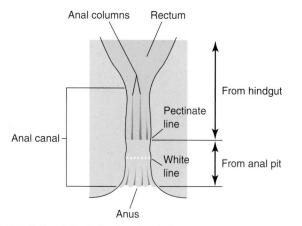

**FIGURE 11–26** Sketch of the rectum and anal canal showing their developmental origins. Note that the superior two thirds of the anal canal are derived from the hindgut, whereas the inferior one third of the canal is derived from the anal pit. Because of their different embryologic origins, the superior and inferior parts of the anal canal are supplied by different arteries and nerves and have different venous and lymphatic drainages.

**FIGURE 11–27** Radiograph of the colon after a barium enema in a 1-month-old infant with congenital megacolon (Hirschsprung disease). The aganglionic distal segment (rectum and distal sigmoid colon) is narrow, with distended normal ganglionic bowel, full of fecal material, proximal to it. Note the transition zone *(arrow).*

## CONGENITAL MEGACOLON

**Congenital megacolon** is a dominantly inherited multigenic disorder with incomplete penetrance and variable expressivity. Of the genes so far identified, the RET protooncogene is the major susceptibility gene and accounts for most cases. This disorder affects 1 in 5000 newborns and is defined as an absence of ganglion cells (**aganglionosis**) in a variable length of distal bowel.

Infants with congenital megacolon (**Hirschsprung disease**) lack autonomic ganglion cells in the myenteric plexus distal to the dilated segment of colon (Fig. 11-27). The enlarged colon, or megacolon, has the normal number of ganglion cells. The dilation results from failure of relaxation of the aganglionic segment, which prevents movement of the intestinal contents, resulting in dilation. In most cases, only the rectum and sigmoid colon are involved; occasionally, ganglia are also absent from more proximal parts of the colon.

*Megacolon is the most common cause of neonatal obstruction of the colon* and accounts for 33% of all neonatal obstructions; males are affected more often than females (4 : 1). Megacolon results from failure of neural crest cells to migrate into the wall of the colon during the fifth to seventh weeks. This results in failure of parasympathetic ganglion cells to develop in the Auerbach and Meissner plexuses.

## ANORECTAL ANOMALIES

Most anorectal anomalies result from abnormal development of the urorectal septum, resulting in incomplete separation of the cloaca into urogenital and anorectal parts (see Fig. 11-29A). *Shh and FGF-10, as well as disruption of β-catenin signaling, have been implicated in birth defects of the hindgut.* There is normally a temporary communication between the rectum and anal canal dorsally from the bladder and urethra ventrally (see Fig. 11-25C). Lesions are classified as low or high depending on whether the rectum ends superior or inferior to the puborectalis muscle, which maintains fecal continence and relaxes to allow defecation.

### Low Birth Defects of Anorectal Region

- **Imperforate anus** occurs in 1 in 5000 neonates and is more common in males than in females (Figs. 11-28 and 11-29C). The anal canal may end blindly or there may be an ectopic anus or an **anoperineal fistula** (**abnormal passage**) that opens into the perineum (see Fig. 11-29D and E). However, the abnormal canal may open into the vagina in females or urethra in males (see Figs. 11-29F and G). More than 90% of low anorectal defects are associated with a **fistula** (e.g., a passage connecting the rectum and urethra).

## ANORECTAL ANOMALIES—cont'd

- In **anal stenosis**, the anus is in the normal position but the anus and anal canal are narrow (see Fig. 11-29*B*). This defect is probably caused by a slight dorsal deviation of the urorectal septum as it grows caudally.

- In **membranous atresia**, the anus is in the normal position but a thin layer of tissue separates the anal canal from the exterior (see Figs. 11-28 and 11-29*C*). The remnant of the epithelial anal plug is thin enough to bulge on straining and appears blue from the presence of **meconium** (feces of neonate) superior to it. This defect results from failure of the epithelial plug to perforate at the end of the eighth week.

### High Birth Defects of Anorectal Region

In **anorectal agenesis**, a high anomaly of the anorectal region, the rectum ends superior to the puborectalis muscle. *This is the most common type of anorectal birth defect.* Although the rectum ends blindly, there is usually a **fistula (abnormal passage)** to the bladder (**rectovesical fistula**) or urethra (**rectourethral fistula**) in males, or to the vagina (**rectovaginal fistula**) or the vestibule of the vagina (**rectovestibular fistula**) in females (see Fig. 11-29*F* and *G*).

**Anorectal agenesis with a fistula** is the result of incomplete separation of the cloaca from the urogenital sinus by the urorectal septum (see Fig. 11-25*C* to *E*). In newborn males with this condition, meconium may be observed in the urine, whereas fistulas in females result in the presence of meconium in the vestibule of the vagina.

In **rectal atresia**, the anal canal and rectum are present but separated (see Fig. 11-29*H* and *I*). Sometimes the two segments of intestine are connected by a fibrous cord, the remnant of an atretic portion of the rectum. The cause of rectal atresia may be abnormal recanalization of the colon or, more likely, a defective blood supply.

**FIGURE 11–28** Imperforate anus. **A,** Female neonate with anal atresia (imperforate anus). In most cases, a thin layer of tissue separates the anal canal from the exterior. Some form of imperforate anus occurs approximately once in every 5000 neonates; it is more common in males. **B,** Radiograph of an infant with an imperforate anus. The dilated end of the radiopaque probe is at the bottom of the blindly ending anal pit. The large intestine is distended with feces and contrast material.

duodenum, liver, pancreas, and biliary apparatus. Because the trachea and esophagus have a common origin from the foregut, incomplete partitioning by the tracheoesophageal septum results in stenoses or atresias, with or without fistulas between them.

- The **hepatic diverticulum**, the primordium of the liver, gallbladder, and biliary duct system, is an outgrowth of the endodermal epithelial lining of the foregut. Epithelial liver cords develop from the hepatic diverticulum and grow into the **septum transversum**. Between the layers of the ventral mesentery, derived from the septum transversum, primordial cells differentiate into hepatic tissues and linings of the ducts of the biliary system.

- **Congenital duodenal atresia** results from failure of the vacuolization and recanalization process to occur after the normal solid developmental stage of the duodenum. Usually the epithelial cells degenerate and the lumen of the duodenum is restored. Obstruction of the duodenum can also be caused by an **annular pancreas** or pyloric stenosis.

- The **pancreas** develops from pancreatic buds that form from the endodermal lining of the foregut. When the duodenum rotates to the right, the **ventral pancreatic bud** moves dorsally and fuses with the dorsal pancreatic bud. The ventral pancreatic bud forms most of the head of the pancreas, including the uncinate process. The **dorsal pancreatic bud** forms the remainder of the pancreas. In some fetuses, the duct systems of the two buds fail to fuse, and an accessory pancreatic duct forms.

- The **midgut** gives rise to the duodenum (the part distal to the entrance of the bile duct), jejunum, ileum, cecum, appendix, ascending colon, and right one half to two thirds of the transverse colon. The midgut forms a U-shaped **umbilical loop of intestine** that herniates into the umbilical cord during the sixth week because there is no room for it in the abdomen. While

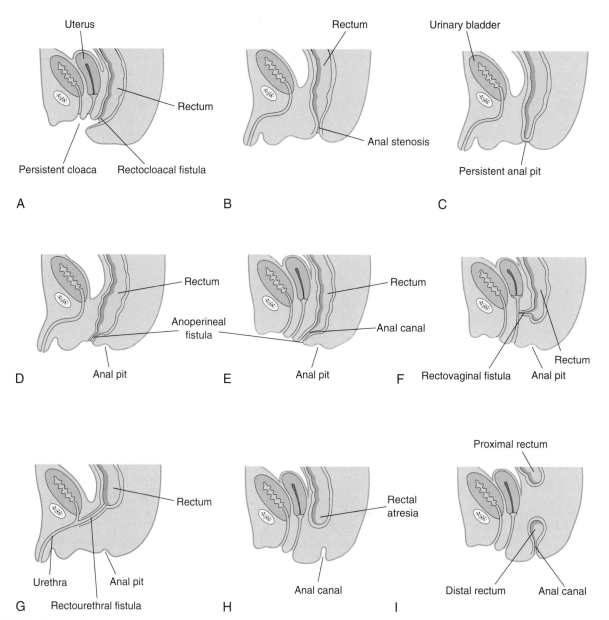

**FIGURE 11–29** Various types of anorectal birth defects. A, Persistent cloaca. Note the common outlet for the intestinal, urinary, and reproductive tracts. B, Anal stenosis. C, Anal atresia. D and E, Anal agenesis with a perineal fistula. F, Anorectal agenesis with a rectovaginal fistula. G, Anorectal agenesis with a rectourethral fistula. H and I, Rectal atresia.

in the umbilical cord, the midgut loop rotates counter-clockwise 90 degrees. During the 10th week, the intestine returns to the abdomen, rotating a further 180 degrees.

- **Omphaloceles, malrotations,** and **abnormal fixation of the gut** result from failure of return or abnormal rotation of the intestine. Because the gut is normally occluded during the fifth and sixth weeks, stenosis (partial obstruction), atresia (complete obstruction), and duplications result if recanalization fails to occur or occurs abnormally. Remnants of the omphaloenteric duct may persist. **Ileal diverticula** are common; however, very few of them become inflamed and produce pain.

- The **hindgut** gives rise to the left one third to one half of the transverse colon, the descending colon and

sigmoid colon, the rectum, and the superior part of the anal canal. The inferior part of the anal canal develops from the anal pit. The caudal part of the hindgut divides the **cloaca** into the urogenital sinus and rectum. The urogenital sinus gives rise to the urinary bladder and urethra. The rectum and superior part of the anal canal are separated from the exterior by the epithelial plug. This mass of epithelial cells breaks down by the end of the eighth week.

- Most **anorectal defects** result from abnormal partitioning of the cloaca into the rectum and anal canal posteriorly and urinary bladder and urethra anteriorly. Arrested growth and/or deviation of the urorectal septum cause most anorectal defects, such as rectal atresia and fistulas between the rectum and urethra, urinary bladder, or vagina.

# CLINICALLY ORIENTED PROBLEMS

## CASE 11–1

*A female infant was born prematurely at 32 weeks' gestation to a 39-year-old woman whose pregnancy was complicated by polyhydramnios. Amniocentesis at 16 weeks showed that the fetus had trisomy 21. The baby began to vomit within a few hours after birth. Marked dilation of the epigastrium was noted. Radiographs of the abdomen showed gas in the stomach and superior part of the duodenum, but no other intestinal gas was observed. A diagnosis of duodenal atresia was made.*

* Where does obstruction of the duodenum usually occur?
* What is the embryologic basis of this congenital defect?
* What caused distention of the infant's epigastrium?
* Is duodenal atresia commonly associated with other defects such as Down syndrome?
* What is the embryologic basis of the polyhydramnios in this case?

## CASE 11–2

*The umbilicus of a neonate failed to heal normally. It was swollen and there was a persistent discharge from the umbilical stump. A sinus tract was outlined with contrast media during fluoroscopy. The tract was resected on the ninth day after birth, and its distal end was found to terminate in a diverticulum of the ileum.*

* What is the embryologic basis of the sinus tract?
* What is the usual clinical name given to this type of ileal diverticulum?
* Is this birth defect common?

## CASE 11–3

*A female infant was born with a small dimple where the anus should have been. Examination of her vagina revealed meconium and an opening of a sinus tract in the posterior wall of the vagina. Radiographic examination using a contrast medium injected through a tiny catheter inserted into the opening revealed a fistulous connection.*

* With which part of the lower bowel would the fistula probably be connected?
* Name this birth defect.
* What is the embryologic basis of this condition?

## CASE 11–4

*A newborn infant was born with a light gray, shiny mass measuring the size of an orange that protruded from the umbilical region. The mass was covered by a thin transparent membrane.*

* What is this birth defect called?
* What is the origin of the membrane covering the mass?
* What would be the composition of the mass?
* What is the embryologic basis of this protrusion?

## CASE 11–5

*A newborn infant appeared normal at birth; however, excessive vomiting and abdominal distention developed after a few hours. The vomitus contained bile, and a little meconium was passed. Radiographic examination showed a gas-filled stomach and dilated, gas-filled loops of small bowel, but no air was present in the large intestine. This indicated a congenital obstruction of the small bowel.*

* What part of the small bowel was probably obstructed?
* What would this condition be called?
* Why was only a little meconium passed?
* What would likely be observed at operation?
* What was the probable embryologic basis of the condition?

Discussion of these problems appears in the Appendix at the back of the book.

## BIBLIOGRAPHY AND SUGGESTED READING

Baxter KJ1, Bhatia AM: Hirschsprung's disease in the preterm infant: implications for diagnosis and outcome, *Am Surg* 79:734, 2013.

Belo J1, Krishnamurthy M, Oakie A, et al: The role of SOX9 transcription factor in pancreatic and duodenal development, *Stem Cells Dev* 22:2935, 2013.

Bishop WP, Ebach DR: The digestive system. In Marcdante KJ, Kliegman KJ, editors: *Nelson essentials of pediatrics*, ed 7, Philadelphia, 2015, Saunders.

Bronshtein M, Blazer S, Zimmer EZ: The fetal gastrointestinal tract and abdominal wall. In Callen PW, editor: *Ultrasonography in obstetrics and gynecology*, ed 5, Philadelphia, 2008, Saunders.

De La Forest A, Duncan SA: Basic science of liver development. In Gumucio DL, Samuelson LC, Spence JR, editors: *Translational research and discovery in gastroenterology: organogenesis to disease*, Hoboken, N.J., 2014, John Wiley & Sons.

Heath JK: Transcriptional networks and signaling pathway that govern vertebrate intestinal development, *Curr Top Dev Biol* 90:159, 2010.

Illig R1, Fritsch H, Schwarzer C: Spatio-temporal expression of HOX genes in human hindgut development, *Dev Dyn* 242:53, 2013.

Keplinger KM, Bloomston M: Anatomy and embryology of the biliary tract, *Surg Clin North Am* 94:203, 2014.

Kluth D, Fiegel HC, Metzger R: Embryology of the hindgut, *Semin Pediatr Surg* 20:152, 2011.

Lade AG, Monga SPS: Beta-catenin signaling in hepatic development and progenitors: which way does WNT blow?, *Dev Dyn* 240:486, 2011.

Lau ST, Caty MG: Hindgut abnormalities, *Surg Clin North Am* 86:285, 2006.

Ledbetter DJ: Gastroschisis and omphalocele, *Surg Clin North Am* 86:249, 2006.

Levitt MA, Pena A: Cloacal malformations: lessons learned from 490 cases, *Semin Pediatr Surg* 9:118, 2010.

Metzger R, Metzger U, Fiegel HC, et al: Embryology of the midgut, *Semin Pediatr Surg* 20:145, 2011.

Metzger R, Wachowiak R, Kluth Dl: Embryology of the early foregut, *Semin Pediatr Surg* 20:136, 2011.

Miyagawa S, Harada M, Matsumaru D: Disruption of the temporally regulated cloaca endodermal β-catenin signaling causes anorectal malformations, *Cell Death Differ* 2014. doi: 10.1038/cdd.2014.21.

Monga SPS: Role and regulation of β-catenin signaling during physiological liver growth, *Gene Expr* 16:51, 2014.

Müller CM, Haase MG, Kemnitz I, et al: Genetic mosaicism of a frameshift mutation in the RET gene in a family with Hirschsprung disease, *Gene* 541:51, 2014.

Mundt E, Bates MD: Genetics of Hirschsprung disease and anorectal malformations, *Semin Pediatr Surg* 19:107, 2010.

Naik-Mathuria B, Olutoye OO: Foregut abnormalities, *Surg Clin North Am* 86:261, 2006.

Vakili K, Pomfret EA: Biliary anatomy and embryology, *Surg Clin North Am* 88:1159, 2008.

Van der Putte SCJ: The development of the human anorectum, *Anat Rec* 292:952, 2009.

Zangen D, Kaufman Y, Banne E, et al: Testicular differentiation factor SF-1 is required for human spleen development, *J Clin Invest* 124:2071, 2014.

# Urogenital System

The **urogenital system** is divided functionally into two different embryologically component parts: the **urinary system** and the **genital system;** however, they are closely interwoven. The urogenital system includes all the organs involved in reproduction and forming and voiding urine. Embryologically, the systems are closely associated, especially during their early stages of development. The urogenital system develops from the **intermediate mesenchyme** (primordial embryonic connective tissue consisting of mesenchymal cells) derived from the dorsal body wall of the embryo (Fig. 12-1A and B). The mesenchyme is primarily responsible for the formation of the kidneys and internal genitalia and their ducts.

During folding of the embryo in the horizontal plane the mesenchyme is carried ventrally and loses its connection with the **somites** (Fig. 12-1B to D). A longitudinal elevation of mesoderm, the **urogenital ridge,** forms on each side of the dorsal aorta (Fig. 12-1D and F). The part of the ridge giving rise to the urinary system is the **nephrogenic cord** (see Fig. 12-1D to F); the part of the ridge giving rise to the genital system is the **gonadal ridge** (see Fig. 12-29C).

*Expression of the following genes is needed for the formation of the urogenital ridge: Wilms tumor suppressor 1 (WT1), steroidogenic factor 1, and DAX1.*

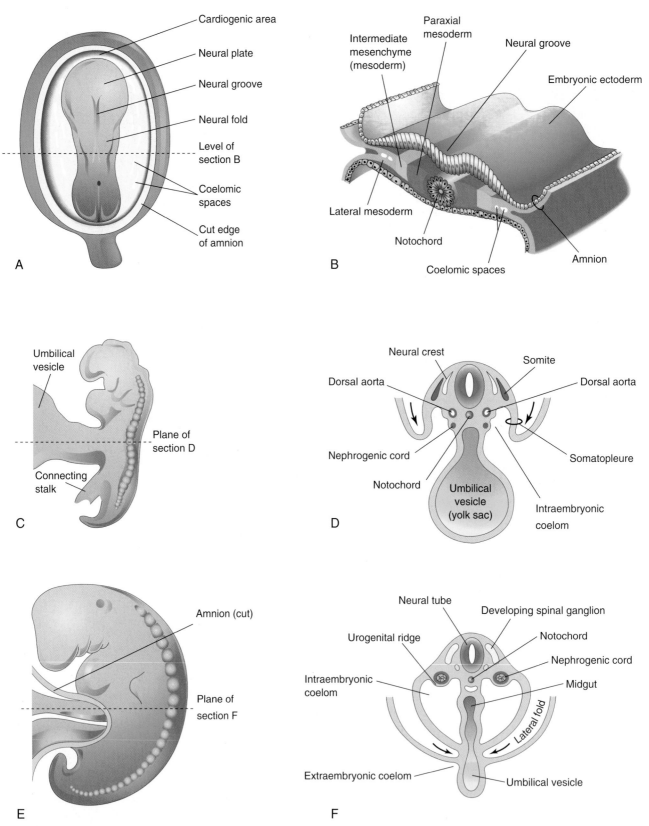

**FIGURE 12–1** A, Dorsal view of an embryo during the third week (approximately 18 days). B, Transverse section of the embryo, showing the position of the intermediate mesenchyme before lateral folding occurs. C, Lateral view of an embryo during the fourth week (approximately 24 days). D, Transverse section of the embryo after the commencement of folding, showing the nephrogenic cords. E, Lateral view of an embryo later in the fourth week (approximately 26 days). F, Transverse section of the embryo, showing the lateral folds meeting each other ventrally.

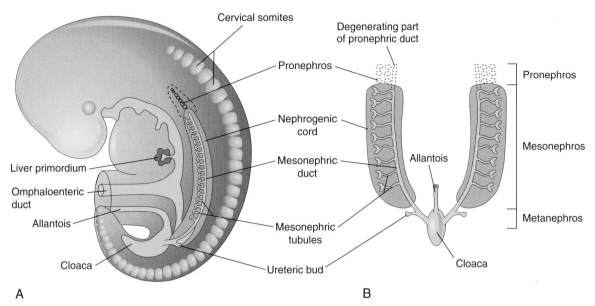

**A**          **B**

**FIGURE 12–2** Illustrations of the three sets of nephric systems in an embryo during the fifth week. **A,** Lateral view. **B,** Ventral view. The mesonephric tubules are pulled laterally; their normal position is shown in **A.**

## DEVELOPMENT OF URINARY SYSTEM

11 The urinary system begins to develop before the genital system and consists of the

- **Kidneys,** which produce and excrete urine
- **Ureters,** which convey urine from the kidneys to the urinary bladder
- **Urinary bladder,** which stores urine temporarily
- **Urethra,** which discharges urine from the bladder externally

### Development of Kidneys and Ureters

*Three sets of successive kidneys develop in the embryos.* The first set, the **pronephroi,** is rudimentary. The second set, the **mesonephroi,** functions briefly during the early fetal period. The third set, the **metanephroi,** forms the permanent kidneys.

#### Pronephroi

**Pronephroi** are bilateral transitory structures that appear early in the fourth week. They are represented by a few cell clusters and tubular structures in the developing neck region (Fig. 12-2*A*). The pronephric ducts run caudally and open into the **cloaca,** the chamber into which the hindgut and allantois emptied (Fig. 12-2*B*). The pronephroi soon degenerate; however, most parts of the ducts persist and are used by the second set of kidneys.

#### Mesonephroi

**Mesonephroi,** which are large, elongated excretory organs, appear late in the fourth week, caudal to the pronephroi (see Fig. 12-2). The mesonephroi function as interim kidneys for approximately 4 weeks, until the permanent kidneys develop and function (Fig. 12-3). The **mesonephric kidneys** consist of **glomeruli** (10–50 per

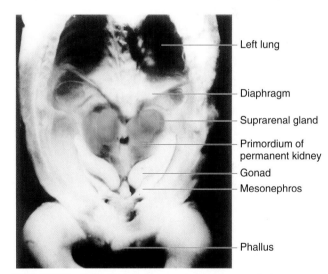

**FIGURE 12–3** Dissection of the thorax, abdomen, and pelvis of an embryo at approximately 54 days. Observe the large suprarenal glands and elongated mesonephroi (interim kidneys). Also observe the gonads (testes or ovaries) and the phallus, the primordium of the penis or clitoris, which develops from the genital tubercle (see Fig. 12-37*A* and *B*) during the indifferent stage of development. *(From Nishimura H, editor: Atlas of human prenatal histology, Tokyo, 1983, Igaku-Shoin.)*

kidney) and **mesonephric tubules** (Figs. 12-4 and 12-5, and see also Fig. 12-3). The tubules open into bilateral **mesonephric ducts,** which were originally the pronephric ducts. The mesonephric ducts open into the **cloaca** (see Fig. 12-2*B* and Chapter 11, Fig. 11-25*A*). The mesonephroi degenerate toward the end of week 12; however, the metanephric tubules become the efferent ductules of the **testes.** The mesonephric ducts have several adult derivatives in males (Table 12-1).

**FIGURE 12–4** Photomicrograph of a transverse section of an embryo at approximately 42 days, showing the mesonephros and developing suprarenal glands. *(From Moore KL, Persaud TVN, Shiota K: Color atlas of clinical embryology, ed 2, Philadelphia, 2000, Saunders.)*

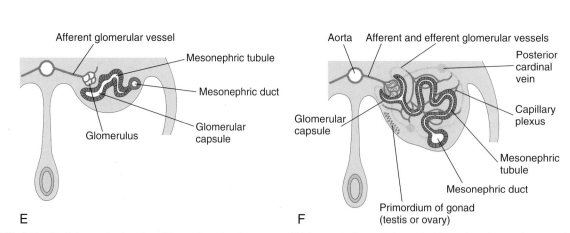

**FIGURE 12–5** Schematic drawings illustrating development of kidneys. A, Lateral view of a 5-week embryo, showing the extent of the early mesonephros and ureteric bud, the primordium of the metanephros (primordium of permanent kidney). B, Transverse section of the embryo, showing the nephrogenic cords from which the mesonephric tubules develop. C to F, Successive stages in the development of mesonephric tubules between the 5th and 11th weeks. The expanded medial end of the mesonephric tubule is invaginated by blood vessels to form a glomerular capsule.

| Table 12–1 | Derivatives and Vestigial Remnants of Embryonic Urogenital Structures* | |
|---|---|---|

| MALE | EMBRYONIC STRUCTURE | FEMALE |
|---|---|---|
| *Testis* | Indifferent gonad | *Ovary* |
| *Seminiferous tubules* | Cortex | *Ovarian follicles* |
| *Rete testis* | Medulla | *Rete ovarii* |
| Gubernaculum testis | Gubernaculum | *Ovarian ligament*<br>*Round ligament of uterus* |
| *Efferent ductules of testis* | Mesonephric tubules | Epoophoron |
| Paradidymis | | Paroophoron |
| Appendix of epididymis | Mesonephric duct | Appendix vesiculosa |
| *Duct of epididymis* | | Duct of epoophoron |
| *Ductus deferens* | | Longitudinal duct (Gartner duct) |
| *Ejaculatory duct and seminal gland* | | |
| *Ureter, pelvis, calices, and collecting tubules* | Stalk of ureteric bud | *Ureter, pelvis, calices, and collecting tubules* |
| Appendix of testis | Paramesonephric duct | Hydatid (of Morgagni) |
| | | *Uterine tube* |
| | | *Uterus* |
| *Urinary bladder* | Urogenital sinus | *Urinary bladder* |
| *Urethra (except navicular fossa)* | | *Urethra* |
| Prostatic utricle | | *Vagina* |
| *Prostate* | | *Urethral and paraurethral glands* |
| *Bulbourethral glands* | | *Greater vestibular glands* |
| Seminal colliculus | Sinus tubercle | Hymen |
| *Penis* | Primordial phallus | *Clitoris* |
| *Glans penis* | | *Glans clitoris* |
| *Corpora cavernosa of penis* | | *Corpora cavernosa of clitoris* |
| *Corpus spongiosum of penis* | | *Bulb of vestibule* |
| *Ventral aspect of penis* | Urogenital folds | *Labia minora* |
| *Scrotum* | Labioscrotal swellings | *Labia majora* |

*Functional derivatives are in italics.

## Metanephroi

**Metanephroi, or the primordia of the permanent kidneys,** begin to develop in the fifth week (Fig. 12-6) and become functional approximately 4 weeks later. Urine formation continues throughout fetal life; the urine is excreted into the amniotic cavity and forms a component of the amniotic fluid. The kidneys develop from two sources (see Fig. 12-6):

● The **ureteric bud** (metanephric diverticulum)
● The **metanephrogenic blastema** (metanephric mass of mesenchyme)

The **ureteric bud** is a diverticulum (outgrowth) from the **mesonephric duct** near its entrance into the cloaca (see Fig. 12-6A and B). The **metanephrogenic blastema** is derived from the caudal part of the **nephrogenic cord**. As

the ureteric bud elongates, it penetrates the **blastema,** a metanephric mass of mesenchyme.

The *stalk of the ureteric bud* becomes the **ureter** (see Fig. 12-6B). The cranial part of the bud undergoes repetitive branching, resulting in the bud differentiating into the **collecting tubules** (Fig. 12-7A and B, and see also Fig. 12-6E). The first four generations of tubules enlarge and become confluent to form the **major calices** (see Fig. 12-6C and D). The second four generations coalesce to form the **minor calices**. The end of each arched collecting tubule induces clusters of mesenchymal cells in the metanephrogenic blastema to form small **metanephric vesicles** (see Fig. 12-7A and B). These vesicles elongate and become **metanephric tubules** (see Fig. 12-7B and C).

As branching occurs, some of the metanephric mesenchyme cells condense and form **cap mesenchyme cells;**

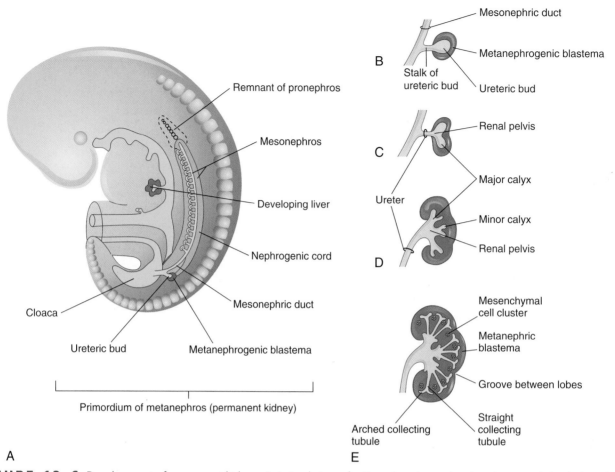

**FIGURE 12–6** Development of permanent kidney. A, Lateral view of a 5-week embryo, showing the ureteric bud, the primordium of the metanephros. B to E, Successive stages in the development of the ureteric bud (fifth to eighth weeks). Observe the development of the kidney: ureter, renal pelvis, calices, and collecting tubules.

these undergo mesenchymal-to-epithelial transition and further develop into the majority of the nephron's epithelium. The proximal ends of the tubules are invaginated by **glomeruli**. The tubules differentiate into proximal and distal convoluted tubules; the **nephron loop (Henle loop)**, together with the **glomerulus** and the **glomerular capsule**, constitute a **nephron** (see Fig. 12-7D).

*Proliferation of the nephron progenitor cells and formation of the nephrons are dependent on BMP7 and Wnt-4 (Notch)/β-catenin signaling.* Each distal convoluted tubule contacts an arched collecting tubule, and the tubules become confluent. A **uriniferous tubule** consists of two embryologically different parts (see Figs. 12-6 and 12-7):

● A **nephron** derived from the metanephrogenic blastema
● A **collecting tubule** derived from the ureteric bud

Between the 10th and 18th weeks, the number of **glomeruli** increases gradually and then increases rapidly until the 36th week, when an upper limit is reached. Nephron formation is complete at birth, with each kidney containing as many as 2 million nephrons, although this number can vary by a factor of 10. The nephrons must last forever because no new nephrons are formed after

this time and limited numbers may result in significant consequences for health in the child and adult.

The **fetal kidneys are subdivided into lobes** (Fig. 12-8). The lobulation usually disappears at the end of the first year of infancy as the nephrons increase and grow. The increase in kidney size after birth results mainly from elongation of the proximal convoluted tubules as well as an increase of interstitial tissue (see Fig. 12-7D). Nephron formation is complete at birth except in premature infants. Although glomerular filtration begins at approximately the ninth fetal week, *functional maturation of the kidneys and increasing rates of filtration occur after birth.*

Branching of the ureteric bud is dependent on induction by the metanephric mesenchyme. Differentiation of the nephrons depends on induction by the collecting tubules. The **ureteric bud** and the **metanephrogenic blastema** interact and induce each other, a process known as **reciprocal induction**, to form the permanent kidneys.

*Molecular studies*, especially knockout and transgenic analyses in the mouse, show that this process involves two principal signaling systems that use conserved molecular pathways. Recent research has provided insight into the complex interrelated molecular events regulating the development of the kidneys (Fig. 12-9). Before induction, a transcription factor, WT1, is expressed in the

Capsule of kidney
Metanephrogenic blastema
Mesenchymal cell cluster
Arched collecting tubule
Metanephric vesicle
Straight collecting tubule

A

Metanephric vesicle
Arched collecting tubule
Site of contact of tubules
Metanephric tubule
Mesenchyme

B

Site of contact
S-shaped metanephric tubule
Site of continuity of tubules
Branch of renal artery
Nephron loop

C

Straight collecting tubule
Distal convoluted tubule
Proximal convoluted tubule
Glomerulus
Glomerular capsule
Descending and ascending limbs of nephron loop

D

**FIGURE 12–7** Development of nephrons. **A,** Nephrogenesis commences around the beginning of the eighth week. **B** and **C,** Note that the metanephric tubules, the primordia of the nephrons, connect with the collecting tubules to form uriniferous tubules. **D,** Observe that nephrons are derived from the metanephrogenic blastema and the collecting tubules are derived from the ureteric bud.

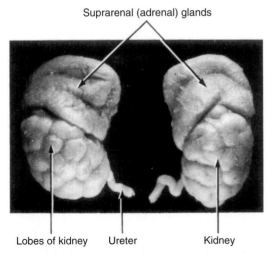

Suprarenal (adrenal) glands

Lobes of kidney   Ureter   Kidney

**FIGURE 12–8** Kidneys and suprarenal glands of a 28-week fetus (×2). The kidneys are subdivided into lobes; this lobulation usually disappears at the end of the first postnatal year. Note that the suprarenal glands are large compared with the kidneys; they will rapidly become smaller during the first year of infancy (see Fig. 12-27).

metanephrogenic blastema supporting the survival of the as yet uninduced mesenchyme. Expression of Pax2, Eya1, and Sall1 is required for the expression of glial-derived neurotropic factor (GDNF) in the metanephric mesenchyme. The transcription factors vHNF1 (HNF1β) and GDNF play an essential role in the induction and branching of the ureteric bud (**branching morphogenesis**). The receptor for GDNF, c-ret, is first expressed in the mesonephric duct but later becomes localized on the tip of the ureteric bud. Subsequent branching is controlled by transcription factors, including Emx2 and Pax2, and growth factor signals of the Wnt, FGF, and BMP families. Transformation of the metanephric mesenchyme to the epithelial cells of the nephron, **mesenchymal–epithelial transition**, is regulated by mesenchyme factors, including Wnt4. Recent studies reveal that mutation of the angiotensin–type 2 receptor gene might account for kidney and urinary tract abnormalities.

## Positional Changes of Kidneys

Initially, the primordial permanent kidneys lie close to each other in the pelvis, ventral to the sacrum (Fig. 12-10A). As the abdomen and pelvis grow, the kidneys

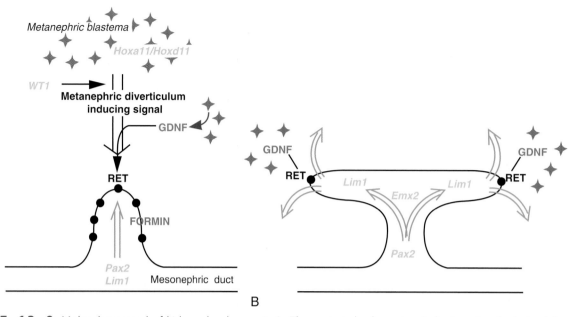

**FIGURE 12–9** Molecular control of kidney development. **A,** The ureteric bud requires inductive signals derived from meta-nephrogenic blastema under control of transcription factors *(yellow text)*, such as WT1 and signaling molecules *(red text)*, including glial-derived neurotropic factor *(GDNF)* and its epithelial receptor, RET. The normal ureteric bud response to these inductive signals is under the control of transcription factors such as Pax2, Lim1, and the *FORMIN* gene. **B,** Branching of the ureteric bud is initiated and maintained by interaction with the mesenchyme under the regulation of genes such as *Emx2* and specified expression of GDNF and RET at the tips of the invading ureteric bud. *(From Piscione TD, Rosenblum ND: The malformed kidney: disruption of glomerular and tubular development, Clin Genet 56:341, 1999.)*

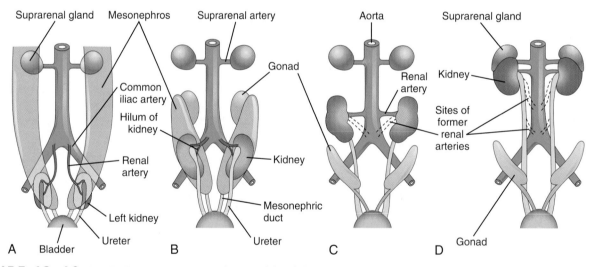

**FIGURE 12–10** A to D, Diagrammatic ventral views of the abdominopelvic region of embryos and fetuses (sixth to ninth weeks), showing medial rotation and relocation of the kidneys from the pelvis to the abdomen. C and D, Note that as the kidneys relocate (ascend), they are supplied by arteries at successively higher levels and that the hila of the kidneys, where the nerves and vessels enter, are directed anteromedially.

gradually relocate to the abdomen and move farther apart (see Fig. 12-10*B* and *C*). The kidneys attain their adult position during the beginning of the fetal period (see Fig. 12-10*D*). This "ascent" results mainly from growth of the embryo's body caudal to the kidneys. In effect, the caudal part of the embryo grows away from the kidneys, so that they progressively occupy their normal position on either side of the vertebral column.

Initially the **hilum** of each kidney (depression on the medial border), where the blood vessels, ureter, and nerves enter and leave, faces ventrally; however, as the kidneys relocate, the hilum rotates medially almost 90 degrees. By the ninth week, the hila are directed antero-medially (see Fig. 12-10*C* and *D*). Eventually, the kidneys become retroperitoneal structures (external to the perito-neum) on the posterior abdominal wall. By this time, the kidneys are in contact with the suprarenal glands (see Fig. 12-10*D*).

## Changes in Blood Supply of Kidneys

During the changes in the kidneys' positions, the kidneys receive their blood supply from vessels that are close to them. Initially, the **renal arteries** are branches of the **common iliac arteries** (see Fig. 12-10*A* and *B*). Later, the kidneys receive their blood supply from the distal end of the **abdominal aorta** (see Fig. 12-10*B*). When the kidneys are located at a higher level, they receive new branches from the aorta (see Fig. 12-10*C* and *D*). Normally, the caudal branches of the renal vessels undergo involution and disappear.

The positions of the kidneys become fixed once the kidneys come into contact with the suprarenal glands in the ninth week. The kidneys receive their most cranial arterial branches from the **abdominal aorta**; these branches become the permanent **renal arteries**. The right renal artery is longer and often in a more superior position than the left renal artery.

*Text continued on p. 255*

## ACCESSORY RENAL ARTERIES

The common variations in the blood supply to the kidneys reflect the manner in which the blood supply continually changes during embryonic and early fetal life (see Fig. 12-10). Approximately 25% of adult kidneys have two to four renal arteries. **Accessory (supernumerary) renal arteries** usually arise from the aorta superior or inferior to the main renal artery and follow it to the hilum of the kidney (Fig. 12-11*A, C,* and *D*). Accessory arteries may also enter the kidneys directly, usually via the superior or inferior pole (see Fig. 12-11*B*). An accessory artery to the inferior pole (polar renal artery) may cross anterior to the ureter and obstruct it, causing **hydronephrosis**, or distention of the renal pelvis and calices with urine. If the artery enters the inferior pole of the right kidney, it usually crosses anterior to the inferior vena cava and ureter.

**Accessory renal arteries** are end arteries; consequently, if an accessory artery is damaged or ligated, the part of the kidney supplied by it will be ischemic. Accessory arteries are approximately twice as common as accessory veins.

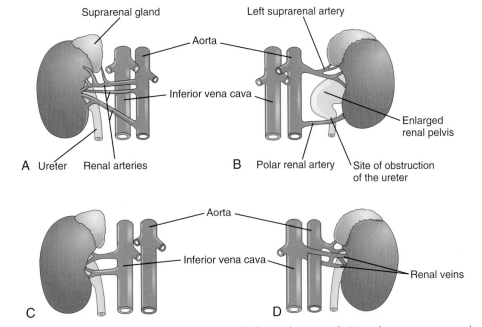

**FIGURE 12–11** Common variations of renal vessels. **A,** Multiple renal arteries. **B,** Note the accessory vessel entering the inferior pole of the kidney and that it is obstructing the ureter and producing an enlarged renal pelvis. **C** and **D,** Supernumerary renal veins.

## CONGENITAL ANOMALIES OF KIDNEYS AND URETERS

Some type of defect of the kidneys and ureters occurs in 3% to 4% of neonates. Defects in shape and position are most common. Many fetal urinary tract defects can be detected before birth by ultrasonography.

### Renal Agenesis

Unilateral renal agenesis (absence) occurs approximately once in every 1000 neonates. Males are affected more often than females, and the left kidney is usually the one that is absent (Figs. 12-12A and B and 12-13A). Unilateral renal agenesis often causes no symptoms and is usually not discovered during infancy because the other kidney usually undergoes compensatory hypertrophy and performs the function of the missing kidney. Unilateral renal agenesis should be suspected in infants with a *single umbilical artery* (see Chapter 7, Fig. 7-18).

Bilateral renal agenesis (see Fig. 12-12C) is associated with oligohydramnios, a condition that develops because little or no urine is excreted into the amniotic cavity. This condition occurs approximately once in 3000 births and is incompatible with postnatal life. About 20% of cases of Potter syndrome are caused by bilateral renal agenesis. These infants have a characteristic facial appearance: the eyes are widely separated and have palpebronasal folds (epicanthic folds), the ears are low set, the nose is broad and flat, the chin is receding, and there are limb and respiratory anomalies. Infants with bilateral renal agenesis usually die shortly after birth from pulmonary hypoplasia leading to respiratory insufficiency.

Renal agenesis results when the ureteric buds do not develop or the primordia (stalks of buds) of the ureters degenerate. Failure of the buds to penetrate the metanephrogenic blastema results in failure of kidney development because no nephrons are induced by the collecting tubules to develop from the blastema. Renal agenesis probably has a multifactorial cause. There is clinical evidence that complete in utero involution of polycystic kidneys (many cysts) could lead to renal agenesis, with a ureter with a blind ending on the same side.

### Malrotated Kidney

If a kidney fails to rotate, the hilum faces anteriorly, that is, the fetal kidney retains its embryonic position (see Figs. 12-10A and 12-13C). If the hilum faces posteriorly, rotation of the kidney proceeded too far; if it faces laterally, lateral instead of medial rotation occurred. Abnormal rotation of the kidneys (malrotation) is often associated with ectopic kidneys.

### Ectopic Kidneys

One or both kidneys may be in an abnormal position (see Fig. 12-13B, E, and F). Most ectopic kidneys are located in the pelvis (Fig. 12-14), but some lie in the inferior part of the abdomen. Pelvic kidneys and other forms of ectopia result from failure of the kidneys to ascend. Pelvic kidneys are close to each other and usually fuse to form a discoid (pancake) kidney (see Fig. 12-13E). Ectopic kidneys receive their blood supply from blood vessels near them (internal or external iliac arteries and/or abdominal aorta). They are often supplied by several vessels. Sometimes a kidney crosses to the other side, resulting in crossed renal ectopia, and 90% of these kidneys are fused (Fig. 12-15). An unusual type of abnormal kidney is unilateral fused kidney. In such cases, the developing kidneys fuse after they leave the pelvis, and one kidney attains its normal position, carrying the other kidney with it (see Fig. 12-13D).

### Horseshoe Kidney

In 0.2% of the population, the poles of the kidneys are fused; usually it is the inferior poles that fuse. The large U-shaped kidney usually lies in the pubic region, anterior to the inferior lumbar vertebrae (Fig. 12-16A). Normal ascent of the fused kidneys is prevented because they are held down by the root of the inferior mesenteric artery (see Fig. 12-16B).

A *horseshoe kidney usually produces no symptoms* because its collecting system develops normally and the ureters enter the bladder. If urinary flow is impeded, signs and symptoms of obstruction and/or infection may appear. Approximately 7% of persons with Turner syndrome have horseshoe kidneys (see Figs. 20-3 and 20-4).

### Duplications of Urinary Tract

Duplications of the abdominal part of the ureter and renal pelvis are common (see Fig. 12-13F). These defects result from abnormal division of the ureteric bud. Incomplete division results in a divided kidney with a bifid ureter (see Fig. 12-13B). Complete division results in a double kidney with a bifid ureter (see Fig. 12-13C) or separate ureters (Fig. 12-17). A supernumerary kidney with its own ureter, which is rare, probably results from the formation of two ureteric buds (see Fig. 12-13F).

### Ectopic Ureter

An ectopic ureter does not enter the urinary bladder. In males, the ureter will open into the *neck of the bladder* or the *prostatic part of the urethra*. The ureter may also enter the *ductus deferens, prostatic utricle,* or *seminal gland*. In females, the ectopic ureter may also open into the neck of the bladder or the *urethra, vagina,* or *vestibule (cavity) of the vagina* (Fig. 12-18). Incontinence is the common complaint resulting from an ectopic ureter because urine flowing from the orifice of the ureter does not enter the bladder; instead it continually dribbles from the urethra in males and the urethra and/or vagina in females.

An ectopic ureter results when the ureter is not incorporated into the trigone between the openings of the ureters

## CONGENITAL ANOMALIES OF KIDNEYS AND URETERS—cont'd

in the posterior part of the urinary bladder. Instead it is carried caudally with the mesonephric duct and is incorporated into the middle pelvic portion of the vesical part of the urogenital sinus. Because this part of the sinus becomes the prostatic urethra in males and urethra in females, the location of ectopic ureteric orifices is understandable. When two ureters form on one side (see Fig. 12-17), they usually open into the urinary bladder (see Fig. 12-13F).

### Cystic Kidney Diseases

In **autosomal recessive polycystic kidney disease** (1 in 20,000 live births), diagnosed at birth or in utero by ultrasonography, both kidneys contain many small cysts (Fig. 12-19A), which result in **renal insufficiency**. Death of the infant may occur shortly after birth, with 25% of cases associated with pulmonary hypoplasia; however, more than 80%

of these infants are surviving beyond 1 year because of postnatal dialysis and kidney transplantation. Most cases have a mutation of the *PKHD1* gene that results in polycystic kidney and congenital hepatic fibrosis.

**Multicystic dysplastic kidney disease** results from dysmorphology, abnormal development of the renal system (see Fig. 12-19B). The outcome for most children with this disease is generally good because the disease is unilateral in 75% of the cases. In this kidney disease, fewer cysts are seen than in autosomal recessive polycystic kidney disease, and they range in size from a few millimeters to many centimeters in the same kidney. It was thought that the cysts were the result of failure of the ureteric bud derivatives to join the tubules derived from the metanephrogenic blastema. It is now believed that the cystic structures are wide dilations of parts of the otherwise continuous nephrons, particularly the **nephron loops** (of Henle).

**FIGURE 12–12** Sonograms of a fetus with unilateral renal agenesis. **A,** Transverse scan at the level of the lumbar region of the vertebral column *(Sp)* showing the right kidney *(RK)* but not the left kidney. **B,** Transverse scan at a slightly higher level showing the left suprarenal gland *(between cursors)* within the left renal fossa. **C,** Dissection of a male fetus of 19.5 weeks with bilateral renal agenesis. *(A and B, From Mahony BS: Ultrasound evaluation of the fetal genitourinary system. In Callen PW, editor: Ultrasonography in obstetrics and gynecology, ed 3, Philadelphia, 1994, Saunders.)*

**FIGURE 12–13** Illustrations of various birth defects of the urinary system. The small sketch to the lower right of each drawing illustrates the probable embryologic basis of the defect. **A,** Unilateral renal agenesis. **B,** *Right side,* pelvic kidney; *left side,* divided kidney with a bifid ureter. **C,** *Right side,* malrotation of the kidney; the hilum is facing laterally. *Left side,* bifid ureter and supernumerary kidney. **D,** Crossed renal ectopia. The left kidney crossed to the right side and fused with the right kidney. **E,** Pelvic kidney (discoid kidney), resulting from fusion of the kidneys while they were in the pelvis. **F,** Supernumerary left kidney resulting from the development of two ureteric buds.

**FIGURE 12–14** Sonogram of the pelvis of a fetus at 29 weeks. Observe the low position of the right kidney *(RK)* near the urinary bladder *(BL)*. This pelvic kidney resulted from its failure to ascend during the sixth to ninth weeks. Observe the normal location of the right suprarenal gland *(AD)*, which develops separately from the kidney.

**FIGURE 12–15** Computed tomography scan showing congenital renal malformation in a 69-year-old woman. Crossed fused renal ectopia is an anomaly in which the kidneys are fused and located on the same side of the midline. *(From Di Muzzio B: Crossed fused renal ectopia. Radiopaedia.org. Accessed October 8, 2014.)*

**FIGURE 12–16** A, Horseshoe kidney in the lower abdomen of a 13-week female fetus. B, Contrast-enhanced computed tomography scan of the abdomen of an infant with a horseshoe kidney. Note the isthmus (vascular) of renal tissue *(thick vertical line)* connecting the right and left kidneys just anterior to the aorta *(arrow)* and inferior vena cava.

**FIGURE 12–17** A duplex kidney with two ureters and renal pelves. **A,** Longitudinal section through the kidney showing two renal pelves and calices. **B,** Anterior surface of the kidney. **C,** Intravenous urography showing duplication of the right kidney and ureter in a 10-year-old male. The distal ends of the right ureter are fused at the level of the first sacral vertebra.

**FIGURE 12–18** Ectopic ureter in a young girl. The ureter enters the vestibule of the vagina near the external urethral orifice. A thin ureteral catheter *(arrow)* with transverse marks has been introduced through the ureteric orifice into the ectopic ureter. This girl had a normal voiding pattern and constant urinary dribbling. *(From Behrman RE, Kliegman RM, Arvin AM, editors: Nelson textbook of pediatrics, ed 15, Philadelphia, 1996, Saunders.)*

**FIGURE 12–19** Cystic kidney disease. **A,** Computed tomography scan (with contrast enhancement) of the abdomen of a 5-month-old male infant with autosomal recessive polycystic kidney disease. Note the linear ectasia (cysts) of collecting tubules. **B,** Ultrasound scan of the left kidney of a 15-day-old male infant showing multiple noncommunicating cysts with no renal tissue (unilateral multicystic dysplastic kidney).

## Development of Urinary Bladder

For descriptive purposes, the **urogenital sinus** is divided into three parts (see Fig. 12-20C):

- A **vesical part** that forms most of the urinary bladder and is continuous with the allantois
- A **pelvic part** that becomes the urethra in the neck of the bladder; the prostatic part of the urethra in males and the entire urethra in females
- A **phallic part** that grows toward the genital tubercle (primordium of the penis or clitoris; see Figs. 12-20C and 12-37)

The bladder develops mainly from the **vesical part of the urogenital sinus** (see Fig. 12-20C). The entire epithelium of the bladder is derived from the endoderm of the vesical part of the **urogenital sinus,** or ventral part of the cloaca (see Fig. 12-20C). The other layers of its wall develop from the adjacent splanchnic mesenchyme.

Initially, the bladder is continuous with the **allantois,** a fetal membrane developed from the hindgut (see Fig. 12-20C). The allantois soon constricts and becomes a thick fibrous cord, the **urachus.** It extends from the apex of the bladder to the umbilicus (Fig. 12-21, and see also Fig. 12-20G and H). In adults, the urachus is represented by the **median umbilical ligament.**

As the bladder enlarges, distal parts of the **mesonephric ducts** are incorporated into its dorsal wall (see Fig. 12-20B to H). These ducts contribute to the formation of the connective tissue in the **trigone of the bladder.** As these ducts are absorbed, the ureters open separately into the urinary bladder (see Fig. 12-20C to H). Partly because of traction exerted by the kidneys as they ascend, the orifices of the ureters move superolaterally and enter obliquely through the base of the bladder (see Fig. 12-20F). In males, the orifices of the ducts move close together and enter the prostatic part of the urethra as the caudal ends of the ducts develop into the **ejaculatory**

ducts (see Fig. 12-33A). In females, the distal ends of the mesonephric ducts degenerate (see Fig. 12-33B).

In infants and children, the urinary bladder, even when empty, is in the abdomen. It begins to enter the greater pelvis at approximately 6 years of age; however, the bladder does not enter the lesser pelvis and become a pelvic organ until after puberty. The **apex of the bladder** in adults is continuous with the **median umbilical ligament,** which extends posteriorly along the posterior surface of the anterior abdominal wall.

### CONGENITAL MEGACYSTIS

A pathologically large urinary bladder, **megacystis (megalocystis),** may result from a congenital disorder of the ureteric bud, which may be associated with dilation of the renal pelvis. The large bladder may also result from posterior urethral valves (Fig. 12-23). Many infants with megacystitis suffer from renal failure in early childhood.

### EXSTROPHY OF BLADDER

Exstrophy of the bladder, a very rare birth defect, occurs approximately once in every 10,000 to 40,000 births. **Exstrophy (eversion) of the bladder** usually occurs in males (Fig. 12-24). Exposure and protrusion of the mucosal surface of the posterior wall of the bladder characterize this defect. The trigone of the bladder and ureteric orifices are exposed, and urine dribbles intermittently from the everted bladder.

**Exstrophy of the bladder,** a deficiency of the anterior abdominal wall, is caused by incomplete median closure of the inferior part of the wall (Fig. 12-25). The defect involves both the abdominal wall and the anterior wall of the urinary bladder. The defect results from failure of mesoderm to migrate between the ectoderm and endoderm of the abdominal wall (see Fig. 12-25B and C). As a result, the inferior parts of the rectus muscles are absent and the external and internal oblique and transversus abdominis muscles are deficient.

No muscle or connective tissue forms in the anterior abdominal wall over the urinary bladder. **Rupture of the cloacal membrane** results in wide communication between the exterior and the mucous membrane of the bladder. Rupture of the membrane before rupture of the cloacal membrane produces **exstrophy of the cloaca,** resulting in exposure of the posterior wall of the bladder (Fig. 12-25F).

### URACHAL BIRTH DEFECTS

In infants, a remnant of the urachal lumen may persist in the inferior part of the urachus. In approximately 50% of cases, the lumen is continuous with the cavity of the bladder. Remnants of the epithelial lining of the urachus may give rise to **urachal cysts** (Fig. 12-22A), which are not usually detected except during a postmortem examination, unless the cysts become infected and enlarged. The patent inferior end of the urachus may dilate to form a **urachal sinus** that opens into the bladder. The lumen in the superior part of the urachus may also remain patent and form a **urachal sinus** that opens at the umbilicus (see Fig. 12-22B). Very rarely, the entire urachus remains patent and forms a **urachal fistula** that allows urine to escape from its umbilical orifice (see Fig. 12-22C).

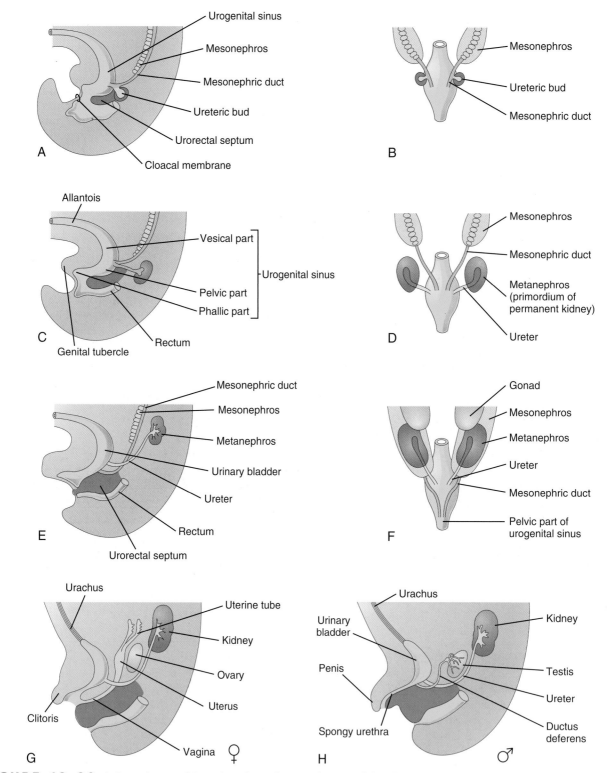

**FIGURE 12-20** A, Lateral view of 5-week embryo showing division of the cloaca by the urorectal septum into the urogenital sinus and rectum. B, D, and F, Dorsal views showing the development of the kidneys and bladder and changes in the location of the kidneys. C, E, G, and H, Lateral views. The stages shown in G and H are reached by the 12th week.

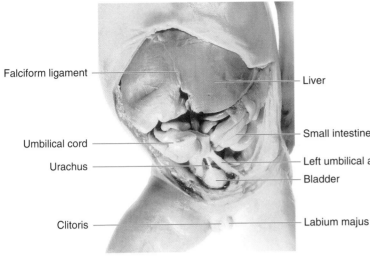

Falciform ligament

Umbilical cord

Urachus

Clitoris

Liver

Small intestine

Left umbilical artery

Bladder

Labium majus

**FIGURE 12–21** Dissection of the abdomen and pelvis of an 18-week female fetus showing the relation of the urachus to the urinary bladder and umbilical arteries.

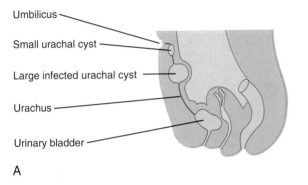

Umbilicus

Small urachal cyst

Large infected urachal cyst

Urachus

Urinary bladder

A

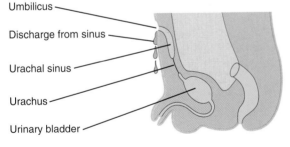

Umbilicus

Discharge from sinus

Urachal sinus

Urachus

Urinary bladder

B

**FIGURE 12–23** Sonogram of an 18-week male fetus with megacystis (enlarged bladder) caused by posterior urethral valves. The *cross* is placed on the fourth intercostal space, the level to which the diaphragm has been elevated by this very large fetal bladder (*arrow*; black = urine). In this case, the fetus survived because of the placement of a pigtail catheter within the fetal bladder, allowing drainage of urine into the amniotic cavity.

Urine dribbling from urachal fistula

Urachal fistula

Urinary bladder

Urethra

C

**FIGURE 12–22** Urachal anomalies. **A,** Urachal cysts; the common site for them is in the superior end of the urachus, just inferior to the umbilicus. **B,** Two types of urachal sinus are shown: one opens into the bladder and the other opens at the umbilicus. **C,** A urachal fistula connects the bladder and umbilicus.

Exstrophy of bladder

Hemipenis

Hemiscrotum

**FIGURE 12–24** Exstrophy (eversion) of bladder and bifid penis in a male neonate. The red bladder mucosa is visible and the halves of the penis and scrotum are widely separated.

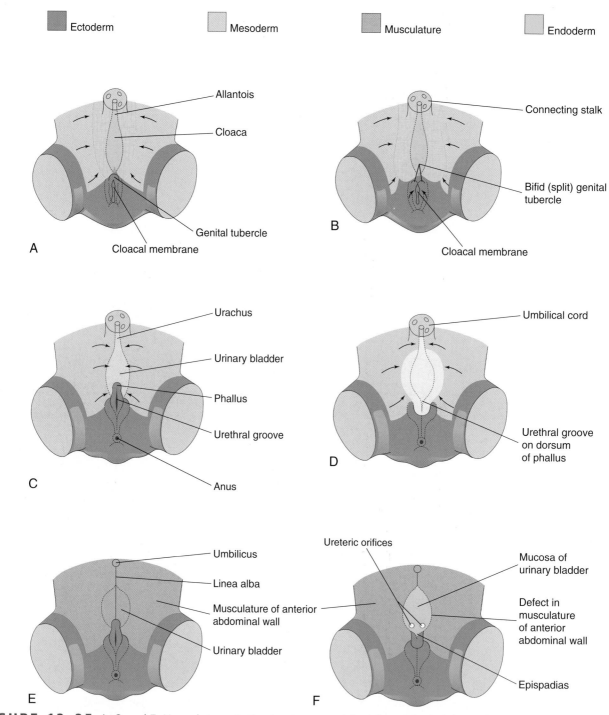

**FIGURE 12–25** A, C, and E, Normal stages in the development of the infraumbilical abdominal wall and the penis during the fourth to eighth weeks. B, D, and F, Probable stages in the development of epispadias and exstrophy of the bladder. B and D, Note that the mesoderm fails to extend into the anterior abdominal wall anterior to the urinary bladder. Also note that the genital tubercle is located in a more caudal position than usual, and the urethral groove has formed on the dorsal surface of the penis. F, The surface ectoderm and anterior wall of the bladder have ruptured, resulting in exposure of the posterior wall of the bladder. Note that the musculature of the anterior abdominal wall is present on each side of the defect. (*Based on Patten BM, Barry A: The genesis of exstrophy of the bladder and epispadias, Am J Anat 90:35, 1952.*)

## Development of Urethra

The epithelium of most of the male urethra and the entire female urethra is derived from endoderm of the **urogenital sinus** (see Figs. 12-20E and H and 12-26). The distal part of the urethra in the **glans penis** is derived from a solid cord of ectodermal cells, which grows inward from the tip of the glans penis and joins the rest of the spongy urethra (Fig. 12-26A to C). Consequently, the epithelium of the terminal part of the urethra is derived from surface ectoderm. The connective tissue and smooth muscle of

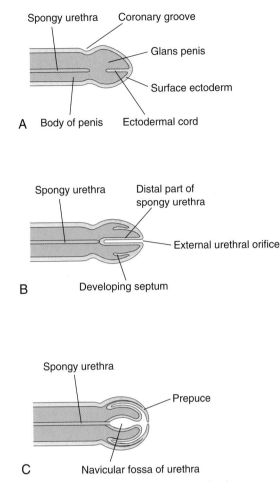

**FIGURE 12–26** Schematic longitudinal sections of the developing penis illustrating development of the prepuce (foreskin) and the distal part of the spongy urethra. **A,** At 11 weeks. **B,** At 12 weeks. **C,** At 14 weeks. The epithelium of the spongy urethra has a dual origin; most of it is derived from endoderm of the phallic part of the urogenital sinus; the distal part of the urethra lining the navicular fossa is derived from surface ectoderm.

the urethra in both sexes are derived from splanchnic mesenchyme.

# DEVELOPMENT OF SUPRARENAL GLANDS

The cortex and medulla of the **suprarenal glands** (adrenal glands) have different origins (Fig. 12-27). The **cortex** develops from mesenchyme and the **medulla** develops from neural crest cells. During the sixth week, the cortex begins as an aggregation of mesenchymal cells on each side of the embryo between the root of the dorsal mesentery and the developing gonad (see Fig. 12-29C). The cells that form the medulla are derived from an adjacent sympathetic ganglion, which is derived from **neural crest cells.**

Initially, the neural crest cells form a mass on the medial side of the embryonic cortex (see Fig. 12-27B). As they are surrounded by the cortex, the cells differentiate into the secretory cells of the suprarenal medulla. Later, more mesenchymal cells arise from the mesothelium (a single layer of flattened cells) and enclose the cortex. These cells give rise to the permanent cortex of the suprarenal gland (see Fig. 12-27C).

Immunohistochemical studies identify a "transitional zone" that is located between the permanent cortex and fetal cortex. It has been suggested that the **zona fasciculata** is derived from this third layer. The **zona glomerulosa** and zona fasciculata are present at birth, but the **zona reticularis** is not recognizable until the end of the third year (see Fig. 12-27H).

Relative to body weight, the **suprarenal glands** of the fetus are 10 to 20 times larger than in the adult glands and are large compared with the kidneys (see Figs. 12-3 and 12-8). These large glands result from the extensive size of the fetal cortex, which produces **steroid precursors** that are used by the placenta for the **synthesis of estrogen.** The suprarenal medulla remains relatively small until after birth.

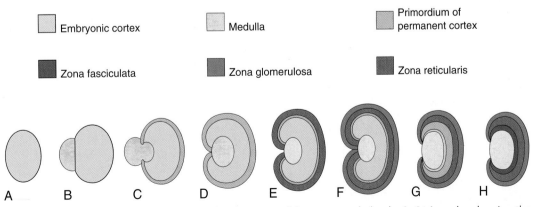

**FIGURE 12–27** Schematic drawings illustrating development of the suprarenal glands. **A,** At 6 weeks, showing the mesodermal primordium of the embryonic cortex. **B,** At 7 weeks, showing the addition of neural crest cells. **C,** At 8 weeks, showing the fetal cortex and early permanent cortex beginning to encapsulate the medulla. **D and E,** Later stages of encapsulation of the medulla by the cortex. **F,** Gland of a neonate showing the fetal cortex and two zones of the permanent cortex. **G,** At 1 year, the cortex has almost disappeared. **H,** At 4 years, showing the adult pattern of cortical zones. Note that the cortex has disappeared and the gland is much smaller than it was at birth (**F**).

The suprarenal glands rapidly become smaller as the fetal cortex regresses during the first year of infancy (see Fig. 12-27H). The glands lose approximately one third of their weight during the 2 to 3 weeks of the neonatal period, and they do not regain their original weight until the end of the second year.

## CONGENITAL ADRENAL HYPERPLASIA AND ADRENOGENITAL SYNDROME

An abnormal increase in the cells of the suprarenal cortex results in **excessive androgen production** during the fetal period. In females, this usually causes masculinization of the external genitalia (Fig. 12-28). Affected male infants have normal external genitalia, and the syndrome may go undetected in early infancy. Later in childhood in both sexes, androgen excess leads to rapid growth and accelerated skeletal maturation.

The **adrenogenital syndrome**, associated with **congenital adrenal hyperplasia (CAH)**, manifests itself in various forms that can be correlated with enzymatic deficiencies of **cortisol biosynthesis**. CAH actually describes a group of **autosomal recessive disorders** that result in **virilization** (formation of masculine characteristics) of female fetuses. CAH is caused by a genetically determined mutation in the cytochrome P450c21–steroid 21–hydroxylase gene, which results in a deficiency of suprarenal cortical enzymes that are necessary for the biosynthesis of various steroid hormones. The reduced hormone output results in an increased release of **adrenocorticotropin** from the anterior pituitary gland, which causes CAH and overproduction of androgens. *Mutations of DAX1 result in X-linked adrenal hypoplasia congenita.*

**FIGURE 12–28** External genitalia of a 6-year-old girl showing an enlarged clitoris and fused labia majora that have formed a scrotum-like structure. The *arrow* indicates the opening into the urogenital sinus. This extreme masculinization is the result of congenital adrenal hyperplasia.

# DEVELOPMENT OF GENITAL SYSTEM

The chromosomal sex of an embryo is determined at fertilization by the kind of sperm (X or Y) that fertilizes the oocyte. Male and female morphologic characteristics do not begin to develop until the seventh week. The early genital systems in the two sexes are similar; therefore, the initial period of genital development is an *indifferent stage of sexual development.*

## Development of Gonads

The **gonads (testes or ovaries)** are the organs that produce sex cells (sperms or oocytes). The gonads are derived from three sources (Fig. 12-29):

- **Mesothelium** (mesodermal epithelium) lining the posterior abdominal wall
- **Underlying mesenchyme** (embryonic connective tissue)
- **Primordial germ cells** (earliest undifferentiated sex cells)

### Indifferent Gonads

The initial stages of gonadal development occur during the fifth week, when a thickened area of mesothelium develops on the medial side of the **mesonephros**, the primordium of a permanent kidney (see Fig. 12-29A). Proliferation of this epithelium and underlying mesenchyme produces a bulge on the medial side of the mesonephros, the **gonadal ridge** (Fig. 12-30). Finger-like epithelial cords, **gonadal cords**, soon grow into the underlying mesenchyme (see Fig. 12-29D). The **indifferent gonads** (primordial organs before differentiation) now consist of an external cortex and an internal medulla.

In embryos with an **XX sex chromosome complex**, the cortex of the indifferent gonad differentiates into an ovary, and the medulla regresses. In embryos with an **XY sex chromosome complex**, the medulla differentiates into a testis, and the cortex regresses.

### Primordial Germ Cells

**Primordial germ cells** are large, spherical sex cells that are first recognizable at 24 days after fertilization among the endodermal cells of the **umbilical vesicle** near the origin of the allantois (see Figs. 12-29A and 12-30). During folding of the embryo (see Chapter 5, Fig. 5-1), the dorsal part of the umbilical vesicle is incorporated into the embryo. As this occurs, the primordial germ cells migrate along the dorsal mesentery of the hindgut to the gonadal ridges (see Fig. 12-29C). During the sixth week, the primordial germ cells enter the underlying mesenchyme and are incorporated in the **gonadal cords** (see Fig. 12-29D). *The migration of primordial germ cells is regulated by the genes* stella, fragilis, *and* BMP-4.

### Sex Determination

Determination of chromosomal and genetic sex depends on whether an X-bearing sperm or a Y-bearing sperm fertilizes the X-bearing oocyte. Before the seventh week, the gonads of the two sexes are identical in appearance and are called **indifferent gonads** (see Figs. 12-29E and 12-30).

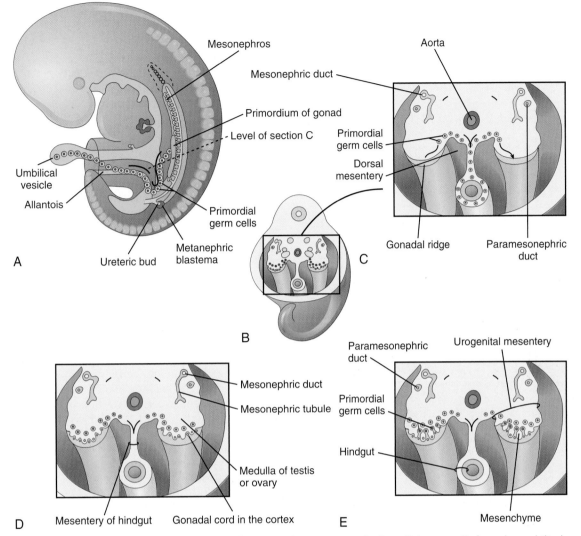

**FIGURE 12–29** A, Sketch of a 5-week embryo illustrating the migration of primordial germ cells from the umbilical vesicle into the embryo. B, Three-dimensional sketch of the caudal region of a 5-week embryo showing the location and extent of the gonadal ridges. C, Transverse section showing the primordium of the suprarenal glands, the gonadal ridges, and the migration of primordial germ cells into the developing gonads. D, Transverse section of a 6-week embryo showing the gonadal cords. E, Similar section at a later stage showing the indifferent gonads and paramesonephric ducts.

Development of a male phenotype (characteristics of an individual) requires a functional Y chromosome. The ***SRY* gene (sex-determining region on the Y chromosome)** for a testis-determining factor has been localized in the short-arm region of the Y chromosome. It is the testis-determining factor regulated by the Y chromosome that determines **testicular differentiation** (Fig. 12-31). Under the influence of this organizing factor, the **gonadal cords** differentiate into **seminiferous cords** (primordia of **seminiferous tubules**). *Sry activates testis-specific enhancers of Sox9. Two gene regulatory networks then prevent ovarian development (Wnt4, Foxl2, Fst, and Rspo1) while enhancing testicular development (Fgf9, Amh, and Dhh).* The absence of a Y chromosome results in the formation of an ovary.

**Development of the female phenotype** requires two X chromosomes. A number of genes and regions of the X chromosome have special roles in sex determination.

Consequently, the type of sex chromosome complex established during fertilization of the oocyte determines the type of gonad that differentiates from the indifferent gonad. The type of gonad then determines the type of sexual differentiation that occurs in the genital ducts and external genitalia.

**Testosterone**, produced by the fetal testes, **dihydrotestosterone** (a metabolite of testosterone), and **antimüllerian hormone (AMH)**, determine normal male sexual differentiation, which begins during the seventh week. **Ovarian development** begins about the 12th week. *Primary female sexual differentiation does not depend on hormones; it occurs even if the ovaries are absent.*

### Development of Testes

Testis-determining factor induces the **seminiferous cords** to condense and extend into the medulla of the **indifferent gonad**, where they branch and anastomose to form the

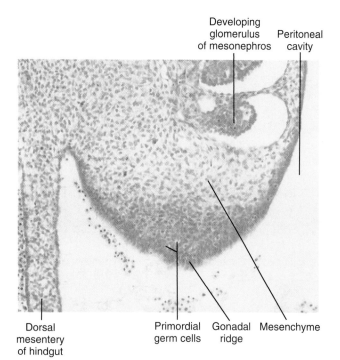

Developing glomerulus of mesonephros — Peritoneal cavity

Dorsal mesentery of hindgut — Primordial germ cells — Gonadal ridge — Mesenchyme

**FIGURE 12-30** Photomicrograph of a transverse section of the abdomen of an embryo at approximately 40 days, showing the gonadal ridge, which will develop into a testis or ovary depending on the chromosomal sex. Most of the developing gonad is composed of mesenchyme derived from the coelomic epithelium of the gonadal ridge. The large round cells in the gonad are primordial germ cells. *(From Moore KL, Persaud TVN, Shiota K: Color atlas of clinical embryology, ed 2, Philadelphia, 2000, Saunders.)*

rete testis, a network of canals (see Fig. 12-31). The connection of the **seminiferous cords** with the surface epithelium is lost when a thick fibrous capsule, the **tunica albuginea**, develops. The development of the dense tunica albuginea is the characteristic feature of testicular development. Gradually, the enlarging testis separates from the degenerating mesonephros and is suspended by its own mesentery, the **mesorchium**.

The seminiferous cords develop into the seminiferous tubules, **tubuli recti** (straight tubules), and **rete testis** (see Fig. 12-31). The **seminiferous tubules** are separated by mesenchyme that gives rise to the **interstitial cells** (Leydig cells). By the eighth week, these cells begin to secrete androgenic hormones, **testosterone** and **androstenedione**, which induce masculine differentiation of the mesonephric ducts and external genitalia.

**Testosterone production** is stimulated by **human chorionic gonadotropin**, which reaches peak amounts during the 8th-week to 12th-week period. In addition to testosterone, the fetal testes produce a glycoprotein, **AMH** or müllerian-inhibiting substance (MIS). AMH is produced by the **sustentacular cells** (Sertoli cells); production continues until puberty, after which the levels of the hormone decrease. *AMH suppresses development of the paramesonephric ducts*, which form the uterus and uterine tubes.

The seminiferous tubules have no lumina until puberty. The walls of the seminiferous tubules are composed of two types of cells (see Fig. 12-31):

- **Sertoli cells** support spermiogenesis; they are derived from the surface epithelium of the testis
- **Spermatogonia**, primordial sperm cells, are derived from primordial germ cells

Sertoli cells constitute most of the seminiferous epithelium in the fetal testis (Fig. 12-32A, and see also Fig. 12-31). During later fetal development, the surface epithelium of the testis flattens to form **mesothelium (a layer of cells)** on the external surface of the testis. The **rete testis** becomes continuous with 15 to 20 **mesonephric tubules** that become **efferent ductules**. These ductules are connected with the mesonephric duct, which becomes the **duct of the epididymis** (Fig. 12-33A, and see also Fig. 12-31).

### Development of Ovaries

Gonadal development occurs slowly in female embryos (see Fig. 12-32). The X chromosome has genes that contribute to ovarian development; an autosomal gene also appears to play a role in ovarian organogenesis. The ovary is not identifiable histologically until approximately the 10th week. **Gonadal cords** are not prominent in the developing ovary, but they extend into the medulla and form a rudimentary **rete ovarii** (see Fig. 12-31). This network of canals and the gonadal cords normally degenerate and disappear (see Fig. 12-31).

**Cortical cords** extend from the surface epithelium of the developing ovary into the underlying mesenchyme during the early fetal period. This epithelium is derived from the mesothelium of the peritoneum. As the cortical cords increase in size, **primordial germ cells** are incorporated in them (see Fig. 12-31). At approximately 16 weeks, these cords begin to break up into isolated cell clusters, or **primordial follicles**, each of which contains an **oogonium (primordial germ cell)**. The follicles are surrounded by a single layer of flattened **follicular cells** derived from the surface epithelium (see Fig. 12-31). Active mitosis of oogonia occurs during fetal life, producing primordial follicles (see Fig. 12-32B).

**No oogonia form postnatally.** Although many oogonia degenerate before birth, the 2 million or so that remain enlarge to become **primary oocytes**. After birth, the surface epithelium of the ovary flattens to a single layer of cells continuous with the mesothelium of the peritoneum at the **hilum of the ovary**, where vessels and nerves enter or leave. The surface epithelium becomes separated from the follicles in the cortex by a thin fibrous capsule, the **tunica albuginea**. As the ovary separates from the regressing mesonephros, it is suspended by a mesentery, the **mesovarium** (see Fig. 12-31).

### Development of Genital Ducts

During the fifth and sixth weeks, the genital system is in an indifferent state, and two pairs of genital ducts are present. The **mesonephric ducts** (wolffian ducts) play an important part in the development of the male reproductive system (see Fig. 12-33A). The **paramesonephric ducts**

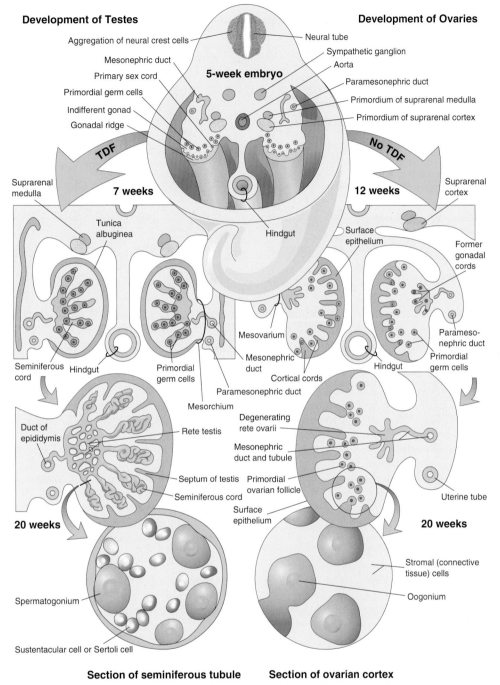

**Development of Testes**

Aggregation of neural crest cells
Mesonephric duct
Primary sex cord
Primordial germ cells
Indifferent gonad
Gonadal ridge

**5-week embryo**

Neural tube
Sympathetic ganglion
Aorta
Paramesonephric duct
Primordium of suprarenal medulla
Primordium of suprarenal cortex

**Development of Ovaries**

TDF

No TDF

**7 weeks**

Suprarenal medulla
Tunica albuginea
Seminiferous cord    Hindgut
Primordial germ cells

Hindgut

Mesovarium
Mesonephric duct
Paramesonephric duct
Mesorchium

**12 weeks**

Surface epithelium
Suprarenal cortex
Former gonadal cords
Parameso-nephric duct
Primordial germ cells
Hindgut
Cortical cords

**20 weeks**

Duct of epididymis
Rete testis
Septum of testis
Seminiferous cord

Degenerating rete ovarii
Mesonephric duct and tubule
Primordial ovarian follicle
Surface epithelium
Uterine tube

**20 weeks**

Spermatogonium
Sustentacular cell or Sertoli cell

Stromal (connective tissue) cells
Oogonium

**Section of seminiferous tubule**     **Section of ovarian cortex**

**FIGURE 12–31** Schematic illustrations showing differentiation of the indifferent gonads in a 5-week embryo *(top)* into ovaries or testes. The left side of the drawing shows the development of testes resulting from the effects of the testis-determining factor *(TDF)* located on the Y chromosome. Note that the gonadal cords become seminiferous cords, the primordia of the seminiferous tubules. The parts of the gonadal cords that enter the medulla of the testis form the rete testis. In the section of the testis at the bottom left, observe that there are two kinds of cells: spermatogonia, derived from the primordial germ cells, and sustentacular or Sertoli cells, derived from mesenchyme. The right side of the drawing shows the development of ovaries in the absence of TDF. Cortical cords have extended from the surface epithelium of the gonad and primordial germ cells have entered them. They are the primordia of the oogonia. Follicular cells are derived from the surface epithelium of the ovary.

(müllerian ducts) have a leading role in the development of the female reproductive system.

The paramesonephric ducts develop lateral to the gonads and mesonephric ducts (see Fig. 12-31) on each side from longitudinal invaginations of the mesothelium on the lateral aspects of the mesonephroi (primordial kidneys). The edges of these grooves approach each other and fuse to form the paramesonephric ducts (Fig. 12-34A, and see also Fig. 12-29C and E). The cranial ends of these ducts open into the peritoneal cavity (see Fig. 12-33B and

**FIGURE 12–32** Transverse sections of gonads of human fetuses. **A,** Section of a testis from a male fetus born prematurely at 21 weeks, showing seminiferous tubules. **B,** Section of an ovary from a 14-day-old female infant that died. Observe the numerous primordial follicles in the cortex, each of which contains a primary oocyte. The *arrow* indicates the relatively thin surface epithelium of the ovary (×275). *(From van Wagenen G, Simpson ME: Embryology of the ovary and testis:* Homo sapiens *and* Macaca mulatta, *New Haven, CT, 1965, Yale University Press. Copyright © Yale University Press.)*

C). Caudally, the paramesonephric ducts run parallel to the mesonephric ducts until they reach the future pelvic region of the embryo. Here they cross ventral to the mesonephric ducts, approach each other in the median plane, and fuse to form a Y-shaped **uterovaginal primordium** (see Fig. 12-34B). This tubular structure projects into the dorsal wall of the urogenital sinus and produces an elevation, the **sinus tubercle.**

## Development of Male Genital Ducts and Glands

The fetal testes produce **masculinizing hormones** (e.g., testosterone) and **MIS.** The Sertoli cells produce MIS at 6 to 7 weeks. The interstitial cells begin producing testosterone in the eighth week. *Testosterone stimulates the mesonephric ducts to form male genital ducts,* whereas AMH causes the paramesonephric ducts to regress. Under the influence of testosterone produced by the fetal testes in the eighth week, the proximal part of each mesonephric duct becomes highly convoluted to form the **epididymis** (see Fig. 12-33A). As the mesonephros degenerates, some mesonephric tubules persist and are transformed into **efferent ductules.** These ductules open into the **duct of the epididymis.** Distal to the epididymis, the mesonephric duct acquires a thick investment of smooth muscle and becomes the **ductus deferens** (see Fig. 12-33A).

### Seminal Glands

Lateral outgrowths from the caudal end of each mesonephric duct become **seminal glands** (vesicles), which produce a secretion that makes up the majority of the fluid in ejaculate and nourishes the sperms (see Fig. 12-33A). The part of the mesonephric duct between the duct of this gland and the urethra becomes the **ejaculatory duct.**

### Prostate

Multiple endodermal outgrowths arise from the prostatic part of the urethra and grow into the surrounding mesenchyme (Fig. 12-35A to C, and see also Fig. 12-33A). The glandular epithelium of the prostate differentiates from these endodermal cells, and the associated mesenchyme differentiates into the dense **stroma** (framework of connective tissue) and smooth muscle of the prostate. *Hox genes control the development of the prostate gland as well as the seminal glands.* Secretions from the prostate contribute to the **semen** (ejaculate).

### Bulbourethral Glands

These pea-sized glands develop from paired outgrowths derived from the spongy part of the urethra (see Fig. 12-33A). The smooth muscle fibers and stroma differentiate from the adjacent mesenchyme. The secretions of these glands also contribute to the semen.

## Development of Female Genital Ducts and Glands

The **mesonephric ducts** of female embryos regress because of the absence of testosterone; only a few nonfunctional remnants persist (see Fig. 12-33B and C and Table 12-1). The **paramesonephric ducts** develop because of the absence of MIS. *Female sexual development during the fetal period does not depend on the presence of ovaries or hormones.* Later, **estrogens** produced by the maternal ovaries and the placenta stimulate development of the uterine tube, uterus, and superior part of the vagina.

The **paramesonephric ducts** form most of the female genital tract. The uterine tubes develop from the unfused cranial parts of these ducts (see Figs. 12-33B and C and 12-34). The caudal fused portions of the paramesonephric ducts form the **uterovaginal primordium,** which gives

12

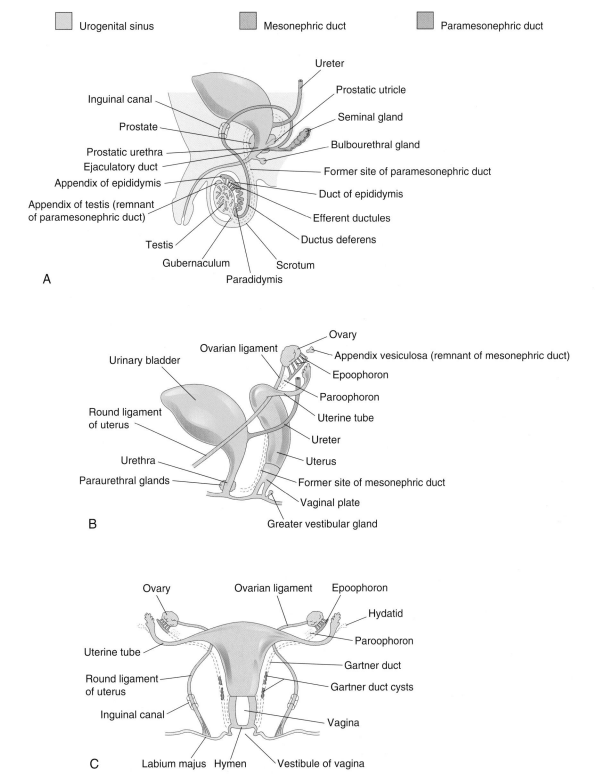

| Urogenital sinus | Mesonephric duct | Paramesonephric duct |

A

Ureter
Prostatic utricle
Seminal gland
Bulbourethral gland
Former site of paramesonephric duct
Duct of epididymis
Efferent ductules
Ductus deferens

Inguinal canal
Prostate
Prostatic urethra
Ejaculatory duct
Appendix of epididymis
Appendix of testis (remnant of paramesonephric duct)
Testis
Gubernaculum
Paradidymis
Scrotum

B

Ovary
Appendix vesiculosa (remnant of mesonephric duct)
Epoophoron
Paroophoron
Uterine tube
Ureter
Uterus
Former site of mesonephric duct
Vaginal plate
Greater vestibular gland

Ovarian ligament
Urinary bladder
Round ligament of uterus
Urethra
Paraurethral glands

C

Ovary
Ovarian ligament
Epoophoron
Hydatid
Paroophoron
Gartner duct
Gartner duct cysts
Vagina

Uterine tube
Round ligament of uterus
Inguinal canal
Labium majus   Hymen   Vestibule of vagina

**FIGURE 12–33** Schematic drawings illustrating development of the male and female reproductive systems from the genital ducts and urogenital sinus. Vestigial structures are also shown. **A,** Reproductive system in a male neonate. **B,** Female reproductive system in a 12-week fetus. **C,** Reproductive system in a female neonate.

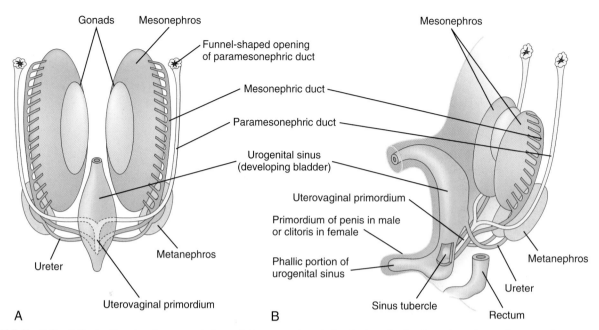

**FIGURE 12–34** A, Sketch of a ventral view of the posterior abdominal wall of a 7-week embryo showing the two pairs of genital ducts present during the indifferent stage of sexual development. B, Lateral view of a 9-week fetus showing the sinus tubercle on the posterior wall of the urogenital sinus. It becomes the hymen in females (see Fig. 12-33C) and the seminal colliculus in males. The colliculus is an elevated part of the urethral crest on the posterior wall of the prostatic urethra (see Fig. 12-33A).

rise to the **uterus** and the superior part of the **vagina** (see Fig. 12-34). The endometrial stroma and myometrium are derived from splanchnic mesenchyme. *Uterine development is regulated by the homeobox gene* HOXA10.

Fusion of the paramesonephric ducts also forms a peritoneal fold that becomes the **broad ligament** and forms two peritoneal compartments, the **rectouterine pouch** and **vesicouterine pouch** (Fig. 12-36A to D). Along the sides of the uterus, between the layers of the broad ligament, the mesenchyme proliferates and differentiates into cellular tissue, or **parametrium**, which is composed of loose connective tissue and smooth muscle.

### Female Auxiliary Genital Glands

Outgrowths from the urethra into the surrounding mesenchyme form the bilateral mucus-secreting **urethral glands** and **paraurethral glands** (see Fig. 12-33B). Outgrowths from the **urogenital sinus** form the **greater vestibular glands** in the lower third of the labia majora (see Fig. 12-34B). These tubuloalveolar glands also secrete mucus and are homologous to the bulbourethral glands in males (see Table 12-1).

### ▶ Development of Vagina

12  The fibromuscular wall of the vagina develops from the surrounding mesenchyme. Contact of the **uterovaginal primordium** with the urogenital sinus, forming the **sinus tubercle** (see Fig. 12-34B), induces the formation of paired endodermal outgrowths, **sinovaginal bulbs** (see Fig. 12-36A). They extend from the urogenital sinus to the caudal end of the uterovaginal primordium. The sinovaginal bulbs fuse to form a **vaginal plate** (see Fig. 12-33B). Later the central cells of this plate break down,

forming the **lumen of the vagina**. The epithelium of the vagina is derived from the peripheral cells of the vaginal plate (see Fig. 12-33C).

Until late fetal life, the lumen of the vagina is separated from the cavity of the urogenital sinus by a membrane, the **hymen** (Fig. 12-37H, and see also Fig. 12-33C). The membrane is formed by invagination of the posterior wall of the urogenital sinus, resulting from expansion of the caudal end of the vagina. The hymen usually ruptures, leaving a small opening during the **perinatal period** (before, during, or after birth), and remains as a thin fold of **mucous membrane** just within the vaginal orifice (see Fig. 12-37H).

### Vestigial Remains of Embryonic Genital Ducts

During conversion of the mesonephric and paramesonephric ducts into adult structures, some parts of the ducts remain as **vestigial structures** (see Fig. 12-33 and Table 12-1). These vestiges are rarely seen unless pathologic changes develop in them (e.g., Gartner duct cysts arising from vestiges of mesonephric ducts; see Fig. 12-33C).

### MESONEPHRIC DUCT REMNANTS IN MALES

The cranial end of the mesonephric duct may persist as an **appendix of the epididymis**, which is usually attached to the head of the epididymis (see Fig. 12-33A). Caudal to the efferent ductules, some mesonephric tubules may persist as a small body, the **paradidymis**.

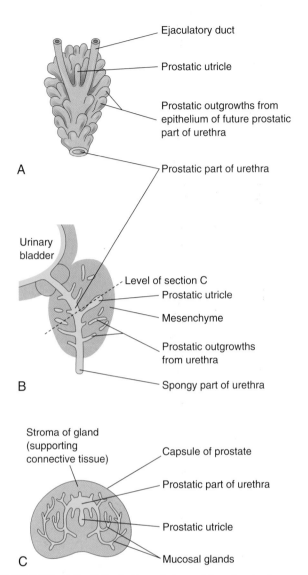

**FIGURE 12–35** A, Dorsal view of the developing prostate in an 11-week fetus. B, Sketch of a median section of the developing urethra and prostate showing numerous endodermal outgrowths from the prostatic urethra. The vestigial prostatic utricle is also shown. C, Section of the prostate (16 weeks) at the level shown in B.

## MESONEPHRIC DUCT REMNANTS IN FEMALES

The cranial end of the mesonephric duct may persist as an **appendix vesiculosa** (see Fig. 12-33B). A few blind tubules and a duct, or **epoophoron**, may persist in the **mesovarium** between the ovary and uterine tube (see Fig. 12-33B and C). Closer to the uterus, some rudimentary tubules may persist as the **paroophoron** (see Fig. 12-33B). Parts of the mesonephric duct, corresponding to the ductus deferens and ejaculatory duct in males, may persist as **Gartner duct cysts** between the layers of the broad ligament along the lateral wall of the uterus and in the wall of the vagina (see Fig. 12-33C).

## PARAMESONEPHRIC DUCT REMNANTS IN MALES

The cranial end of the **paramesonephric duct** may persist as a vesicular **appendix of the testis**, which is attached to the superior pole of the testis (see Fig. 12-33A). The **prostatic utricle**, a small saclike structure arising from the paramesonephric duct, opens into the prostatic urethra. The lining of the prostatic utricle is derived from the epithelium of the urogenital sinus. Within its epithelium, endocrine cells containing neuron-specific enolase and serotonin have been detected. The **seminal colliculus**, a small elevation in the posterior wall of the prostatic urethra, is the adult derivative of the sinus tubercle (see Fig. 12-34B).

## PARAMESONEPHRIC DUCT REMNANTS IN FEMALES

Part of the cranial end of the paramesonephric duct that does not contribute to the infundibulum of the uterine tube may persist as a **vesicular appendage** (see Fig. 12-33C), called a **hydatid** (of Morgagni).

## DEVELOPMENT OF EXTERNAL GENITALIA

Up to the seventh week, the external genitalia are similar in both sexes (see Fig. 12-37A and B). Distinguishing sexual characteristics begin to appear during the 9th week, but the external genitalia are not fully differentiated until the 12th week. Early in the fourth week, proliferating mesenchyme produces a **genital tubercle** (primordium of the penis or clitoris) in both sexes at the cranial end of the **cloacal membrane** (see Fig. 12-37A). *The cloacal ectoderm is believed to be the source of the genital initiation signal that involves Fgf8 expression.*

**Labioscrotal swellings** and **urogenital folds** soon develop on each side of the cloacal membrane. The genital tubercle elongates to form a **primordial phallus** (penis or clitoris). The **urogenital membrane** lies in the floor of a median cleft, the **urethral groove**, which is bounded by the **urethral folds** (see Fig. 12-37A to D). In female fetuses, the urethra and vagina open into a common cavity, the **vestibule of the vagina** (see Fig. 12-37H).

### Development of Male External Genitalia

Masculinization of the indifferent external genitalia is induced by **testosterone** produced by the interstitial cells of the fetal testes (see Fig. 12-37C, E, and G). As the **primordial phallus** enlarges and elongates to form the **penis**, the urethral folds form the lateral walls of the

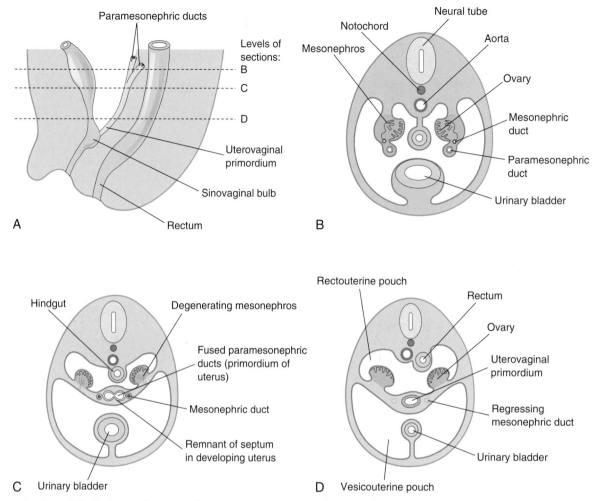

**FIGURE 12–36** Early development of ovaries and uterus. **A,** Schematic drawing of a sagittal section of the caudal region of an 8-week female embryo. **B,** Transverse section showing the paramesonephric ducts approaching each other. **C,** Similar section at a more caudal level illustrating fusion of the paramesonephric ducts. A remnant of the septum in the developing uterus that separates the paramesonephric ducts is shown. **D,** Similar section showing the uterovaginal primordium, broad ligament, and pouches in the pelvic cavity. Note that the mesonephric ducts have regressed.

**urethral groove** on the ventral surface of the penis (Fig. 12-38*A* and *B*, and see also Fig. 12-37*C*). This groove is lined by a proliferation of endodermal cells, the **urethral plate** (see Fig. 12-37*C*), which extends from the phallic portion of the urogenital sinus. The **urethral folds** fuse with each other along the ventral surface of the penis to form the **spongy urethra** (see Figs. 12-37*E* and *G* and 12-38*C₁* and *C₃*). The surface ectoderm fuses in the median plane of the penis, forming the **penile raphe** and enclosing the spongy urethra within the penis (see Fig. 12-37*G*).

At the tip of the **glans penis**, an ectodermal ingrowth forms a cellular **ectodermal cord**, which grows toward the root of the penis to meet the spongy urethra (see Figs. 12-26*A* and 12-38*C*). As this cord canalizes, its lumen joins the previously formed spongy urethra. This juncture completes the terminal part of the urethra and moves the **external urethral orifice** to the tip of the glans penis (see Figs. 12-26*B* and *C* and 12-37*G*). HOX, FGF, *and* Shh *genes regulate the development of the penis.*

During the 12th week, a circular ingrowth of ectoderm occurs at the periphery of the glans penis (see Fig. 12-26*B*). When this ingrowth breaks down, it forms the **prepuce** (foreskin), a covering fold of skin (see Fig. 12-26*C*). The **corpus cavernosum penis** (one of two columns of erectile tissue) and **corpus spongiosum penis** (median column of erectile tissue between the two corpora cavernosa) develop from mesenchyme in the phallus. The two **labioscrotal swellings** grow toward each other and fuse to form the **scrotum** (see Fig. 12-37*A*, *E*, and *G*). The line of fusion of these folds is clearly visible as the **scrotal raphe** (see Figs. 12-37*G* and 12-38*C*).

## Development of Female External Genitalia

The **primordial phallus** in the female fetus gradually becomes the clitoris (see Figs. 12-20*G*, 12-37*B* to *D*, *F*, and *H*, and 12-38*B*). The clitoris is still relatively large at 18 weeks (see Fig. 12-21). The **urethral folds** do not

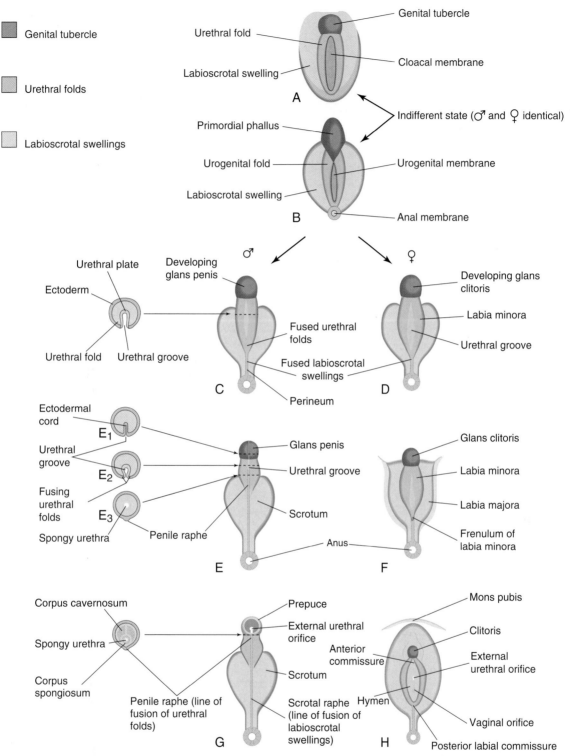

**FIGURE 12-37** Development of external genitalia. **A** and **B,** Diagrams illustrating the appearance of the genitalia during the indifferent stage (fourth to seventh weeks). **C, E,** and **G,** Stages in the development of male external genitalia at 9, 11, and 12 weeks, respectively. To the left are schematic transverse sections of the developing penis illustrating formation of the spongy urethra. **D, F,** and **H,** Stages in the development of female external genitalia at 9, 11, and 12 weeks, respectively. The mons pubis is a pad of fatty tissue over the symphysis pubis.

**FIGURE 12–38** Scanning electron micrographs of the developing external genitalia. **A,** The perineum during the indifferent stage of a 17-mm, 7-week embryo (×100). *1,* Developing glans penis with the ectodermal cord; *2,* urethral groove continuous with the urogenital sinus; *3,* urethral folds; *4,* labioscrotal swellings; *5,* anus. **B,** The external genitalia of a 7.2-cm, 10-week female fetus (×45). *1,* Glans clitoris; *2,* external urethral orifice; *3,* opening into urogenital sinus; *4,* urethral fold (primordium of labium minora); *5,* labioscrotal swelling (labium majora); *6,* anus. **C,** The external genitalia of a 5.5-cm, 10-week male fetus (×40). *1,* Glans penis with ectodermal cord; *2,* remains of urethral groove; *3,* urethral folds in the process of closing; *4,* labioscrotal swellings fusing to form the scrotal raphe; *5,* anus. *(From Hinrichsen KV: Embryologische Grundlagen. In Sohn C, Holzgreve W, editors:* Ultraschall in Gynäkologie und Geburtshilfe, *New York, 1995, Georg Thieme Verlag.)*

fuse, except posteriorly, where they join to form the **frenulum of the labia minora** (see Fig. 12-37*F*). The unfused parts of the urogenital folds form the **labia minora.** The labioscrotal folds fuse posteriorly to form the **posterior labial commissure** and anteriorly to form the

**anterior labial commissure** and **mons pubis** (Fig. 12-37*H*). Most parts of the **labioscrotal folds** remain unfused but develop into two large folds of skin, the **labia majora.**

*Text continued on p. 276*

## DETERMINATION OF FETAL SEX

*Visualization of external genitalia during ultrasonography* is clinically important for several reasons, including detection of fetuses at risk of severe X-linked disorders (Fig. 12-39). Careful examination of the perineum may detect **ambiguous genitalia** (Fig. 12-40*B*). Ultrasonographic confirmation of testes in the scrotum provides the only 100% gender determination, which is not possible in utero until 22 to 36 weeks. In 30% of fetuses, fetal position prevents good visualization of the **perineum** (area between the thighs).

When there is normal sexual differentiation, the appearance of the external and internal genitalia is consistent with the **sex chromosome complement.** Errors in sex determination and differentiation result in various degrees of intermediate sex. Advances in molecular genetics have led to a better understanding of abnormal sexual development and **ambiguous genitalia.**

Because of psychosocial stigma and in order to provide better clinical management for infants born with atypical chromosomal constitution or gonads, a new nomenclature has been introduced to describe these conditions that are now called **disorders of sex development (DSD)** (see Lee et al, 2006).

**DSD** implies a discrepancy between the morphology of the gonads (testes or ovaries) and the appearance of the external genitalia. Intersexual conditions are classified according to the histologic appearance of the gonads:

● **Ovotesticular DSD:** ovarian and testicular tissue is found either in the same gonad or in opposite gonads
● **46,XX DSD:** ovaries are present
● **46,XY DSD:** testicular tissue is present

## DETERMINATION OF FETAL SEX—cont'd

### Ovotesticular DSD (True Gonadal Intersex)

Persons with **ovotesticular DSD**, a rare intersexual condition, usually have **chromatin-positive nuclei** (sex chromatin in cells observed in a buccal smear). Approximately 70% of these persons have a 46,XX chromosome constitution; approximately 20% have 46,XX/46,XY **mosaicism** (the presence of two or more cell lines), and approximately 10% have a 46,XY chromosome constitution. The causes of ovotesticular DSD are still poorly understood.

Most persons with this condition have both testicular and ovarian tissue and an **ovotestis** (gonad in which both testicular and ovarian components are present). These tissues are not usually functional. An ovotestis forms if both the medulla and cortex of the indifferent gonads develop. Ovotesticular DSD results from an error in sex determination. The phenotype may be male or female, but the external genitalia are always ambiguous.

### 46,XX DSD

Persons with **46,XX DSD** have chromatin-positive nuclei and a 46,XX chromosome constitution. This anomaly results from exposure of a female fetus to **excessive androgens**, causing virilization of the external genitalia (clitoral enlargement and labial fusion; see Figs. 12-28 and 12-40). A common cause of 46,XX DSD is **CAH**. There is no ovarian abnormality; however, excessive production of androgens by the fetal suprarenal glands causes varying degrees of masculinization of the external genitalia. Commonly, there is **clitoral hypertrophy**, partial fusion of the labia majora, and a persistent urogenital sinus (see Fig. 12-40).

In rare cases, the masculinization may be so intense that a complete clitoral urethra results. The administration of androgenic agents to women during early pregnancy may cause similar anomalies of the fetal external genitalia. Most cases have resulted from the use of certain progestational compounds for treatment of a threatened abortion. **Masculinizing maternal tumors** can also cause virilization of female fetuses.

### 46,XY DSD

Persons with this intersexual condition have **chromatin-negative nuclei** (no sex chromatin) and a 46,XY chromosome constitution. The external genitalia are developmentally variable, as is the development of the internal genitalia, due to varying degrees of development of the paramesonephric ducts.

*These anomalies are caused by inadequate production of testosterone and MIS by the fetal testes.* Testicular development in these individuals ranges from rudimentary to normal. Genetic defects in the enzymatic synthesis of testosterone by the fetal testes and in interstitial cells produce 46,XY DSD through inadequate virilization of the male fetus.

**FIGURE 12–39** Sonogram of a 33-week male fetus showing normal external genitalia. Observe the penis *(arrow)* and scrotum *(S)*. Also note the testes in the scrotum.

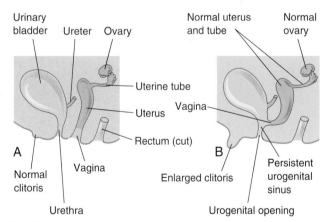

**FIGURE 12–40** Schematic lateral views of the female urogenital system. **A,** Normal. **B,** Female with 46,XX disorder of sex development caused by congenital adrenal hyperplasia. Note the enlarged clitoris and persistent urogenital sinus that were induced by androgens produced by the hyperplastic suprarenal glands.

## ANDROGEN INSENSITIVITY SYNDROME

Persons with androgen insensitivity syndrome, previously called **testicular feminization syndrome**, which occurs in 1 in 20,000 live births, are **normal-appearing females**, despite the presence of testes and a 46,XY chromosome constitution (Fig. 12-41). **The external genitalia are female**; however, the vagina usually ends in a blind pouch and the uterus and uterine tubes are absent or rudimentary. At puberty, there is normal development of breasts and female characteristics; however, menstruation does not occur.

The testes are usually in the abdomen or inguinal canals, but they may be within the labia majora. The failure of masculinization to occur in these persons results from a resistance to the action of testosterone at the cellular level in the genital tubercle and labioscrotal and urethral folds (see Fig. 12-37*A*, *B*, *D*, *F*, and *H*).

Persons with **partial androgen insensitivity syndrome** exhibit some masculinization at birth, such as ambiguous external genitalia, and they may have an enlarged clitoris. The vagina ends blindly and the uterus is absent. Testes are in the inguinal canals or *labia majora*. There are usually point mutations in the sequence that codes for the **androgen receptor**. Usually, the testes of these persons are removed as soon as they are discovered because, in approximately one third of these individuals, malignant tumors develop by 50 years of age. Androgen insensitivity syndrome follows X-linked recessive inheritance, and the gene encoding the androgen receptor has been localized.

**FIGURE 12–41** A, Photograph of a 17-year-old woman with androgen insensitivity syndrome. The external genitalia are female; however, she has a 46,XY karyotype and testes in the inguinal region. B, Photomicrograph of a section through a testis removed from the inguinal region of this woman showing seminiferous tubules lined by Sertoli cells. There are no germ cells, and the interstitial cells are hypoplastic. (*From Jones HW, Scott WW:* Hermaphroditism, genital anomalies and related endocrine disorders, *Baltimore, 1958, Williams & Wilkins.*)

## MIXED GONADAL DYSGENESIS

Persons with this rare condition usually have a 46,XY chromosomal complement, with a testis on one side and an undifferentiated gonad on the other side. The internal genitalia are female; however, male derivatives of the mesonephric ducts are sometimes present (e.g., an appendix of the epididymis; see Fig. 12-33A). The external genitalia range from normal female through intermediate states to normal male. At puberty, neither breast development nor menstruation occurs; however, varying degrees of virilization (masculine characteristics) are common.

## HYPOSPADIAS

Hypospadias is the most common defect of the penis. There are four main types:
- Glanular hypospadias, the most common type
- Penile hypospadias
- Penoscrotal hypospadias
- Perineal hypospadias

In 1 of every 125 male neonates, the **external urethral orifice** is on the ventral surface of the glans penis (**glanular hypospadias**) or on the ventral surface of the body of the penis (**penile hypospadias**). Usually, the penis is underdeveloped and curved ventrally (**chordee**; Fig. 12-42).

Glanular hypospadias and penile hypospadias constitute approximately 80% of cases. In **penoscrotal hypospadias**, the urethral orifice is at the junction of the penis and scrotum. In **perineal hypospadias**, the labioscrotal folds (swellings) fail to fuse (see Figs. 12-37 and 12-38) and the external urethral orifice is located between the unfused halves of the scrotum. Because the external genitalia in this severe type of hypospadias are ambiguous, persons with perineal hypospadias and cryptorchidism (undescended testes) are sometimes misdiagnosed as having 46,XY DSD.

*Hypospadias results from inadequate production of androgens by the fetal testes and/or inadequate receptor sites for the hormones.* Most likely, both genomic and environmental factors are involved. It has been suggested that the expression of testosterone-related genes is affected. These defects result in failure of canalization of the ectodermal cord in the glans penis and/or failure of fusion of the urethral folds; as a consequence, there is incomplete formation of the spongy urethra.

**FIGURE 12–42** Glanular hypospadias in an infant. The external urethral orifice is on the ventral surface of the glans penis (*arrow*).

## EPISPADIAS

In one of every 30,000 male infants, the urethra opens on the dorsal surface of the penis; note that when the penis is flaccid, its dorsal surface is directed anteriorly. Although epispadias may occur as a separate entity, it is often associated with **exstrophy of the bladder** (see Figs. 12-24 and 12-25F). Epispadias may result from *inadequate ectodermal–mesenchymal interactions* during development of the genital tubercle (see Fig. 12-37A). As a consequence, the genital tubercle develops more dorsally than in normal embryos. Consequently, when the **urogenital membrane** ruptures, the urogenital sinus opens on the dorsal surface of the penis (see Fig. 12-37B and C). Urine is expelled at the root of the malformed penis, which is located in the superficial perineal pouch.

## AGENESIS OF EXTERNAL GENITALIA

Congenital absence of the penis or clitoris is an extremely rare condition (Fig. 12-43). Failure of the **genital tubercle** to develop (see Fig. 12-37A and B) may result from inadequate ectodermal–mesenchymal interactions during the seventh week. The urethra usually opens into the perineum near the anus.

**FIGURE 12–43** Perineum of an infant with agenesis of the external genitalia. There are no external genitalia.

## BIFID PENIS AND DIPHALLIA

These defects are very rare. **Bifid penis** is usually associated with **exstrophy of the bladder** (see Fig. 12-24). It may also be associated with urinary tract abnormalities and imperforate anus. **Diphallia** (double penis) results when two genital tubercles develop; fewer than 100 cases have been reported worldwide.

## MICROPENIS

In this condition, the penis is so small that it is almost hidden by the suprapubic fat pad. **Micropenis** results from fetal testicular failure and is commonly associated with hypopituitarism (diminished activity of the anterior lobe of the hypophysis).

## ANOMALIES OF UTERINE TUBES, UTERUS, AND VAGINA

Defects of the uterine tubes are rare; there are only a few irregularities, including hydatid cysts, accessory ostia (openings), complete and segmental absence of the tubes, duplication of a uterine tube, lack of the muscular layer, and failure of the tube to canalize. Various types of uterine duplications and vaginal anomalies result from arrests of development of the uterovaginal primordium during the eighth week (Fig. 12-44) by:

- Incomplete development of a paramesonephric duct
- Failure of parts of one or both paramesonephric ducts to develop
- Incomplete fusion of the paramesonephric ducts
- Incomplete canalization of the vaginal plate to form the vagina

**Double uterus** (uterus didelphys) results from failure of fusion of the inferior parts of the paramesonephric ducts. It may be associated with a double or a single vagina (see Fig. 12-44B to D). In some cases, the uterus appears normal externally but is divided internally by a thin septum (see Fig. 12-44F). If the duplication involves only the superior part of the body of the uterus, the condition is called **bicornuate uterus** (Fig. 12-45, and see also Fig. 12-44D and E).

If growth of one paramesonephric duct is retarded and the duct does not fuse with the second duct, a **bicornuate uterus with a rudimentary horn** (cornu) develops (see Fig. 12-44E). The rudimentary horn may not communicate with the cavity of the uterus. A **unicornuate uterus** develops when one paramesonephric duct fails to develop; this results in a uterus with one uterine tube (see Fig. 12-44G). In many cases, the individuals are fertile but may have an increased incidence of preterm delivery or recurrent pregnancy loss.

### Absence of Vagina and Uterus

Once in approximately every 5000 births, absence of the vagina occurs. This results from failure of the **sinovaginal bulbs** to develop and form the vaginal plate (see Figs. 12-33B and 12-36A). When the vagina is absent, the uterus is usually absent because the developing uterus (uterovaginal primordium) induces the formation of sinovaginal bulbs, which fuse to form the vaginal plate.

### Other Vaginal Anomalies

Failure of canalization of the vaginal plate results in **atresia** (blockage) of the vagina. A transverse **vaginal septum** occurs in approximately one in 80,000 women. Usually the septum is located at the junction of the middle and superior thirds of the vagina. Failure of the inferior end of the vaginal plate to perforate results in an **imperforate hymen**, the most common anomaly of the female reproductive tract that results in obstruction. Variations in the appearance of the hymen are common (Fig. 12-46). The vaginal orifice varies in diameter from very small to large, and there may be more than one orifice.

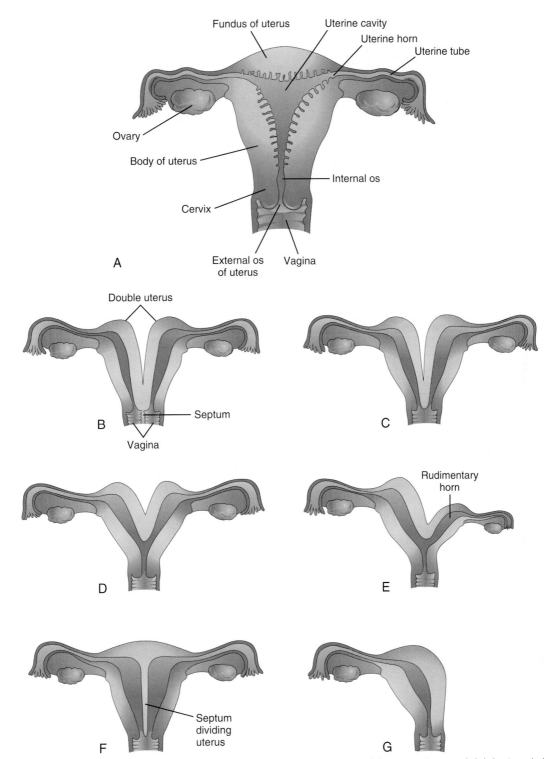

**FIGURE 12–44** Uterine birth defects. **A,** Normal uterus and vagina. **B,** Double uterus (uterus didelphys) and double vagina (vagina duplex). Note the septum separating the vagina into two parts. **C,** Double uterus with single vagina. **D,** Bicornuate uterus (two uterine horns). **E,** Bicornuate uterus with a rudimentary left horn. **F,** Septate uterus; the septum separates the body of the uterus. **G,** Unicorn uterus; only one lateral horn exists.

**FIGURE 12–45** Sonogram of bicornuate uterus. **A,** Axial sonogram of the fundus of uterus showing two separate endometrial canals with a 1-week chorionic (gestational) sac *(arrow)*. **B,** A three-dimensional ultrasound scan of the same patient with a 4-week chorionic sac *(arrow)* on the right of a uterine septum *(S)*. **C,** Coronal ultrasound scan of a uterus with a large septum *(S)* extending down to the cervix.

**FIGURE 12–46** A to F, Congenital anomalies of the hymen. The normal appearance of the hymen is illustrated in A and in the black-and-white photograph *(left)*, which is a normal crescentic hymen in a prepubertal child.

# DEVELOPMENT OF INGUINAL CANALS

12 The **inguinal canals** form pathways for the testes to descend from the dorsal abdominal wall through the anterior abdominal wall into the scrotum. *Inguinal canals develop in both sexes* because of the morphologically indifferent stage of sexual development. As the mesonephros degenerates, a ligament, the **gubernaculum**, develops on each side of the abdomen from the caudal pole of the gonad (Fig. 12-47A). The gubernaculum passes obliquely through the developing anterior abdominal wall at the site of the future inguinal canal (Fig. 12-47B to D) and attaches caudally to the internal surface of the **labioscrotal swellings** (future halves of the scrotum or labia majora).

The **processus vaginalis,** an evagination of peritoneum, develops ventral to the gubernaculum (a fibrous cord connecting two structures, e.g., the testis and scrotum) and herniates through the abdominal wall along the path formed by this cord (see Fig. 12-47B). The processus vaginalis carries extensions of the layers of the abdominal wall before it, which form the walls of the inguinal canal. These layers also form the coverings of the spermatic cord and testis (see Fig. 12-47D to F). The opening in the transversalis fascia produced by the processus vaginalis becomes the **deep inguinal ring,** and the opening created in the external oblique aponeurosis (broad, flat tendinous portion of the external abdominal oblique muscle) forms the **superficial inguinal ring.**

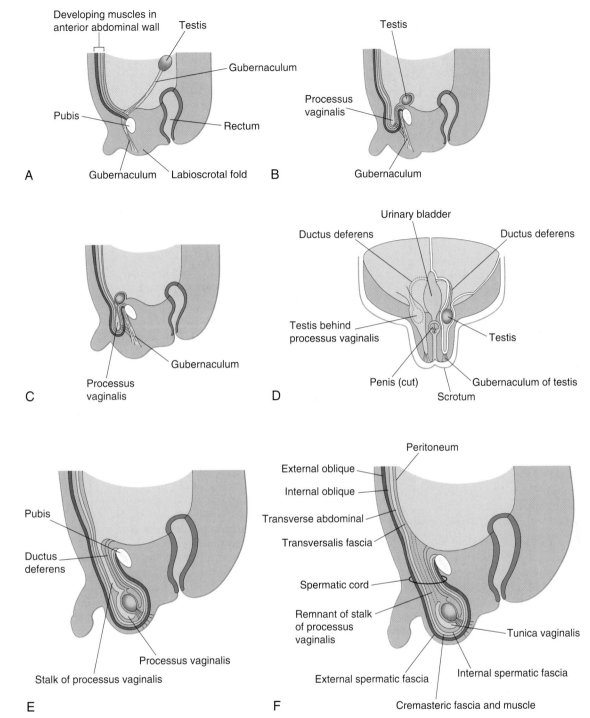

**FIGURE 12–47** Formation of the inguinal canals and descent of the testes. **A,** Sagittal section of a 7-week embryo showing the testis before its descent from the dorsal abdominal wall. **B** and **C,** Similar sections at approximately 28 weeks showing the processus vaginalis and testis beginning to pass through the inguinal canal. Note that the processus vaginalis carries fascial layers of the abdominal wall before it. **D,** Frontal section of a fetus approximately 3 days later, illustrating descent of the testis posterior to the processus vaginalis. The processus has been cut away on the left side to show the testis and ductus deferens. **E,** Sagittal section of a male neonate showing the processus vaginalis communicating with the peritoneal cavity by a narrow stalk. **F,** Similar section of a 1-month-old male infant after obliteration of the stalk of the processus vaginalis. Note that the extended fascial layers of the abdominal wall now form the coverings of the spermatic cord.

## COMPLEX OR UNDETERMINED INTERSEX DISORDERS OF SEXUAL DEVELOPMENT

In embryos with **abnormal sex chromosome complexes**, such as XXX or XXY, the number of X chromosomes appears to be unimportant in sex determination. If a normal Y chromosome is present, the embryo develops as a male. If no Y chromosome is present or the testis-determining region of the Y chromosome is absent, female development occurs. The loss of an X chromosome does not appear to interfere with the migration of primordial germ cells to the gonadal ridges, because some germ cells have been observed in the fetal gonads of 45,XO females with **Turner syndrome** (see Figs. 20-3 and 20-4). Two X chromosomes are needed, however, to bring about normal ovarian development.

## RELOCATION OF TESTES AND OVARIES

### Testicular Descent

This descent is associated with:

- Enlargement of the testes and atrophy of the **mesonephroi** (mesonephric kidneys), allowing movement of the testes caudally along the posterior abdominal wall
- Atrophy of the **paramesonephric ducts** induced by MIS, enabling the testes to move transabdominally to the deep inguinal rings
- Enlargement of the **processus vaginalis** guiding the testis through the inguinal canal into the scrotum

By 26 weeks, the testes have usually descended retroperitoneally (external to the peritoneum) from the superior lumbar region to the posterior abdominal wall to the deep inguinal rings (Fig. 12-47B and C). This change in position occurs as the fetal pelvis enlarges and the body or trunk of the embryo elongates. **Transabdominal relocation of the testes** is largely a relative movement that results from growth of the cranial part of the abdomen away from the future pelvic region. The descent of the testes through the inguinal canals into the scrotum is controlled by androgens (e.g., testosterone) produced by the fetal testes (see Fig. 12-33A). The **gubernaculum** forms a path through the anterior abdominal wall for the processus vaginalis to follow during formation of the inguinal canal (see Fig. 12-47B to E). The gubernaculum anchors the testis to the scrotum and guides its descent into the scrotum. Passage of the testis through the inguinal canal may also be aided by the increase in *intra-abdominal pressure* resulting from the growth of abdominal viscera.

Descent of the testes through the inguinal canals into the scrotum usually begins during the 26th week, and in some fetuses, it takes 2 or 3 days. By 32 weeks, both testes are present in the scrotum in most cases. The testes pass external to the peritoneum and processus vaginalis.

After the testes enter the scrotum, the inguinal canal contracts around the spermatic cord. More than 97% of full-term neonates have both testes in the scrotum. During the first 3 months after birth, most undescended testes descend into the scrotum.

The mode of descent of the testis explains why the **ductus deferens** crosses anterior to the ureter (see Fig. 12-33A); it also explains the course of the **testicular vessels**. These vessels form when the testes are located high on the posterior abdominal wall. As the testes descend, they carry the ductus deferens and vessels with them and they are ensheathed by the fascial extensions of the abdominal wall (see Fig. 12-47F).

- The extension of the transversalis fascia becomes the **internal spermatic fascia**.
- The extensions of the internal oblique muscle and fascia become the **cremasteric muscle** and **fascia**.
- The extension of the transversalis fascia becomes the **internal spermatic fascia**.

Within the scrotum, the testis projects into the distal end of the **processus vaginalis**. During the perinatal period, the connecting stalk of the processus normally obliterates, forming a serous membrane, the **tunica vaginalis**, which covers the front and sides of the testis (see Fig. 12-47F).

### Ovarian Descent

The ovaries also descend from the lumbar region of the posterior abdominal wall and relocate to the lateral wall of the pelvis; however, they do not pass from the pelvis and enter the inguinal canals. The **gubernaculum** is attached to the uterus near the attachment of the uterine tube. The cranial part of the gubernaculum becomes the **ovarian ligament**, and the caudal part forms the **round ligament of the uterus** (see Fig. 12-33C). The round ligaments pass through the inguinal canals and terminate in the **labia majora**. The relatively small **processus vaginalis** in the female usually obliterates and disappears long before birth. A persistent processus in the fetus is known as the **processus vaginalis of the peritoneum** or vaginal process of the peritoneum (canal of Nuck).

## SUMMARY OF UROGENITAL SYSTEM

- Development of the urinary and genital systems is intimately associated.
- The urinary system develops before the genital system.
- Three successive kidney systems develop: **pronephroi** (nonfunctional), **mesonephroi** (temporary excretory organs), and **metanephroi** (primordia of permanent kidneys).
- The **metanephroi** develop from two sources: the **ureteric buds**, which give rise to the **ureter**, renal pelvis, calices, and collecting tubules, and the metanephrogenic blastema, which gives rise to the **nephrons**.
- At first, the **kidneys** are located in the pelvis; however, they gradually shift position to the abdomen. This apparent migration results from disproportionate growth of the fetal lumbar and sacral regions.

## CRYPTORCHIDISM

**Cryptorchidism** (hidden testes) is the most common defect in neonates; it occurs in about 30% of premature males and 3% to 5% of full-term males. This reflects the fact that the testes begin to descend into the scrotum by the end of the second trimester. Cryptorchidism may be unilateral or bilateral. In most cases, undescended testes descend into the scrotum by the end of the first year. If both testes remain within or just outside the abdominal cavity, they fail to mature and sterility is common.

If cryptorchidism is uncorrected, these males have a significantly higher risk of developing **germ cell tumors**, especially in cases of *abdominal cryptorchidism*. Undescended testes are often histologically normal at birth, but failure of development and atrophy are detectable by the end of the first year. Cryptorchid testes may be in the abdominal cavity or anywhere along the usual path of descent of the testis, but they are usually in the inguinal canal (Fig. 12-48A). The cause of most cases of cryptorchidism is unknown; however, a deficiency of androgen production by the fetal testes is an important factor.

## ECTOPIC TESTES

As the fetus passes through the inguinal canal, the testes may deviate from their usual path of descent and arrive in various abnormal locations (see Fig. 12-48B):

- **Interstitial** (external to the aponeurosis of the external oblique muscle)
- In the **proximal part of the medial thigh**
- **Dorsal to the penis**
- On the opposite side (**crossed ectopia**)

All types of ectopic testes are rare, but **interstitial ectopia** occurs most frequently. An ectopic testis occurs when a part of the gubernaculum passes to an abnormal location and the testis follows it.

## CONGENITAL INGUINAL HERNIA

If the communication between the tunica vaginalis and the peritoneal cavity fails to close (Fig. 12-49A and B), a **persistent processus vaginalis** exists. A loop of intestine may herniate through it into the scrotum or labium majora (see Fig. 12-49B).

Embryonic remnants resembling the ductus deferens or epididymis are often found in **inguinal hernial sacs**. Congenital inguinal hernia is much more common in males, especially when there are undescended testes. These hernias are also common with ectopic testes and in **androgen insensitivity syndrome** (see Fig. 12-41).

## HYDROCELE

Occasionally, the abdominal end of the **processus vaginalis** remains open; however, it is too small to permit herniation of intestine. Peritoneal fluid passes into the **patent processus vaginalis** and forms a **scrotal hydrocele** (see Fig. 12-49D). If only the middle part of the processus vaginalis remains open, fluid may accumulate and give rise to a **hydrocele of the spermatic cord** (see Fig. 12-49C).

- Birth defects of the kidneys and ureters are common. Incomplete division of the ureteric bud results in a **double ureter** and **supernumerary kidney**. An ectopic kidney that is abnormally rotated results if the developing kidney remains in its embryonic position in the pelvis.
- The **urinary bladder** develops from the **urogenital sinus** and the surrounding splanchnic mesenchyme. The female urethra and most of the male urethra have a similar origin.
- **Exstrophy of the bladder** results from a rare ventral body wall defect through which the posterior wall of the urinary bladder protrudes onto the abdominal wall. **Epispadias** is a common associated defect in males; the urethra opens on the dorsum of the penis.
- The **genital system** develops in close association with the urinary system. **Chromosomal sex** is established at fertilization; however, the gonads do not attain sexual characteristics until the seventh week.
- **Primordial germ cells** form in the wall of the **umbilical vesicle** during the fourth week and migrate into the developing gonads, where they differentiate into germ cells (oogonia/spermatogonia).
- The **external genitalia** do not acquire distinct masculine or feminine characteristics until the 12th week. The genitalia develop from primordia that are identical in both sexes.

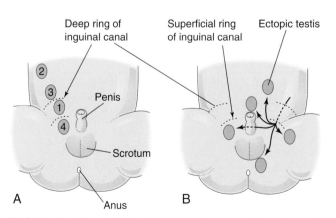

**FIGURE 12-48** Possible sites of cryptorchid and ectopic testes. A, Positions of cryptorchid testes, numbered (1 to 4) in order of frequency. B, Usual locations of ectopic testes.

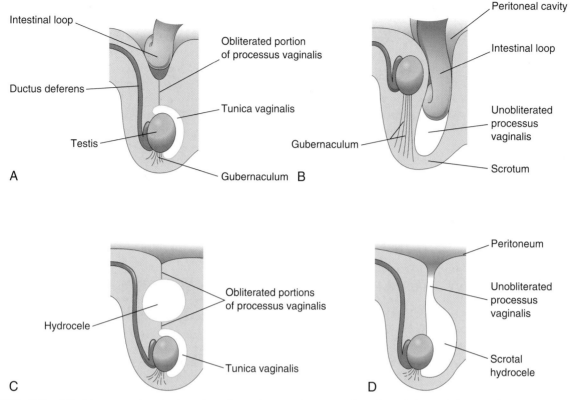

**FIGURE 12–49** Diagrams of sagittal sections illustrating conditions resulting from failure of closure of the processus vaginalis. **A,** Incomplete congenital inguinal hernia resulting from persistence of the proximal part of the processus vaginalis. **B,** Complete congenital inguinal hernia into the scrotum resulting from persistence of the processus vaginalis. Cryptorchidism, a commonly associated defect, is also illustrated. **C,** Large hydrocele that resulted from an unobliterated portion of the processus vaginalis. **D,** Hydrocele of the testis and spermatic cord resulting from peritoneal fluid passing into an unobliterated processus vaginalis.

- **Gonadal sex** is determined by **testes-determining factor,** which is located on the Y chromosome. Testes-determining factor directs testicular differentiation. The **interstitial cells** (Leydig cells) produce **testosterone,** which stimulates development of the **mesonephric ducts** into male genital ducts. Testosterone also stimulates development of the indifferent external genitalia into the penis and scrotum. **MIS,** produced by the **Sertoli cells,** inhibits development of the **paramesonephric ducts** (primordia of the female genital ducts).

- In the absence of a Y chromosome and the presence of two X chromosomes, ovaries develop, the **mesonephric ducts** regress, and the **paramesonephric ducts** develop into the uterus and uterine tubes. The vagina develops from the **vaginal plate** derived from the **urogenital sinus,** and the indifferent external genitalia develop into the clitoris and labia majora and minora.

- Persons with **ovotesticular DSD** have both ovarian and testicular tissue and variable internal and external genitalia. In the 46,XY disorder of sex development, the fetal testes fail to produce adequate amounts of masculinizing hormones or there is tissue insensitivity of the sexual structures. In the 46,XX disorder of sex development, the cause is usually **congenital adrenal hyperplasia,** *a disorder of the fetal suprarenal glands*

that causes excessive production of androgens and masculinization of the external genitalia.

- Most defects of the female genital tract, such as **double uterus,** result from incomplete fusion of the paramesonephric ducts. **Cryptorchidism** and **ectopic testes** result from abnormalities of testicular descent.

- **Congenital inguinal hernia** and **hydrocele** result from persistence of the **processus vaginalis.** Failure of the urethral folds to fuse in males results in various types of **hypospadias.**

## CLINICALLY ORIENTED PROBLEMS

### CASE 12–1

*A 4-year-old girl was still in diapers because she was continually wet. The pediatrician saw urine coming from the infant's vagina. An intravenous urogram showed two renal pelves and two ureters on the right side. One ureter was clearly observed to enter the bladder, but the termination of the other one was not clearly seen. A pediatric urologist examined the child under general anesthesia and observed a small opening in the posterior wall of the vagina. The urologist passed a tiny catheter into it and injected contrast media. This procedure showed that the opening in the vagina was the orifice of the second ureter.*

* What is the embryologic basis for the two renal pelves and ureters?
* Describe the embryologic basis of an ectopic ureteric orifice.
* What is the anatomic basis of the continual dribbling of urine into the vagina?

### CASE 12–2

*A radiologist carried out femoral artery catheterization and aortography (radiographic visualization of the aorta and its branches) on a patient that had no brain activity because of having been injured in a motor vehicle collision. The patient's family had agreed to organ donation. The examination showed a single large renal artery on the right but one normal and one small renal artery on the left. Only the right kidney was used for transplantation. Grafting of the small accessory renal artery into the aorta would be difficult because of its size, and part of the kidney would die if one of the arteries was not successfully grafted.*

* Are accessory renal arteries common?
* What is the embryologic basis of the two left renal arteries?
* In what other circumstance might an accessory renal artery be of clinical significance?

### CASE 12–3

*A 32-year-old woman with a short history of cramping, lower abdominal pain, and tenderness underwent a laparotomy because of a suspected ectopic pregnancy. The operation revealed a pregnancy in a rudimentary right uterine horn.*

* Is this type of uterine birth defect common?
* What is the embryologic basis of the rudimentary uterine horn?

### CASE 12–4

*During the physical examination of a male neonate, it was observed that the urethra opened on the ventral surface of the penis at the junction of the glans penis and the body of the penis. The penis was curved toward the undersurface of the penis.*

* Give the medical terms for the birth defects described.
* What is the embryologic basis of the abnormal urethral orifice?
* Is this anomaly common? Discuss its etiologic basis.

### CASE 12–5

*A woman had previously been prevented from competing in the Olympics because genetic testing revealed an XY chromosome complement.*

* Is she a male or a female?
* What is the probable basis for the results of this test?
* Is there an anatomic basis for not allowing her to compete in the Olympics?

### CASE 12–6

*A 10-year-old boy suffered pain in his left groin while attempting to lift a heavy box. Later he noticed a lump in his groin. When he told his mother about the lump, she arranged an appointment with the family physician. After a physical examination, a diagnosis of indirect inguinal hernia was made.*

* Explain the embryologic basis of this type of inguinal hernia.
* Based on your embryologic knowledge, list the layers of the spermatic cord that would cover the hernial sac.

Discussion of problems appears in the Appendix at the back of the book.

## BIBLIOGRAPHY AND SUGGESTED READING

Ashley RA, Barthold JS, Kolon TF: Cryptorchidism: pathogenesis, diagnosis and prognosis, *Urol Clin North Am* 37:183, 2010.

Avni FE, Maugey-Laulom B, Cassart M, et al: The fetal genitourinary tract. In Callen PW, editor: *Ultrasonography in obstetrics and gynecology*, ed 5, Philadelphia, 2008, Saunders.

Bendon RW: Oligohydramnios, *Front Fetal Health* 2:10, 2000.

Billmire DF: Germ cell tumors, *Surg Clin North Am* 86:489, 2006.

Elder JS: Urologic disorders in infants and children. In Behrman RE, Kliegman RM, Jenson HB, editors: *Nelson textbook of pediatrics*, ed 17, Philadelphia, 2004, Saunders.

Faa G, Gerosa C, Fanni D, et al: Morphogenesis and molecular mechanisms involved in human kidney development, *J Cell Physiol* 227:1257, 2012.

Fiegel HC, Rolle U, Metzger R, et al: Embryology of testicular descent, *Semin Pediatr Surg* 20:161, 2011.

Haynes JH: Inguinal and scrotal disorders, *Surg Clin North Am* 86:371, 2006.

Hecht NB: Molecular mechanism of male germ cell differentiation, *Bioessays* 20:555, 1998.

Kluth D, Fiegel HC, Geyer C: Embryology of the distal urethra and external genitals, *Semin Pediatr Surg* 20:176, 2011.

Kraft KH, Shukla AR, Canning DA: Hypospadia, *Urol Clin North Am* 37:167, 2010.

Kuure S, Vuolteenaho R, Vainio S: Kidney morphogenesis: cellular and molecular regulation, *Mech Dev* 92:19, 2000.

Lambert SM, Vilain EJ, Kolon TF: A practical approach to ambiguous genitalia in the newborn period, *Urol Clin North Am* 37:195, 2010.

Lancaster MA, Gleeson JG: Cystic kidney disease: the role of Wnt signaling, *Trends Mol Med* 16:349, 2010.

Larney C, Bailey TYL, Koopman P: Switching on sex: transcriptional regulation of the testis-determining gene Sry, *Development* 141:2195, 2014.

Lee PA, Houk CP, Ahmed SF, et al: Consensus statement on management of intersex disorders, *Pediatrics* 118:e4888, 2006.

Little M, Georgas K, Pennisi D, et al: Kidney development: two tales of tubulogenesis, *Curr Top Dev Biol* 90:193, 2010.

Meeks J, Schaeffer EM: Genetic regulation of prostate development, *J Androl* 32:210, 2011.

Moore KL, Dalley AF, Agur AMR: *Clinically oriented anatomy*, ed 7, Baltimore, 2014, Williams & Wilkins.

Nebot-Cegarra J, Fàbregas PJ, Sánchez-Pérez I: Cellular proliferation in the urorectal septation complex of the human embryo at Carnegie stages 13–18: a nuclear area-based morphometric analysis, *J Anat* 207:353, 2005.

Nishida H, Miyagawa S, Matsumaru D, et al: Gene expression analyses on embryonic external genitalia: identification of regulatory genes possibly involved in masculinization process, *Congenit Anom* 48:63, 2008.

Palmert MR, Dahms WT: Abnormalities of sexual differentiation. In Martin RJ, Fanaroff AA, Walsh MC, editors: *Fanaroff and Martin's neonatal–perinatal medicine: diseases of the fetus and infant*, ed 8, Philadelphia, 2006, Mosby.

Persaud TVN: Embryology of the female genital tract and gonads. In Copeland LJ, Jarrell J, editors: *Textbook of gynecology*, ed 2, Philadelphia, 2000, Saunders.

Poder L: Ultrasound evaluation of the uterus. In Callen PW, editor: *Ultrasonography in obstetrics and gynecology*, ed 5, Philadelphia, 2008, Saunders.

Powell DM, Newman KD, Randolph J: A proposed classification of vaginal anomalies and their surgical correction, *J Pediatr Surg* 30:271, 1995.

Sobel V, Zhu Y-S, Imperato-McGinley J: Fetal hormones and sexual differentiation, *Obstet Gynecol Clin North Am* 31:837, 2004.

Stec AA: Embryology and bony and pelvic floor anatomy in the bladder and exstrophy-epispadias complex, *Semin Pediatr Surg* 20:66, 2011.

Telega G, Cronin D, Avner ED: New approaches to the ARKPD patient with dual kidney–liver complications, *Pediatr Transplant* 17:328, 2013.

Vogt BA, Dell KM, Davis ID: The kidney and urinary tract. In Martin RJ, Fanaroff AA, Walsh MC, editors: *Fanaroff and Martin's neonatal–perinatal medicine: diseases of the fetus and infant*, ed 8, Philadelphia, 2006, Mosby.

Witschi E: Migration of the germ cells of human embryos from the yolk sac to the primitive gonadal folds, *Contr Embryol Carnegie Inst* 32:67, 1948.

Woolf AS: A molecular and genetic view of human renal and urinary tract malformations, *Kidney Int* 58:500, 2000.

Yiee JH, Baskin LS: Environmental factors in genitourinary development, *J Urol* 184:34, 2010.

# Cardiovascular System

*T*he cardiovascular system is the first major system to function in the embryo. The primordial heart and vascular system appear in the middle of the third week (Fig. 13-1). This precocious cardiac development occurs because the rapidly growing embryo can no longer satisfy its nutritional and oxygen requirements by diffusion alone. Consequently, there is a need for an efficient method of acquiring oxygen and nutrients from the maternal blood and disposing of carbon dioxide and waste products.

Multipotential cardiac progenitor cells from several sources contribute to the formation of the heart. These include two distinct mesodermal populations of cardiac precursor cells, a primary (first) heart field and a second heart field. Neural crest cells also contribute to the heart. Mesodermal cells from the primitive streak migrate to form bilateral paired strands

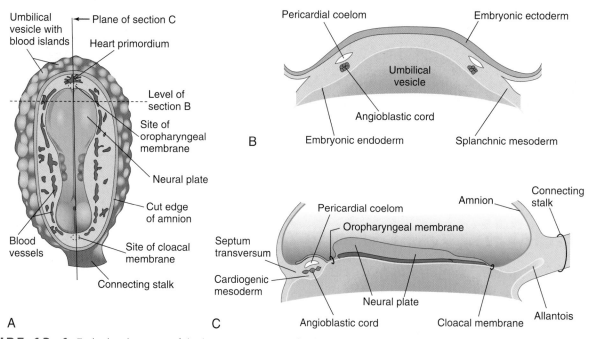

**FIGURE 13-1** Early development of the heart. **A,** Drawing of a dorsal view of an embryo (approximately 18 days). **B,** Transverse section of the embryo showing the angioblastic cords in the cardiogenic mesoderm and their relationship to the pericardial coelom. **C,** Longitudinal section of the embryo illustrating the relationship of the angioblastic cords to the oropharyngeal membrane, pericardial coelom, and septum transversum.

of the *primary heart field.* Cardiac progenitor cells from the pharyngeal mesoderm are constituted as the *second heart field,* which is located medial to the first heart field.

Successive stages in the development of blood and blood vessels (**angiogenesis**) are described in Chapter 4, Figure 4-11. Primordial blood vessels cannot be distinguished structurally as arteries or veins; however, they are named according to their future fates and relationship to the heart.

# EARLY DEVELOPMENT OF HEART AND BLOOD VESSELS

By day 18, the lateral mesoderm has somatopleure and splanchnopleure components; the latter gives rise to almost all of the heart components. These early endocardial cells separate from the mesoderm to create paired heart tubes. As lateral embryonic folding occurs, the **endocardial heart tubes** approach each other and fuse to form a single **heart tube** (see Figs. 13-7C and 13-9C). Fusion of the heart tubes begins at the cranial end of the developing heart and extends caudally. *The heart begins to beat at 22 to 23 days* (Fig. 13-2). Blood flow begins during the fourth week, and heartbeats can be visualized by Doppler ultrasonography (Fig. 13-3).

*Molecular studies* show that more than 500 genes are involved in the development of the mammalian heart. Several members of the T-box family of genes play an essential role in lineage determination, specification of the cardiac chambers, valvuloseptal development, and formation of the conducting system.

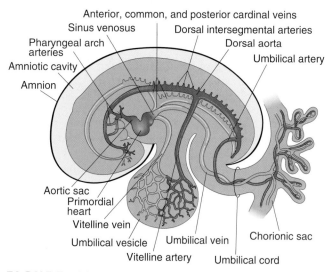

**FIGURE 13-2** Drawing of the embryonic cardiovascular system (approximately 26 days), showing vessels on the left side. The umbilical vein carries well-oxygenated blood and nutrients from the chorionic sac to the embryo. The umbilical arteries carry poorly oxygenated blood and waste products from the embryo to the chorionic sac (outermost embryonic membrane).

Gene expression analysis and lineage tracing experiments suggest that progenitor cells from the pharyngeal mesoderm, located anterior to the early heart tube (**anterior heart field**), gives rise to ventricular myocardium and the myocardial wall of the outflow tract. Moreover,

**FIGURE 13–3** Endovaginal scan of a 4-week embryo. A, Bright (echogenic) 2.4-mm embryo *(calipers)*. B, Cardiac activity of 116 beats/min demonstrated with motion mode. Calipers used to encompass two beats.

another wave of progenitor cells from the pharyngeal mesoderm (**second heart field**) also contributes to the rapid growth and elongation of the heart tube. The myocardium of the left ventricle and the anterior pole of the heart tube are derived mostly from the second field. *Expression of Hes-1 in pharyngeal endoderm and mesoderm (second heart field) plays an essential role for the development of the outflow tract.*

*The basic helix–loop–helix genes, dHAND and eHAND, are expressed in the paired primordial endocardial tubes and in later stages of cardiac morphogenesis. The MEF2C and Pitx-2 genes, which are expressed in cardiogenic precursor cells emerging from the primitive streak before formation of the heart tubes (Wnt 3a–mediated), also appear to be essential regulators in early cardiac development.*

## Development of Veins Associated with Embryonic Heart

Three paired veins drain into the primordial heart of a 4-week embryo (see Fig. 13-2):

- **Vitelline veins** return poorly oxygenated blood from the umbilical vesicle.
- **Umbilical veins** carry well-oxygenated blood from the chorionic sac.
- **Common cardinal veins** return poorly oxygenated blood from the body of the embryo to the heart.

The **vitelline veins** follow the omphaloenteric duct into the embryo. This duct is the narrow tube connecting the umbilical vesicle with the midgut (see Fig. 11-1). After passing through the septum transversum, which provides a pathway for blood vessels, the vitelline veins enter the venous end of the heart, the **sinus venosus** (Fig. 13-4A, and see also Fig. 13-2). The left vitelline vein regresses, and the right vitelline vein forms most of the **hepatic portal system** (see Fig. 13-5B and C), as well as a portion of the inferior vena cava (IVC). As the **liver primordium** grows into the septum transversum, the **hepatic cords** anastomose around preexisting endothelium-lined spaces. These spaces, the primordia of the **hepatic sinusoids**, later become linked to the vitelline veins.

The **umbilical veins** run on each side of the liver and carry well-oxygenated blood from the placenta to the sinus venosus (see Fig. 13-2). As the liver develops, the umbilical veins lose their connection with the heart and empty into the liver. The right umbilical vein disappears during the seventh week, leaving the left umbilical vein as the only vessel carrying well-oxygenated blood from the placenta to the embryo.

Transformation of the umbilical veins may be summarized as follows (Fig. 13-5):

- The right umbilical vein and the cranial part of the left umbilical vein between the liver and the sinus venosus degenerate.
- The persistent caudal part of the left umbilical vein becomes the **umbilical vein**, which carries all the blood from the placenta to the embryo.
- A large venous shunt, the **ductus venosus**, develops within the liver (see Fig. 13-5B) and connects the umbilical vein with the IVC. The ductus venosus forms a bypass through the liver, enabling most of the blood from the placenta to pass directly to the heart without passing through the capillary networks of the liver.

The **cardinal veins** constitute the main venous drainage system of the embryo (see Figs. 13-2 and 13-4A). The **anterior and posterior cardinal veins**, the earliest veins to develop, drain cranial and caudal parts of the embryo, respectively. They join the **common cardinal veins**, which enter the sinus venosus (see Fig. 13-2). During the eighth week, the **anterior cardinal veins** are connected by an **anastomosis** (see Fig. 13-5A and B), which shunts blood from the left to the right anterior cardinal vein. This anastomotic shunt becomes the **left brachiocephalic vein** when the caudal part of the left anterior cardinal vein

**FIGURE 13–4** Illustrations of the primordial veins of bodies (trunks) of embryos (ventral views). Initially, three systems of veins are present: the umbilical veins from the chorion, vitelline veins from the umbilical vesicle, and cardinal veins from the body of the embryos. Next the subcardinal veins appear, and finally the supracardinal veins develop. **A,** At 6 weeks. **B,** At 7 weeks. **C,** At 8 weeks. **D,** Adult. This drawing illustrates the transformations that produce the adult venous pattern. *IVC,* Inferior vena cava; *L.,* left; *R.,* right; *v.,* vein; *vv.,* veins. *(Modified from Arey LB: Developmental anatomy, revised ed 7, Philadelphia, 1974, Saunders.)*

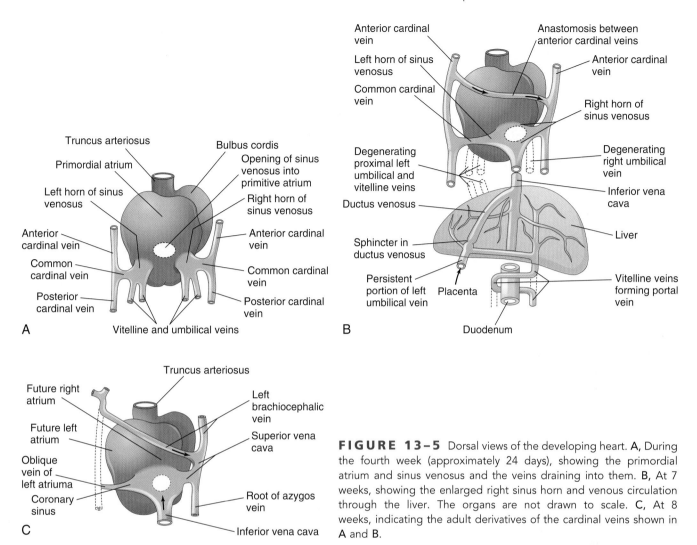

**FIGURE 13-5** Dorsal views of the developing heart. **A,** During the fourth week (approximately 24 days), showing the primordial atrium and sinus venosus and the veins draining into them. **B,** At 7 weeks, showing the enlarged right sinus horn and venous circulation through the liver. The organs are not drawn to scale. **C,** At 8 weeks, indicating the adult derivatives of the cardinal veins shown in **A** and **B.**

degenerates (see Figs. 13-4*D* and 13-5*C*). The **superior vena cava (SVC)** forms from the right anterior cardinal vein and the right common cardinal vein.

The **posterior cardinal veins** develop primarily as the vessels of the **mesonephroi** (interim kidneys) and largely disappear with these transitory kidneys (see Chapter 12, Fig. 12-5*F*). The only adult derivatives of these veins are the root of the azygos vein and common iliac veins (see Fig. 13-4*D*). The subcardinal and supracardinal veins gradually develop and replace and supplement the posterior cardinal veins (see Fig. 13-4*A* to *D*).

The **subcardinal veins** appear first (see Fig. 13-4*A*). They are connected with each other through the **subcardinal anastomosis** and with the posterior cardinal veins through the mesonephric sinusoids. The subcardinal veins form the stem of the left renal vein, the suprarenal veins, the gonadal veins (testicular and ovarian), and a segment of the IVC (see Fig. 13-4*D*). The subcardinal veins become disrupted in the region of the kidneys (see Fig. 13-4*C*). Cranial to this region, they are united by an anastomosis that is represented in the adult by the **azygos**

and **hemiazygos veins** (see Figs. 13-4*D* and 13-5*C*). Caudal to the kidneys, the left supracardinal vein degenerates; however, the right supracardinal vein becomes the inferior part of the IVC (see Fig. 13-4*D*).

## Development of Inferior Vena Cava

The **IVC** forms during a series of changes in the primordial veins of the trunk of the body, which occur when blood, returning from the caudal part of the embryo, is shifted from the left to the right side of the body. The IVC is composed of four main segments (Fig. 13-4*C*):

- A *hepatic segment* derived from the hepatic vein (proximal part of the right vitelline vein) and hepatic sinusoids
- A *prerenal segment* derived from the right subcardinal vein
- A *renal segment* derived from the subcardinal–supracardinal anastomosis
- A *postrenal segment* derived from the right supracardinal vein

## ANOMALIES OF VENAE CAVAE

Because of the many transformations that occur during the formation of the SVC and IVC, variations in their adult forms may occur. The most common anomaly of the IVC is for its abdominal course to be interrupted; as a result, blood drains from the lower limbs, abdomen, and pelvis to the heart through the azygos system of veins.

### Double Superior Venae Cavae

Persistence of the left anterior cardinal vein results in a **persistent left SVC**; hence, there are two superior venae cavae (Fig. 13-6). The anastomosis that usually forms the left brachiocephalic vein is small or absent. The abnormal left SVC, derived from the left anterior cardinal and common cardinal veins, opens into the right atrium through the coronary sinus.

### Left Superior Vena Cava

The left anterior cardinal vein and common cardinal vein may form a left SVC, and the right anterior cardinal vein and common cardinal vein, which usually form the SVC, degenerate. As a result, blood from the right side is carried by the brachiocephalic vein to the unusual left SVC, which empties into the coronary sinus.

### Absence of Hepatic Segment of Inferior Vena Cava

Occasionally, the hepatic segment of the IVC fails to form. As a result, blood from inferior parts of the body drains into the right atrium through the azygos and hemiazygos veins. The hepatic veins open separately into the right atrium.

### Double Inferior Venae Cavae

In unusual cases, the IVC inferior to the renal veins is represented by two vessels; usually, the left one is much smaller. This condition probably results from failure of an anastomosis to develop between the veins of the trunk (see Fig. 13-4B). As a result, the inferior part of the left supracardinal vein persists as a second IVC.

## Pharyngeal Arch Arteries and Other Branches of Dorsal Aortae

As the pharyngeal arches form during the fourth and fifth weeks, they are supplied by arteries, the **pharyngeal arch arteries,** that arise from the **aortic sac** and terminate in the **dorsal aortae** (see Fig. 13-2). Neural crest cells delaminate from the neural tube and contribute to the formation of the outflow tract of the heart and to the pharyngeal arch arteries. Initially, the paired dorsal aortae run through the entire length of the embryo. Later, the caudal portions of the aortae fuse to form a single lower thoracic/abdominal aorta. Of the remaining paired dorsal aortae, the right one regresses and the left one becomes the primordial aorta.

### Intersegmental Arteries

Thirty or so branches of the dorsal aorta, the **intersegmental arteries,** pass between and carry blood to the somites and their derivatives (see Fig. 13-2). These arteries in the neck join to form a longitudinal artery on each side, the **vertebral artery.** Most of the original connections of the arteries to the dorsal aorta disappear.

In the thorax, the intersegmental arteries persist as **intercostal arteries.** Most of the intersegmental arteries in the abdomen become **lumbar arteries;** however, the fifth pair of lumbar intersegmental arteries remains as the **common iliac arteries.** In the sacral region, the intersegmental arteries form the **lateral sacral arteries.**

## Fate of Vitelline and Umbilical Arteries

The unpaired ventral branches of the **dorsal aorta** supply the umbilical vesicle, allantois, and chorion (see Fig. 13-2). The **vitelline arteries** pass to the umbilical vesicle and later to the primordial gut, which forms from the incorporated part of the umbilical vesicle. Only three vitelline artery derivatives remain: the celiac arterial trunk to the foregut, the superior mesenteric artery to the midgut, and the inferior mesenteric artery to the hindgut.

**FIGURE 13-6** Computed tomography scan showing a duplicated superior vena cava. Note the aorta (A), the right superior vena cava (R, unopacified), and the left superior vena cava (L, with contrast from left arm injection).

The paired **umbilical arteries** pass through the *connecting stalk* (primordial umbilical cord) and become continuous with vessels in the **chorion**, the embryonic part of the placenta (see Chapter 7, Fig. 7-5). The umbilical arteries carry poorly oxygenated blood to the placenta (see Fig. 13-2). The proximal parts of these arteries become **internal iliac arteries** and **superior vesical arteries**. The distal parts of the umbilical arteries become modified and form the **medial umbilical ligaments**.

## LATER DEVELOPMENT OF HEART

The external layer of the embryonic heart tube, the primordial **myocardium**, is formed from splanchnic mesoderm surrounding the pericardial cavity (cardiac precursors of the anterior, or second, heart field; Figs. 13-7A and B and 13-8B). At this stage, the developing heart is composed of a thin endothelial tube, separated from a thick myocardium by a gelatinous matrix of connective tissue, cardiac jelly (Fig. 13-8C and D).

The **endothelial tube** becomes the internal endothelial lining of the heart, or **endocardium**, and the primordial myocardium becomes the muscular wall of the heart, or **myocardium**. The visceral pericardium, or **epicardium**, is derived from mesothelial cells that arise from the external surface of the **sinus venosus** and spread over the myocardium (Fig. 13-7D and F).

As folding of the head region occurs, the heart and pericardial cavity come to lie ventral to the foregut

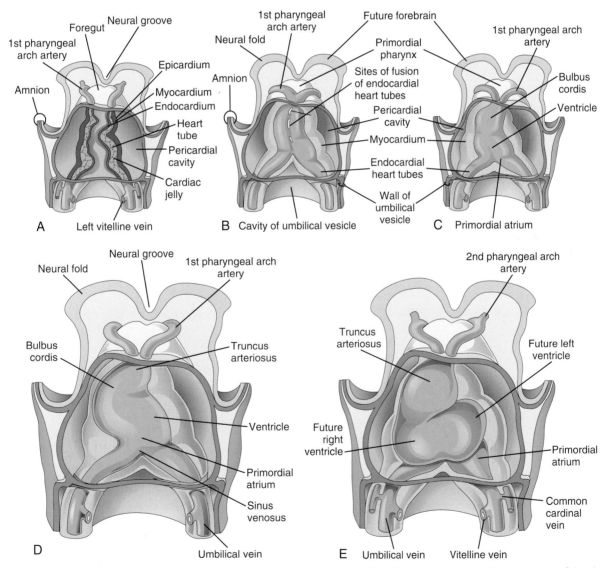

**FIGURE 13–7** Drawings showing fusion of the heart tubes and looping of the tubular heart. **A** to **C**, Ventral views of the developing heart and pericardial region (22 to 35 days). The ventral pericardial wall has been removed to show the developing myocardium and fusion of the two heart tubes to form a tubular heart. The endothelium of the heart tube forms the endocardium of the heart. **D** and **E**, As the straight tubular heart elongates, it bends and undergoes looping, which forms a D-loop (D, dextro; rightward) that produces an S-shaped heart.

**FIGURE 13–8** A, Dorsal view of an embryo (approximately 20 days). B, Schematic transverse section of the heart region of the embryo illustrated in A, showing the two heart tubes and lateral folds of the body. C, Transverse section of a slightly older embryo showing the formation of the pericardial cavity and fusion of the heart tubes. D, Similar section (approximately 22 days) showing the tubular heart suspended by the dorsal mesocardium. E, Schematic drawing of the heart (approximately 28 days) showing degeneration of the central part of the dorsal mesocardium and formation of the transverse pericardial sinus. The *arrow* shows the bending of the primordial heart. The tubular heart now has a D-loop (D, dextro; rightward). F, Transverse section of the embryo at the level seen in E, showing the layers of the heart wall.

and caudal to the **oropharyngeal membrane** (Fig. 13-9*A* to *C*). Concurrently, the tubular heart elongates and develops alternate dilations and constrictions (see Fig. 13-7*C* to *E*): the **bulbus cordis** (composed of the *truncus arteriosus, conus arteriosus,* and *conus cordis*), ventricle, atrium, and **sinus venosus**. The growth of the heart tube results from the addition of cells, cardiomyocytes, differentiating from mesoderm at the dorsal wall of the pericardium. Progenitor cells added to the rostral and caudal poles of the heart tube form a proliferative pool of mesodermal cells located in the dorsal wall of the pericardial cavity and the pharyngeal arches.

The **truncus arteriosus** is continuous cranially with the aortic sac from which the pharyngeal arch arteries arise (Fig. 13-10*A*). Progenitor cells from the **second heart field** contribute to the formation of the arterial and venous ends of the developing heart. The **sinus venosus** receives the umbilical, vitelline, and common cardinal veins from the chorion, umbilical vesicle, and embryo, respectively (Fig. 13-10*B*). The arterial and venous ends of the heart are fixed by the pharyngeal arches and septum transversum, respectively. Before the formation of the heart tube, the homeobox transcription factor (Pitx2c) is expressed in the left heart-forming field and plays an important role in the left–right patterning of the heart tube during formation of the cardiac loop. The tubular heart undergoes a dextral (right-handed) looping at approximately 23 to 28 days, forming a U-shaped D-loop (**bulboventricular loop**) that results in a heart with its apex pointing to the left (see Figs. 13-7*D* and *E* and 13-8*E*).

*The signaling molecule(s) and cellular mechanisms responsible for cardiac looping are complex and involve pathways including the BMP, Notch, Wnt, and SHH pathways; all are required in heat tube remodeling.* As the primordial heart bends, the atrium and sinus venosus come to lie dorsal to the truncus arteriosus, bulbus cordis, and ventricle (see Fig. 13-10*B* and *C*). By this stage, the sinus venosus has developed lateral expansions, the right and left **sinus horns** (see Fig. 13-5*A*).

As the heart elongates and bends, it gradually invaginates into the pericardial cavity (see Figs. 13-7*B* to *D* and 13-8*C* and *D*). The heart is initially suspended from the dorsal wall by a mesentery (double layer of peritoneum), the dorsal mesocardium. The central part of the mesentery soon degenerates, forming a communication, the **transverse pericardial sinus**, between the right and left sides of the pericardial cavity (see Fig. 13-8*E* and *F*). The heart is now attached only at its cranial and caudal ends.

## Circulation through Primordial Heart

The initial contractions of the heart are of myogenic origin (in or starting from muscle). The muscle layers of the atrium and ventricle outflow tract are continuous, and contractions occur in peristalsis-like waves that begin in the sinus venosus. At first, circulation through the primordial heart is an ebb-and-flow type; however, by the end of the fourth week, coordinated contractions of

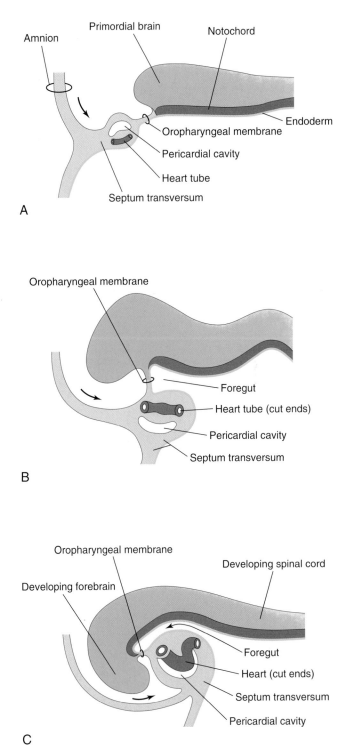

**FIGURE 13–9** Illustrations of longitudinal sections through the cranial half of embryos during the fourth week, showing the effect of the head fold *(arrows)* on the position of the heart and other structures. A and B, As the head fold develops, the tubular heart and pericardial cavity move ventral to the foregut and caudal to the oropharyngeal membrane. C, Note that the positions of the pericardial cavity and septum transversum have reversed with respect to each other. The septum transversum now lies posterior to the pericardial cavity, where it will form the central tendon of the diaphragm.

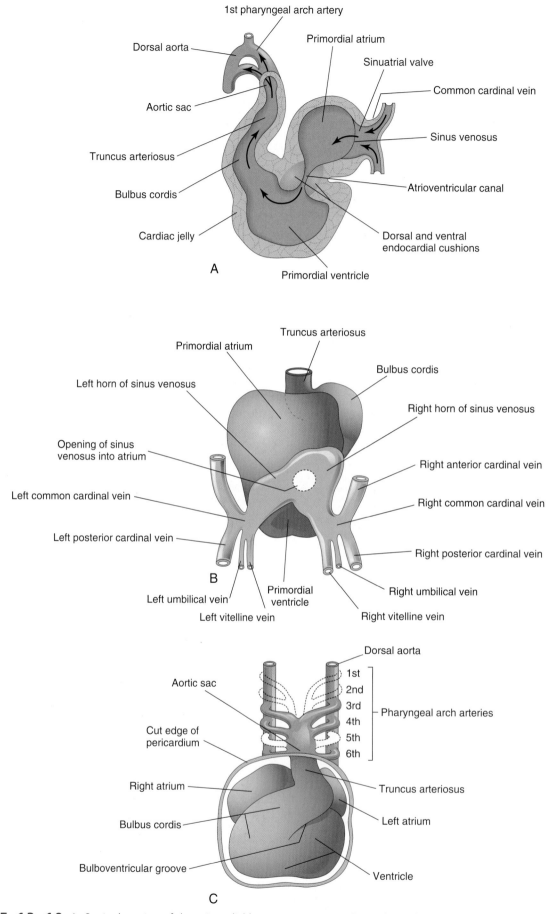

**FIGURE 13–10** A, Sagittal section of the primordial heart at approximately 24 days, showing blood flow through it *(arrows)*. B, Dorsal view of the heart at approximately 26 days showing the horns of the sinus venosus and the dorsal location of the primordial atrium. C, Ventral view of the heart and pharyngeal arch arteries at approximately 35 days. The ventral wall of the pericardial sac has been removed to show the heart in the pericardial cavity.

**FIGURE 13-11** A and B, Sagittal sections of the heart during the fourth and fifth weeks, illustrating blood flow through the heart and division of the atrioventricular canal. The *arrows* are passing through the sinuatrial orifice. **C**, Fusion of the atrioventricular endocardial cushions. **D**, Coronal section of the heart at the plane shown in **C**. Note that the septum primum and interventricular septa have started to develop.

the heart result in unidirectional flow. Blood enters the **sinus venosus** (see Fig. 13-10*A* and *B*) from the:

- Embryo through the common cardinal veins
- Developing placenta through the umbilical veins
- Umbilical vesicle through the vitelline veins

Blood from the sinus venosus enters the **primordial atrium**; flow from it is controlled by sinuatrial (SA) valves (Fig. 13-11*A* to *D*). The blood then passes through the **atrioventricular (AV) canal** into the primordial ventricle. When the ventricle contracts, blood is pumped through the **bulbus cordis** and **truncus arteriosus** into the **aortic sac**, from which it is distributed to the pharyngeal arch arteries in the pharyngeal arches (see Fig. 13-10*C*). The blood then passes into the **dorsal aortae** for distribution to the embryo, umbilical vesicle, and placenta (see Fig. 13-2).

## Partitioning of Primordial Heart

Partitioning of the AV canal, primordial atrium, ventricle, and outflow tract begins during the middle of the fourth week. Partitioning is essentially completed by the end of

the eighth week. Although described separately, these processes occur concurrently.

### Partitioning of Atrioventricular Canal

Toward the end of the fourth week, **AV endocardial cushions** form on the dorsal and ventral walls of the AV canal (see Fig. 13-11*A* and *B*). The AV endocardial cushions develop from a specialized extracellular matrix (**cardiac jelly**), as well as neural crest cells (see Fig. 13-8*C* and *D*). As these masses of tissue are invaded by mesenchymal cells during the fifth week, the AV endocardial cushions approach each other and fuse, dividing the AV canal into **right and left canals** (see Fig. 13-11*C* and *D*). These canals partially separate the primordial atrium from the primordial ventricle, and the endocardial cushions function as **AV valves**. The septal valves are derived from the fused superior and inferior endocardial cushions. The mural leaflets (thin, flattened layers of wall) are mesenchymal in origin.

After **inductive signals** emanate from the myocardium of the AV canal, a segment of the inner endocardial cells undergoes **epithelial–mesenchymal transformation**, and the resulting cells then invade the extracellular matrix.

The transformed AV cushions contribute to the formation of the valves and membranous septa of the heart.

*Transforming growth factor-β (TGF-β₁ and TGF-β₂), bone morphogenetic proteins (BMP-2A and BMP-4), the zinc finger protein Slug, and an activin receptor–like kinase (ChALK2) have been reported to be involved in the epithelial–mesenchymal transformation and formation of the endocardial cushions.*

### Partitioning of Primordial Atrium

Beginning at the end of the fourth week, the primordial atrium is divided into right and left atria by the formation of, and subsequent modification and fusion of, two septa: the septum primum and septum secundum (Figs. 13-12 and 13-13).

The **septum primum**, a thin crescent-shaped membrane, grows toward the fusing endocardial cushions from the roof of the **primordial atrium**, partially dividing the common atrium into right and left halves. As the curtain-like muscular septum primum grows, a large opening, or **foramen primum**, is located between its crescentic free edge and the endocardial cushions (see Figs. 13-12C and 13-13A to C). This foramen (perforation) serves as a shunt, enabling oxygenated blood to pass from the right to the left atrium. The foramen becomes progressively smaller and disappears as the mesenchymal cap of the septum primum fuses with the fused AV endocardial cushions to form a **primordial AV septum** (see Fig. 13-13D and D₁). *Molecular studies have revealed that a distinct population of extracardiac progenitor cells from the second heart field migrates through the dorsal mesocardium to complete the lateral septum; Shh signaling plays a critical role in this process.*

Before the foramen primum disappears, perforations produced by **apoptosis** (programmed cell death) appear in the central part of the septum primum. As the septum fuses with the fused endocardial cushions, these perforations coalesce to form another opening in the septum primum, the **foramen secundum**. Concurrently, the free edge of the septum primum fuses with the left side of the fused endocardial cushions, obliterating the foramen primum (see Figs. 13-12D and 13-13D). The foramen secundum ensures continued shunting of oxygenated blood from the right to the left atrium.

The **septum secundum**, a thick crescentic muscular fold, grows from the muscular ventrocranial wall of the right atrium, immediately adjacent to the septum primum (see Fig. 13-13D₁). As this thick septum grows during the fifth and sixth weeks, it gradually overlaps the foramen secundum in the septum primum (see Fig. 13-13E). The septum secundum forms an incomplete partition between the atria; consequently, a **foramen ovale** forms. The cranial part of the septum primum, initially attached to the roof of the left atrium, gradually disappears (see Fig. 13-13G₁ and H₁). The remaining part of the septum, attached to the fused endocardial cushions, forms the flap-like valve of the foramen ovale.

*Before birth*, the foramen ovale allows most of the oxygenated blood entering the right atrium from the IVC to pass into the left atrium (Fig. 13-14A, and see also Fig. 13-13H). It also prevents the passage of blood in the opposite direction because the septum primum closes against the relatively rigid septum secundum (see Fig. 13-14B).

*After birth*, the foramen ovale functionally closes because the pressure in the left atrium is higher than that in the right atrium. At approximately 3 months, the valve of the foramen ovale fuses with the septum secundum, forming the **oval fossa** (fossa ovalis; see Fig. 13-14B). As a result, the interatrial septum becomes a complete partition between the atria.

### Changes in Sinus Venosus

Initially, the sinus venosus opens into the center of the dorsal wall of the **primordial atrium**, and its right and left horns are approximately the same size (see Fig. 13-5A). Progressive enlargement of the right horn results from two **left-to-right shunts of blood**:

- The first shunt results from transformation of the vitelline and umbilical veins.
- The second shunt occurs when the anterior cardinal veins are connected by an anastomosis (see Fig. 13-5B and C). This communication shunts blood from the left to the right anterior cardinal vein; this shunt becomes the **left brachiocephalic vein**. The right anterior cardinal vein and right common cardinal vein become the **SVC** (Fig. 13-15C).

By the end of the fourth week, the right horn of the sinus venosus is noticeably larger than the left horn (Fig. 13-15A). As this occurs, the **SA orifice** moves to the right and opens in the part of the primordial atrium that will become the adult right atrium (see Figs. 13-11 and 13-15C). As the right horn of the sinus enlarges, it receives all the blood from the head and neck through the SVC and from the placenta and caudal regions of the body through the IVC. Initially, the **sinus venosus** is a separate chamber of the heart and opens into the dorsal wall of the right atrium (see Fig. 13-10A and B). The left horn becomes the **coronary sinus**, and the right horn is incorporated into the wall of the right atrium (see Fig. 13-15B and C).

Because it is derived from the sinus venosus, the smooth part of the wall of the right atrium is called the **sinus venarum of the right atrium** (see Fig. 13-15B and C). The remainder of the anterior internal surface of the atrial wall and the conical muscular pouch, the **right auricle**, has a rough trabeculated appearance. These two parts are derived from the primordial atrium. The smooth part and the rough part are demarcated internally in the right atrium by a vertical ridge, the **crista terminalis**, and externally by a shallow groove, the **sulcus terminalis** (see Fig. 13-15B). The crista terminalis represents the cranial part of the right SA valve (see Fig. 13-15C). The caudal part of the SA valve forms the valves of the IVC and coronary sinus. The left SA valve fuses with the septum secundum and is incorporated with it into the interatrial septum.

### Primordial Pulmonary Vein and Formation of Left Atrium

Most of the wall of the left atrium is smooth because it is formed by incorporation of the **primordial pulmonary**

**FIGURE 13–12** Drawings of the heart showing partitioning of the atrioventricular canal, primordial atrium, and ventricle. **A,** Sketch showing the plane of the sections B to E. **B,** Frontal section of the heart during the fourth week (approximately 28 days) showing the early appearance of the septum primum, interventricular septum, and dorsal atrioventricular endocardial cushion. **C,** Frontal section of the heart (approximately 32 days) showing perforations in the dorsal part of the septum primum. **D,** Section of the heart (approximately 35 days) showing the foramen secundum. **E,** Section of the heart (at approximately 8 weeks) showing the heart after it is partitioned into four chambers. The *arrow* indicates the flow of well-oxygenated blood from the right into the left atrium. **F,** Sonogram of a second-trimester fetus showing the four chambers of the heart. Note the septum secundum *(arrow)*. *SVC,* Superior vena cava.

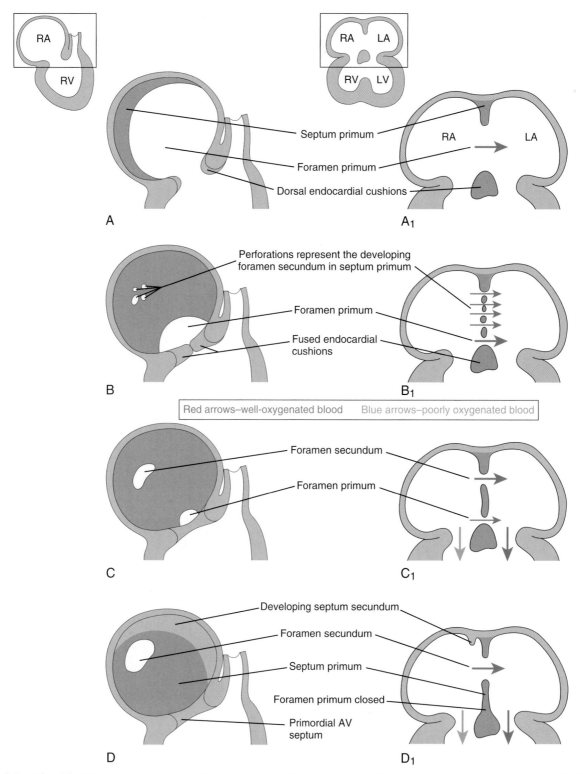

**FIGURE 13–13** Diagrammatic sketches illustrating progressive stages in partitioning of the primordial atrium. **A** to **H**, Sketches of the developing interatrial septum as viewed from the right side. **A₁** to **H₁** are coronal sections of the developing interatrial septum. Note that as the septum secundum grows, it overlaps the opening in the septum primum, the foramen secundum. Observe the valve of the foramen ovale in **G₁** and **H₁**. When pressure in the right atrium *(RA)* exceeds that in the left atrium *(LA)*, blood passes from the right to the left side of the heart. When the pressures are equal or higher in the left atrium, the valve closes the foramen ovale (**G₁**). *AV*, Atrioventricular; *LV*, left ventricle; *RV*, right ventricle.

**FIGURE 13-13, cont'd**

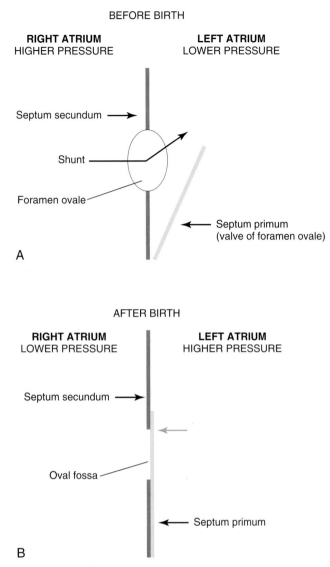

BEFORE BIRTH

**RIGHT ATRIUM**
HIGHER PRESSURE

**LEFT ATRIUM**
LOWER PRESSURE

Septum secundum

Shunt

Foramen ovale

Septum primum
(valve of foramen ovale)

A

AFTER BIRTH

**RIGHT ATRIUM**
LOWER PRESSURE

**LEFT ATRIUM**
HIGHER PRESSURE

Septum secundum

Oval fossa

Septum primum

B

**FIGURE 13–14** Diagrams illustrating the relationship of the septum primum to the foramen ovale and septum secundum. **A,** Before birth, well-oxygenated blood is shunted from the right atrium through the foramen ovale into the left atrium when the pressure increases. When the pressure decreases in the right atrium, the flap-like valve of the foramen ovale is pressed against the relatively rigid septum secundum. This closes the foramen ovale. **B,** After birth, the pressure in the left atrium increases as the blood returns from the lungs. Eventually the septum primum is pressed against the septum secundum and adheres to it, permanently closing the foramen ovale and forming the oval fossa.

vein (Fig. 13-16*A*). This vein develops as an outgrowth of the dorsal atrial wall, just to the left of the septum primum. As the atrium expands, the primordial pulmonary vein and its main branches are incorporated into the wall of the left atrium. As a result, four pulmonary veins are formed (Fig. 13-16*C* and *D*).

Molecular studies have confirmed that atrial myoblasts migrate into the walls of the pulmonary veins.

The functional significance of this **pulmonary cardiac muscle** (pulmonary myocardium) is uncertain. The small left auricle is derived from the primordial atrium; its internal surface has a rough trabeculated appearance.

## ANOMALOUS PULMONARY VENOUS CONNECTIONS

In the disorder involving total anomalous pulmonary venous connections, none of the pulmonary veins connect with the left atrium. Most commonly, the veins coalesce into a confluence of one of the systemic veins posterior to the left atrium and then drain into this chamber of the heart. In the disorder involving partial anomalous pulmonary venous connections, one or more pulmonary veins have similar anomalous connections but the others have normal connections.

### Partitioning of Primordial Ventricle

Division of the ventricle is indicated by a median ridge, the muscular **interventricular septum**, in the floor of the ventricle near its apex (see Fig. 13-12*B*). Myocytes (muscles) from both the left and right primordial ventricles contribute to the formation of the **muscular part of the interventricular septum**. The septum has a concave free edge (Fig. 13-17*A*). Initially, it attains most of its height from dilation of the ventricles on each side of the muscular interventricular septum (Fig. 13-17*B*). Later, there is active proliferation of myoblasts in the septum, which increases the size of the septum.

Until the seventh week, there is a crescent-shaped **interventricular foramen** between the free edge of the interventricular septum and the fused endocardial cushions. The foramen permits communication between the right and left ventricles (Fig. 13-18*B*, and see also Fig. 13-17). The foramen usually closes by the end of the seventh week as the **bulbar ridges** fuse with the endocardial cushion (Fig. 13-18*C* to *E*).

Closure of the interventricular foramen and formation of the membranous part of the interventricular septum result from the fusion of tissues from three sources: the right bulbar ridge, the left bulbar ridge, and the endocardial cushion. The **membranous part of the interventricular septum** is derived from an extension of tissue from the right side of the endocardial cushion to the muscular part of the septum as well as neural crest cells. This tissue merges with the **aorticopulmonary septum** and the thick muscular part of the interventricular septum (Fig. 13-19*C*, and see also Fig. 13-18*E*). After closure of the interventricular foramen and formation of the membranous part of the interventricular septum, the pulmonary trunk is in communication with the right ventricle and the aorta communicates with the left ventricle (see Fig. 13-18*E*).

Cavitation of the ventricular walls forms a spongy mass of muscular bundles, **trabeculae carneae**. Some of

☐ Left horn of sinus venosus    ☐ Right horn of sinus venosus

A

Primordial atrium

Left anterior cardinal vein

Future superior vena cava

Right horn of sinus venosus

Left common cardinal vein

Site of opening of sinus venosus into right atrium

Left horn of sinus venosus

Inferior vena cava

B

Aorta

Superior vena cava

Pulmonary artery

Sinus venarum of right atrium

Pulmonary veins

Sulcus terminalis

Oblique vein of left atrium

Right auricle

Coronary sinus

Inferior vena cava

Middle cardiac vein

C

Superior vena cava

Crista terminalis

Septum secundum

Sinus venarum
(smooth part
of atrial wall)

Foramen ovale

Septum primum

Rough part
of atrial wall

Valve of coronary sinus

Right auricle

Valve of inferior vena cava

**FIGURE 13–15** Diagrams illustrating the fate of the sinus venosus. **A,** Dorsal view of the heart (approximately 26 days) showing the primordial atrium and sinus venosus. **B,** Dorsal view at 8 weeks after incorporation of the right horn of the sinus venosus into the right atrium. The left horn of the sinus horn becomes the coronary sinus. **C,** Internal view of the fetal right atrium showing: (1) the smooth part of the wall of the right atrium (sinus venarum) derived from the right horn of the sinus venosus and (2) the crista terminalis and valves of the inferior vena cava and coronary sinus that are derived from the right sinuatrial valve. The primordial right atrium becomes the right auricle, a conical muscular pouch. The *arrows* indicate the flow of blood.

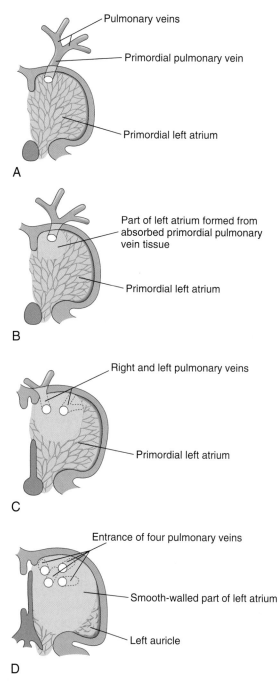

**FIGURE 13–16** Diagrammatic sketches illustrating absorption of the pulmonary vein into the left atrium. **A**, At 5 weeks, showing the primordial pulmonary vein opening into the primordial left atrium. **B**, Later stage showing partial absorption of the primordial pulmonary vein. **C**, At 6 weeks, showing the openings of two pulmonary veins into the left atrium resulting from absorption of the primordial pulmonary vein. **D**, At 8 weeks, showing four pulmonary veins with separate atrial orifices. The primordial left atrium becomes the left auricle, a tubular appendage of the atrium. Most of the left atrium is formed by absorption of the primordial pulmonary vein and its branches.

these bundles become **papillary muscles** and **tendinous cords (chordae tendineae)**. The cords run from the papillary muscles to the AV valves (see Fig. 13-19C and D).

---

## FETAL CARDIAC ULTRASONOGRAPHY

Cardiac screening using high-resolution real-time ultrasonography is usually first performed between 18 and 22 weeks of gestation (Fig. 13-20), when the heart is large enough to examine. Based on international convention, a four-chamber view of the heart is obtained (see Fig. 13-20) and the great vessels are also examined for anomalies.

---

### Partitioning of Bulbus Cordis and Truncus Arteriosus

During the fifth week, active proliferation of mesenchymal cells in the walls of the **bulbus cordis** results in the formation of **bulbar ridges** (Fig. 13-21B and C, and see also Fig. 13-18C and D). Similar ridges that are continuous with the bulbar ridges form in the **truncus arteriosus**. The **bulbar** and **truncal ridges** are derived largely from neural crest mesenchyme (see Fig. 13-21B and C).

**Neural crest cells** migrate through the primordial pharynx and pharyngeal arches to reach the ridges. As this occurs, the bulbar and truncal ridges undergo a 180-degree spiraling. The spiral orientation of the ridges, caused in part by streaming of blood from the ventricles, results in the formation of a spiral **aorticopulmonary septum** when the ridges fuse (see Fig. 13-21D to G). This septum divides the bulbus cordis and truncus arteriosus into two arterial channels, the ascending aorta and pulmonary trunk. Because of the spiraling of the aorticopulmonary septum, the **pulmonary trunk** twists around the **ascending aorta** (see Fig. 13-21H).

The **bulbus cordis** is incorporated into the walls of the definitive ventricles (see Fig. 13-18A and B):

- In the right ventricle, the bulbus cordis is represented by the **conus arteriosus** (infundibulum), which is the origin of the pulmonary trunk.
- In the left ventricle, the bulbus cordis forms the walls of the **aortic vestibule**, the part of the ventricular cavity just inferior to the aortic valve.

### Development of Cardiac Valves

When partitioning of the **truncus arteriosus** is nearly completed (see Fig. 13-21A to C), the **semilunar valves** begin to develop from three swellings of subendocardial tissue around the orifices of the aorta and pulmonary trunk. Cardiac precursor neural crest cells also contribute to this tissue. These swellings are hollowed out and reshaped to form three thin-walled cusps (Fig. 13-22, and see also Fig. 13-19C and D). The **AV valves** (tricuspid and mitral valves) develop similarly from localized proliferations of tissue around the AV canals.

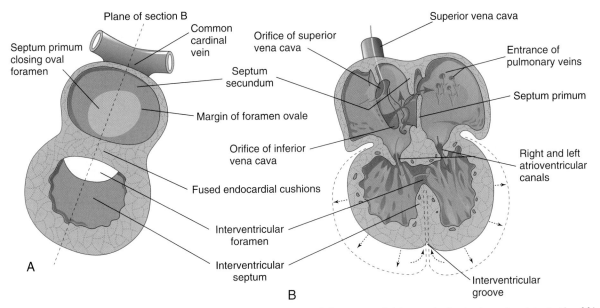

**FIGURE 13–17** Schematic diagrams illustrating partitioning of the primordial heart. A, Sagittal section late in the fifth week showing the cardiac septa and foramina. B, Coronal section at a slightly later stage illustrating the directions of blood flow through the heart (*blue arrows*) and expansion of the ventricles (*black arrows*).

## Conducting System of Heart

Initially, the muscle in the primordial atrium and ventricle is continuous. As the chambers of the heart form, their myocardium conducts the wave of depolarization faster than the remaining myocardium. Throughout development, this impulse wave moves from the venous pole to the arterial pole of the heart. *The atrium acts as the interim pacemaker of the heart*, but the sinus venosus soon takes over this function. The **SA node** develops during the fifth week. This node is located in the right wall of the sinus venosus, but it becomes incorporated into the wall of the right atrium with the sinus venosus (see Fig. 13-19*A* and *D*). The SA node is located high in the right atrium, near the entrance of the **SVC**.

After incorporation of the sinus venosus, cells from its left wall are found in the base of the interatrial septum just anterior to the opening of the coronary sinus. Together with cells from the AV region, they form the **AV node** and **bundle**, which are located just superior to the endocardial cushions. The fibers arising from the **AV bundle** pass from the atrium into the ventricle and split into right and left **bundle branches**. These branches are distributed throughout the **ventricular myocardium** (see Fig. 13-19*D*). The two chambers (atrial and ventricular) become electrically isolated by fibrous tissue; only the AV node and bundle can conduct.

*The SA node, AV node, and AV bundle are richly supplied by nerves*; however, the conducting system is well developed before these nerves enter the heart. This specialized tissue is normally the only signal pathway from the atria to the ventricles. As the four chambers of the heart develop, a band of connective tissue grows in from the epicardium (visceral layer of the serous pericardium), subsequently separating the muscle of the atria from that of the ventricles. The connective tissue forms part of the **cardiac skeleton** (fibrous skeleton of the heart). The parasympathetic innervation of the heart is formed by neural crest cells that also play an essential role in the development of the conducting system of the heart.

## BIRTH DEFECTS OF HEART AND GREAT VESSELS

Congenital heart defects (CHDs) are relatively common, with a frequency of six to eight cases per 1000 live births, and are a leading cause of neonatal morbidity. Some CHDs are caused by single-gene or chromosomal mechanisms. Other defects result from exposure to teratogens such as the **rubella virus** (see Chapter 20, Table 20-6); however, in many cases the cause is unknown. Most CHDs are thought to be caused by multiple factors that are genetic and environmental (i.e., **multifactorial inheritance**), each of which has a minor effect.

The molecular aspects of abnormal cardiac development are poorly understood, and gene therapy for infants with CHDs is at present a remote prospect. Imaging technology, such as real-time two-dimensional echocardiography, permits detection of fetal CHDs as early as the 16th week.

Most CHDs are well tolerated during fetal life; however, at birth, when the fetus loses contact with the maternal circulation, the impact of CHDs becomes apparent. Some types of CHDs cause very little disability; others are incompatible with extrauterine life. Because of recent advances in cardiovascular surgery, many types of CHDs can be palliated or corrected surgically, and fetal cardiac surgery may soon be possible for complex CHDs.

*Text continued on p. 317*

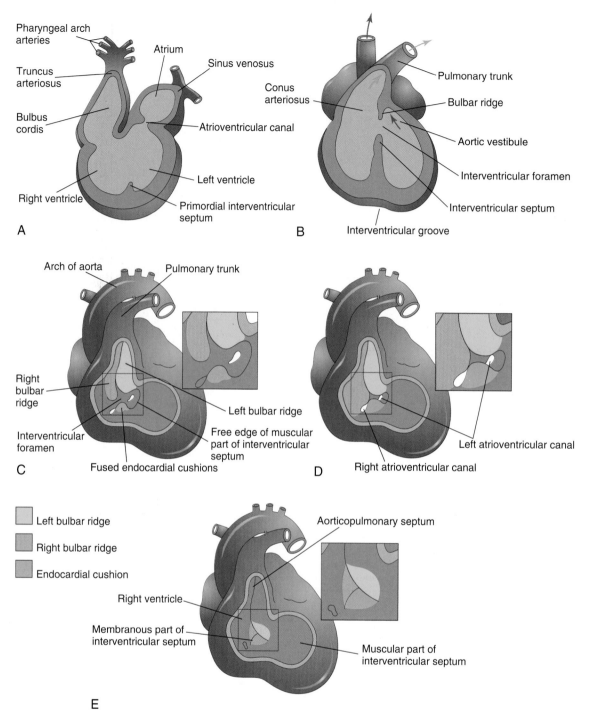

**FIGURE 13–18** Sketches illustrating incorporation of the bulbus cordis into the ventricles and partitioning of the bulbus cordis and truncus arteriosus into the aorta and pulmonary trunk. **A,** Sagittal section at 5 weeks showing the bulbus cordis as one of the chambers of the primordial heart. **B,** Schematic coronal section at 6 weeks, after the bulbus cordis has been incorporated into the ventricles to become the conus arteriosus of the right ventricle, which is the origin of the pulmonary trunk and aortic vestibule of the left ventricle. The *arrow* indicates blood flow. **C to E,** Schematic drawings illustrating closure of the interventricular foramen and formation of the membranous part of the interventricular septum. The walls of the truncus arteriosus, bulbus cordis, and right ventricle have been removed. **C,** At 5 weeks, showing the bulbar ridges and fused atrioventricular endocardial cushions. **D,** At 6 weeks, showing how proliferation of subendocardial tissue diminishes the interventricular foramen. **E,** At 7 weeks, showing the fused bulbar ridges, the membranous part of the interventricular septum formed by extensions of tissue from the right side of the atrioventricular endocardial cushions, and closure of the interventricular foramen.

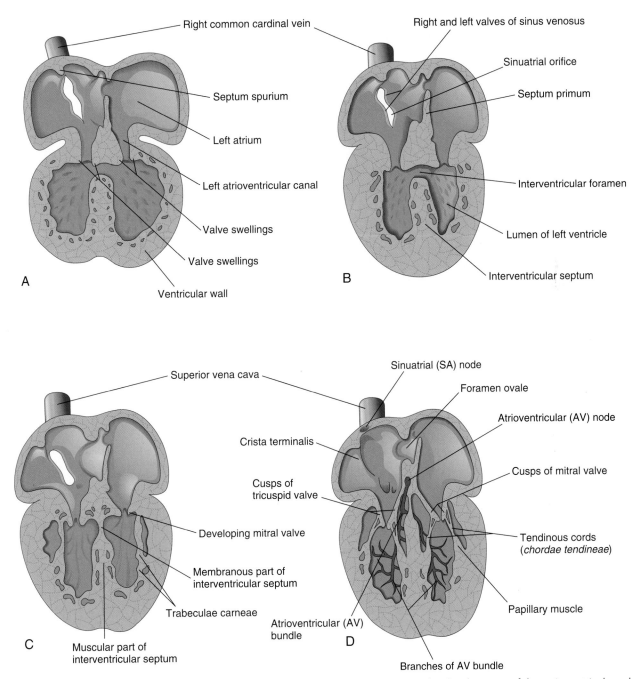

**FIGURE 13–19** Schematic sections of the heart illustrating successive stages in the development of the atrioventricular valves, tendinous cords (Latin *chordae tendineae*), and papillary muscles. **A,** At 5 weeks. **B,** At 6 weeks. **C,** At 7 weeks. **D,** At 20 weeks, showing the conducting system of the heart.

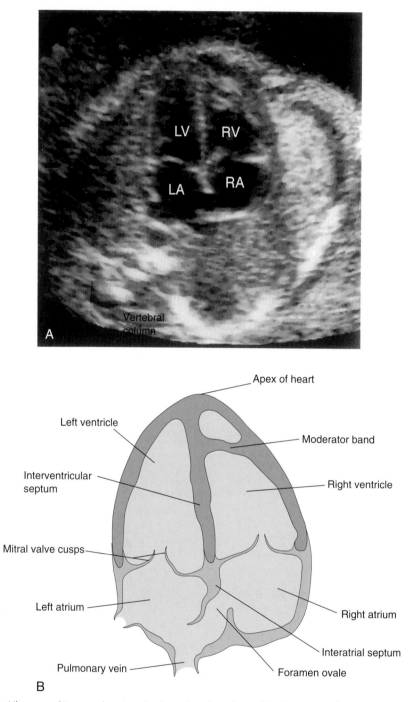

**FIGURE 13–20** A, Ultrasound image showing the four-chamber view of the heart in a fetus of approximately 20 weeks' gestation. B, Orientation sketch (modified from the American Institute of Ultrasound in Medicine Technical Bulletin, Performance of the Basic Fetal Cardiac Ultrasound Examination). The scan was obtained across the fetal thorax. The ventricles and atria are well formed, and two atrioventricular valves are present. The moderator band is one of the trabeculae carneae that carries part of the right branch of the atrioventricular bundle. *LA,* Left atrium; *LV,* left ventricle; *RA,* right atrium; *RV,* right ventricle.

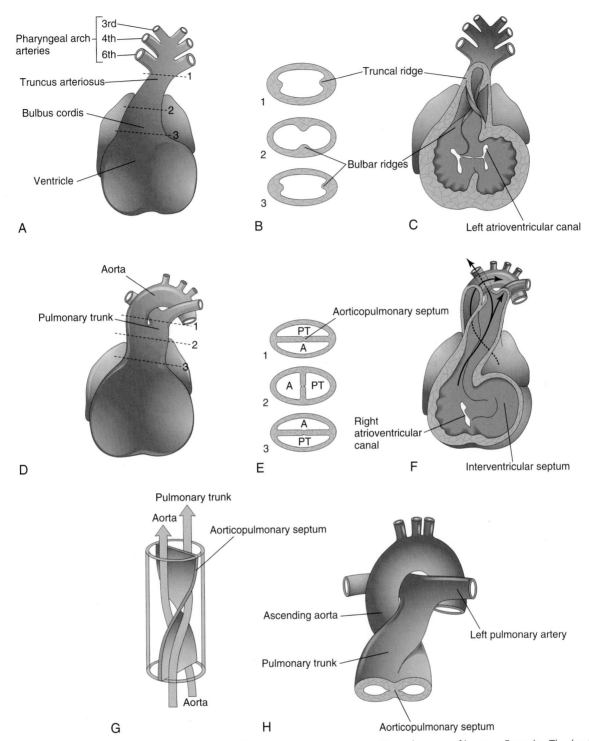

**FIGURE 13–21** Partitioning of the bulbus cordis and truncus arteriosus. **A,** Ventral aspect of heart at 5 weeks. The *broken lines* and *arrows* indicate the levels of the sections shown in **A. B,** Transverse sections of the truncus arteriosus and bulbus cordis, illustrating the truncal and bulbar ridges. **C,** The ventral wall of the heart and truncus arteriosus have been removed to demonstrate these ridges. **D,** Ventral aspect of heart after partitioning of the truncus arteriosus. The *broken lines* and *arrows* indicate the levels of the sections shown in **E. E,** Sections through the newly formed aorta *(A)* and pulmonary trunk *(PT)*, showing the aorticopulmonary septum. **F,** At 6 weeks. The ventral wall of the heart and pulmonary trunk have been removed to show the aorticopulmonary septum. **G,** Diagram illustrating the spiral form of the aorticopulmonary septum. **H,** Drawing showing the great arteries (ascending aorta and pulmonary trunk) twisting around each other as they leave the heart.

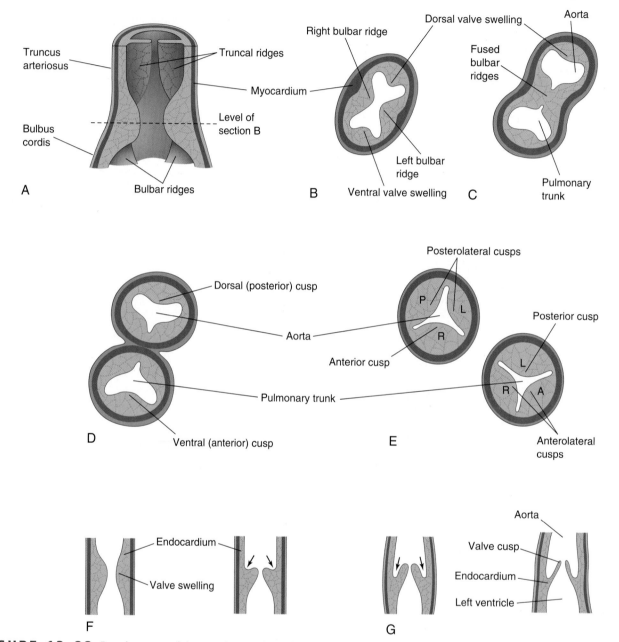

**FIGURE 13–22** Development of the semilunar valves of the aorta and pulmonary trunk. **A,** Sketch of a section of the truncus arteriosus and bulbus cordis showing the valve swellings. **B,** Transverse section of the bulbus cordis. **C,** Similar section after fusion of the bulbar ridges. **D,** Formation of the walls and valves of the aorta and pulmonary trunk. **E,** Rotation of the vessels has established the adult relations of the valves. **F** and **G,** Longitudinal sections of the aorticoventricular junction illustrating successive stages in the hollowing (arrows) and thinning of the valve swellings to form the valve cusps. *L,* Left; *P,* posterior; *R,* right.

## DEXTROCARDIA

If the embryonic heart tube bends to the left instead of to the right (Fig. 13-23B), the heart is displaced to the right and the heart and its vessels are reversed left to right as in a mirror image of their normal configuration. *Dextrocardia is the most frequent positional defect of the heart.* In **dextrocardia with situs inversus** (transposition of the abdominal viscera), the incidence of accompanying cardiac defects is low. If there is no other associated vascular abnormality, the heart functions normally.

In **isolated dextrocardia**, the abnormal position of the heart is not accompanied by displacement of other viscera. This defect is usually complicated by severe cardiac defects (e.g., a single ventricle and transposition of the great vessels). *The TGF-β factor Nodal is involved in looping of the heart tube, but its role in dextrocardia is unclear.*

## ECTOPIA CORDIS

In **ectopia cordis**, a rare condition, the heart is in an abnormal location (Fig. 13-24). *In the thoracic form of ectopia cordis*, the heart is partly or completely exposed on the thoracic wall. Ectopia cordis is usually associated with widely separated halves of the sternum (nonfusion) and an open pericardial sac. Death occurs in most cases during the first few days after birth, usually from infection, cardiac failure, or hypoxemia. If there are no severe cardiac defects, surgical therapy usually consists of covering the heart with skin. In some cases of ectopia cordis, the heart protrudes through the diaphragm into the abdomen.

The clinical outcome for patients with ectopia cordis has improved, and many children have survived to adulthood. The most common thoracic form of ectopia cordis results from faulty development of the sternum and pericardium because of failure of complete fusion of the lateral folds in the formation of the thoracic wall during the fourth week (see Chapter 5, Fig. 5-1).

NORMAL

Truncus arteriosus
Bulbus cordis
Ventricle
Atrium
Sinus venosus

A

DEXTROCARDIA

Truncus arteriosus
Bulbus cordis
Ventricle
Atrium
Sinus venosus

B

**FIGURE 13–23** The embryonic heart tube during the fourth week. **A,** Normal looping of the tubular heart to the right. **B,** Abnormal looping of the tubular heart to the left.

**FIGURE 13–24** A, Fetal magnetic resonance image using single-shot turbo spin echo shows the heart in an ectopic position *(asterisk)* and eventration of a part of the liver at the midline *(arrow)*. Notice the small thoracic cavity *(t)*. No malformation of the central nervous system could be seen. **B1,** Two-dimensional ultrasound shows a transposition of the great arteries with a hypoplastic right outlet and a partial evisceration of the liver *(arrow)* through a midline supraumbilical abdominal wall defect **(B2). B3,** Three-dimensional reconstruction shows the heart protruding through the sternum. *Ao,* Aortic outflow tract; *LV,* left ventricle; *Po,* pulmonary outflow tract; *RV,* right ventricle. *(From Leyder M, van Berkel E, Done K, et al: Ultrasound meets magnetic resonance imaging in the diagnosis of pentalogy of Cantrell with complete ectopy of the heart, Gynecol Obstet (Sunnyvale) 4:200, 2014.)*

## ATRIAL SEPTAL DEFECTS

An **atrial septal defect (ASD)** is a common CHD and occurs more frequently in females than males. The most common form of ASD is **patent foramen ovale** (Fig. 13-25*B*). A **probe patent foramen ovale** is present in up to 25% of people (see Fig. 13-25*B*). In this circumstance, a probe can be passed from one atrium to the other through the superior part of the floor of the oval fossa.

*This form of ASD is not clinically significant,* but a probe patent foramen ovale may be forced open because of other cardiac defects and contribute to the functional pathology of the heart. Probe patent foramen ovale results from incomplete adhesion between the flap-like valve of the foramen ovale and the *septum secundum* after birth.

There are four clinically significant **types of ASD** (Figs. 13-26 and 13-27): ostium secundum defect, endocardial cushion defect with ostium primum defect, sinus venosus defect, and common atrium. The first two types of ASD are relatively common.

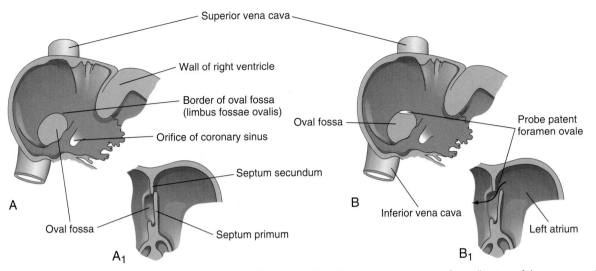

**FIGURE 13–25** A, Normal postnatal appearance of the right side of the interatrial septum after adhesion of the septum primum to the septum secundum. $A_1$, Sketch of a section of the interatrial septum illustrating formation of the oval fossa in the right atrium. Note that the floor of the oval fossa is formed by the septum primum. B and $B_1$, Similar views of a probe patent foramen ovale resulting from incomplete adhesion of the septum primum to the septum secundum. Some well-oxygenated blood can enter the right atrium via a patent foramen ovale; however, if the opening is small it is usually of no hemodynamic significance.

## ATRIAL SEPTAL DEFECTS—cont'd

Ostium secundum ASDs (see Figs. 13-26A to D and 13-27) are in the area of the oval fossa and include defects of the septum primum and septum secundum. Ostium secundum ASDs are well tolerated during childhood; symptoms such as **pulmonary hypertension** (e.g., fibrosis of the lung) usually appear in the 30s or later. Closure of the ASD has traditionally been carried out at open heart surgery, but more recently, endovascular catheter-based closures have been accomplished; mortality rates for either approach have been less than 1%. The defects may be multiple, and in symptomatic older children, defects of 2 cm or more in diameter are not unusual. Females with ASD outnumber males 3 to 1. Ostium secundum ASDs are one of the most common types of CHDs yet are the least severe.

A **patent foramen ovale** usually results from abnormal resorption of the septum primum during the formation of the foramen secundum. If resorption occurs in abnormal locations, the septum primum is fenestrated or net-like (see Fig. 13-26A). If excessive resorption of the septum primum occurs, the resulting short septum primum will not close the foramen ovale (see Fig. 13-26B). If an abnormally large foramen ovale occurs because of defective development of the septum secundum, a normal septum primum will not close the abnormal foramen ovale at birth (see Fig. 13-26C).

A small isolated patent foramen ovale is of no hemodynamic significance; however, if there are other defects (e.g., pulmonary stenosis or atresia), blood is shunted through the ovale into the left atrium and produces **cyanosis** (deficient oxygenation of blood). Large ostium secundum ASDs may also occur because of a combination of excessive resorption of the septum primum and a large foramen ovale (see Figs. 13-26D and 13-27).

Endocardial cushion defects with ostium primum ASDs are less common forms of ASDs (see Fig. 13-26E). Several cardiac defects are grouped together under this heading because they result from the same developmental defect, a deficiency of the endocardial cushions and the AV septum. The septum primum does not fuse with the endocardial cushions; as a result, there is a **patent foramen primum–ostium primum defect**. Usually, there is also a cleft in the anterior cusp of the mitral valve. In the less common complete type of endocardial cushion and AV septal defects, fusion of the endocardial cushions fails to occur. As a result, there is a large defect in the center of the heart, an **AV septal defect** (Fig. 13-28A). This type of ASD occurs in approximately 20% of persons with Down syndrome; otherwise, it is a relatively uncommon cardiac defect. It consists of a continuous interatrial and interventricular defect with markedly abnormal AV valves.

All **sinus venosus ASDs** (high ASDs) are located in the superior part of the interatrial septum close to the entry of the SVC (see Fig. 13-26F). A sinus venosus defect is a rare type of ASD. It results from incomplete absorption of the sinus venosus into the right atrium and/or abnormal development of the septum secundum. This type of ASD is commonly associated with partial anomalous pulmonary venous connections.

**Common atrium** is a rare cardiac defect in which the interatrial septum is absent. This defect is the result of failure of the septum primum and septum secundum to develop (combination of ostium secundum, ostium primum, and sinus venosus defects).

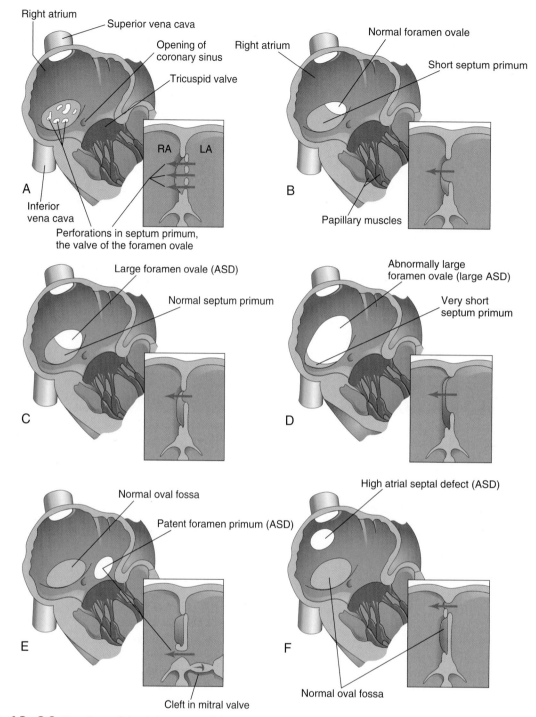

**FIGURE 13–26** Drawings of the right aspect of the interatrial septum. The adjacent sketches of sections of the septa illustrate various types of atrial septal defect (ASD). **A,** Patent foramen ovale resulting from resorption of the septum primum in abnormal locations. **B,** Patent foramen ovale caused by excessive resorption of the septum primum (short flap defect). **C,** Patent foramen ovale resulting from an abnormally large foramen ovale. **D,** Patent foramen ovale resulting from an abnormally large foramen ovale and excessive resorption of the septum primum. **E,** Endocardial cushion defect with primum-type ASD. The adjacent section shows the cleft in the anterior cusp of the mitral valve. **F,** Sinus venosus ASD. The high septal defect resulted from abnormal absorption of the sinus venosus into the right atrium. In **E** and **F,** note that the oval fossa has formed normally. Arrows indicate the direction of the flow of blood.

## VENTRICULAR SEPTAL DEFECTS

Ventricular septal defects (VSDs) *are the most common types of CHDs*, accounting for approximately 25% of heart defects. VSDs occur more frequently in males than in females. VSDs may occur in any part of the interventricular septum (see Fig. 13-28B), but **membranous VSD** is the most common type (Fig. 13-29A, and see also Fig. 13-28B). Frequently, during the first year, 30% to 50% of small VSDs close spontaneously.

Incomplete closure of the interventricular foramen results from failure of the membranous part of the interventicular septum to develop. This results from failure of an extension of subendocardial tissue to grow from the right side of the **endocardial cushion** and fuse with the aorticopulmonary septum and the muscular part of the interventricular septum (see Fig. 13-18C to E). Large VSDs with excessive pulmonary blood flow (Fig. 13-30) and pulmonary hypertension result in **dyspnea** (difficult breathing) and cardiac failure early in infancy.

**Muscular VSD** is a less common type of defect and may appear anywhere in the muscular part of the interventricular septum. Sometimes there are multiple small defects, producing what is sometimes called the "Swiss cheese" VSD. Muscular VSDs probably occur because of excessive cavitation of myocardial tissue during formation of the ventricular walls and the muscular part of the interventricular septum.

Absence of the interventricular septum (**single ventricle**, or common ventricle), resulting from failure of the interventricular septum to form, is extremely rare and results in a **three-chambered heart** (Latin, *cor triloculare biatriatum*). When there is a single ventricle, the atria empty through a single common valve or two separate AV valves into a single ventricular chamber. The aorta and pulmonary trunk arise from the ventricle. **Transposition of the great arteries** (**TGA**; see Fig. 13-32) and a rudimentary outlet chamber are present in most infants with a single ventricle. Some children die during infancy from **congestive heart failure**.

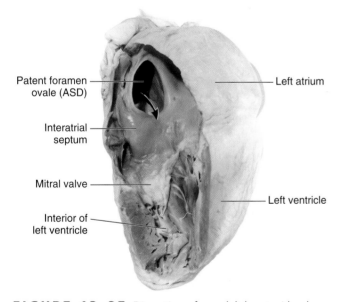

Patent foramen ovale (ASD)
Interatrial septum
Mitral valve
Interior of left ventricle
Left atrium
Left ventricle

**FIGURE 13–27** Dissection of an adult heart with a large patent foramen ovale. The *arrow* passes through a large atrial septal defect *(ASD)*, which resulted from an abnormally large foramen ovale and excessive resorption of the septum primum. This is referred to as a secundum-type ASD, and it is one of the most common types of congenital heart diseases.

## PERSISTENT TRUNCUS ARTERIOSUS

**Persistent truncus arteriosus** results from failure of the truncal ridges and the aorticopulmonary septum to develop normally and divide the truncus arteriosus into the aorta and pulmonary trunk (Fig. 13-31A and B). A **single arterial trunk**, the truncus arteriosus, arises from the heart and supplies the systemic, pulmonary, and coronary circulations. A VSD is always present with a truncus arteriosus defect; the truncus arteriosus straddles the VSD (see Fig. 13-31B).

Recent studies indicate that developmental arrest of the outflow tract, **semilunar valves**, and aortic sac in the early embryo (days 31–32) is involved in the pathogenesis of truncus arteriosus defects. The common type of truncus arteriosus defect is a single arterial vessel that branches to form the **pulmonary trunk** and **ascending aorta** (see Fig. 13-31A and B). In the next most common type of truncus arteriosus defect, the right and left pulmonary arteries arise close together from the dorsal wall of the truncus arteriosus (Fig. 13-31C). Less common types are illustrated in Figure 13-31D and E.

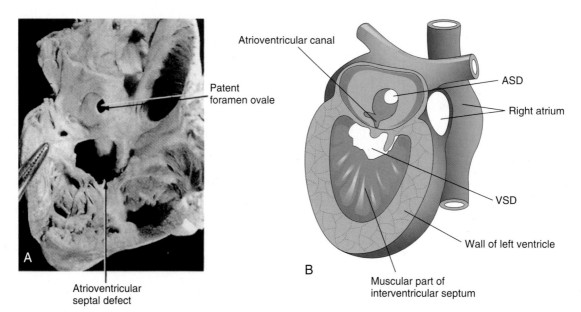

**FIGURE 13–28** A, An infant's heart sectioned and viewed from the right side, showing a patent foramen ovale and an atrioventricular septal defect. B, Schematic drawing of a heart illustrating various septal defects. *ASD,* Atrial septal defect; *VSD,* ventricular septal defect. (*A, From Lev M:* Autopsy diagnosis of congenitally malformed hearts, *Springfield, IL, 1953, Charles C. Thomas.*)

**FIGURE 13–29** A, Ultrasound image of the heart of a second-trimester fetus with an atrioventricular *(AV)* canal (atrioventricular septal) defect. An atrial septal defect and a ventricular septal defect are also present. *Ao,* Aorta. B, Orientation drawing.

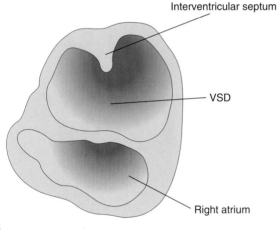

**FIGURE 13–30** A, Ultrasound scan of a fetal heart at 23 weeks with an atrioventricular septal defect and a large ventricular septal defect *(VSD)*. B, Orientation drawing.

## AORTICOPULMONARY SEPTAL DEFECT

Aorticopulmonary septal defect is a rare condition in which there is an opening (**aortic window**) between the aorta and pulmonary trunk near the aortic valve. The aorticopulmonary defect results from a localized defect in the formation of the **aorticopulmonary septum**. The presence of pulmonary and aortic valves and an intact interventricular septum distinguishes this defect from the persistent truncus arteriosus defect.

## TRANSPOSITION OF THE GREAT ARTERIES

Transposition of the great arteries (TGA) is the common cause of cyanotic heart disease in neonates (Fig. 13-32). TGA is often associated with other cardiac defects (e.g., ASD and VSD). In typical cases, the aorta lies anterior and to the right of the pulmonary trunk and arises from the morphologic right ventricle, whereas the pulmonary trunk arises from the morphologic left ventricle. The associated ASD and VSD defects permit some interchange between the pulmonary and systemic circulations.

Because of these anatomic defects, **deoxygenated systemic venous blood** returning to the right atrium enters the right ventricle and then passes to the body through the aorta. Oxygenated pulmonary venous blood passes through the left ventricle back into the pulmonary circulation. With a patent foramen ovale and patency of the ductus arteriosus, there is some mixing of blood. However, in the absence of a patent foramen ovale, a balloon atrial septoplasty (creation of a hole between the atria) is lifesaving by permitting blood to flow from left to right while awaiting definitive surgical correction. Without surgical correction of the TGA, these infants usually die within a few months.

Many attempts have been made to explain the basis of TGA, but the **conal growth hypothesis** is favored by most investigators. According to this explanation, the **aorticopulmonary septum** fails to pursue a spiral course during partitioning of the bulbus cordis and truncus arteriosus. This defect is thought to result from failure of the **conus arteriosus** to develop normally during incorporation of the bulbus cordis into the ventricles. Defective migration of neural crest cells is involved.

## UNEQUAL DIVISION OF THE TRUNCUS ARTERIOSUS

Unequal division of the truncus arteriosus results when partitioning of the truncus arteriosus superior to the valves is unequal (Figs. 13-33A and 13-34B and C). One of the great arteries is large and the other is small. As a result, the **aorticopulmonary septum** is not aligned with the interventricular septum and a VSD develops; of the two vessels, the one with the larger diameter usually straddles the VSD (see Fig. 13-33B).

In **pulmonary valve stenosis**, the cusps of the pulmonary valve are fused to form a dome with a narrow central opening (see Fig. 13-34D).

In **infundibular stenosis**, the conus arteriosus (infundibulum) of the right ventricle is underdeveloped. The two types of pulmonary stenosis may occur. Depending on the degree of obstruction to blood flow, there is a variable degree of hypertrophy (greater bulk) of the right ventricle (see Fig. 13-33A and B).

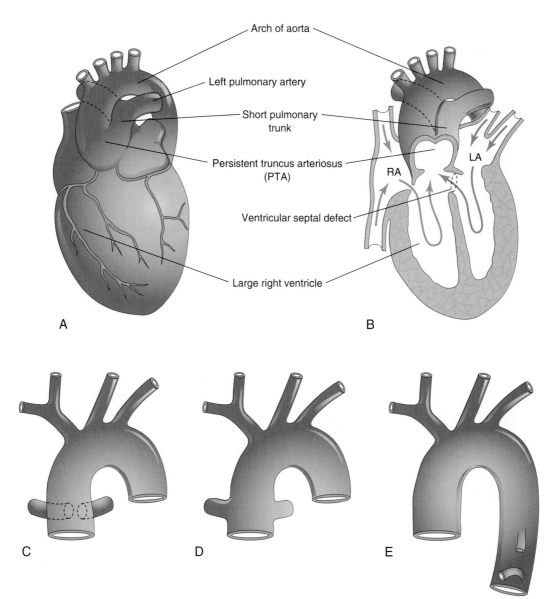

FIGURE 13-31 Illustrations of common types of persistent truncus arteriosus. A, The common trunk divides into the aorta and a short pulmonary trunk. B, Coronal section of the heart shown in A. Observe the circulation of blood in this heart *(arrows)* and the ventricular septal defect. *LA,* Left atrium; *RA,* right atrium. C, The right and left pulmonary arteries arise close together from the truncus arteriosus. D, The pulmonary arteries arise independently from the sides of the truncus arteriosus. E, No pulmonary arteries are present; the lungs are supplied by the bronchial arteries.

**FIGURE 13-32** Drawing of a heart illustrating transposition of the great arteries (TGA). The ventricular and atrial septal defects allow mixing of the arterial and venous blood. TGA is the most common single cause of cyanotic heart disease in neonates. This birth defect is often associated with other cardiac defects as shown (i.e., ventricular septal defect and atrial septal defect).

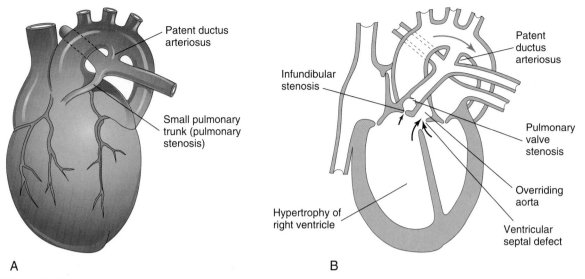

A                                                    B

**FIGURE 13–33** A, Drawing of an infant's heart showing a small pulmonary trunk (pulmonary stenosis), and a large aorta resulting from unequal partitioning of the truncus arteriosus. There is also hypertrophy of the right ventricle and a patent ductus arteriosus. B, Frontal section of this heart illustrating the tetralogy of Fallot. Observe the four cardiac defects of this tetralogy: pulmonary valve stenosis, ventricular septal defect, overriding aorta, and hypertrophy of right ventricle. The *arrows* indicate the flow of blood into the great vessels (aorta and pulmonary trunk).

## TETRALOGY OF FALLOT

Tetralogy of Fallot is a classic group of four cardiac defects (Figs. 13-35 and 13-36, and see also Fig. 13-33B) consisting of:

● Pulmonary artery stenosis (obstruction of right ventricular outflow)
● Ventricular septal defect
● Dextroposition of the aorta (overriding or straddling the aorta)
● Right ventricular hypertrophy

In these defects, the pulmonary trunk is usually small (see Fig. 13-33A) and there may be various degrees of pulmonary artery stenosis. Cyanosis *(deficient oxygenation of blood),* is an obvious sign of the tetralogy, but it is not usually present at birth.

The tetralogy results when division of the truncus arteriosus is unequal and the pulmonary trunk is stenotic. **Pulmonary atresia with VSD** is an extreme form of tetralogy of Fallot; the entire right ventricular output is through the aorta. Pulmonary blood flow is dependent on a patent ductus arteriosus or bronchial collateral vessels. Initial treatment may require surgical placement of a temporary shunt, but in many cases, primary surgical repair is the treatment of choice in early infancy.

## AORTIC STENOSIS AND AORTIC ATRESIA

In **aortic valve stenosis,** the edges of the valve are usually fused to form a dome with a narrow opening (see Fig. 13-34D). This defect may be congenital or develop after birth. The valvular stenosis causes extra work for the heart and results in **hypertrophy of the left ventricle** and abnormal **heart sounds (heart murmurs).**

In subaortic stenosis, there is often a band of fibrous tissue just inferior to the aortic valve. The narrowing of the aorta results from persistence of tissue that normally degenerates as the valve forms. **Aortic atresia** is present when obstruction of the aorta or its valve is complete.

## HYPOPLASTIC LEFT HEART SYNDROME

The left ventricle is small and nonfunctional (Fig. 13-37); the right ventricle maintains both pulmonary and systemic circulations. The blood passes through an **ASD** or a dilated foramen ovale from the left to the right side of the heart, where it mixes with the systemic venous blood.

In addition to the underdeveloped left ventricle, there is atresia of the aortic or mitral orifice and hypoplasia of the ascending aorta. Infants with this severe defect usually die during the first few weeks after birth. Disturbances in the migration of neural crest cells, in hemodynamic function, and in apoptosis and the proliferation of the extracellular matrix are likely responsible for the pathogenesis of many CHDs such as this syndrome.

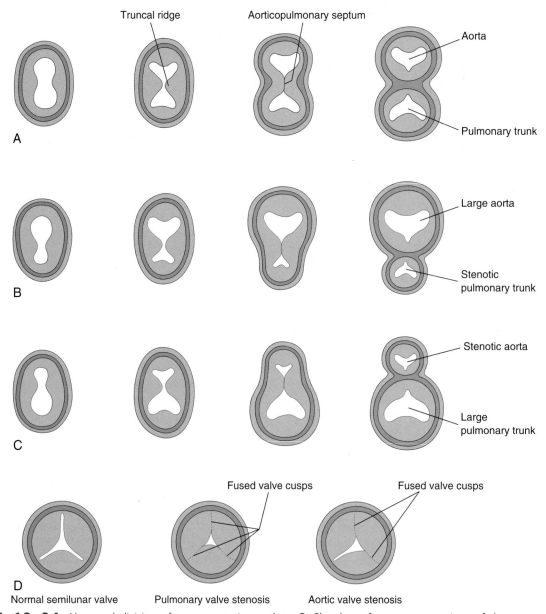

**FIGURE 13–34** Abnormal division of truncus arteriosus. A to C, Sketches of transverse sections of the truncus arteriosus, illustrating normal and abnormal partitioning of the truncus arteriosus. **A,** Normal. **B,** Unequal partitioning of the truncus arteriosus resulting in a small pulmonary trunk. **C,** Unequal partitioning resulting in a small aorta. **D,** Sketches illustrating a normal semilunar valve and stenotic pulmonary and aortic valves.

**FIGURE 13–35** A, Ultrasound image of the heart of a 20-week fetus with tetralogy of Fallot. Note that the large overriding aorta *(Ao)* straddles the interventricular septum. As a result, it receives blood from the left ventricle *(LV)* and right ventricle *(RV)*. IVS, Interventricular septum; *LA,* left atrium. **B,** Orientation drawing.

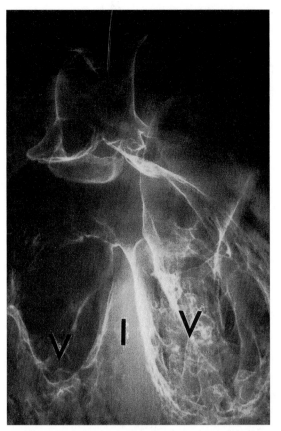

**FIGURE 13–36** Tetralogy of Fallot. Fine barium powder was injected into the heart. Note the two ventricles (V), interventricular septum (I), interventricular septal defect at the superior margin, and origin of the aorta above the right ventricle (overriding aorta). The main pulmonary artery is not visualized.

# DERIVATIVES OF PHARYNGEAL ARCH ARTERIES

As the pharyngeal arches develop during the fourth week, they are supplied by pharyngeal arch arteries from the **aortic sac** (Fig. 13-38B). Mesodermal cells migrate from the arches to the aortic sac, connecting the pharyngeal arch arteries to the outflow tract. These arteries terminate in the dorsal aorta on the ipsilateral side. Although six pairs of arch arteries usually develop, they are not present at the same time (see Fig. 13-38B and C). By the time the sixth pair of arch arteries has formed, the first two pairs have disappeared (see Fig. 13-38C). During the eighth week, the primordial **pharyngeal arch arterial pattern** is transformed into the final fetal arterial arrangement (Fig. 13-39C).

*Molecular studies indicate that the transcription factor Tbx1 regulates migration of the neural crest cells that contribute to the formation of the pharyngeal arch arteries.*

## Derivatives of First Pair of Pharyngeal Arch Arteries

Most of these arteries disappear, but remnants of them form part of the **maxillary arteries**, which supply the ears, teeth, and muscles of the eye and face. These arteries may also contribute to the formation of the **external carotid arteries** (see Fig. 13-39B).

## Derivatives of Second Pair of Pharyngeal Arch Arteries

Dorsal parts of these arteries persist and form the stems of the **stapedial arteries**; these small vessels run through

**FIGURE 13–37** A, Ultrasound image of the heart of a second-trimester fetus with a hypoplastic left heart. Note that the left ventricle (LV) is much smaller than the right ventricle (RV). This is an oblique scan of the fetal thorax through the long axis of the ventricles. B, Orientation drawing.

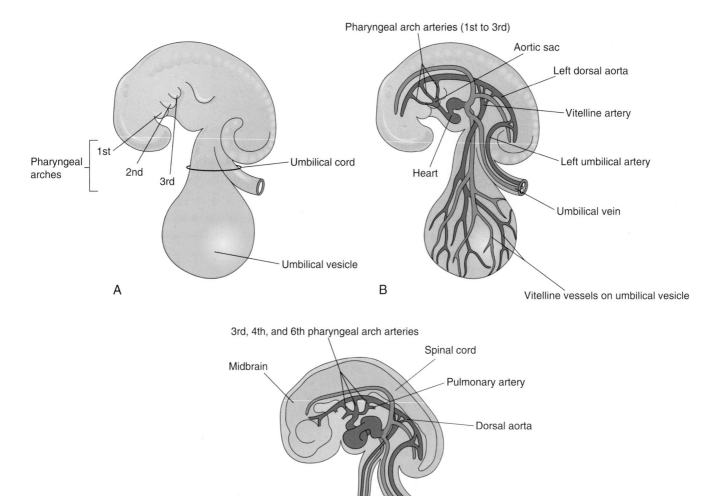

**FIGURE 13-38** Pharyngeal arches and pharyngeal arch arteries. **A,** Left side of an embryo (approximately 26 days). **B,** Schematic drawing of this embryo showing the left pharyngeal arch arteries arising from the aortic sac, running through the pharyngeal arches, and terminating in the left dorsal aorta. **C,** An embryo (approximately 37 days) showing the single dorsal aorta and that most of the first two pairs of pharyngeal arch arteries have degenerated.

the ring of the stapes, a small bone in the middle ear (see Fig. 18-18C).

## Derivatives of Third Pair of Pharyngeal Arch Arteries

Proximal parts of these arteries form the **common carotid arteries,** which supply structures in the head (see Fig. 13-39D). Distal parts of these arteries join with the dorsal **aortae** to form the **internal carotid arteries,** which supply

the middle ears, orbits, brain, meninges, and pituitary gland.

## Derivatives of Fourth Pair of Pharyngeal Arch Arteries

The *left fourth arch artery* forms **part of the arch of the aorta** (see Fig. 13-39C). The proximal part of the artery develops from the **aortic sac** and the distal part is derived from the **left dorsal aorta.** The *right fourth arch artery*

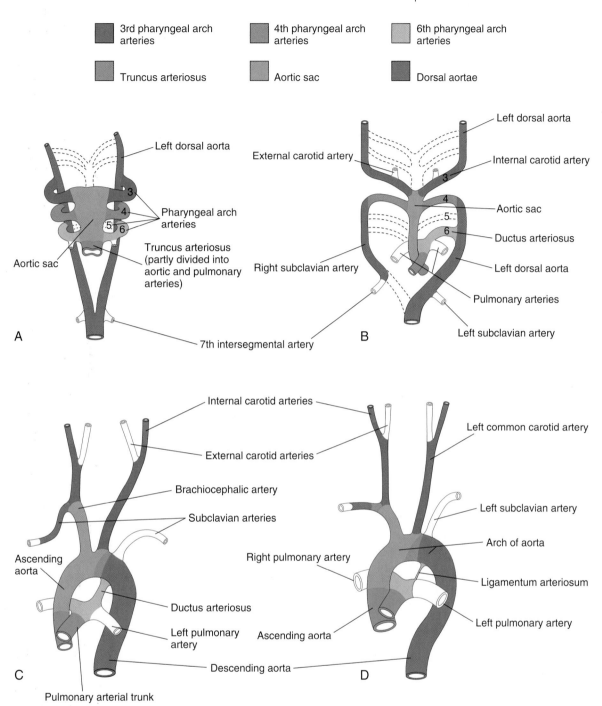

**FIGURE 13–39** Schematic drawings illustrating the arterial changes that result during transformation of the truncus arteriosus, aortic sac, pharyngeal arch arteries, and dorsal aortae into the adult arterial pattern. The vessels that are not colored are not derived from these structures. **A,** Pharyngeal arch arteries at 6 weeks; by this stage, the first two pairs of arteries have largely disappeared. **B,** Pharyngeal arch arteries at 7 weeks; the parts of the dorsal aortae and pharyngeal arch arteries that normally disappear are indicated with *broken lines.* **C,** Arterial arrangement at 8 weeks. **D,** Sketch of the arterial vessels of a 6-month-old infant. Note that the ascending aorta and pulmonary arteries are considerably smaller in **C** than in **D**. This represents the relative flow through these vessels at the different stages of development. Observe the large size of the ductus arteriosus in **C** and that it is essentially a direct continuation of the pulmonary trunk. The ductus arteriosus normally becomes functionally closed within the first few days after birth. Eventually the ductus arteriosus becomes the ligamentum arteriosum, as shown in **D**.

becomes the **proximal part of the right subclavian artery.** The distal part of the right subclavian artery forms from the **right dorsal aorta** and **right seventh intersegmental artery.**

The left subclavian artery is not derived from a pharyngeal arch artery; it is formed from the **left seventh intersegmental artery** (see Fig. 13-39*A*). As development proceeds, differential growth shifts the origin of the left subclavian artery cranially. Consequently, it lies close to the origin of the left common carotid artery (see Fig. 13-39*D*).

## Fate of Fifth Pair of Pharyngeal Arch Arteries

Approximately 50% of the time, the fifth pair of arteries consists of rudimentary vessels that soon degenerate, leaving no vascular derivatives. In the other 50% of persons, these arteries do not develop.

## Derivatives of Sixth Pair of Pharyngeal Arch Arteries

The **left sixth artery** develops as follows (see Fig. 13-39*B* and *C*):

- The proximal part of the artery persists as the proximal part of the **left pulmonary artery.**
- The distal part of the artery passes from the left pulmonary artery to the dorsal aorta and forms a prenatal shunt, the **ductus arteriosus.**

The **right sixth artery** develops as follows:

- The proximal part of the artery persists as the proximal part of the **right pulmonary artery.**
- The distal part of the artery degenerates.

The transformation of the sixth pair of arteries explains why the course of the **recurrent laryngeal nerves** differs on the two sides. These nerves supply the sixth pair of pharyngeal arches and hook around the sixth pair of arteries on their way to the developing larynx (Fig. 13-40*A*).

**On the right,** because the distal part of the right sixth artery degenerates, the right recurrent laryngeal nerve moves superiorly and hooks around the proximal part of the **right subclavian artery,** the derivative of the fourth artery (Fig. 13-40*B*). **On the left,** the left recurrent laryngeal nerve hooks around the **ductus arteriosus** formed by the distal part of the sixth artery. When this arterial shunt involutes after birth, the nerve remains around the **ligamentum arteriosum** (remnant of the ductus arteriosus) and the arch of the aorta (Fig. 13-40*C*).

## Pharyngeal Arch Arterial Birth Defects

Because of the many changes involved in transformation of the pharyngeal arch arterial system into the adult arterial pattern, arterial birth defects may occur. Most defects result from the persistence of parts of the pharyngeal arch arteries that usually disappear, or from disappearance of parts that normally persist.

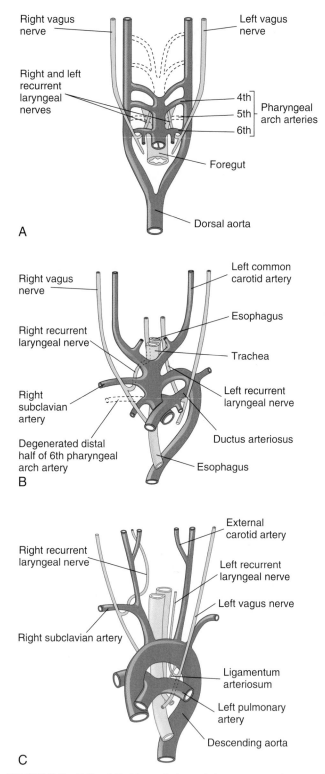

**FIGURE 13–40** The relation of the recurrent laryngeal nerves to the pharyngeal arch arteries. **A,** At 6 weeks, showing the recurrent laryngeal nerves hooked around the sixth pair of pharyngeal arch arteries. **B,** At 8 weeks, showing the right recurrent laryngeal nerve hooked around the right subclavian artery, and the left recurrent laryngeal nerve hooked around the ductus arteriosus and the arch of the aorta. **C,** After birth, showing the left recurrent nerve hooked around the ligamentum arteriosum and the arch of the aorta.

## COARCTATION OF AORTA

Aortic coarctation (constriction) occurs in approximately 10% of children with CHDs. Coarctation is characterized by an aortic constriction of varying length (Fig. 13-41). Most coarctations occur distal to the origin of the left subclavian artery at the entrance of the ductus arteriosus (juxtaductal coarctation).

The classification into preductal and postductal coarctations is commonly used; however, in 90% of instances, the coarctation is directly opposite the ductus arteriosus. Coarctation occurs twice as often in males as in females and is associated with a mitral (bicuspid) aortic valve in 70% of cases (see Fig. 13-12E).

In **postductal coarctation**, the constriction is just distal to the ductus arteriosus (see Fig. 13-41A and B). This permits development of a collateral circulation during the fetal period (see Fig. 13-41B), thereby assisting with passage of blood to inferior parts of the body.

In **preductal coarctation**, the constriction is proximal to the ductus arteriosus (see Fig. 13-41C). The narrowed segment may be extensive (see Fig. 13-41D); before birth, blood flows through the ductus arteriosus to the descending aorta for distribution to the lower body.

In an infant with severe **aortic coarctation**, closure of the ductus arteriosus results in **hypoperfusion** and rapid deterioration of the infant. These babies usually receive prostaglandin $E_2$ in an attempt to reopen the ductus arteriosus and establish an adequate blood flow to the lower limbs. Aortic coarctation may be a feature of Turner syndrome (see Chapter 20, Figs. 20-3 and 20-4). This and other observations suggest that genetic and/or environmental factors cause coarctation.

There are three main views about the embryologic basis of coarctation of the aorta:

- During formation of the arch of the aorta, muscle tissue of the ductus arteriosus may be incorporated into the wall of the aorta; then, when the ductus arteriosus constricts at birth, the ductal muscle in the aorta also constricts, forming a coarctation.
- There may be abnormal involution of a small segment of the left dorsal aorta (see Fig. 13-41F). Later, this stenotic segment (area of coarctation) moves cranially with the left subclavian artery (see Fig. 13-41G).
- During fetal life, the segment of the arch of the aorta between the left subclavian artery and the ductus arteriosus is normally narrow because it carries very little blood. After closure of the ductus arteriosus, this narrow area (isthmus) normally enlarges until it is the same diameter as the aorta. If the isthmus persists, a coarctation forms.

## DOUBLE PHARYNGEAL ARCH ARTERY

**Double pharyngeal arch artery** is a rare anomaly that is characterized by a **vascular ring** around the trachea and esophagus (Fig. 13-42B). Varying degrees of compression of these structures may occur in infants. If the compression is significant, it causes wheezing respirations that are aggravated by crying, feeding, and flexion of the neck. The vascular ring results from failure of the distal part of the right dorsal aorta to disappear (Fig. 13-42A); as a result, right and left arches form. Usually, the right arch of the aorta is larger and passes posterior to the trachea and esophagus (see Fig. 13-42B).

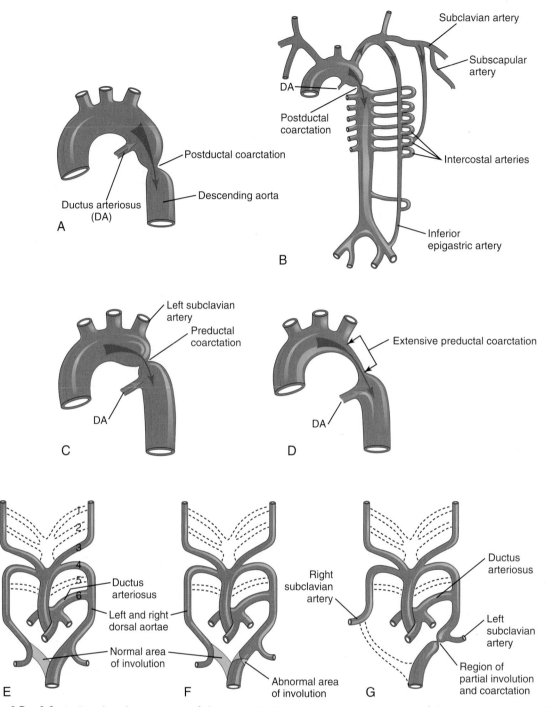

**FIGURE 13–41** A, Postductal coarctation of the aorta. B, Diagrammatic representation of the common routes of collateral circulation that develop in association with postductal coarctation of the aorta. C and D, Preductal coarctation. E, Sketch of the pharyngeal arch arterial pattern in a 7-week embryo, showing the areas that normally involute (see dotted branches of arteries). Note that the distal segment of the right dorsal aorta normally involutes as the right subclavian artery develops. F, Abnormal involution of a small distal segment of the left dorsal aorta. G, Later stage showing the abnormally involuted segment appearing as a coarctation of the aorta. This moves to the region of the ductus arteriosus with the left subclavian artery. These drawings (E to G) illustrate one hypothesis about the embryologic basis of coarctation of the aorta.

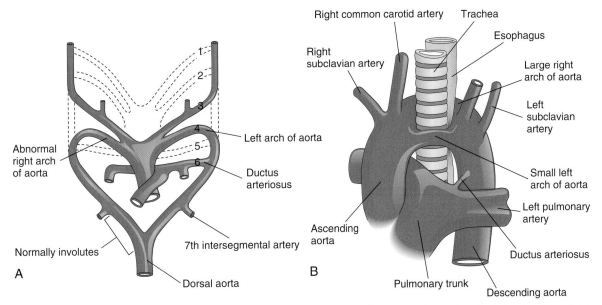

**FIGURE 13–42** A, Drawing of the embryonic pharyngeal arch arteries illustrating the embryologic basis of the right and left arches of the aorta (double arch of aorta). B, A large right arch of the aorta and a small left arch of the aorta arise from the ascending aorta, forming a vascular ring around the trachea and esophagus. Observe that there is compression of the esophagus and trachea. The right common carotid and subclavian arteries arise separately from the large right arch of the aorta.

## RIGHT ARCH OF AORTA

When the entire right dorsal aorta persists (Fig. 13-43A and B) and the distal part of the left dorsal aorta involutes, a right arch of the aorta results. There are two main types:

- **Right arch of the aorta without a retroesophageal component** (see Fig. 13-43B). The ductus arteriosus or ligamentum arteriosum passes from the right pulmonary artery to the right arch of the aorta. Because no vascular ring is formed, this condition is usually asymptomatic.
- **Right arch of the aorta with a retroesophageal component** (Fig. 13-43C). Originally, a small left arch of the aorta probably involuted, leaving the right arch of the aorta posterior to the esophagus. The ductus arteriosus (ligamentum arteriosum) attaches to the distal part of the arch of the aorta and forms a ring, which may constrict the esophagus and trachea.

## ANOMALOUS RIGHT SUBCLAVIAN ARTERY

The right subclavian artery arises from the distal part of the arch of the aorta and passes posterior to the trachea and esophagus to supply the right upper limb (Figs. 13-44 and 13-45). A **retroesophageal right subclavian artery** occurs when the right fourth pharyngeal arch artery and the right dorsal aorta disappear cranial to the seventh intersegmental artery. As a result, the right subclavian artery forms from the right seventh intersegmental artery and the distal part of the right dorsal aorta. As development proceeds, differential growth shifts the origin of the right subclavian artery cranially until it comes to lie close to the origin of the left subclavian artery.

Although an anomalous right subclavian artery is fairly common and always forms a vascular ring, it is rarely clinically significant because the ring is usually not tight enough to constrict the esophagus and trachea very much.

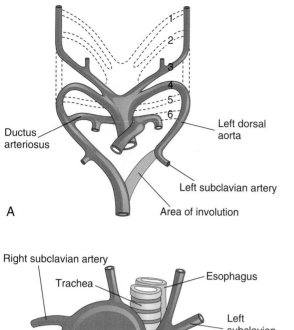

Ductus arteriosus

Left dorsal aorta

Left subclavian artery

Area of involution

A

Right subclavian artery

Trachea

Esophagus

Left subclavian artery

Ligamentum arteriosum

Right arch of aorta

Descending aorta

B

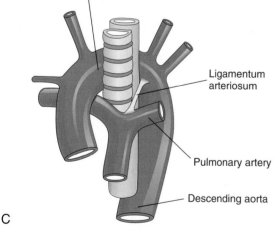

Retroesophageal right arch of aorta

Ligamentum arteriosum

Pulmonary artery

Descending aorta

C

**FIGURE 13–43** A, Sketch of the pharyngeal arch arteries showing the normal involution of the distal portion of the left dorsal aorta. There is also persistence of the entire right dorsal aorta and the distal part of the right sixth pharyngeal arch artery. B, Right pharyngeal arch artery without a retroesophageal component. C, Right arch of the aorta with a retroesophageal component. The abnormal right arch of the aorta and the ligamentum arteriosum (postnatal remnant of the ductus arteriosus) form a ring that compresses the esophagus and trachea.

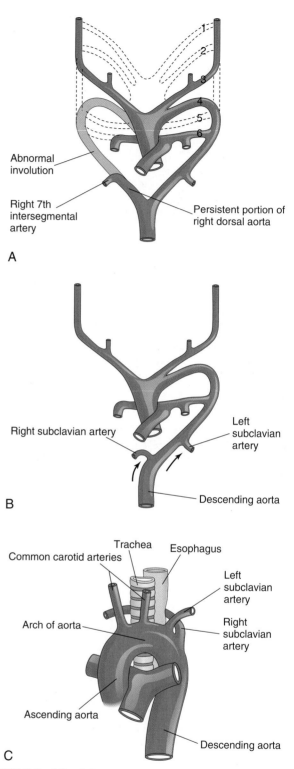

Abnormal involution

Right 7th intersegmental artery

Persistent portion of right dorsal aorta

A

Right subclavian artery

Left subclavian artery

Descending aorta

B

Common carotid arteries

Trachea

Esophagus

Left subclavian artery

Arch of aorta

Right subclavian artery

Ascending aorta

Descending aorta

C

**FIGURE 13–44** Sketches illustrating the possible embryologic basis of abnormal origin of the right subclavian artery. A, The right fourth pharyngeal arch artery and the cranial part of the right dorsal aorta have involuted. As a result, the right subclavian artery forms from the right seventh intersegmental artery and the distal segment of the right dorsal aorta. B, As the arch of the aorta forms, the right subclavian artery is carried cranially (arrows) with the left subclavian artery. C, The abnormal right subclavian artery arises from the aorta and passes posterior to the trachea and esophagus.

**FIGURE 13–45** Abnormal origin of right subclavian artery. This left anterior oblique view of an aortic arch arteriogram shows both common carotid arteries arising from a common stem (*BT*) of the arch of the aorta. The origin of the right subclavian artery (*RS*) is distal to the separate origin of the left subclavian artery (*LS*) but is superimposed in this view. The right subclavian artery then courses cranially and to the right, posterior to the esophagus and trachea. *AA*, Arch of aorta; *BT*, brachiocephalic trunk; *LCC*, left common carotid (artery); *LT#2*, left side, number 2 view; *LV*, left vertebral artery; *RCC*, right common carotid artery.

## FETAL AND NEONATAL CIRCULATION

The **fetal cardiovascular system** is designed to serve prenatal needs and permit modifications at birth that establish the neonatal circulatory pattern (Figs. 13-46 and 13-47). Good respiration in the neonatal period (1 to 28 days) is dependent on normal circulatory changes occurring at birth, which result in oxygenation of the blood in the lungs when fetal blood flow through the placenta ceases. In prenatal life, the lungs do not provide gas exchange and the pulmonary vessels are **vasoconstricted** (narrowed). The three vascular structures most important in the transitional circulation are the ductus venosus, foramen ovale, and ductus arteriosus.

### Fetal Circulation

**Highly oxygenated, nutrient-rich blood** returns under high pressure from the placenta in the **umbilical vein** (see Fig. 13-46). On approaching the liver, approximately half of the blood passes directly into the **ductus venosus**, a fetal vessel connecting the umbilical vein to the IVC (Figs. 13-48 and 13-49); consequently, this blood bypasses the liver. The other half of the blood in the umbilical vein flows into the sinusoids of the liver and enters the IVC through the **hepatic veins**.

Blood flow through the ductus venosus is regulated by a sphincter mechanism close to the umbilical vein. When the sphincter contracts, more blood is diverted to the portal vein and hepatic sinusoids and less to the ductus venosus (see Fig. 13-49). Although an anatomic sphincter in the ductus venosus has been described, its presence is not universally accepted. However, it is generally agreed that there is a physiologic sphincter that prevents overloading of the heart when venous flow in the umbilical vein is high (e.g., during uterine contractions).

After a short course in the IVC, the blood enters the right atrium of the heart. Because the IVC also contains poorly oxygenated blood from the lower limbs, abdomen, and pelvis, the blood entering the right atrium is not as well oxygenated as that in the umbilical vein, but it still has high oxygen content (see Fig. 13-46). Most blood from the IVC is directed by the **crista dividens** (inferior border of the septum secundum) through the foramen ovale into the left atrium (Fig. 13-50). Here it mixes with the relatively small amount of poorly oxygenated blood returning from the lungs through the pulmonary veins. The fetal lungs use oxygen from the blood instead of replenishing it. From the left atrium, the blood then passes to the left ventricle and leaves through the ascending aorta.

The arteries to the heart, neck, head, and upper limbs receive well-oxygenated blood from the ascending aorta. The liver also receives well-oxygenated blood from the umbilical vein (see Figs. 13-48 and 13-49). The small amount of well-oxygenated blood from the IVC in the right atrium that does not enter the foramen ovale mixes with poorly oxygenated blood from the SVC and coronary sinus and passes into the right ventricle. This blood, which has a medium oxygen content, leaves through the pulmonary trunk.

Approximately 10% of this blood flow goes to the lungs; most blood passes through the **ductus arteriosus** into the descending aorta of the fetus and returns to the placenta through the umbilical arteries (see Fig. 13-46). The ductus arteriosus protects the lungs from circulatory overloading and allows the right ventricle to strengthen in preparation for functioning at full capacity at birth. Because of the high pulmonary vascular resistance in fetal life, pulmonary blood flow is low. Approximately 10% of blood from the ascending aorta enters the descending aorta; 65% of the blood in the descending aorta passes into the umbilical arteries and is returned to the placenta for reoxygenation. The remaining 35% of the blood in the descending aorta supplies the viscera and the inferior part of the body.

### Transitional Neonatal Circulation

Important circulatory adjustments occur at birth, when the circulation of fetal blood through the placenta ceases and the neonate's lungs expand and begin to function (see Fig. 13-47). As soon as the baby is born, the foramen ovale, ductus arteriosus, ductus venosus, and umbilical vessels are no longer needed. The sphincter in the ductus venosus constricts, so that all blood entering the liver

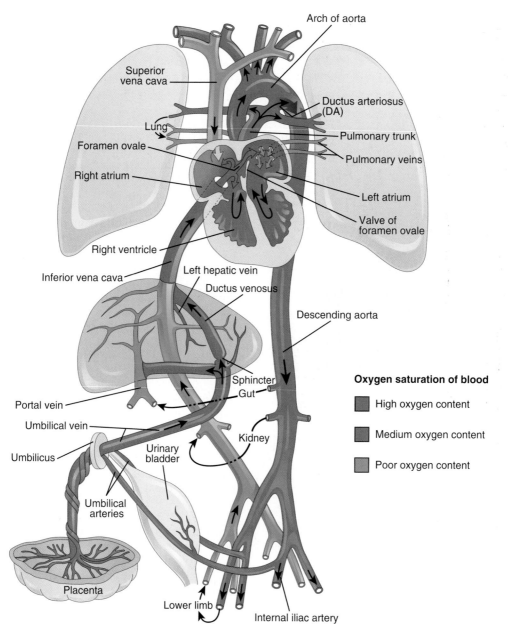

**FIGURE 13–46** Fetal circulation. The *colors* indicate the oxygen saturation of the blood, and the *arrows* show the course of the blood from the placenta to the heart. The organs are not drawn to scale. A small amount of highly oxygenated blood from the inferior vena cava remains in the right atrium and mixes with poorly oxygenated blood from the superior vena cava. Blood with medium oxygenation then passes into the right ventricle. Observe that three shunts permit most of the blood to bypass the liver and lungs: (1) ductus venosus, (2) foramen ovale, and (3) ductus arteriosus. The poorly oxygenated blood returns to the placenta for oxygenation and nutrients through the umbilical arteries.

passes through the hepatic sinusoids. Occlusion of the placental circulation causes an immediate decrease in blood pressure in the IVC and right atrium.

Aeration of the lungs at birth is associated with a:

- Dramatic decrease in pulmonary vascular resistance
- Marked increase in pulmonary blood flow
- Progressive thinning of the walls of the pulmonary arteries

The thinning of the arterial walls results mainly from stretching of the lungs at birth.

Because of increased pulmonary blood flow and loss of flow from the umbilical vein, the pressure in the left atrium is higher than that in the right atrium. The increased left atrial pressure functionally closes the **foramen ovale** by pressing the valve of the foramen against the septum secundum (see Fig. 13-47). The output from the right ventricle now flows into the pulmonary trunk. Because the pulmonary vascular resistance is lower than the systemic vascular resistance, blood flow in the ductus arteriosus reverses, passing from the descending aorta to the pulmonary trunk.

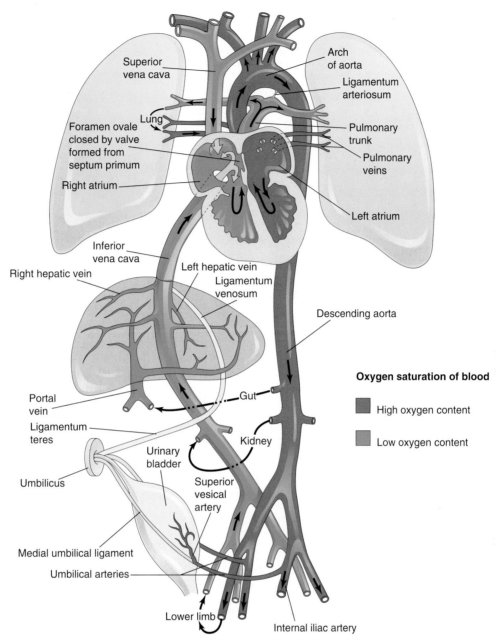

**FIGURE 13-47** Neonatal circulation. The adult derivatives of the fetal vessels and structures that become nonfunctional at birth are shown. The *arrows* indicate the course of the blood in the neonate. The organs are not drawn to scale. After birth, the three shunts that short-circuited the blood during fetal life cease to function, and the pulmonary and systemic circulations become separated.

The right ventricular wall is thicker than the left ventricular wall in fetuses and neonates because the right ventricle has been working harder in utero. By the end of the first month, the left ventricular wall is thicker than the right ventricular wall because the left ventricle is now working harder. The right ventricular wall becomes thinner because of the atrophy associated with its lighter workload.

*The ductus arteriosus constricts at birth*, but a small amount of blood may continue to be shunted via the ductus arteriosus from the aorta to the pulmonary trunk for 24 to 48 hours in a normal full-term neonate. At the

end of 24 hours, 20% of ducts are functionally closed; by 48 hours, about 80% are closed; and by 96 hours, 100% are closed. In premature neonates and in those with **persistent hypoxia** (**decreased oxygen**), the ductus arteriosus may remain open much longer.

In full-term neonates, oxygen is the most important factor in controlling closure of the ductus arteriosus; the oxygen appears to be mediated by **bradykinin**, a substance released from the lungs during initial inflation. Bradykinin has potent contractile effects on smooth muscle. The action of this substance appears to be dependent on the high oxygen content of the blood in the aorta,

**FIGURE 13–48** *A,* Schematic illustration of the course of the umbilical vein from the umbilical cord to the liver. *B,* Ultrasound scan showing the umbilical cord and the course of its vessels in the embryo. *b,* Bladder; *c,* umbilical cord; *DV,* ductus venosus; *UA,* umbilical artery; *UV,* umbilical vein. *C,* Schematic presentation of the relationship among the ductus venosus, umbilical vein, hepatic veins, and inferior vena cava. The oxygenated blood is coded with *red.* (*B, From Goldstein RB: Ultrasound evaluation of the fetal abdomen. In Callen PW, editor: Ultrasonography in obstetrics and gynecology, ed 3, Philadelphia, 1996, Saunders. C, From Tekay A, Campbell S: Doppler ultrasonography in obstetrics. In Callen PW, editor: Ultrasonography in obstetrics and gynecology, ed 4, Philadelphia, 2000, Saunders.*)

**FIGURE 13–49** Dissection of the visceral surface of the fetal liver. Approximately 50% of umbilical venous blood bypasses the liver and joins the inferior vena cava through the ductus venosus.

resulting from aeration of the lungs at birth. When the pO₂ of the blood passing through the ductus arteriosus reaches approximately 50 mm Hg, the wall of the ductus arteriosus constricts. The mechanisms by which oxygen causes ductal constriction are not well understood.

The effects of oxygen on the ductal smooth muscle may be direct or be mediated by its effects on prostaglandin E₂ secretion. *TGF-β* is probably involved in the anatomic closure of the ductus arteriosus after birth. During fetal life, the patency of the ductus arteriosus is controlled by the lower content of oxygen in the blood passing through it and by endogenously produced **prostaglandins** that act on the smooth muscle in the wall of the ductus arteriosus. The prostaglandins cause the ductus arteriosus to relax. **Hypoxia** and other ill-defined influences cause the local production of prostaglandin E₂ and prostacyclin I₂, which keeps the ductus arteriosus open. Inhibitors of prostaglandin synthesis, such as **indomethacin**, can cause constriction of a patent ductus arteriosus in premature neonates.

*The umbilical arteries constrict at birth*, preventing loss of the neonate's blood. Because the umbilical cord is not tied for a minute or so, blood flow through the umbilical vein continues, transferring well-oxygenated fetal blood from the placenta to the neonate. *The change from the fetal to the adult pattern of blood circulation is not a sudden occurrence.* Some changes occur with the first breath; others take place over hours and days. During the transitional stage, there may be a right-to-left flow through the foramen ovale. The closure of fetal vessels and the foramen ovale is initially a functional change.

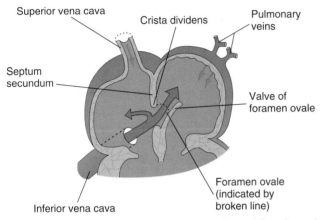

**FIGURE 13–50** Schematic diagram of blood flow through the fetal atria illustrating how the crista dividens (lower edge of septum secundum) separates the blood coming from the inferior vena cava into two streams. The larger stream passes through the foramen ovale into the left atrium, where it mixes with the small amount of poorly oxygenated blood coming from the lungs through the pulmonary veins. The smaller stream of blood from the inferior vena cava remains in the right atrium and mixes with poorly oxygenated blood from the superior vena cava and coronary sinus.

Later, anatomic closure results from proliferation of fibrous tissues.

## Derivatives of Fetal Vessels and Structures

Because of the changes in the cardiovascular system at birth, some vessels and structures are no longer required. Over a period of months, these fetal vessels form nonfunctional ligaments. Fetal structures, such as the foramen ovale, persist as anatomic vestiges (e.g., oval fossa; see Fig. 13-52).

### Umbilical Vein and Round Ligament of Liver

The umbilical vein remains patent for a considerable period and may be used for exchange transfusions of blood during the early neonatal period (first 4 weeks). These transfusions are often done to prevent brain damage and death in neonates with anemia (in which the blood is deficient in red blood cells) resulting from *erythroblastosis fetalis* (a grave hemolytic anemia). In exchange transfusions, most of the neonate's blood is replaced with donor blood.

The lumen of the umbilical vein usually does not disappear completely; in these neonates, the round ligament can be cannulated, if necessary, for the injection of contrast media or chemotherapeutic drugs. The intra-abdominal part of the umbilical vein eventually becomes the **round ligament of the liver** (ligamentum teres) (see Fig. 13-47), which passes from the umbilicus to the **porta hepatis** (fissure on the visceral surface of the liver); here it is attached to the left branch of the portal vein (Fig. 13-51).

### Ductus Venosus and Ligamentum Venosum

The ductus venosus becomes the **ligamentum venosum**; this ligament passes through the liver from the left branch of the portal vein and attaches to the **IVC** (see Fig. 13-51).

**FIGURE 13–51** Dissection of the visceral surface of an adult liver. Note that the umbilical vein is represented by the round ligament of the liver and the ductus venosus by the ligamentum venosum.

## Umbilical Arteries and Abdominal Ligaments

Most of the intra-abdominal parts of the umbilical arteries become **medial umbilical ligaments** (see Fig. 13-47). The proximal parts of these vessels persist as the **superior vesical arteries**, which supply the urinary bladder.

## Foramen Ovale and Oval Fossa

The foramen ovale usually closes functionally at birth. Anatomic closure occurs by the third month and results from tissue proliferation and adhesion of the septum primum to the left margin of the septum secundum. The **septum primum** forms the floor of the oval fossa

(Fig. 13-52). The inferior edge of the **septum secundum** forms a rounded fold, the border of the oval fossa (limbus fossa ovalis), which marks the former boundary of the foramen ovale.

## Ductus Arteriosus and Ligamentum Arteriosum

Functional closure of the ductus arteriosus in healthy term neonates is usually completed within the first few days after birth (Fig. 13-53A). Anatomic closure of the ductus arteriosus and formation of the ligamentum arteriosum normally occur by the 12th postnatal week (Fig. 13-53C). The short, thick ligamentum arteriosum extends from the left pulmonary artery to the arch of the aorta.

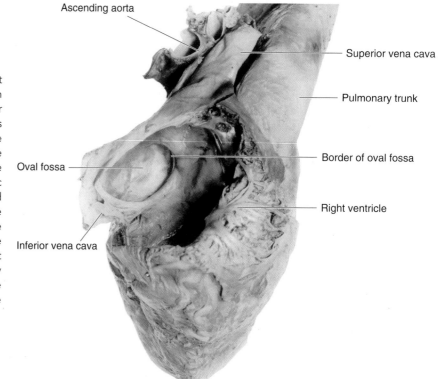

**FIGURE 13–52** Dissection of the right atrial aspect of the interatrial septum of an adult heart. Observe the oval fossa and border of the oval fossa. The floor of the oval fossa is formed by the septum primum, whereas the border of the fossa is formed by the free edge of the septum secundum. Aeration of the lungs at birth is associated with a dramatic decrease in pulmonary vascular resistance and a marked increase in pulmonary flow. Because of the increased pulmonary blood flow, the pressure in the left atrium is increased above that in the right atrium. This increased left atrial pressure closes the foramen ovale by pressing the valve of the foramen ovale against the septum secundum. This forms the oval fossa.

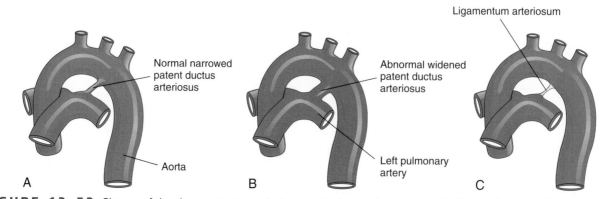

**FIGURE 13–53** Closure of the ductus arteriosus. **A,** Ductus arteriosus of a neonate. **B,** Abnormal patent ductus arteriosus in a 6-month-old infant. **C,** Ligamentum arteriosum in a 6-month-old infant.

*Apelin signaling, Prox1, Sox18, and COUP-TF11 appear to influence the migration and proliferation of these precursor lymphatic cells.*

## Development of Lymph Sacs and Lymphatic Ducts

*There are six primary lymph sacs present at the end of the embryonic period (see Fig. 13-54A):*

- *Two jugular lymph sacs* near the junction of the subclavian veins with the anterior cardinal veins (the future internal jugular veins)
- *Two iliac lymph sacs* near the junction of the iliac veins with the posterior cardinal veins
- *One retroperitoneal lymph sac* in the root of the mesentery on the posterior abdominal wall
- *One cisterna chyli (chyle cistern)* located dorsal to the retroperitoneal lymph sac

Lymphatic vessels soon connect to the lymph sacs and pass along main veins to the head, neck, and upper limbs from the jugular lymph sacs; to the lower trunk and lower limbs from the iliac lymph sacs; and to the primordial gut from the retroperitoneal lymph sac and the **cisterna chyli.** Two large channels (right and left thoracic ducts) connect the jugular lymph sacs with this cistern. Soon a large anastomosis forms between these channels (Fig. 13-54B).

## Development of Thoracic Duct

The **thoracic duct** is formed by the caudal part of the **right thoracic duct,** the anastomosis between the left and right thoracic ducts, and the cranial part of the **left thoracic duct.** As a result, there are many variations in the origin, course, and termination of the thoracic duct. The **right lymphatic duct** is derived from the cranial part of the right thoracic duct (Fig. 13-54C). The **thoracic duct** and right lymphatic duct connect with the venous system at the **venous angle** between the internal jugular vein and subclavian vein (see Fig. 13-54B).

## Development of Lymph Nodes

Except for the superior part of the **cisterna chyli,** the lymph sacs are transformed into groups of lymph nodes during the early fetal period. Mesenchymal cells invade each lymph sac and break up its cavity into a network of lymphatic channels, the **primordia of the lymph sinuses.** Other mesenchymal cells give rise to the capsule and connective tissue framework of the lymph nodes.

## Development of Lymphocytes

The lymphocytes are derived originally from **primordial stem cells** in the umbilical vesicle mesenchyme and later from the liver and spleen. These early lymphocytes eventually enter the bone marrow, where they divide to form **lymphoblasts.** The lymphocytes that appear in lymph nodes before birth are derived from the **thymus,** a derivative of the third pair of pharyngeal pouches (see Chapter 9, Fig. 9-8B and C). Small lymphocytes leave the thymus

## PATENT DUCTUS ARTERIOSUS

Patent ductus arteriosus, a common birth defect, is two to three times more frequent in females than in males (Fig. 13-53B). Functional closure of the ductus arteriosus usually occurs soon after birth; however, if it remains patent, aortic blood is shunted into the pulmonary trunk. *It has been suggested that persistent patency of the ductus arteriosus may result from failure of TGF-β induction after birth.*

Patent ductus arteriosus is commonly associated with **maternal rubella infection** during early pregnancy (see Chapter 20, Table 20-6). Preterm neonates and infants living at a high altitude may have a patent ductus arteriosus; the patency is the result of **hypoxia** (a decreased level of oxygen) and immaturity. Virtually all preterm neonates (≤28 weeks) whose birth weight is less than 1750 g have a patent ductus arteriosus in the first 24 hours of postnatal life.

*The embryologic basis of patent ductus arteriosus is* failure of the ductus arteriosus to involute after birth and form the ligamentum arteriosum. Failure of contraction of the muscular wall of the ductus arteriosus after birth is the primary cause of patency. There is some evidence that low oxygen content of the blood in neonates with **respiratory distress syndrome** can adversely affect closure of the ductus arteriosus. For example, patent ductus arteriosus commonly occurs in small premature neonates with respiratory difficulties associated with a deficiency of **surfactant** (a phospholipid that reduces surface tension in alveoli in the lungs).

Patent ductus arteriosus may occur as an isolated defect or in infants with certain **chromosomal anomalies** or **cardiac defects.** Large differences between aortic and pulmonary blood pressures can cause a heavy flow of blood through the ductus arteriosus, thereby preventing normal constriction. Such pressure differences may be caused by **coarctation of the aorta** (see Fig. 13-41A to D), **TGA** (see Fig. 13-32), or **pulmonary stenosis** and **atresia** (see Fig. 13-34).

## DEVELOPMENT OF LYMPHATIC SYSTEM

The lymphatic system begins to develop at the end of the sixth week, approximately 2 weeks after the primordia of the cardiovascular system are recognizable. Lymphatic vessels develop in a manner similar to that previously described for blood vessels (see Chapter 4, Fig. 4-11) and make connections with the venous system. The early lymphatic capillaries join each other to form a network of lymphatics (Fig. 13-54A). Recent studies have shown that the precursor endothelial cells of the lymphatic vessels are derived from the cardinal veins. *Podoplanin, LYVE-1, and VEGFR3 delineate the progenitor endothelial cells.*

**FIGURE 13–54** Development of lymphatic system. **A,** Left side of a 7.5-week embryo showing the primary lymph sacs. **B,** Ventral view of the lymphatic system at 9 weeks showing the paired thoracic ducts. **C,** Later in the fetal period, illustrating formation of the thoracic duct and right lymphatic duct.

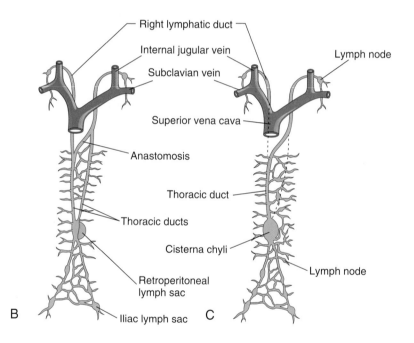

and circulate to other lymphoid organs. Later, some mesenchymal cells in the lymph nodes also differentiate into lymphocytes. Lymph nodules do not appear in the lymph nodes until just before and/or after birth.

## Development of Spleen and Tonsils

The **spleen** develops from an aggregation of mesenchymal cells in the dorsal mesogastrium (see Chapter 11). The **palatine tonsils** develop from the endoderm of the second pair of pharyngeal pouches and nearby mesenchyme. The **tubal tonsils** develop from aggregations of lymph nodules around the pharyngeal openings of the pharyngotympanic tubes. The **pharyngeal tonsils (adenoids)** develop from an aggregation of lymph **nodules** in the wall of the nasopharynx. The **lingual tonsil** lymph develops from an aggregation of lymph nodules in the root of the tongue.

Lymph nodules also develop in the mucosa of the respiratory and alimentary systems.

## SUMMARY OF CARDIOVASCULAR SYSTEM

- The cardiovascular system begins to develop at the end of the third week. *The primordial heart starts to beat at the beginning of the fourth week.* Mesenchymal cells derived from splanchnic mesoderm proliferate and form isolated cell clusters, which soon develop into *two heart tubes* that join to form the **primordial vascular system.** Splanchnic mesoderm surrounding the heart tube forms the primordial myocardium.
- The **heart primordium** consists of four chambers: the bulbus cordis, ventricle, atrium, and sinus venosus.

**FIGURE 13-55** Cystic hygroma. **A,** Transverse axial sonogram of the neck of a fetus with a large cystic hygroma. **B,** Photograph of a neck dissection. The hygroma was demonstrated from this cross-sectional view of the posterior fetal neck at 18.5 weeks. The lesion was characterized by multiple, septated cystic areas within the mass itself as shown in the pathology specimen. *Post,* Posterior.

## ANOMALIES OF LYMPHATIC SYSTEM

Congenital anomalies of the lymphatic system are rare. There may be a diffuse swelling of part of the body, **congenital lymphedema**. This condition may result from dilation of primordial lymphatic channels or from congenital hypoplasia of lymphatic vessels. More rarely, diffuse cystic dilation of lymphatic channels involves widespread portions of the body.

In **cystic hygroma**, large swellings usually appear in the inferolateral part of the neck and consist of large single or multilocular, fluid-filled cavities (Fig. 13-55). Hygromas may be present at birth, but they often enlarge and become evident during infancy, especially after infection or hemorrhage. Most hygromas appear to be derived from *abnormal transformation of the jugular lymph sacs.* **Hygromas** are believed to arise from parts of a jugular lymph sac that are pinched off or from lymphatic spaces that fail to establish connections with the main lymphatic channels. Hygromas diagnosed in utero in the first trimester of development are associated with chromosomal abnormalities in about 50% of cases. The fetal outcome in these cases is poor.

- The **truncus arteriosus** (primordium of the ascending aorta and pulmonary trunk) is continuous caudally with the **bulbus cordis,** which becomes part of the ventricles. As the heart grows, it bends to the right and soon acquires the general external appearance of the adult heart. The heart becomes partitioned into four chambers between the fourth and seventh weeks.

- *Three systems of paired veins drain into the primordial heart*: the vitelline system, which becomes the portal system; the cardinal veins, which form the **caval system**; and the umbilical veins, which involute after birth.

- As the **pharyngeal arches** form during the fourth and fifth weeks, they are penetrated by **pharyngeal arteries** that arise from the aortic sac. During the sixth to eight weeks, the pharyngeal arch arteries are transformed into the adult arterial arrangement of the carotid, subclavian, and pulmonary arteries.

- *The critical period of heart development is from day 20 to day 50 after fertilization.* Numerous events occur during cardiac development, and deviation from the normal pattern at any time may produce one or more CHDs. Because partitioning of the primordial heart results from complex cellular and molecular processes, defects of the cardiac septa are relatively common, particularly **VSDs**. Some birth defects result from abnormal transformation of the pharyngeal arch arteries into the adult arterial pattern.

- Because the lungs are nonfunctional during prenatal life, the fetal cardiovascular system is structurally designed so that *blood is oxygenated in the placenta* and most of it bypasses the lungs. The modifications that establish the postnatal circulatory pattern are not abrupt but extend into infancy. Failure of these changes in the circulatory system to occur at birth results in two of the most common congenital anomalies of the heart and great vessels: **patent foramen ovale** and **patent ductus arteriosus**.

- The lymphatic system begins to develop late in the sixth week in close association with the venous system. Six primary lymph sacs develop, which later become interconnected by lymphatic vessels. *Lymph nodes develop along the network of lymphatic vessels*; lymph nodules do not appear until just before or after birth.

# CLINICALLY ORIENTED PROBLEMS

### CASE 13–1

*A pediatrician detected a congenital cardiac defect in an infant, and he explained to the baby's mother that this is a common birth defect.*

* What is the most common type of congenital cardiac defect?
* What percentage of congenital heart disease results from this defect?
* Discuss blood flow in infants with this defect.
* What problems would you likely encounter if the cardiac defect were large?

### CASE 13–2

*A female infant was born after a pregnancy complicated by a rubella infection during the first trimester. She had congenital cataracts and congenital heart disease. A radiograph of the infant's chest at 3 weeks showed generalized cardiac enlargement with some increase in pulmonary vascularity.*

* What congenital cardiovascular defect is commonly associated with maternal rubella infection during early pregnancy?
* What probably caused the cardiac enlargement?

### CASE 13–3

*A male neonate was referred to a pediatrician because of the blue color of his skin (cyanosis). An ultrasound examination was ordered to confirm the preliminary diagnosis of tetralogy of Fallot.*

* In tetralogy of Fallot, there are four cardiac defects. What are they?
* What is one of the most obvious clinical signs of tetralogy of Fallot?
* What radiographic technique might be used to confirm a tentative diagnosis of this type of congenital heart defect?
* What do you think would be the main aim of therapy in this case?

### CASE 13–4

*A male neonate was born after a full-term normal pregnancy. Severe generalized cyanosis was observed on the first day. A chest radiograph revealed a slightly enlarged heart with a narrow base and increased pulmonary vascularity. A clinical diagnosis of transformation of the great arteries was made.*

* What radiographic technique would likely be used to verify the diagnosis?
* What would this technique reveal in the present case?
* How was the infant able to survive with this severe heart defect?

### CASE 13–5

*During an autopsy of a 72-year-old man who died from chronic heart failure, it was observed that his heart was very large and that the pulmonary artery and its main branches were dilated. Opening the heart revealed a very large atrial septal defect.*

* What type of atrial septal defect was probably present?
* Where would the defect likely be located?
* Explain why the pulmonary artery and its main branches were dilated.
* Why might this have not been diagnosed earlier?

Discussion of these problems appears in the Appendix at the back of the book.

## BIBLIOGRAPHY AND SUGGESTED READING

Adams SM, Good MW, De Franco GM: Sudden infant death syndrome, *Am Fam Physician* 79:870, 2009.

Anderson RH, Brown NA, Moorman AFM: Development and structures of the venous pole of the heart, *Dev Dyn* 235:2, 2006.

Bajolle F, Zaffran S, Bonnet D: Genetics and embryological mechanisms of congenital heart disease, *Arch Cardiovasc Dis* 102:59, 2009.

Baschat AA: Examination of the fetal cardiovascular system, *Semin Fetal Neonatal Med* 16:2, 2011.

Bentham J, Bhattacharya S: Genetic mechanisms controlling cardiovascular development, *Ann N Y Acad Sci* 1123:10, 2008.

Bernstein E: The cardiovascular system. In Behrman RE, Kliegman RM, Jenson HB, editors: *Nelson textbook of pediatrics*, ed 17, Philadelphia, 2004, Saunders.

Camp E, Munsterberg A: Ingression, migration and early differentiation of cardiac progenitors, *Front Biosci* 17:2416, 2011.

Chappell JC, Bautch VL: Vascular development: genetic mechanisms and links to vascular disease, *Curr Top Dev Biol* 90:43, 2010.

Combs MD, Yutzey KE: Heart valve development: regulatory networks in development and disease, *Circ Res* 105:408, 2009.

Conte G, Pellegrini A: On the development of the coronary arteries in human embryos, stages 13–19, *Anat Embryol* 169:209, 1984.

Dyer LA, Kirby ML: The role of secondary heart field in cardiac development, *Dev Dyn* 336:137, 2009.

Gessert S, Kuhl M: The multiple phases and faces of Wnt signaling during cardiac differentiation and development, *Circ Res* 107:186, 2010.

Gloviczki P, Duncan A, Kaira M, et al: Vascular malformations: an update, *Perspect Vasc Surg Endovasc Ther* 21:133, 2009.

Harvey RP, Meilhac SM, Buckingham M: Landmarks and lineages in the developing heart, *Circ Res* 104:1235, 2009.

Hildreth V, Anderson RH, Henderson DJH: Autonomic innervations of the developing heart: origins and function, *Clin Anat* 22:36, 2009.

Horsthuis T, Christoffels VM, Anderson RH, et al: Can recent insights into cardiac development improve our understanding of congenitally malformed heart, *Clin Anat* 22:4, 2009.

Jones PN, Showengerdt KO Jr: Prenatal diagnosis of congenital heart disease, *Pediatr Clin North Am* 56:709, 2009.

Kamedia Y: Hoxa3 and signaling molecules involved in aortic arch patterning and remodeling, *Cell Tissue Res* 336:165, 2010.

Kodo K, Yamagishi H: A decade of advances in the molecular embryology and genetics underlying congenital heart defects, *Circ J* 75:2296, 2011.

Loukas M, Bilinsky C, Bilinski E, et al: The normal and abnormal anatomy of the coronary arteries, *Clin Anat* 22:114, 2009.

Loukas M, Groat C, Khangura R, et al: Cardiac veins: a review of the literature, *Clin Anat* 22:129, 2009.

Männer J: The anatomy of cardiac looping: a step towards the understanding of the morphogenesis of several forms of congenital cardiac malformations, *Clin Anat* 22:21, 2009.

Martinsen BJ, Lohr JL: Cardiac development. In Iaizzo PA, editor: *Handbook of cardiac anatomy, physiology, and devices*, ed 2, Totowa, N.J., 2009, Humana Press, pp 15–23.

Moore KL, Dalley AF, Agur AMR: *Clinically oriented anatomy*, ed 7, Baltimore, 2014, Williams & Wilkins.

Moorman AFM, Brown N, Anderson RH: Embryology of the heart. In Anderson RH, Baker EJ, Penny DJ, et al, editors: *Pediatric cardiology*, ed 3, Philadelphia, 2009, Elsevier.

Nemer M: Genetic insights into normal and abnormal heart development, *Cardiovasc Pathol* 17:48, 2008.

O'Rahilly R: The timing and sequence of events in human cardiogenesis, *Acta Anat* 79:70, 1971.

Penny DJ, Vick GW: Ventricular septal defect, *Lancet* 377:1103, 2011.

Pierpont MEM, Markwald RR, Lin AE: Genetic aspects of atrioventricular septal defects, *Am J Med Genet* 97:289–296, 2000.

Solloway M, Harvey RP: Molecular pathways in myocardial development: a stem cell perspective, *Cardiovasc Res* 58:264, 2006.

Srivastava D: Genetic regulation of cardiogenesis and congenital heart disease, *Ann Rev Pathol* 1:199, 2006.

Sylva M, van den Hoff MJB, Moorman AFM: Development of the human heart, *Am J Med Genet* 164A(6):1347, 2014.

Vincent SD, Buckingham ME: How to make a heart: the origin and regulation of cardiac progenitor cells, *Curr Top Dev Biol* 90:1, 2010.

Watanabe M, Schaefer KS: Cardiac embryology. In Martin RJ, Fanaroff AA, Walsh MC, editors: *Fanaroff and Martin's neonatal–perinatal medicine: diseases of the fetus and infant*, ed 8, Philadelphia, 2006, Mosby.

Yoo S-J, Jaeggi E: Ultrasound evaluation of the fetal heart. In Callen PW, editor: *Ultrasonography in obstetrics and gynecology*, ed 5, Philadelphia, 2008, Saunders.

Zavos PM: Stem cells and cellular therapy: potential treatment for cardiovascular diseases, *Int J Cardiol* 107:1, 2006.

# 14

# Skeletal System

**A**s the notochord and neural tube form in the third week, the **intraembryonic mesoderm** lateral to these structures thickens to form two longitudinal columns of **paraxial mesoderm** (Fig. 14-1A and B). Toward the end of the third week, these dorsolateral columns, located in the body (trunk), become segmented into blocks of mesoderm (somites) (see Fig. 14-1C). Externally, the somites appear as bead-like elevations along the dorsolateral surface of the embryo (see Chapter 5, Fig. 5-6A to D). Each somite differentiates into two parts (see Fig. 14-1D and E):

- The ventromedial part is the **sclerotome**. Its cells form the vertebrae and ribs.
- The dorsolateral part is the **dermomyotome.** Cells from its myotome region form **myoblasts** (primordial muscle cells), and those from its dermatome region form the dermis (**fibroblasts**).

## DEVELOPMENT OF BONE AND CARTILAGE

At the end of the fourth week, the **sclerotome cells** form a loosely woven tissue called **mesenchyme** (embryonic connective tissue), which has bone-forming capacity. Bones first appear as condensations of mesenchymal cells that form bone models. **Condensation** (dense packing) marks the beginning of selective gene activity, which precedes cell differentiation (Fig. 14-2). Most flat bones develop in mesenchyme within preexisting membranous sheaths; this type

**337**

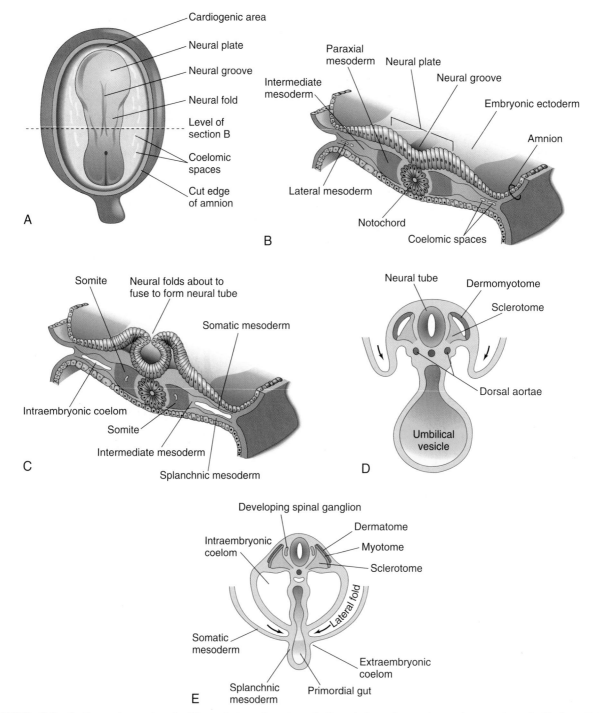

**FIGURE 14–1** Formation and early differentiation of somites. **A,** Dorsal view of an embryo of approximately 18 days. **B,** Transverse section of the embryo shown in **A** shows the paraxial mesoderm from which the somites are derived. **C,** Transverse section of an embryo of approximately 22 days shows the appearance of early somites. The neural folds are about to fuse to form the neural tube. **D,** Transverse section of an embryo of approximately 24 days shows folding of the embryo in the horizontal plane (*arrows*). The dermomyotome region of the somite gives rise to the dermatome and myotome. **E,** Transverse section of an embryo of approximately 26 days shows the dermatome, myotome, and sclerotome regions of a somite.

of **osteogenesis** is called **membranous (intramembranous) bone formation.** Mesenchymal models of most limb bones are transformed into cartilage bone models, which later become ossified by **endochondral bone formation.**

Proteins encoded by the HOX genes, bone morphogenetic proteins (BMP5 and BMP7), growth factor GDF5,

*members of the transforming growth factor-β (TGF-β) superfamily, and other signaling molecules are endogenous regulators of chondrogenesis and skeletal development. Lineage commitment of skeletal precursor cells to chondrocytes and osteoblasts is determined by β-catenin levels. β-Catenin in the canonical Wnt signaling*

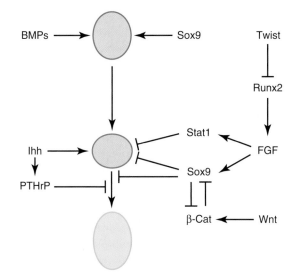

**FIGURE 14–2** Schematic representation of secreted molecules and transcription factors that regulate the initial differentiation, proliferation, and terminal differentiation of chondrocytes. From *top to bottom*: mesenchymal cells *(blue)*, resting and proliferating (nonhypertrophic) chondrocytes *(red)*, and hypertrophic chondrocytes *(yellow)*. Lines with *arrowheads* indicate a positive action, and lines with *bars* indicate an inhibition. *β-Cat*, β-catenin; *BMPs*, bone morphogenic proteins; *FGF*, fibroblast growth factor; *PTHrP*, parathyroid hormone–related protein. *(From Karsenty G, Kronenberg HM, Settembre C: Genetic control of bone formation, Annu Rev Cell Dev Biol 25:629, 2009.)*

**FIGURE 14–3** Light micrograph of intramembranous ossification (×132). The trabeculae of bone are being formed by the osteoblasts lining their surface *(arrows)*. Osteocytes are trapped in lacunae *(arrowheads)*, and primordial osteons are beginning to form. The osteons (canals) contain blood capillaries. *(From Gartner LP, Hiatt JL: Color textbook of histology, ed 2, Philadelphia, 2001, Saunders.)*

*pathway plays a critical role in the formation of cartilage and bone.*

## Histogenesis of Cartilage

Cartilage develops from mesenchyme during the fifth week. In areas where cartilage is programmed to develop, the mesenchyme condenses to form **chondrification centers**. The mesenchymal cells differentiate into **prechondrocytes** and then into **chondroblasts**, which secrete collagenous fibrils and ground substance (**extracellular matrix**). Subsequently, collagenous or elastic fibers, or both, are deposited in the intercellular substance or matrix. *Three types of cartilage are distinguished* according to the type of matrix that is formed:

- **Hyaline cartilage**, the most widely distributed type (e.g., joints)
- **Fibrocartilage** (e.g., intervertebral discs)
- **Elastic cartilage** (e.g., auricles of the external ears)

## Histogenesis of Bone

Bone primarily develops in two types of connective tissue, mesenchyme and cartilage, but it can also develop in other connective tissues (e.g., patella develops in a tendon). Like cartilage, bone consists of cells and an organic intercellular substance (**bone matrix**) that comprises collagen fibrils embedded in an amorphous component. Studies of the cellular and molecular events during embryonic bone formation suggest that **osteogenesis** and **chondrogenesis** are programmed early in development and are independent events under the influence of vascular changes.

## Intramembranous Ossification

Intramembranous ossification occurs in mesenchyme that has formed a membranous sheath (Fig. 14-3) and produces osseous tissue without prior cartilage formation. The mesenchyme condenses and becomes highly vascular. Precursor cells differentiate into **osteoblasts** (bone-forming cells) and begin to deposit unmineralized matrix (**osteoid**). *Wnt signaling is a key factor in osteoblast differentiation.* Calcium phosphate is then deposited in **osteoid tissue** as it is organized into bone. **Bone osteoblasts** are trapped in the matrix and become **osteocytes**.

At first, new bone has no organized pattern. Spicules of bone soon become organized and coalesce into lamellae (layers). **Concentric lamellae** develop around blood vessels, forming **osteons** (Haversian systems). Some osteoblasts remain at the periphery of the developing bone and continue to lay down lamellae, forming plates of compact bone on the surfaces. Between the surface plates, the intervening bone remains spiculated or spongy. This spongy environment is somewhat accentuated by the action of cells (**osteoclasts**) that reabsorb bone. Osteoclasts are multinucleated cells with a hematopoietic origin. In the interstices of spongy bone, the mesenchyme differentiates into **bone marrow**. Hormones and cytokines regulate remodeling of bone by the coordinated action of osteoclasts and osteoblasts.

## Endochondral Ossification

Endochondral ossification (cartilaginous bone formation) is a type of bone formation that occurs in preexisting cartilaginous models (Fig. 14-4). In a long bone, for example, the **primary center of ossification** appears in the **diaphysis** (part of a long bone between its ends), which forms the **shaft of a bone** (e.g., humerus). At this center of ossification, chondrocytes (cartilage cells) increase in size (hypertrophy), the matrix becomes calcified, and the cells die.

Concurrently, a thin layer of bone is deposited under the **perichondrium** surrounding the diaphysis, and the

**Cartilage Model of Bone**

Cartilage / Calcified cartilage / Bone / Arteries

**Intracartilaginous Ossification**

Mesenchymal cell
Perichondrium
Chondroblast
Cartilage matrix
Enlarged area

Diaphyseal (primary) center of ossification
Uncalcified hyaline cartilage
Calcified hyaline cartilage
Chondrocyte
Periosteum
Subperiosteal bone
Periosteal capillary

Epiphyseal artery
Epiphyseal cartilage plate
Metaphyseal artery
Nutrient artery
Medullary cavity of long bone

Epiphyseal (secondary) center of ossification
Epiphyseal artery
Epiphysis
Nutrient artery
Diaphysis
Epiphysis
Epiphyseal center of ossification

**FIGURE 14–4** A to E, Schematic longitudinal sections of a 5-week embryo show endochondral ossification in a developing long bone.

perichondrium becomes the **periosteum**. Invasion by vascular connective tissue from blood vessels surrounding the periosteum also breaks up the cartilage. **Osteoblasts** reach the developing bone from these blood vessels. Some invading cells differentiate into **hemopoietic cells** (blood cells of bone marrow). This process continues toward the **epiphyses** (ends of the bones). The spicules of bone are remodeled by the action of osteoclasts and osteoblasts. *The transcription factor SOX9 and the coactivator-associated arginine methyltransferase 1 (CARM1) regulate osteochondral ossification.*

Lengthening of long bones occurs at the **diaphyseal-epiphyseal junction**. Lengthening of bone depends on the **epiphyseal cartilage plates** (growth plates), whose chondrocytes proliferate and participate in endochondral bone formation (see Fig. 14-4*E*). Toward the diaphysis, the cartilage cells hypertrophy (increase in size), and the matrix becomes calcified. The spicules of the bone are isolated from each other by vascular invasion from the marrow or **medullary cavity** of long bone (see Fig. 14-4*E*). Bone is deposited on these spicules by osteoblasts; resorption of the bone keeps the spongy bone masses relatively constant in length and enlarges the medullary cavity.

**Ossification of limb bones** begins at the end of the embryonic period (56 days after fertilization). Thereafter, it makes demands on the maternal supply of calcium and phosphorus. Pregnant women are advised to maintain an adequate intake of these elements to preserve healthy bones and teeth.

At birth, the diaphyses are largely ossified, but most of the epiphyses are still cartilaginous. **Secondary ossification centers** appear in the epiphyses in most bones during the first few years after birth. The epiphyseal cartilage cells hypertrophy, and there is invasion by vascular connective tissue. Ossification spreads radially, and only the articular cartilage and a transverse plate of cartilage (**epiphyseal cartilage plate**) remain cartilaginous (see Fig. 14-4*E*). On completion of growth, the cartilage plate is replaced by spongy bone, the epiphyses and diaphysis are united, and no further elongation of the bone occurs.

In most bones, the epiphyses fuse with the diaphysis by the age of 20 years. Growth in the diameter of a bone results from deposition of bone at the periosteum (see Fig.

14-4*B*) and from resorption on the internal medullary surface. The rate of deposition and resorption is balanced to regulate the thickness of the compact bone and the size of the medullary cavity. The internal reorganization of bone continues throughout life. The development of irregular bones is similar to that of the epiphyses of long bones. Ossification begins centrally and spreads in all directions.

## DEVELOPMENT OF JOINTS

Joints begin to develop with the appearance of **condensed mesenchyme** in the joint interzone during the sixth week, and by the end of the eighth week, they resemble adult joints (Fig. 14-5). Joints are classified as **fibrous joints**, **cartilaginous joints**, and **synovial joints**. Joints with little or no movement are classified according to the type of material holding the bones together; for example, the bones of fibrous joints are joined by fibrous tissue. Molecular studies show that a distinct cohort of progenitor cells expressing TGF-β receptor 2 at prospective joint sites

**FIGURE 14–5** Development of joints during the sixth and seventh weeks. **A,** Condensed interzonal mesenchyme is seen in the gap between developing bones. This primordial joint may differentiate into a synovial joint (**B**), a cartilaginous joint (**C**), or a fibrous joint (**D**).

contributes to formation of the synovial joints and articular cartilages.

## Fibrous Joints

During the development of fibrous joints, the **interzonal mesenchyme** between the developing bones differentiates into dense fibrous tissue (see Fig. 14-5D). For example, the sutures of the cranium are fibrous joints (see Fig. 14-9).

## Cartilaginous Joints

During the development of cartilaginous joints, the **interzonal mesenchyme** between the developing bones differentiates into **hyaline cartilage** (e.g., costochondral joints) or **fibrocartilage** (pubic symphysis) (see Fig. 14-5C).

## Synovial Joints

During the development of synovial joints (e.g., knee joint), the interzonal mesenchyme between the developing bones differentiates as follows (see Fig. 14-5B):

- Peripherally, the interzonal mesenchyme forms the **joint capsule** and other ligaments.
- Centrally, the mesenchyme disappears, and the resulting space becomes the **joint cavity** (synovial cavity).
- Where it lines the joint capsule and articular surfaces, the mesenchyme forms the **synovial membrane**, which secretes synovial fluid and is a part of the joint capsule (fibrous capsule lined with synovial membrane)

Probably as a result of joint movements, the mesenchymal cells subsequently disappear from the surfaces of the articular cartilages. An abnormal intrauterine environment restricting embryonic and fetal movements may interfere with limb development and cause joint fixation.

# DEVELOPMENT OF AXIAL SKELETON

The axial skeleton is composed of the cranium (skull), vertebral column, ribs, and sternum. During the fourth week, cells in the **sclerotomes** surround the **neural tube** (primordium of spinal cord) and **notochord**, the structure around which the primordia of the vertebrae develop (Fig. 14-6A). This positional change of the sclerotomal cells is effected by differential growth of the surrounding structures and not by active migration of sclerotomal cells. *The HOX and PAX genes regulate the patterning and regional development of the vertebrae along the anterior-posterior axis.*

## Development of Vertebral Column

During the **precartilaginous or mesenchymal stage**, mesenchymal cells from the **sclerotomes** are found in three main areas (see Fig. 14-6A): around the **notochord**, surrounding the neural tube, and in the body wall. In a frontal section of a 4-week embryo, the **sclerotomes**

appear as paired condensations of mesenchymal cells around the notochord (see Fig. 14-6B). Each sclerotome consists of loosely arranged cells cranially and densely packed cells caudally.

Some densely packed cells move cranially, opposite the center of the **myotome** (muscle plate), where they form the **intervertebral disc** (Fig. 14-6C and D). The remaining densely packed cells fuse with the loosely arranged cells of the immediately caudal sclerotome to form the mesenchymal **centrum**, the primordium of the body of a vertebra. Thus, each centrum develops from two adjacent sclerotomes and becomes an intersegmental structure.

The nerves lie close to the intervertebral discs, and the **intersegmental arteries** lie on each side of the vertebral bodies. In the thorax, the dorsal intersegmental arteries become the **intercostal arteries**.

The *notochord degenerates* and disappears where it is surrounded by the developing vertebral bodies. Between the vertebrae, the **notochord** expands to form the *gelatinous center of the* intervertebral disc, the **nucleus pulposus** (see Fig. 14-6D). This nucleus is later surrounded by circularly arranged fibers that form the **annulus fibrosus**. *The nucleus pulposus and annulus fibrosus form the intervertebral disc.* The mesenchymal cells that surround the neural tube form the **neural arch**, which is the **primordium of the vertebral arch** (see Fig. 14-6C). The mesenchymal cells in the body wall form **costal processes**, which form the ribs in the thoracic region.

## CHORDOMA

Remnants of the notochord may persist and form a **chordoma**, a rare neoplasm (tumor). Approximately one third of these slow-growing malignant tumors occurs at the base of the cranium and extends to the nasopharynx. Chordomas infiltrate bone and are difficult to remove. Chordomas also develop in the lumbosacral region. Surgical resection has provided long-term, disease-free survival for many patients.

## Cartilaginous Stage of Vertebral Development

During the sixth week, **chondrification centers** appear in each mesenchymal vertebra (Fig. 14-7A and B). The two centers in each **centrum** fuse at the end of the embryonic period to form a cartilaginous centrum. Concomitantly, the centers in the neural arches fuse with each other and the centrum. The spinous and transverse processes develop from extensions of chondrification centers in the neural arch. Chondrification spreads until a cartilaginous vertebral column is formed.

## Bony Stage of Vertebral Development

Ossification of typical vertebrae begins during the seventh week and ends by the 25th year. There are two **primary ossification centers**, ventral and dorsal, for the centrum (Fig. 14-7C). These centers soon fuse to form one center.

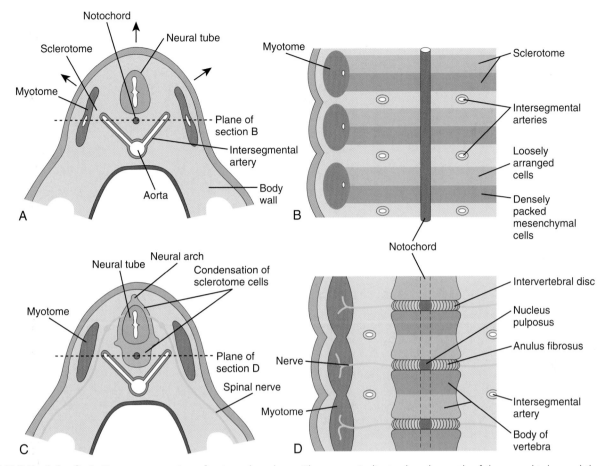

**FIGURE 14–6** A, Transverse section of a 4-week embryo. The *arrows* indicate dorsal growth of the neural tube and the simultaneous dorsolateral movement of the somite remnant, leaving behind a trail of sclerotomal cells. B, Diagrammatic frontal section of the same embryo as in A shows that the condensation of sclerotomal cells around the notochord consists of a cranial area of loosely packed cells and a caudal area of densely packed cells. C, Transverse section through a 5-week embryo shows the condensation of sclerotomal cells around the notochord and neural tube, which forms a mesenchymal vertebra. D, Diagrammatic frontal section of the same embryo as in C illustrates vertebral body formation from the cranial and caudal halves of two successive sclerotomal masses. The intersegmental arteries cross the bodies of the vertebrae, and the spinal nerves lie between the vertebrae. The notochord is degenerating except in the region of the intervertebral disc, where it forms the nucleus pulposus.

Three primary centers are present by the eighth week: one in the centrum and one in each half of the neural arch.

Ossification becomes evident in the **neural arches** during the eighth week. Each typical vertebra consists of three bony parts connected by cartilage: a vertebral arch, a body, and transverse processes (see Fig. 14-7D). The bony halves of the **vertebral arch** usually fuse during the first 3 to 5 years. The arches first unite in the lumbar region, and union progresses cranially. The vertebral arch articulates with the **centrum** at cartilaginous **neurocentral joints**, which permit the vertebral arches to grow as the spinal cord enlarges. These joints disappear when the vertebral arch fuses with the centrum during the third to sixth years.

*Five secondary ossification centers* appear in the vertebrae after puberty:

- One for the tip of the spinous process
- One for the tip of each transverse process

- Two **anular epiphyses**, one on the superior and one on the inferior rim of the vertebral body (see Fig. 14-7E and F)

The **vertebral body** is a composite of the anular epiphyses and the mass of bone between them. The vertebral body includes the centrum, parts of the vertebral arch, and the facets for the heads of the ribs. All secondary centers unite with the rest of the vertebrae at approximately 25 years of age. Exceptions to the typical ossification of vertebrae occur in the atlas or C1 vertebra, axis or C2 vertebra, C7 vertebra, lumbar vertebrae, sacrum, and coccyx.

The Notch signaling pathways are involved in the patterning of the vertebral column. Severe congenital birth defects, including the **VACTERL syndrome** (*v*ertebral, *a*nal, *c*ardiac, *t*racheal, *e*sophageal, *r*enal, and *l*imb birth defects) and **CHARGE syndrome** (coloboma of the eye, heart defects, including tetralogy of Fallot, patent ductus

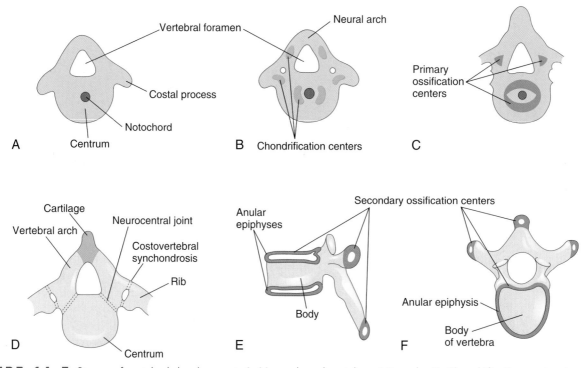

**FIGURE 14–7** Stages of vertebral development. **A,** Mesenchymal vertebra at 5 weeks. **B,** Chondrification centers in a mesenchymal vertebra at 6 weeks. The neural arch is the primordium of the vertebral arch of the vertebra. **C,** Primary ossification centers in a cartilaginous vertebra at 7 weeks. **D,** Thoracic vertebra at birth consists of three bony parts: vertebral arch, body of vertebra, and transverse processes. Notice the cartilage between the halves of the vertebral arch and between the arch and the centrum (neurocentral joint). **E** and **F,** Two views of a typical thoracic vertebra at puberty show the locations of the secondary centers of ossification.

arteriosus, and ventricular or atrial septal defect) are associated with mutation in Notch pathway genes. Minor defects of the vertebrae are common but usually have little clinical importance.

### VARIATION IN THE NUMBER OF VERTEBRAE

Most people have 7 cervical, 12 thoracic, 5 lumbar, and 5 sacral vertebrae. A few have one or two additional vertebrae or one less. To determine the number of vertebrae, it is necessary to examine the entire vertebral column because an apparent extra (or absent) vertebra in one segment of the column may be compensated for by an absent (or extra) vertebra in an adjacent segment, such as 11 thoracic vertebrae with 6 lumbar vertebrae.

## Development of Ribs

Ribs develop from the mesenchymal **costal processes** of the thoracic vertebrae (see Fig. 14-7A). They become cartilaginous during the embryonic period and ossify during the fetal period. The original site of union of the costal processes with the vertebra is replaced by **costovertebral synovial joints** (see Fig. 14-7D). Seven pairs of ribs (1–7; **true ribs**) attach through their own cartilages

to the sternum. Five pairs of ribs (8–12; **false ribs**) attach to the sternum through the cartilage of another rib or ribs. The last two pairs of ribs (11 and 12; **floating ribs**) do not attach to the sternum.

## Development of Sternum

A pair of vertical mesenchymal bands, the **sternal bars,** develops ventrolaterally in the body wall. **Chondrification** occurs in these bars as they move medially. By 10 weeks, they fuse craniocaudally in the median plane to form cartilaginous models of the manubrium, sternebrae (segments of sternal body), and xiphoid process. The manubrium develops from the mesenchyme between the clavicles with contributions from neural crest cells in the region of endochondral ossification. Centers of ossification appear craniocaudally in the sternum before birth, except that for the **xiphoid process,** which appears during childhood. The xiphoid process may never completely ossify.

## Development of Cranium

The cranium (skull) develops from mesenchyme around the developing brain. The growth of the **neurocranium** (bones of cranium enclosing the brain) is initiated from ossification centers within the **desmocranium mesenchyme,** which is the primordium of the cranium. *TGF-β plays a critical role in the development of the cranium by regulating osteoblast differentiation.*

The cranium consists of two parts:

- **Neurocranium**, a bony case that encloses the brain
- **Viscerocranium**, the facial skeleton that is derived from the pharyngeal arches

## Cartilaginous Neurocranium

Initially, the cartilaginous neurocranium (**chondrocranium**) consists of the cartilaginous base of the developing cranium, which forms by fusion of several cartilages (Fig. 14-8A to D). Later, endochondral ossification of the chondrocranium forms the bones in the base of the cranium. The ossification pattern of these bones has a definite sequence, beginning with the occipital bone, body of sphenoid, and ethmoid bone.

The **parachordal cartilage**, or basal plate, forms around the cranial end of the notochord (see Fig. 14-8A) and fuses with the cartilages derived from the sclerotome regions of the occipital somites. This cartilaginous mass contributes to the **base of the occipital bone**; later, extensions grow around the cranial end of the spinal cord and form the boundaries of the **foramen magnum**, which is a large opening in the basal part of the occipital bone (see Fig. 14-8C).

The **hypophyseal cartilage** forms around the developing **pituitary gland** (*hypophysis cerebri*) and fuses to form the body of the sphenoid bone. The **trabeculae cranii** fuse to form the body of the ethmoid bone, and the **ala orbitalis** forms the lesser wing of the sphenoid bone.

**FIGURE 14-8** Superior views show the developmental stages of the cranial base. **A,** At 6 weeks, various cartilages begin to fuse and form the chondrocranium. **B,** At 7 weeks, some of the paired cartilages have fused. **C,** At 12 weeks, the cartilaginous base of the cranium is formed by the fusion of various cartilages. **D,** Derivation of the bones of the fetal cranium is indicated at 20 weeks.

**Otic capsules** develop around the **otic vesicles**, which are the primordia of the internal ears (see Chapter 18, Fig. 18-15), and form the petrous and mastoid parts of the temporal bone. **Nasal capsules** develop around the nasal sacs and contribute to the formation of the ethmoid bone.

## Membranous Neurocranium

Intramembranous ossification occurs in the head mesenchyme at the sides and top of the brain, forming the **calvaria** (skullcap). During fetal life, the flat bones of the calvaria are separated by dense connective tissue membranes that form fibrous joints, the **sutures of calvaria** (Fig. 14-9).

Six large fibrous areas (fontanelles) are found where several sutures meet. The softness of the bones and their loose connections at the sutures enable the calvaria to undergo changes of shape during birth. During **molding of the fetal cranium** (adaptation of the fetal head to pressure in the birth canal), the frontal bones become flat, the occipital bone is lengthened, and one parietal bone slightly overrides the other one. Within a few days after birth, the shape of the calvaria returns to normal.

## Cartilaginous Viscerocranium

Most mesenchyme in the head region is derived from the neural crest. **Neural crest cells** migrate into the pharyngeal arches and form the bones and connective tissue of **craniofacial structures**. Homeobox *(HOX)* genes regulate the migration and subsequent differentiation of the neural crest cells, which are crucial for the complex patterning of the head and face. These parts of the fetal cranium are derived from the cartilaginous skeleton of the first two pairs of **pharyngeal arches** (see Chapter 9, Fig. 9-5 and Table 9-1).

● The dorsal end of the first arch cartilage forms two middle ear bones, the malleus and incus of the middle ear.
● The dorsal end of the second arch cartilage forms a portion of the stapes of the middle ear and the styloid process of the temporal bone. Its ventral end ossifies to form the **lesser horn** *(cornu)* of the hyoid.
● The third, fourth, and sixth arch cartilages form only in the ventral parts of the arches. The third arch cartilages form the greater horns of the hyoid bone.
● The fourth arch cartilages fuse to form the **laryngeal cartilages**, except for the epiglottis (see Chapter 9, Table 9-1).

## Membranous Viscerocranium

Intramembranous ossification occurs in the maxillary prominence of the first pharyngeal arch (see Chapter 9, Figs. 9-4 and 9-5) and subsequently forms the squamous temporal, maxillary, and zygomatic bones. The **squamous temporal bones** become part of the **neurocranium** (cranial bones enclosing the brain rather than the face). The mesenchyme in the **mandibular prominence** of the first arch condenses around its cartilage and undergoes **intramembranous ossification** to form the mandible (see Chapter 9, Fig. 9-4B). Some **endochondral ossification** (replacement of calcified cartilage by osseous tissue) occurs in the median plane of the chin and mandibular condyle.

**FIGURE 14–9** Bones, fontanelles, and sutures of the fetal cranium (skull). **A,** Lateral view. **B,** Superior view. Because of growth of the surrounding bones, the posterior and anterolateral fontanelles disappear within 2 to 3 months after birth, but they remain as sutures for several years. The posterolateral fontanelles disappear in a similar manner by the end of the first year, and the anterior fontanelle disappears by the end of the second year. The halves of the frontal bone normally begin to fuse during the second year, and the frontal suture is usually obliterated by the eighth year. The other sutures disappear during adult life, with wide variation in timing among individuals. **C,** In this three-dimensional ultrasound rendering of the fetal head at 22 weeks, notice the anterior fontanelle *(asterisk)* and the frontal suture *(arrow)*. The coronal and sagittal sutures are also shown.

## Cranium of Neonate

After recovering from molding during birth, the neonate's cranium is round, and its bones are thin. Like the fetal cranium (see Fig. 14-9), it is large in proportion to the rest of the skeleton, and the face is relatively small compared with the **calvaria** (roof of cranium). The small facial region of the cranium results from the small size of the jaws, virtual absence of paranasal (air) sinuses, and underdevelopment of the facial bones.

## Postnatal Growth of Cranium

The fibrous sutures of the neonate's calvaria permit the brain to enlarge during infancy and childhood. The increase in size of the **calvaria** is greatest during the first 2 years, the period of most rapid postnatal growth of the brain. The calvaria normally increases in capacity until approximately 16 years. After this, it usually increases slightly for 3 to 4 years because of thickening of the bones.

Rapid growth of the face and jaws coincides with eruption of the primary (deciduous) teeth. These facial changes are more marked after the secondary (permanent) teeth erupt (see Chapter 19, Fig. 19-14*H*). Concurrent enlargement of the frontal and facial regions is associated with the increase in the size of the **paranasal sinuses** (frontal, maxillary, sphenoid, and ethmoid). Most paranasal sinuses are rudimentary or absent at birth. Growth of the sinuses alters the shape of the face and adds resonance to the voice.

### KLIPPEL-FEIL SYNDROME (BREVICOLLIS)

The main features of Klippel-Feil syndrome are short neck, low hairline, restricted neck movements, fusion of one or more cervical motion segments, and abnormalities of the brainstem and cerebellum. In most cases, the reduced number of cervical vertebral bodies results from fusion of vertebrae before birth. In some cases, there is a lack of segmentation of several elements of the cervical region of the vertebral column. The number of cervical nerve roots may be normal, but they are small, as are the intervertebral foramina. Individuals with this syndrome may have other birth defects, including **scoliosis** (abnormal lateral and rotational curvature of the vertebral column) and urinary tract disorders.

### SPINA BIFIDA

Failure of the halves of the embryonic cartilaginous neural arch to fuse results in various types of spina bifida, which are major birth defects (see Chapter 17, Fig. 17-12). The incidence of these vertebral defects ranges from 0.04% to 0.15%; they occur more frequently in girls than boys. About 80% of spina bifida cases are *open* and covered by a thin membrane of exposed neural tissue. The types of spina bifida are described in Chapter 17 (see Figs. 17-14 to 17-17).

### ACCESSORY RIBS

Accessory ribs, which usually are rudimentary, result from development of the costal processes of cervical or lumbar vertebrae (Fig. 14-10*A*). These processes usually form ribs only in the thoracic region. The most common accessory rib is a **lumbar rib**, but it usually is clinically insignificant. A **cervical rib** occurs in 0.5% to 1% of people. This supernumerary rib is usually attached to the manubrium of the sternum (see Fig. 14-10*A*) or the seventh cervical vertebra and may be fused with the first rib. Pressure of a cervical rib on the brachial plexus of nerves that are located partly in the neck and axilla or on the subclavian artery often produces neurovascular symptoms (e.g., paralysis, anesthesia of the upper limb). Accessory ribs may be unilateral or bilateral.

### FUSED RIBS

Fusion of ribs occasionally occurs posteriorly when two or more ribs arise from a single vertebra (see Fig. 14-10*C*). Fused ribs are often associated with a hemivertebra (one side of a vertebra fails to develop).

### HEMIVERTEBRA

In normal circumstances, the developing vertebral bodies have two chondrification centers that soon unite. A hemivertebra results from *failure of one of the chondrification centers to appear* and subsequent failure of one half of the vertebra to form (see Fig. 14-10*B*). Hemivertebrae are the most common cause of **congenital scoliosis** (lateral and rotational curvature) of the vertebral column (see Fig. 14-10*C*). Less common causes of scoliosis include **myopathic scoliosis** resulting from weakness of the back muscles.

### RACHISCHISIS

Rachischisis (cleft vertebral column) refers to vertebral abnormalities in a complex group of defects (**spinal dysraphism**) that primarily affect axial structures (Fig. 14-11). In these infants, the neural folds fail to fuse because of faulty induction by the underlying notochord or from the action of **teratogenic agents** on the neuroepithelial cells in the neural folds. The neural and vertebral defects may be extensive or be restricted to a small area.

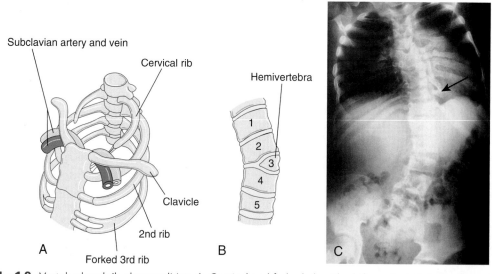

**FIGURE 14–10** Vertebral and rib abnormalities. **A,** Cervical and forked ribs. The left cervical rib has a fibrous band that passes posterior to the subclavian vessels and attaches to the manubrium of the sternum. **B,** Anterior view of the vertebral column shows a hemivertebra. The right half of the third thoracic vertebra is absent. Notice the associated lateral curvature (scoliosis) of the vertebral column. **C,** Radiograph of a child with the kyphoscoliotic deformity of the lumbar region of the vertebral column shows multiple anomalies of the vertebrae and ribs. Notice the fused ribs *(arrow)*.

**FIGURE 14–11 A,** Second-trimester fetus with holoacrania (absence of cranium or acrania). A cyst-like structure surrounds the intact fetal brain. **B,** Lateral view of a neonate with acrania, meroencephaly (partial absence of brain), and rachischisis (extensive clefts in vertebral arches of the vertebral column), which is not clearly visible.

## ANOMALIES OF STERNUM

A concave depression of the lower sternum (**pectus excavatum**) accounts for 90% of thoracic wall defects. Boys are more often affected (1 in 400 to 1000 live births). It is probably caused by overgrowth of the costal cartilage, which displaces the lower sternum inward. *Minor sternal clefts* (notch or foramen in the xiphoid process) are common and are of no clinical concern. Various sizes and forms of the **sternal foramen** occasionally occur at the junction of the third and fourth sternebrae (segments of primordial sternum). This insignificant foramen is the result of incomplete fusion of the cartilaginous sternal bars during the embryonic period.

## CRANIAL BIRTH DEFECTS

Cranial birth defects range from major defects that are incompatible with life (see Fig. 14-11) to those that are minor and insignificant. With large defects, there is often *herniation of the meninges or brain, or both* (see Chapter 17, Figs. 17-33 and 17-34).

## ACRANIA

Acrania is complete or partial absence of the neurocranium (brain box) that may be accompanied by extensive defects of the vertebral column (see Fig. 14-11). **Acrania** associated with **meroencephaly** (partial absence of the brain) occurs in approximately 1 of 1000 births and is incompatible with life. **Meroencephaly** results from failure of the cranial end of the neural tube to close during the fourth week and causes failure of the neurocranium to form (see Fig. 14-11*B*).

## CRANIOSYNOSTOSIS

Prenatal fusion of the cranial sutures results in several birth defects. The cause of craniosynostosis is unclear. *Mutations of the homeobox genes MSX2, ALX4, FGFR1, FGFR2, and TWIST have been implicated in the molecular mechanisms of craniosynostosis and other cranial defects.* A strong association between maternal valproic acid use during early pregnancy and infant craniosynostosis has been reported; a linkage to maternal smoking and thyroid disease has also been suggested. These birth defects are more common in boys than girls, and they are often associated with other skeletal defects.

*The type of deformed cranium produced depends on which sutures close prematurely.* If the sagittal suture closes early, the cranium becomes long, narrow, and wedge shaped (**scaphocephaly**) (Fig. 14-12*A* and *B*). This type of cranial deformity constitutes about one half the cases of craniosynostosis. Another 30% of cases involve premature closure of the coronal suture, which results in a high, tower-like cranium (**brachycephaly**) (see Fig. 14-12*C*). If the coronal suture closes prematurely on one side only, the cranium is twisted and asymmetric (**plagiocephaly**). Premature closure of the frontal (metopic) suture results in a deformity of the frontal and orbital bones in addition to other anomalies (**trigonocephaly**) (see Fig. 14-12*D*).

## MICROCEPHALY

Neonates with microcephaly are born with normal-sized or slightly small calvaria. The **fontanelles** close during early infancy, and the other sutures close during the first year. However, this defect is not caused by premature closure of sutures. **Microcephaly** is the result of abnormal development of the central nervous system, in which the brain and neurocranium fail to grow. Infants with microcephaly have small heads and are mentally deficient (see Chapter 17, Fig. 17-36).

## ANOMALIES AT CRANIOVERTEBRAL JUNCTION

Congenital abnormalities at the craniovertebral junction occur in approximately 1% of neonates, but they may not produce symptoms until adult life. Examples of these anomalies are **basilar invagination** (superior displacement of bone around the foramen magnum), **assimilation of the atlas** (nonsegmentation at the junction of the atlas and occipital bone), **atlantoaxial dislocation** (disarrangement of atlantoaxial joint), **Chiari malformation** (see Chapter 17, Fig. 17-42*A* and *B*), and a **separate dens** (failure of the centers in the dens to fuse with the centrum of the axis).

# DEVELOPMENT OF APPENDICULAR SKELETON

The appendicular skeleton consists of the pectoral and pelvic girdles and limb bones. Mesenchymal bones form during the fifth week as **condensations of mesenchyme** appear in the limb buds (Fig. 14-13*A* to *C*). During the sixth week, the **mesenchymal bone models** in the limbs undergo chondrification to form **hyaline cartilage bone models** (see Fig. 14-13*D* and *E*).

The **clavicle** initially develops by intramembranous ossification, and it later forms growth cartilages at both ends. The models of the pectoral girdle and upper limb bones appear slightly before those of the pelvic girdle and lower limb bones. The bone models appear in a proximodistal sequence. *Patterning in the developing limbs is regulated by* HOX *genes.*

Ossification begins in the long bones by the eighth week and initially occurs in the diaphyses of the bones from **primary ossification centers** (see Fig. 14-4*B* to *D*). By 12 weeks, primary ossification centers have appeared in most bones of the limbs (Fig. 14-14*A*).

The clavicles begin to ossify before other bones in the body. The **femora** are the next bones to show traces of ossification (see Fig. 14-14*B*). The first indication of the primary center of ossification in the cartilaginous model of a long bone is visible near the center of its future shaft,

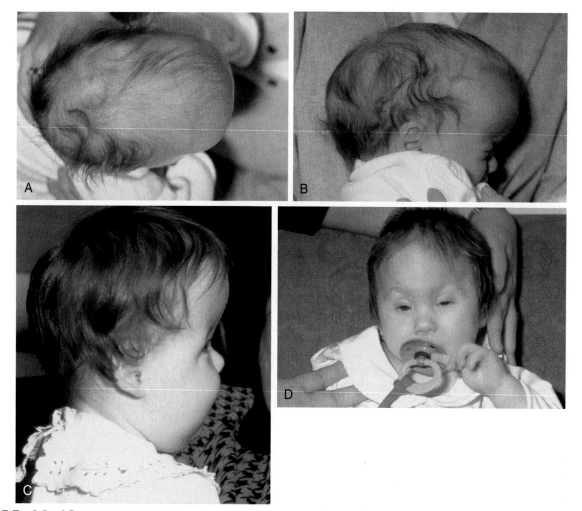

**FIGURE 14–12** Craniosynostosis. **A** and **B,** The infant has scaphocephaly, a condition that results from premature closure (synostosis) of the sagittal suture. The elongated, wedge-shaped cranium is seen from above (**A**) and from the side (**B**). **C,** In an infant with bilateral premature closure of the coronal suture (brachycephaly), notice the high, markedly elevated forehead. **D,** In an infant with premature closure of the frontal suture (trigonocephaly), notice the hypertelorism (abnormal distance between the eyes) and the prominent midline ridging of the forehead.

the diaphysis (see Fig. 14-4C). Primary centers appear at different times in different bones, but most of them appear between the 7th and 12th weeks. Virtually all primary centers of ossification are present at birth.

The **secondary ossification centers** of the bones at the knee are the first to appear in utero. The centers for the distal end of the femur and the proximal end of the tibia usually appear during the last month of intrauterine life (34–38 weeks). These centers are usually present at birth, but most secondary centers appear after birth. The part of a bone ossified from a secondary center is the **epiphysis** (see Fig. 14-4C). The bone formed from the primary center in the **diaphysis** does not fuse with that formed from the secondary centers in the epiphyses until the bone grows to its adult length. This delay enables lengthening of the bone to continue until the final size is reached. During bone growth, a plate of cartilage (**epiphyseal cartilage plate**) intervenes between the diaphysis and epiphysis (see Fig. 14-4E). The epiphyseal plate is eventually replaced by bone development on each of its two sides, *diaphyseal* and *epiphyseal*. When this occurs, growth of the bone ceases.

## BONE AGE

Bone age is a good index of general maturation. Determination of the number, size, and fusion of epiphyseal centers from **radiographs** is a commonly used method. A radiologist determines the bone age by assessing the ossification centers using two criteria:

- The time of appearance of calcified material in the diaphysis or epiphysis, or both, is specific for each diaphysis and epiphysis and for each bone and sex.
- The disappearance of the dark line representing the epiphyseal cartilage plate indicates that the epiphysis has fused with the diaphysis.

Fusion of the diaphyseal-epiphyseal centers, which occurs at specific times for each epiphysis, happens 1 to 2 years earlier in girls than in boys. Individual variation also occurs. Fetal ultrasonography is used for evaluation and measurement of bones and for determination of fertilization age.

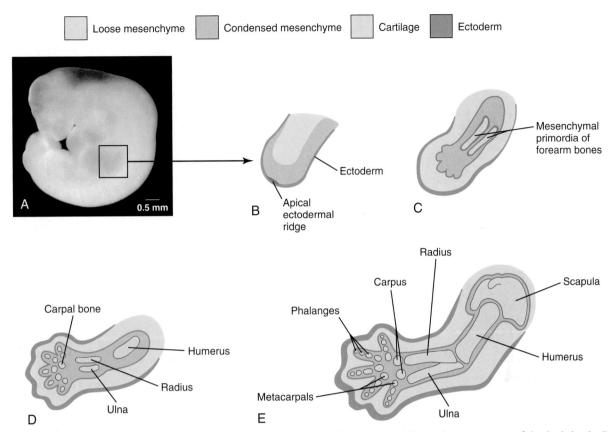

| Loose mesenchyme | Condensed mesenchyme | Cartilage | Ectoderm |

**FIGURE 14–13** A, Photograph of an embryo at approximately 28 days shows the early appearance of the limb buds. B, Longitudinal section through an upper limb bud shows the apical ectodermal ridge, which has an inductive influence on the mesenchyme. This ridge promotes growth of the mesenchyme and imparts the ability to form specific cartilaginous elements. C, Similar sketch of an upper limb bud at approximately 33 days shows the mesenchymal primordia of the forearm bones. The digital rays are mesenchymal condensations that undergo chondrification and ossification to form the bones of the hand. D, Section of the upper limb at 6 weeks shows the cartilage models of the bones. E, Later in the sixth week, the cartilaginous models of the bones of the upper limb are completed.

## GENERALIZED SKELETAL MALFORMATIONS

**Achondroplasia** is the most common cause of dwarfism *(short stature)* (see Chapter 20, Fig. 20-13). This rare defect occurs in approximately 1 of 15,000 births. The limbs become bowed and short (Fig. 14-15) because of disturbance of endochondral ossification during fetal life at the epiphyseal cartilage plates, particularly of the long bones. The trunk of the body is usually short, and the head is enlarged with a bulging forehead and "scooped-out" nose (flat nasal bridge).

**Achondroplasia** is an autosomal dominant disorder. Approximately 80% of cases arise from new mutations, and the rate increases with paternal age. Most cases are caused by a point mutation (G380R) in the fibroblast growth factor receptor 3 gene *(FGFR3)* that amplifies the normal inhibiting effect of endochondral ossification, specifically in the zone of chondrocyte proliferation. This results in shortened bones but does not affect growth of bone width (periosteal bone growth).

**Thanatophoric dysplasia** is the most common type of lethal skeletal dysplasia, with distinct tubular bones, flattened vertebral bodies, and shortened ribs. It occurs in approximately 1 of 20,000 births. The affected infants die of respiratory failure within minutes or days of birth. This lethal disorder is associated with mutations in FGFR3.

Parietal bone

Frontal bone

Occipital bone

Cervical vertebrae

Maxilla

Mandible

Metacarpals

Scapula
Humerus

Radius

Ulna
Ribs

Thoracic vertebrae

Femur

Metatarsal bone

Ilium

Tibia
Fibula

A

B    C

**FIGURE 14–14** Alizarin-stained and cleared human fetuses. **A,** In a 12-week fetus, ossification has progressed from the primary centers of ossification and is endochondral in the appendicular and axial parts of the skeleton except for most of the cranial bones, which form the neurocranium. The carpus and tarsus are wholly cartilaginous at this stage, as are the epiphyses of all long bones. **B and C,** Ossification in a fetus of approximately 20 weeks.

**FIGURE 14–15** Radiograph of the upper limb of a 2-year-old child with achondroplasia. Notice the shortened femur with metaphyseal flaring.

## HYPERPITUITARISM

*Congenital hyperpituitarism*, which causes an infant to grow at an abnormally rapid rate, is rare. It may result in **gigantism** (excessive height and body proportions) or **acromegaly** in an adult (enlargement of soft tissues, visceral organs, and bones of the face, hands, and feet). Gigantism and acromegaly result from an excessive secretion of growth hormone.

## HYPOTHYROIDISM AND CRETINISM

*A severe deficiency of fetal thyroid hormone production* results in **cretinism**, a condition characterized by growth retardation, mental deficiency, skeletal abnormalities, and auditory and neurologic disorders. Bone age appears as less than chronologic age because epiphyseal development is delayed. Cretinism is rare except in areas where there is a lack of iodine in the soil and water. **Agenesis** (absence) of the thyroid gland also results in cretinism.

## SUMMARY OF SKELETAL SYSTEM

- The skeletal system develops from mesenchyme, which is derived from mesoderm and the neural crest. In most bones, such as the long bones in the limbs, the condensed mesenchyme undergoes chondrification to form cartilage models for bone formation. Ossification centers appear in the models by the end of the embryonic period (56 days), and the bones ossify later by endochondral ossification. Some bones (e.g., flat bones of the cranium) develop by intramembranous ossification.
- The vertebral column and ribs develop from mesenchymal cells derived from the sclerotomes of somites. Each vertebra is formed by fusion of a condensation of the caudal half of one pair of sclerotomes with the cranial half of the subjacent pair of sclerotomes.
- The developing cranium (skull) consists of a neurocranium and a viscerocranium, each of which has membranous and cartilaginous components. *The neurocranium forms the calvaria*, and the *viscerocranium forms the skeleton of the face.*
- The appendicular skeleton develops from endochondral ossification of the cartilaginous bone models, which form from mesenchyme in the developing limbs.
- Joints are classified as fibrous joints, cartilaginous joints, and synovial joints. They develop from interzonal mesenchyme between the primordia of bones. In a **fibrous joint**, the intervening mesenchyme differentiates into dense fibrous connective tissue. In a **cartilaginous joint**, the mesenchyme between the bones differentiates into cartilage. In a **synovial joint**, a synovial cavity is formed within the intervening mesenchyme by breakdown of the cells. Mesenchyme also gives rise to the synovial membrane, capsule, and ligaments of the joint.

## CLINICALLY ORIENTED PROBLEMS

### CASE 14-1

*A neonate presented with a lesion in his lower back, which was thought to be a neural arch defect.*

- What is the most common birth defect of the vertebral column?
- Where is the defect usually located?
- Does this birth defect usually cause symptoms (e.g., back problems)?

### CASE 14-2

*A young girl presented with pain in her upper limb, which worsened when she lifted heavy objects. After a radiographic examination, the physician told her parents that she had an accessory rib in her neck.*

- Are accessory ribs clinically important?
- What is the embryologic basis of an accessory rib?

### CASE 14-3

*A mother of a girl with a "crooked spine" was told that her daughter had scoliosis.*

- What vertebral defect can produce scoliosis?
- What is the embryologic basis of the vertebral defect?

### CASE 14-4

*A boy had a long, thin head. His mother was concerned that it might have cognitive consequences for her son.*

- What is meant by the term *craniosynostosis*?
- What results from this developmental abnormality?
- Give a common example, and describe it.

### CASE 14-5

*A child had characteristics of Klippel-Feil syndrome.*

- What are the main features of this condition?
- What vertebral anomalies are usually detected?

Discussion of these problems appears in the Appendix at the back of the book.

## BIBLIOGRAPHY AND SUGGESTED READING

Alexander PG, Tuan RS: Role of environmental factors in axial skeletal dysmorphogenesis, *Birth Defects Res C Embryo Today* 90:118, 2010.

Bamshad M, Van Heest AE, Pleasure D: Arthrogryposis: a review and update, *J Bone Joint Surg Am* 91(Suppl 4):40, 2009.

Brewin J, Hill M, Ellis H: The prevalence of cervical ribs in a London population, *Clin Anat* 22:331, 2009.

Buckingham M: Myogenic progenitor cells and skeletal myogenesis in vertebrates, *Curr Opin Genet Dev* 16:525, 2006.

Cohen MM Jr: Perspectives on craniosynostosis: sutural biology, some well-known syndromes and some unusual syndromes, *J Craniofac Surg* 20:646, 2009.

Cooperman DR, Thompson GH: Musculoskeletal disorders. In Martin RJ, Fanaroff AA, Walsh MC, editors: *Fanaroff and Martin's neonatal–perinatal medicine: diseases of the fetus and infant,* ed 8, Philadelphia, 2006, Mosby.

Dallas SL, Bonewald LF: Dynamics of the transition from osteoblast to osteocyte, *Ann N Y Acad Sci* 1192:437, 2010.

Dunwoodie SL: The role of Notch in patterning the human vertebral column, *Curr Opin Genet Dev* 19:329, 2009.

Franz-Odendaal TA, Hall BK, Witten PE: Buried alive: how osteoblasts become osteocytes, *Dev Dyn* 235:176, 2006.

Gardner LP, Hiatt JL: *Color textbook of histology,* ed 3, Philadelphia, 2007, Saunders.

Gibb S, Maroto M, Dale JK: The segmentation clock mechanism moves up a notch, *Trends Cell Biol* 20:593, 2010.

Hall BK: *Bones and cartilage: developmental skeletal biology,* Philadelphia, 2005, Elsevier.

Hinrichsen KV, Jacob HJ, Jacob M, et al: Principles of ontogenesis of leg and foot in man, *Ann Anat* 176:121, 1994.

Iimura T, Denans N, Pourquie O: Establishment of Hox vertebral identities in the embryonic spine precursors, *Curr Top Dev Biol* 88:201, 2009.

Javed A, Chen H, Ghori FY: Genetic and transcriptional control of bone formation, *Oral Maxillofac Surg Clin North Am* 22:283, 2010.

Karsenty G, Kronenberg HM, Settembre C: Genetic control of bone formation, *Annu Rev Cell Dev Biol* 25:629, 2009.

Keller B, Yang T, Munivez E, et al: Interaction of TGF-beta and BMP signaling pathways during chondrogenesis, *PLoS One* 6:e16421, 2011.

Kubota T, Michigami T, Ozono K: Wnt signaling in bone, *Clin Pediatr Endocrinol* 19:49, 2010.

Lefebvre V, Bhattaram P: Vertebrate skeletogenesis, *Curr Top Dev Biol* 90:291, 2010.

Lewis J, Hanisch A, Holder M: Notch signaling, the segmentation clock, and the patterning of vertebrate somites, *J Biol* 8:44, 2009.

Mackie EJ, Tatarczuch L, Mirams M: The skeleton: a multi-functional complex organ: the growth plate chondrocyte and endochondral ossification, *J Endocrinol* 211:109, 2011.

Rodríguez-Vázquez JF, Verdugo-López S, Garrido JM, et al: Morphogenesis of the manubrium of sternum in human embryos: a new concept, *Anat Rec* 296:279, 2013.

Seo HS, Serra R: Tgfbr2 is required for development of the skull vault, *Dev Biol* 334:481, 2009.

Thornton GK, Woods CG: Primary microcephaly: do all roads lead to Rome? *Trends Genet* 25:501, 2009.

Wellik DM: Hox patterning of the vertebrate axial skeleton, *Dev Dyn* 236:2454, 2007.

C H A P T E R

# Muscular System

The muscular system develops from **mesoderm**, except for muscles of the iris of the eye, which develop from **neuroectoderm**, and muscles of the esophagus, which are thought to develop by transdifferentiation from smooth muscle. **Myoblasts** (embryonic muscle cells) are derived from **mesenchyme** (embryonic connective tissue). Three types of muscle—skeletal, cardiac, and smooth—are formed during the embryonic period.

MYOD, a member of the family of myogenic regulatory factors, activates transcription of muscle-specific genes, and *MYOD* is considered an important regulatory gene for the induction of myogenic differentiation. The **induction of myogenesis** in mesenchymal cells by MYOD depends on the degree of mesenchymal cell differentiation.

Most of the mesenchyme in the head is derived from the neural crest (see Chapter 4, Fig. 4-10), particularly the tissues derived from the pharyngeal arches (see Chapter 9, Figs. *9-1H* and *I* and 9-2). However, the original mesenchyme in these arches gives rise to the musculature of the face and neck (see Chapter 9, Table 9-1).

## DEVELOPMENT OF SKELETAL MUSCLE

Limb and axial muscles of the trunk and head develop by **epitheliomesenchymal transformation** from myogenic precursor cells. Studies show that **myogenic precursor cells** originate from the somatic mesoderm and from the ventral dermomyotome of somites in response to molecular signals from nearby tissues (Figs. 15-1 and 15-2).

The first indication of **myogenesis** (muscle formation) is elongation of the nuclei and cell bodies of mesenchymal cells as they differentiate into myoblasts. These primordial muscle cells soon fuse to form myotubes: elongated, multinucleated, cylindrical structures.

At the molecular level, these events are preceded by activation and expression of the genes of the MYOD family of muscle-specific, basic helix-loop-helix transcription factors (including MYOD, myogenin *[MYOG]*, MYF5, myogenic factor 6 *[MYF6]*, formerly called

**355**

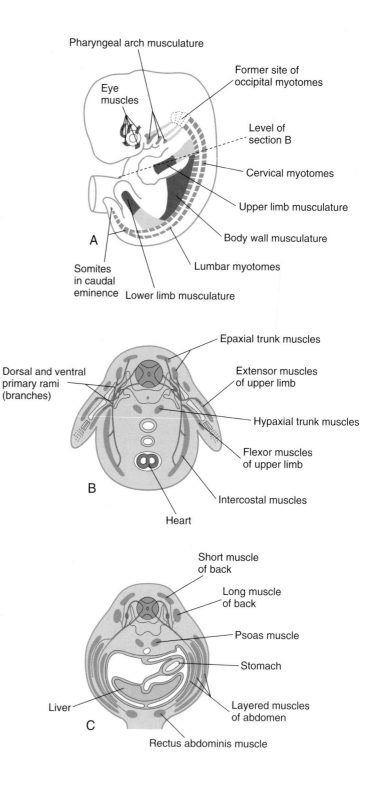

**FIGURE 15–1** A, Sketch of an embryo at approximately 41 days shows the myotomes and developing muscular system. B, Transverse section of the embryo illustrates the epaxial and hypaxial derivatives of a myotome. C, Similar section of a 7-week embryo shows the muscle layers formed from the myotomes.

myogenic regulatory factor 4 *[MRF4])* in the precursor myogenic cells. *Retinoic acid enhances skeletal myogenesis by upregulating the expression of mesodermal markers and myogenic regulatory factors. It has been suggested that signaling molecules from the ventral neural tube and notochord (e.g., SHH) and others from the dorsal neural tube (e.g., WNTs, bone morphogenetic protein 4 [BMP4]) and from overlying ectoderm (e.g., WNTs, BMP4) regulate the beginning of myogenesis and* *the induction of the myotome* (Fig. 15-3). Further muscle growth in the fetus results from the ongoing fusion of myoblasts and myotubes.

During or after fusion of the myoblasts, **myofilaments** develop in the cytoplasm of the myotubes. Other organelles characteristic of striated muscle cells, such as **myofibrils**, also form. As the myotubes develop, they become invested with external laminae (layers), which segregate them from the surrounding connective tissue. **Fibroblasts**

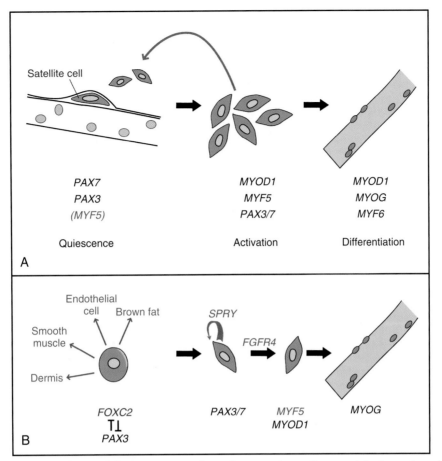

**FIGURE 15–2** Genetic regulation of the progression of muscle progenitor cells toward the formation of differentiated skeletal muscle. **A,** Adult muscle satellite cells progress to form new muscle fiber. *MYF5* is shown in the quiescent state *(red)* to indicate that transcripts are present but not the protein. **B,** During the progression of somatic cells in myogenesis, expression of *PAX3* activates target genes *(red)* that regulate various stages of this process. *(From Buckingham M, Rigby PW: Gene regulatory networks and transcriptional mechanisms that control myogenesis, Dev Cell 28:225, 2014.)*

produce the **perimysium** and **epimysium layers** of the fibrous sheath of the muscle; the **endomysium** is formed by the external lamina and reticular fibers.

Most skeletal muscles develop before birth, and almost all remaining muscles are formed by the end of the first year. The increase in size of a muscle after the first year results from increased fiber diameter from formation of more myofilaments. Muscles increase in length and width to grow with the skeleton. Their ultimate size depends on the amount of exercise that is performed. Not all embryonic muscle fibers persist; many of them fail to establish themselves as necessary units of the muscle and soon degenerate.

## Myotomes

Each typical myotome part of a somite divides into a **dorsal epaxial division** and a **ventral hypaxial division** (see Fig. 15-1*B*). Every developing spinal nerve divides and sends a branch to each myotome division. The dorsal primary ramus supplies the epaxial division, and the ventral primary ramus supplies the hypaxial division. The myoblasts that form the skeletal muscles of the trunk are derived from mesenchyme in the myotome regions of the somites (see Fig. 15-1). Some muscles, such as the intercostal muscles, remain segmentally arranged like the somites, but most myoblasts migrate away from the myotome and form nonsegmented muscles.

Gene-targeting studies in the mouse embryo show that myogenic regulatory factors (MYOD, MYF6, MYF5, and MYOG) are essential for development of the hypaxial, epaxial, abdominal, and intercostal muscles.

Myoblasts from epaxial divisions of the myotomes form the extensor muscles of the neck and vertebral column (Fig. 15-4). The embryonic extensor muscles derived from the sacral and coccygeal myotomes degenerate; their adult derivatives are the dorsal **sacrococcygeal ligaments.** Myoblasts from the hypaxial divisions of the cervical myotomes form the scalene, prevertebral, geniohyoid, and infrahyoid muscles (see Fig. 15-4). The **thoracic myotomes** form the lateral and ventral flexor muscles of the vertebral column, and the **lumbar myotomes** form the quadratus lumborum muscle. The **sacrococcygeal myotomes** form the muscles of the pelvic diaphragm and probably the striated muscles of the anus and sex organs.

A  Epaxial myogenesis | Later myogenesis from the central dermomyotome | Hypaxial myogenesis

B  Extraocular muscles | Masticatory muscles (1st branchial arch derivatives)

C  Migration | Prevent premature activation

**FIGURE 15–3** Gene regulatory networks govern myogenesis in the trunk (**A**), the head (**B**), and cells that migrate from the hypaxial somite to the forelimb (**C**). (*From Buckingham M, Rigby PW: Gene regulatory networks and transcriptional mechanisms that control myogenesis, Dev Cell 28:225, 2014.*)

## Pharyngeal Arch Muscles

Myoblasts from the pharyngeal arches, which originate from the unsegmented paraxial mesoderm and **prechordal plate,** form the muscles of mastication, facial expression, pharynx, and larynx as described elsewhere (see Chapter 9, Fig. 9-6 and Table 9-1). These muscles are innervated by pharyngeal arch nerves.

## Ocular Muscles

The origin of the extrinsic eye muscles is unclear. They may be derived from mesenchymal cells near the prechordal plate (see Figs. 15-1 and 15-4). The mesenchyme in this area is thought to give rise to three preotic myotomes. Myoblasts differentiate from mesenchymal cells derived from these myotomes. Groups of myoblasts, each supplied by its own nerve (cranial nerve [CN] III, CN IV, or CN VI), form the extrinsic muscles of the eye.

## Tongue Muscles

Initially there are four *occipital (postotic) myotomes;* the first pair disappears. Myoblasts from the remaining myotomes form the tongue muscles, which are innervated by the hypoglossal nerve (CN XII).

## Limb Muscles

The musculature of the limbs develops from myoblasts surrounding the developing bones (see Fig. 15-1). The myoblasts form a mass of tissue on the dorsal (extensor) and ventral (flexor) aspects of the limbs. Grafting and gene targeting studies in birds and mammals have demonstrated that the precursor myogenic cells in the limb buds originate from the somites. These cells are first located in the ventral part of the dermomyotome and are epithelial in nature (see Chapter 14, Fig. 14-1*D*). The cells then migrate into the primordium of the limb.

Molecular signals from the neural tube and notochord induce PAX3, MYOD, and MYF5 expression in the somites. In the limb bud, PAX3 regulates the expression of MET (a migratory peptide growth factor), which regulates migration of the precursor myogenic cells.

## DEVELOPMENT OF SMOOTH MUSCLE

Smooth muscle fibers differentiate from **splanchnic mesenchyme** surrounding the endoderm of the primordial gut and its derivatives (see Fig. 15-1). The somatic mesoderm provides smooth muscle in the walls of many blood and lymphatic vessels. The muscles of the iris (sphincter and dilator pupillae) and the myoepithelial cells in mammary and sweat glands are thought to be derived from mesenchymal cells that originate from ectoderm.

The first sign of differentiation of smooth muscle is development of elongated nuclei in spindle-shaped myoblasts. During early development, additional myoblasts continue to differentiate from mesenchymal cells but do not fuse as in skeletal muscle; they remain mononucleated.

During later development, division of existing myoblasts gradually replaces the differentiation of new myoblasts in the production of new smooth muscle tissue. As smooth muscle cells differentiate, filamentous but nonsarcomeric contractile elements develop in their cytoplasm, and the external surface of each cell acquires a surrounding external lamina. As smooth muscle fibers develop into sheets or bundles, they receive autonomic innervation. Muscle cells and fibroblasts synthesize and lay down collagenous, elastic, and reticular fibers.

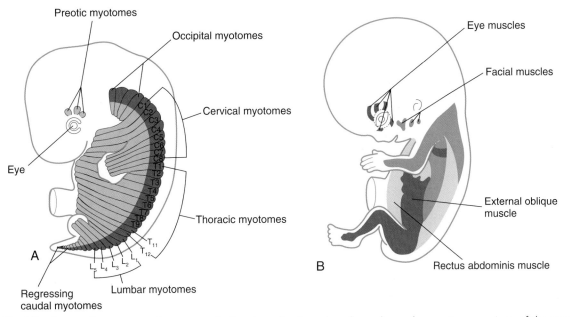

**FIGURE 15–4** Developing muscular system. **A,** Drawing of a 6-week embryo shows the myotome regions of the somites that give rise to skeletal muscles. **B,** Drawing of an 8-week embryo shows the developing trunk and limb musculature.

## DEVELOPMENT OF CARDIAC MUSCLE

Cardiac muscle develops from the lateral splanchnic mesoderm, which gives rise to the mesenchyme surrounding the developing heart tube (see Chapter 13, Figs. 13-1*B* and 13-7*C* to *E*). **Cardiac myoblasts** differentiate from the primordial myocardium. *Heart muscle is recognizable in the fourth week.* It likely develops through expression of cardiac-specific genes. *Studies suggest that PBX proteins interacting with the transcription factor HAND2 promote cardiac muscle differentiation.* Immunohistochemical studies have revealed a spatial distribution of tissue-specific antigens (myosin heavy-chain isoforms) in the embryonic heart between the fourth and eighth weeks.

**Cardiac muscle fibers** arise by differentiation and growth of single cells, unlike striated skeletal muscle fibers, which develop by fusion of cells. Growth of cardiac muscle fibers results from the formation of new myofilaments. The myoblasts adhere to each other as in developing skeletal muscle, but the intervening cell membranes do not disintegrate. These areas of adhesion give rise to **intercalated disks** (intercellular locations of attachment of cardiac muscles). Late in the embryonic period, special bundles of muscle cells develop from original trabeculated myocardium that has fast-conducting gap junctions with relatively few myofibrils and relatively larger diameters than typical cardiac muscle fibers. These atypical cardiac muscle cells (**Purkinje fibers**) *form the conducting system of the heart* (see Chapter 13, Figs. 13-18*E* and 13-19*C* and *D*).

## ANOMALIES OF MUSCLES

Absence of one or more skeletal muscles is more common than is generally recognized. Common examples are the sternocostal head of the pectoralis major, palmaris longus, trapezius, serratus anterior, and quadratus femoris. Usually, only a single muscle is absent on one side of the body, or only part of the muscle fails to develop. Occasionally, the same muscle or muscles may be absent on both sides of the body.

**Absence of the pectoralis major** (often its sternal part) is usually associated with **syndactyly** (fusion of digits). These birth defects are part of the **Poland syndrome** (absence of pectoralis major and minor muscles, ipsilateral breast hypoplasia, and absence of two to four ribs) (Fig. 15-5). Absence

of the pectoralis major is occasionally associated with absence of the mammary gland in the breast and/or hypoplasia of the nipple.

Some muscular birth defects, such as congenital absence of the diaphragm, cause difficulty in breathing, which is usually associated with incomplete expansion of the lungs or part of a lung (**pulmonary atelectasis**) and pneumonitis (pneumonia). Absence of muscles of the anterior abdominal wall may be associated with severe gastrointestinal and genitourinary defects such as **exstrophy of the bladder** (see Chapter 12, Fig. 12-24). Muscle development and muscle repair depend on expression of muscle regulatory genes.

**FIGURE 15–5** A young girl with a severe Poland syndrome with absence of the pectoralis muscles and the nipple. *(From Al-Quattan MM, Kozin SH: Update on embryology of the upper limb,* J Hand Surg Am *38:1835, 2013.)*

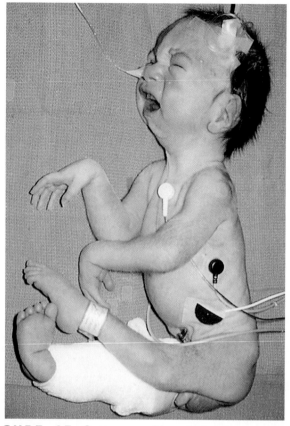

**FIGURE 15–6** Neonate with multiple joint contractures due to arthrogryposis. Infants with this syndrome have stiffness of the joints associated with hypoplasia of the associated muscles.

## ARTHROGRYPOSIS

The term *arthrogryposis* (arthrogryposis multiplex congenita) is used clinically to describe multiple **congenital joint contractures** that affect different parts of the body (Fig. 15-6). Arthrogryposis occurs in 1 in 3000 live births. It includes more than 300 heterogeneous disorders. The causes of arthrogryposis are unclear. In about 30% of cases, genetic factors are involved. Neuropathic disorders and muscle and connective tissue abnormalities restrict intrauterine movement and may lead to **fetal akinesia** (absence or loss of the power of voluntary movement) and joint contractures. The involvement of contractures around certain joints and not others may offer clues to the underlying cause. For instance, **amyoplasia** typically includes bilateral flexion contractures of the wrist, extension of the knees, and talipes equinovarus, but it spares other joints (see Chapter 16, Fig. 16-15).

## VARIATIONS IN MUSCLES

All muscles are subject to a certain amount of variation; however, some are affected more often than others. Certain muscles are functionally vestigial (rudimentary), such as those of the external ear and scalp. Some muscles present in other primates appear in only some humans (e.g., sternalis muscle, a band sometimes found parallel to the sternum). Variations in the form, position, and attachments of muscles are common and are usually functionally insignificant.

**FIGURE 15-7** An 11-year-old boy with untreated left congenital muscular torticollis with restricted lateral flexion to the right and limited neck rotation to the right. *(From Graham J: Smith's recognizable patterns of human deformation, ed 3, Philadelphia, 2007, Elsevier.)*

## CONGENITAL TORTICOLLIS

Some cases of torticollis (wry neck) may result from tearing of fibers of the sternocleidomastoid (SCM) muscle during childbirth. Bleeding into the muscle occurs in a localized area, forming a **hematoma**. A solid mass develops later because of **necrosis** of muscle fibers and fibrosis. Shortening of the muscle usually follows, which causes lateral bending of the head to the affected side and a slight turning of the head away from the side of the short muscle (Fig. 15-7).

Although birth trauma may be a cause of torticollis, the condition has been observed in infants delivered by cesarean section, suggesting that there are other causes, including intrauterine crowding and primary SCM **myopathy**.

## PRUNE-BELLY SYNDROME

Abdominal muscle deficiency and hypotonia are signs of prune-belly syndrome. Male neonates with this syndrome have associated **cryptorchidism** (failure of one or both testes to descend), and **megaureters** (dilation of ureters) are common. The abdominal wall usually is so thin that the viscera (e.g., intestines) are visible and easily palpated. The cause of prune-belly syndrome appears to be related to transient urethral obstruction in the embryo or failure of development of specific mesodermal tissues.

## ACCESSORY MUSCLES

Accessory muscles occasionally develop. For example, an accessory soleus muscle occurs in approximately 3% of people. The primordium of the soleus muscle may undergo early splitting to form an accessory soleus. An accessory flexor muscle of the foot (quadratus plantae muscle) occasionally may develop. In some cases, accessory muscles cause clinically significant symptoms.

## SUMMARY OF MUSCULAR SYSTEM

- Muscle development occurs through the formation of myoblasts, which undergo proliferation to form myocytes.
- Skeletal muscle is derived from the myotome regions of somites.
- Some head and neck muscles are derived from pharyngeal arch mesenchyme.
- The limb muscles develop from myogenic precursor cells surrounding bones in the limbs.
- Cardiac muscle and most smooth muscle are derived from splanchnic mesoderm.
- Absence or variation of some muscles is common and is usually of little consequence.

## CLINICALLY ORIENTED PROBLEMS

### CASE 15-1

*An infant with absence of the left anterior axillary fold also had a left nipple that was much lower than usual.*

- Absence of which muscle probably caused these unusual observations?
- What syndrome do you suspect?
- What features would you look for?
- Would the infant be likely to suffer any disability if absence of this muscle was the only birth defect?

### CASE 15-2

*A medical student discovered hat she had only one palmaris longus muscle.*

- Is this a common occurrence?
- What is its incidence?
- Does the absence of this muscle cause a disability?

### CASE 15-3

*The parents of a 4-year-old girl observed that she always held her head slightly tilted to the right side and that one of her neck muscles was more prominent than the others. The clinical history revealed that her delivery had been a breech birth, one in which the buttocks presented.*

* Name the muscle that was likely prominent.
* Did this muscle pull the child's head to the right side?
* What is this deformity called?
* What likely caused the muscle shortening that resulted in this condition?

*CASE 15–4*

*A neonate had an abdominal wall defect. Failure of striated muscle to develop in the median plane of the anterior abdominal wall is associated with the formation of a severe congenital birth defect of the urinary system.*

* What is this defect called?
* What is the probable embryologic basis of the failure of muscle to form in this neonate?

Discussion of these problems appears in the Appendix at the back of the book.

## BIBLIOGRAPHY AND SUGGESTED READING

Bamshad M, Van Heest AE, Pleasure D: Arthrogryposis: a review and update, *J Bone Joint Surg Am* 91(Suppl 4):40, 2009.

Bonnet A, Dai F, Brand-Saberi B, et al: Vestigial-like 2 acts downstream of MyoD activation and is associated with skeletal muscle differentiation in chick myogenesis, *Mech Dev* 127:120, 2010.

Bothe I, Tenin G, Oseni A, et al: Dynamic control of head mesoderm patterning, *Development* 138:2807, 2011.

Buckingham M: Myogenic progenitor cells and skeletal myogenesis in vertebrates, *Curr Opin Genet Dev* 16:525, 2006.

Cheng JC, Tang SP, Chen TM, et al: The clinical presentation and outcome of treatment of congenital muscular torticollis in infants—a study of 1,086 cases, *J Pediatr Surg* 35:1091, 2000.

Cooperman DR, Thompson GH: Musculoskeletal disorders. In Martin RJ, Fanaroff AA, Walsh MC, editors: *Fanaroff and Martin's neonatal-perinatal medicine: diseases of the fetus and infant*, ed 8, Philadelphia, 2006, Mosby.

Gasser RF: The development of the facial muscle in man, *Am J Anat* 120:357, 1967.

Giacinti C, Giodano A: Cell cycle regulation in myogenesis. In Giordano A, Galderisi U, editors: *Cell cycle regulation and differentiation in cardiovascular and neural systems*, New York, 2010, Springer.

Gibb S, Maroto M, Dale JK: The segmentation clock mechanism moves up a notch, *Trends Cell Biol* 20:593, 2010.

Goncalves LF, Kusanovic JP, Gotsch F, et al: The fetal musculoskeletal system. In Callen PW, editor: *Ultrasonography in obstetrics and gynecology*, ed 5, Philadelphia, 2008, Elsevier.

Kablar B, Krastel K, Ying C, et al: Myogenic determination occurs independently in somites and limb buds, *Dev Biol* 206:219, 1999.

Kablar B, Tajbakhsh S, Rudnick MA: Transdifferentiation of esophageal smooth muscle is myogenic bHLH factor-dependent, *Development* 127:1627, 2000.

Kalcheim C, Ben-Yair R: Cell rearrangements during development of the somite and its derivatives, *Curr Opin Genet Dev* 15:371, 2005.

Martin J, Afouda BA, Hoppler S: Wnt/beta-catenin signaling regulates cardiomyogenesis via GATA transcription factors, *J Anat* 216:92, 2010.

Mathew SJ, Hansen JM, Merrell AJ, et al: Connective tissue fibroblasts and Tcf4 regulate myogenesis, *Development* 138:371, 2011.

Maves L, Tyler A, Moens CB, et al: Pbx acts with Hand 2 in early myocardial differentiation, *Dev Biol* 333:409, 2009.

Messina G, Biressi S, Monteverde S, et al: Nfix regulates fetal-specific transcription in developing skeletal muscle, *Cell* 140:554, 2010.

Moore KL, Dalley AF, Agur AMR: *Clinically oriented anatomy*, ed 7, Baltimore, 2014, Lippincott Williams & Wilkins.

Noden DM: Vertebrate craniofacial development—the relation between ontogenetic process and morphological outcome, *Brain Behav Evol* 38:190, 1991.

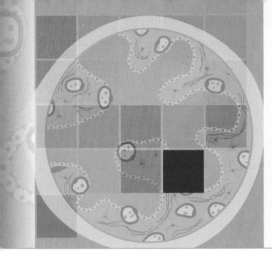

## CHAPTER 16

# Development of Limbs

## EARLY STAGES OF LIMB DEVELOPMENT

The upper limbs of the embryo appear at 26 days' gestation. The lower limb buds become visible at the end of the fourth week with the activation of a group of mesenchymal cells in the somatic lateral mesoderm (Fig. 16-1*A*). Homeobox (Hox) genes regulate patterning in the formation of the limbs. The **limb buds** form deep to a thick band of ectoderm, the **apical ectodermal ridge** (**AER**) (Fig. 16-2*A*). The buds first appear as small bulges on the ventro-lateral body wall (see Fig. 16-1). The upper limb buds are visible by day 24, and the lower limb buds appear 1 or 2 days later. Each limb bud consists of a mesenchymal core of mesoderm covered by a layer of ectoderm.

The limb buds elongate by proliferation of the mesenchyme. The upper limb buds appear disproportionately low on the embryo's trunk because of the early development of the cranial half of the embryo (see Fig. 16-1). The earliest stages of limb development are alike for the upper and lower limbs (see Figs. 16-1*B* and 16-4). Later, distinct differences arise because of differences in form and function of the hands and feet.

The **upper limb buds** develop opposite the caudal cervical segments and the **lower limb buds** form opposite the lumbar and upper sacral segments. At the apex of each limb bud, the ectoderm thickens to form the AER. This ridge is a specialized, multilayered epithelial structure (see Fig. 16-2) that is induced by the paracrine factor, fibroblast growth factor 10 (FGF10), from the underlying mesenchyme. Bone morphogenetic protein (BMP) signaling is required for its formation.

*FGF8, secreted by the AER, exerts an inductive influence on the limb mesenchyme that initiates growth and development of the limbs in a proximodistal axis. Retinoic acid promotes formation of the limb bud by inhibiting FGF signaling.* Mesenchymal cells aggregate at the posterior margin of the limb bud to form the **zone of polarizing activity**, an important signaling center in limb development. *FGFs from the AER activate the zone of polarizing activity, which causes expression of the sonic hedgehog (SHH genes).*

*SHH secretions (morphogens) control the normal patterning of the limbs along the anterior-posterior axis. Expression of WNT7A from the dorsal non-AER ectoderm of the*

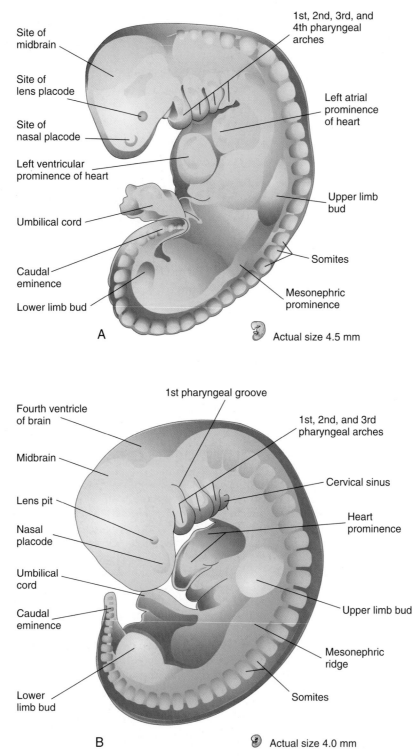

Site of midbrain

1st, 2nd, 3rd, and 4th pharyngeal arches

Site of lens placode

Site of nasal placode

Left atrial prominence of heart

Left ventricular prominence of heart

Umbilical cord

Upper limb bud

Caudal eminence

Somites

Lower limb bud

Mesonephric prominence

A

Actual size 4.5 mm

Fourth ventricle of brain

1st pharyngeal groove

Midbrain

1st, 2nd, and 3rd pharyngeal arches

Lens pit

Cervical sinus

Nasal placode

Heart prominence

Umbilical cord

Caudal eminence

Upper limb bud

Lower limb bud

Mesonephric ridge

Somites

B

Actual size 4.0 mm

**FIGURE 16–1** Drawings of human embryos show development of the limbs. **A,** Lateral view of an embryo at approximately 28 days. The upper limb bud appears as a swelling or bulge on the ventrolateral body wall. The lower limb bud is much smaller than the upper limb bud. **B,** Lateral view of an embryo at approximately 32 days. The upper limb buds are paddle-shaped, and the lower limb buds are flipper-like. *(Modified from Nishimura H, Semba R, Tanimura T, Tanaka O: Prenatal development of the human with special reference to craniofacial structures: an atlas, Washington, DC, 1977, National Institutes of Health.)*

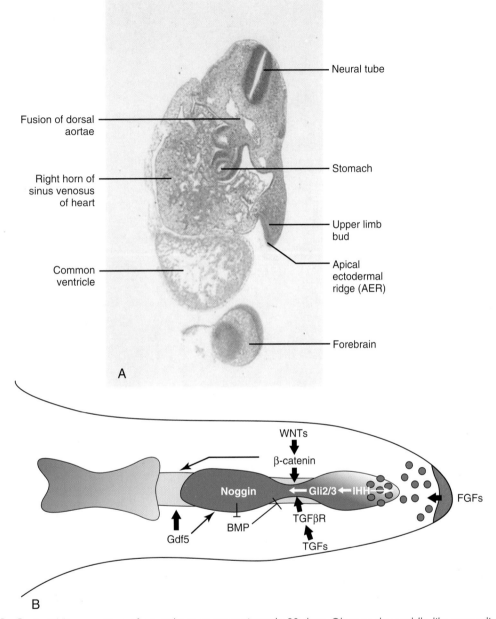

**FIGURE 16-2** A, Oblique section of an embryo at approximately 28 days. Observe the paddle-like upper limb bud lateral to the embryonic heart and the apical epidermal ridge *(AER)*. B, Signaling pathways regulate the elongation and segmentation of the digit ray. In the AER, fibroblast growth factor *(FGF)* signaling *(red)* maintains a small population of subridge undifferentiated mesenchymal cells, which are actively incorporated into the digital condensation *(blue)*. At the presumptive joint site, the newly differentiated chondrogenic cells dedifferentiate to interzone status under the regulation of multiple signaling pathways. *WNTs* promote chondrocyte dedifferentiation through canonical WNT signaling. Indian hedgehog *(IHH)* signals to the interzone region through localized expression of the transcription factors *Gli2* and *Gli3*. Transforming growth factors signal to the interzone cells through the type II receptor. Growth differentiation factor 5 *(Gdf5)* regulates the progression of the joint and skeletogenesis of the digit elements. *BMP,* Bone morphogenetic protein; *TGFβR,* transforming growth factor-β receptor. (*A, From Moore KL, Persaud TVN, Shiota K: Color atlas of clinical embryology, ed 2, Philadelphia, 2000, Saunders. B, From Hu J, He L: Patterning mechanisms controlling digit development, J Genet Genomics 35:517–524, 2008.)*

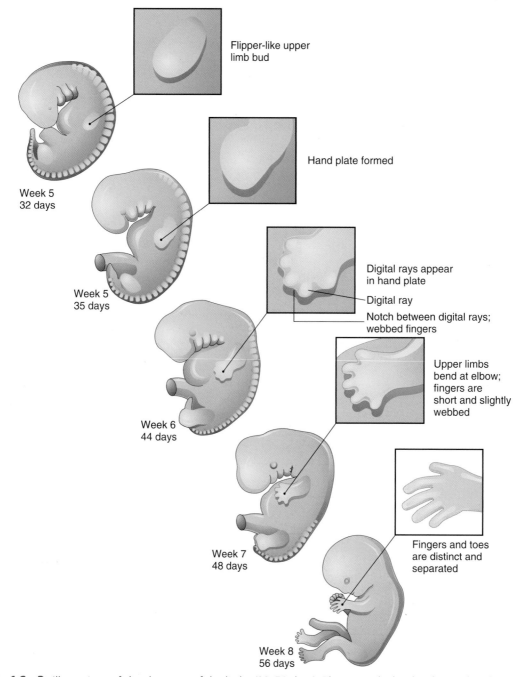

Flipper-like upper limb bud

Hand plate formed

Week 5
32 days

Week 5
35 days

Digital rays appear in hand plate

Digital ray

Notch between digital rays; webbed fingers

Upper limbs bend at elbow; fingers are short and slightly webbed

Week 6
44 days

Week 7
48 days

Fingers and toes are distinct and separated

Week 8
56 days

**FIGURE 16–3** Illustrations of development of the limbs (32–56 days). The upper limbs develop earlier than the lower limbs.

*limb bud and engrailed homeobox 1 (EN1) from the ventral aspect are involved in specifying the dorsal-ventral axis. The AER itself is maintained by inductive signals from SHH and WNT7. It has been suggested that epiprofin, a zinc finger transcription factor, regulates WNT signaling in the limb bud (see Fig. 16-2B).*

The mesenchyme adjacent to the AER consists of undifferentiated, rapidly proliferating cells, whereas mesenchymal cells proximal to it differentiate into blood vessels and cartilage bone models. The distal ends of the limb buds flatten into *hand plates* and *foot plates* (Fig. 16-3 and Fig. 16-4B and H). Studies have shown

that endogenous retinoic acid is also involved in limb development and pattern formation.

By the end of the sixth week, mesenchymal tissue in the **hand plates** has condensed to form **digital rays** (see Figs. 16-3 and 16-4C). These mesenchymal condensations outline the pattern of the digits (fingers) in the hand plates. During the seventh week, similar condensations of mesenchyme condense to form digital rays and digits (toes) in the footplates (see Fig. 16-4I).

At the tip of each digital ray, a part of the AER induces development of the mesenchyme into the mesenchymal **primordia of the bones** (phalanges) in the digits (see

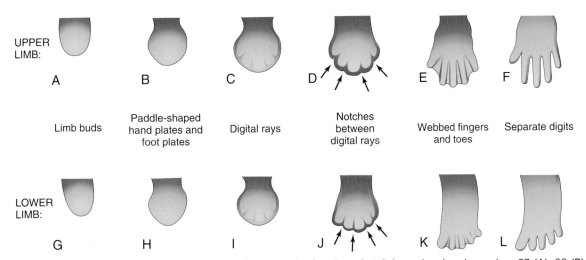

**FIGURE 16–4** Illustrations of limb development between the fourth and eighth weeks—hands on days 27 (A), 32 (B), 41 (C), 46 (D), 50 (E), and 52 (F); feet on days 28 (G), 36 (H), 46 (I), 49 (J), 52 (K), and 56 (L). The early stages are alike except that development of the hands precedes that of the feet by a day or two. The *arrows* in D and J indicate the tissue breakdown process (apoptosis) that separates the fingers and toes.

Fig. 16-6*C* and *D*). The intervals between the digital rays are occupied by loose mesenchyme. These intervening regions of mesenchyme soon break down, forming *notches between the digital rays* (Fig. 16-5; see Fig. 16-3 and Fig. 16-4*D* and *F*). As the tissue breakdown progresses, separate digits (fingers and toes) are formed by the end of the eighth week (Fig. 16-6; see Fig. 16-4*E*, *F*, *K*, and *L*).

*Molecular studies* indicate that the earliest stages of limb patterning and digit formation involve expression of the patched 1 gene (*PTCH1*), which is essential for the downstream regulation of the SHH pathway. **Programmed cell death** *(apoptosis)* is responsible for the tissue breakdown in the interdigital regions. Antagonism between retinoic acid and transforming growth factor-β (TGF-β) appears to control the interdigital apoptosis. Blockade of these cellular and molecular events could account for **syndactyly** or webbing of the fingers or toes (see Fig. 16-14*C* and *D*).

## FINAL STAGES OF LIMB DEVELOPMENT

As the limbs elongate, mesenchymal models of the bones are formed by cellular aggregations (see Fig. 16-7*B*). **Chondrification centers** appear in the fifth week. By the end of the sixth week, the entire limb skeleton is cartilaginous (Fig. 16-7; see Chapter 14, Fig. 14-13*D* and *E*). **Osteogenesis of long bones** begins in the seventh week from primary ossification centers in the middle of the cartilaginous models of the long bones. **Ossification centers** are present in all long bones by the 12th week (see Chapter 14, Fig. 14-14*A*).

From the **dermomyotome regions** of the somites, myogenic precursor cells migrate into the limb buds and later differentiate into **myoblasts**, precursors of muscle cells. *The c-Met receptor tyrosine kinase (encoded by the gene MET) plays an essential role in regulating this process.*

As the long bones form, the myoblasts aggregate and form a large muscle mass in each limb bud (see Chapter 15, Fig. 15-1). In general, this muscle mass separates into dorsal (extensor) and ventral (flexor) components. The mesenchyme in the limb bud also gives rise to ligaments and blood vessels.

Early in the seventh week, the limbs extend ventrally. Originally, the flexor aspect of the limbs is ventral and the extensor aspect is dorsal; the preaxial and postaxial borders are cranial and caudal, respectively (see Fig. 16-10*A* and *D*). The developing upper and lower limbs rotate in opposite directions and to different degrees (Figs. 16-8 and 16-9):

- *The upper limbs rotate laterally* through 90 degrees on their longitudinal axis; as a result, the future elbows come to point dorsally, and the extensor muscles lie on the lateral and posterior aspects of the limb.
- *The lower limbs rotate medially* through almost 90 degrees; therefore, the future knees come to face ventrally, and the extensor muscles lie on the anterior aspect of the limb.

Developmentally, the radius and tibia are homologous bones, as are the ulna and fibula; likewise, the thumb and great toe are homologous digits. **Synovial joints** appear at the beginning of the fetal period (ninth week), coinciding with functional differentiation of the limb muscles and their innervation.

### Cutaneous Innervation of Limbs

There is a strong relationship between the growth and rotation of the limbs and their cutaneous segmental nerve supply. **Motor axons** arising from the spinal cord enter the limb buds during the fifth week and grow into the dorsal and ventral muscle masses. **Sensory axons** enter the limb buds after the motor axons and use them for guidance. Neural crest cells, the precursors of Schwann cells, surround the motor and sensory nerve fibers in the

**FIGURE 16–5** Scanning electron micrographs show dorsal (A) and plantar (B) views of the right foot of an embryo at approximately 48 days. The toe buds (*arrowheads* in A) and the heel cushion and metatarsal tactile elevation (*asterisks* in B) have just appeared. Dorsal (C) and distal (D) views of the right foot of embryos at approximately 55 days show that the tips of the toes are separated and interdigital degeneration has begun. Notice the dorsiflexion of the metatarsus and toes (C) as well as the thickened heel cushion (D). *(From Hinrichsen KV, Jacob HJ, Jacob M, et al: Principles of ontogenesis of leg and foot in man. Ann Anat 176:121, 1994.)*

**FIGURE 16–6** Scanning electron micrographs show a dorsal view of the left foot (**A**) and a plantar view of the right foot (**B**) of an 8-week embryo. Although the foot is supinated, dorsiflexion is distinct. **C** and **D**, Paraffin sections of the tarsus and metatarsus of a young fetus, stained with hematoxylin and eosin, show metatarsal cartilages (*1–5*), cubital cartilage (*6*), and calcaneus (*7*). The separation between the interosseous muscles (*IM*) and the short flexor muscles of the big toe (*SFH*) is clearly seen. The plantar crossing (*Cr*) of the tendons of the long flexors of the digits and the hallux (great toe) is shown in **D**. *(From Hinrichsen KV, Jacob HJ, Jacob M, et al: Principles of ontogenesis of leg and foot in man. Ann Anat 176:121, 1994.)*

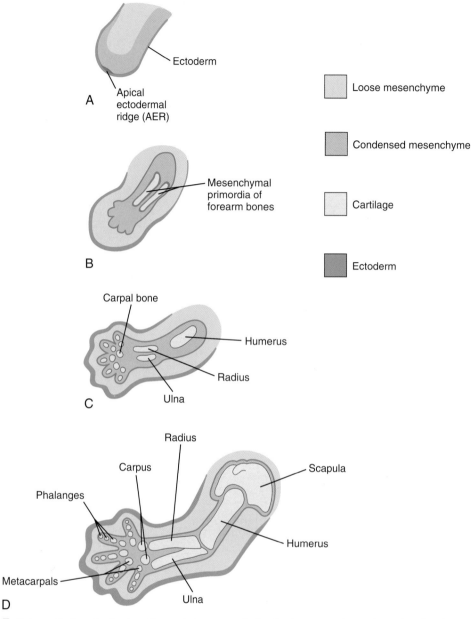

**FIGURE 16–7** Schematic longitudinal sections of the upper limb of a human embryo show the development of cartilaginous bones at 28 (**A**), 44 (**B**), 48 (**C**), and 56 (**D**) days.

limbs and form the **neurolemma** (sheath of Schwann) and **myelin sheaths** (see Chapter 17, Fig. 17-11).

During the fifth week, peripheral nerves grow from the developing brachial and lumbosacral **limb plexuses** into the mesenchyme of the limbs (Fig. 16-10*B* and *E*). The **spinal nerves** are distributed in segmental bands, supplying both dorsal and ventral surfaces of the limbs. A **dermatome** is the area of skin supplied by a single spinal nerve and its spinal ganglion; however, cutaneous nerve areas and dermatomes show considerable overlap.

As the limbs elongate, the cutaneous distribution of the spinal nerves migrates along the limbs and no longer reaches the surface in the distal parts of the limbs. Although the original dermatomal pattern changes during growth of the limbs, an orderly sequence of distribution can still be recognized in the adult (see Fig. 16-10*C* and *F*). In the upper limb, the areas supplied by spinal nerves C5 and C6 adjoin the areas supplied by T2, T1, and C8, but the overlap between them is minimal at the ventral axial line.

A **cutaneous nerve area** is the area of skin supplied by a peripheral nerve. If the dorsal root supplying the area is cut, the dermatomal patterns indicate that there may be a slight deficit in the area indicated. However, because there is overlapping of dermatomes, a particular area of skin is not exclusively innervated by a single segmental nerve. The limb dermatomes may be traced progressively down the lateral aspect of the upper limb and back up its medial aspect. A comparable distribution of dermatomes occurs in the lower limbs, which may be traced

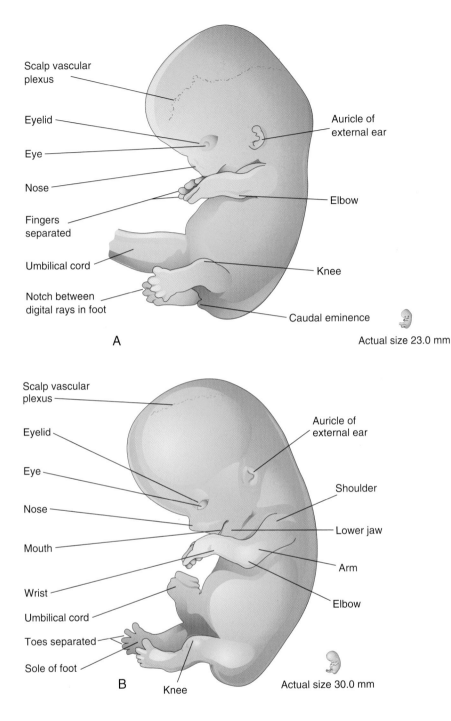

Scalp vascular plexus

Eyelid

Eye

Nose

Fingers separated

Umbilical cord

Notch between digital rays in foot

Auricle of external ear

Elbow

Knee

Caudal eminence

A

Actual size 23.0 mm

Scalp vascular plexus

Eyelid

Eye

Nose

Mouth

Wrist

Umbilical cord

Toes separated

Sole of foot

Auricle of external ear

Shoulder

Lower jaw

Arm

Elbow

B Knee

Actual size 30.0 mm

**FIGURE 16–8** Drawings of lateral views of embryos. **A,** At approximately 52 days, the fingers are separated, and the toes are beginning to separate. Notice that the feet are fan shaped. **B,** At approximately 56 days, all regions of the limbs are apparent, and the digits of the hands and feet are separated. *(Modified from Nishimura H, Semba R, Tanimura T, Tanaka O: Prenatal development of the human with special reference to craniofacial structures: an atlas, Washington, DC, 1977, National Institutes of Health.)*

down the ventral aspect and then up the dorsal aspect. As the limbs descend, they carry their nerves with them; this explains the oblique courses of the nerves arising from the brachial and lumbosacral plexuses.

## Blood Supply of Limbs

The limb buds are supplied by branches of the **intersegmental arteries** (Fig. 16-11A), which arise from the **dorsal aorta** and form a fine capillary network throughout the mesenchyme. The primordial vascular pattern consists of a **primary axial artery** and its branches (see Fig. 16-11B and C), which drain into a peripheral marginal sinus.

Blood in the **marginal sinus** drains into a peripheral vein. The vascular patterns change as the limbs develop, chiefly by **angiogenesis**. The new vessels coalesce with other sprouts to form new vessels.

The primary axial artery becomes the **brachial artery** in the arm and the common interosseous artery in the forearm (see Fig. 16-11B), which has anterior and posterior interosseous branches. The ulnar and radial arteries are terminal branches of the brachial artery. As the digits form, the marginal sinus breaks up and the final venous pattern, represented by the basilic and cephalic veins and their tributaries, develops. In the lower limb, the primary axial artery becomes the **deep artery of the thigh**

**FIGURE 16–9** Illustrations of positional changes of the developing limbs of embryos. **A,** At approximately 48 days, the limbs extend ventrally, and the hand plates and foot plates face each other. **B,** At approximately 51 days, the upper limbs are bent at the elbow, and the hands are curved over the thorax. **C,** At approximately 54 days, the soles of the feet face medially. **D,** At approximately 56 days (end of embryonic stage), the elbows point caudally and the knees cranially.

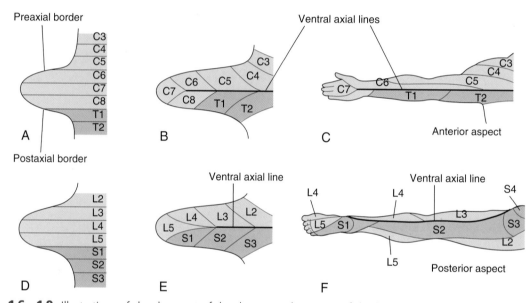

**FIGURE 16–10** Illustrations of development of the dermatomal patterns of the limbs. The axial lines indicate areas in which there is no sensory overlap. **A** and **D,** Ventral aspect of the limb buds early in the fifth week. At this stage, the dermatomal patterns show the primordial segmental arrangement. **B** and **E,** Similar views later in the fifth week show the modified arrangement of dermatomes. **C** and **F,** The dermatomal patterns in the adult upper and lower limbs. The primordial dermatomal pattern has disappeared, but an orderly sequence of dermatomes can still be recognized. Notice in **F** that most of the original ventral surface of the lower limb lies on the back of the adult limb. This arrangement results from the medial rotation of the lower limb that occurs toward the end of the embryonic period. In the upper limb (**C**), the ventral axial line extends along the anterior surface of the arm and forearm. In the lower limb (**F**), the ventral axial line extends along the medial side of the thigh and knee and down the posteromedial aspect of the leg to the heel.

(*profunda femoris artery*), and the anterior and posterior **tibial arteries** in the leg.

## BIRTH DEFECTS OF LIMBS

Minor birth defects involving the limbs are relatively common and can usually be corrected surgically. Although these defects are often of no serious medical consequence, they may serve as indicators of more serious defects, which may be part of a recognizable pattern.

*The critical period of limb development is from 24 to 36 days after fertilization.* This statement is based on clinical studies of neonates who were exposed in utero to the drug **thalidomide,** a potent human **teratogen** during the embryonic period. Exposure to this teratogen before day 36 can cause severe limb defects such as **amelia** (absence of limbs; Fig. 16-12A). For a teratogen to cause amelia or **meromelia** (partial absence of limbs), it must be taken before the end of the critical period of limb development. Many severe limb defects occurred from 1957 to 1962 as a result of *maternal ingestion of*

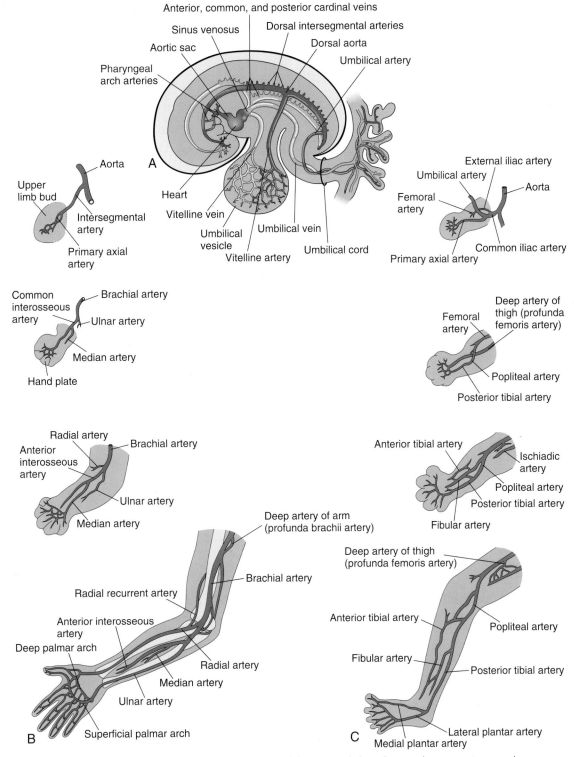

**FIGURE 16–11** Development of limb arteries. **A,** Sketch of the primordial cardiovascular system in an embryo at approximately 26 days. **B,** Development of arteries in the upper limb. **C,** Development of arteries in the lower limb.

**FIGURE 16–12** Birth defects of limbs caused by maternal ingestion of thalidomide. **A,** Quadruple amelia: absence of upper and lower limbs. **B,** Meromelia of the upper limbs; the limbs are represented by rudimentary stumps. **C,** Meromelia with the rudimentary upper limbs attached directly to the trunk. *(From Lenz W, Knapp K: Foetal malformation due to thalidomide. Geriatr Med Monthly 7:253, 1962.)*

*thalidomide.* This hypnotic drug, widely used as a sedative and antinauseant, was withdrawn from the market in December 1961. Since that time, similar limb defects have rarely been observed. Although thalidomide is now used for the treatment of leprosy and other disorders, it is *absolutely contraindicated in women of childbearing age.*

Major limb defects appear approximately 1 in 500 neonates. Most of these defects are caused by genetic factors. *Molecular studies have implicated gene mutations (in Hox genes, BMP, SHH, WNT7, EN1, and others) in some cases of limb defects.* Several unrelated birth defects of the lower limb have been found to be associated with an aberrant arterial pattern, which might be of some importance in the pathogenesis of these defects. *Experimental studies indicate that thalidomide affects the formation of early blood vessels in the limb buds.*

## LIMB ANOMALIES

There are two main types of limb anomalies or defects:
- **Amelia,** absence of a limb or limbs (Fig. 16-13A; see Fig. 16-12A)
- **Meromelia,** absence of part of a limb (see Figs. 16-12B and C and 16-13B and C); it includes **hemimelia,** such as absence of the fibula in the leg, and **phocomelia,** in which the hands and/or feet are attached close to the body

## CAUSES OF LIMB DEFECTS

Birth defects of the limbs originate at different stages of development. Suppression of limb bud development during the early part of the fourth week results in absence of the limb (amelia). Arrest or disturbance of differentiation or growth of a limb during the fifth week results in various types of meromelia.

Like other congenital anomalies, limb defects may be caused by several factors:
- **Genetic factors,** such as chromosomal abnormalities associated with trisomy 18 (see Chapter 20, Fig. 20-7)
- **Mutant genes,** as in brachydactyly, abnormal shortness of the fingers, or osteogenesis imperfecta, a severe limb defect with fractures occurring before birth
- **Environmental factors,** such as teratogens (e.g., thalidomide, alcohol)
- A combination of genetic and environmental factors (*multifactorial inheritance*), as in developmental dysplasia of the hip
- Vascular disruption and **ischemia** (diminished blood supply), as in limb reduction defects

Experimental studies support the suggestion that mechanical influences during intrauterine development may cause some fetal limb defects. A reduced quantity of amniotic fluid (*oligohydramnios*) is commonly associated with limb deformations; however, the significance of in utero mechanical influences on congenital postural deformation is still open to question.

**FIGURE 16–13** Various types of birth defects. **A,** Female neonate with amelia, complete absence of the upper limbs. **B,** Radiograph of a female fetus shows absence of the right fibula. Notice also that the right leg is shorter than the left, and the femur and tibia are bowed and hypoplastic (underdeveloped). **C,** Radiograph shows partial absence and fusion of the lower ends of the tibia and fibula in a 5-year-old child. **D,** Absence of the central digits of the hands results in a defect called bifurcate (forked) hand or split hand. **E,** Absence of the second to fourth toes results in a bifurcate or split foot.

## SPLIT-HAND/FOOT MALFORMATIONS

In severe birth defects such as bifurcate (forked) hand or cleft foot, which clinically are called **split-hand/foot malformations (SHFMs)**, there is absence of one or more central digits (fingers or toes) due to failure of development of one or more digital rays (see Fig. 16-13D and E). The hand or foot is divided into two parts that oppose and curve inward. This is a rare condition affecting approximately 1 in 20,000 live births.

The **split hand syndrome** is an autosomal dominant abnormality with incomplete penetrance. The malformation originates in the fifth to sixth week of development, when the hands are forming. This disorder has 70% penetrance; that is, only 70% of the people who have the defective gene(s) exhibit the defect.

## CONGENITAL ABSENCE OF THE RADIUS

The radius is partially or completely absent. The hand deviates laterally, and the ulna bows with the concavity on the lateral side of the forearm. This defect results from failure of the mesenchymal primordium of the radius to form during the fifth week of development. Absence of the radius is usually caused by genetic factors and may be associated with other abnormalities in the newborn, such as thrombocytopenia (a condition known as thrombocytopenia absent radii [TAR] syndrome).

## BRACHYDACTYLY

Brachydactyly, or shortness of the digits (fingers or toes), is caused by reduction in the length of the phalanges. This birth defect is usually inherited as a dominant trait and is often associated with shortness of stature (see Chapter 20, Fig. 20-13).

## POLYDACTYLY

Polydactyly is the presence of **supernumerary digits**; that is, more than five digits on the hands or feet (Fig. 16-14*A* and *B*). Often, the extra digit is incompletely formed and lacks normal muscular development. If the hand is affected, the extra digit is most commonly medial or lateral rather than central. In the foot, the extra toe is usually on the lateral side. Polydactyly is inherited as a dominant trait.

## SYNDACTYLY

Syndactyly is a common birth defect of the hand or foot. **Cutaneous syndactyly** (simple webbing between digits) is more frequent in the foot than in the hand (see Fig. 16-14*C* and *D*). Cutaneous syndactyly results from failure of the webs to degenerate between two or more digits. **Apoptosis** is responsible for the tissue breakdown between the digits. Blockade of these cellular and molecular events is likely responsible for the defects.

**Osseous syndactyly** (fusion of bones, *synostosis*) occurs when the notches between the digital rays fail to develop and as a result, separation of the digits does not occur. This defect is most frequently observed between the third and fourth fingers and between the second and third toes (**SD type I**). It is inherited as a simple autosomal dominant. A case of syndactyly and polydactyly (synpolydactyly, or **SD type II**), caused by mutations in the amino-terminal, non–DNA binding part of *HoxD13*, has been reported.

**FIGURE 16–14** Types of digital birth defects. Polydactyly: more than five digits on the hands (**A**) or feet (**B**). Syndactyly (webbing or fusion) of the fingers (**C**) or toes (**D**).

## CONGENITAL CLUBFOOT

Talipes equinovarus (clubfoot) is a relatively common birth defect (occurring in approximately 1 in 1000 births), and it is the most common musculoskeletal deformation. It is characterized by multiple components that lead to an abnormal position of the foot, preventing normal weight bearing. The sole of the foot is turned medially, and the foot is inverted (Fig. 16-15). Clubfoot is bilateral in approximately 50% of cases, and it occurs approximately twice as frequently in males.

Although it is commonly stated that clubfoot results from abnormal positioning or restricted movement of the lower limbs of the fetus in utero, the evidence for this is inconclusive. Clubfoot appears to be caused by **multifactorial inheritance**, with genetic and environmental factors acting together. In this condition, all anatomical structures are present, so the majority of cases can be treated with casting or taping. In other cases, the deformity is flexible and is amenable to physiotherapy alone to resolve the deformation.

**FIGURE 16–15** Neonate with bilateral talipes equinovarus (clubfeet). Observe the hyperextension and incurving of the feet.

## DEVELOPMENTAL DYSPLASIA OF THE HIP

Developmental dysplasia of the hip occurs in approximately 1 in 1500 neonates, and it is more common in females than in males. The joint capsule is very relaxed at birth, and there is underdevelopment of the acetabulum of the hip bone and the head of the femur. Dislocation almost always occurs after birth. There are two causative factors:

- **Abnormal development of the acetabulum** occurs in approximately 15% of neonates with congenital dislocation of the hip, which is common after breech deliveries. This suggests that the breech posture during the terminal months of pregnancy may result in abnormal development of the acetabulum and the head of the femur.
- **Generalized joint laxity** is often a dominantly inherited condition that appears to be associated with congenital dislocation of the hip. It follows a multifactorial pattern of inheritance.

## ▶ SUMMARY OF LIMB DEVELOPMENT

- **Limb buds** appear toward the end of the fourth week of gestation as slight bulges of the ventrolateral body wall. Development of the upper limb buds proceeds approximately 2 days ahead of development of the lower limb buds. The tissues of the limb buds are derived from two main sources, mesoderm and ectoderm.
- The **AER** (apical ectodermal ridge) exerts an inductive influence on the limb mesenchyme (see Fig. 16-2), promoting growth and development of the limbs. The limb buds elongate by proliferation of the mesenchyme within them. **Apoptosis** is an important mechanism in limb development; for example, in the breakdown of the tissue in the notches between the digital rays.
- Limb muscles are derived from mesenchyme (myogenic precursor cells) originating in the somites. The muscle-forming cells (**myoblasts**) form dorsal and ventral muscle masses. Nerves grow into the limb buds after the muscle masses have formed. Most blood vessels in the limb buds arise as buds from the intersegmental arteries.
- Initially, the developing limbs are directed caudally; later, they project ventrally; and finally, they rotate on their longitudinal axes. The upper and lower limbs rotate in opposite directions and to different degrees (see Fig. 16-9).
- Most birth defects of the limbs are caused by genetic factors; however, many defects probably result from an interaction of genetic and environmental factors (**multifactorial inheritance**).

## CLINICALLY ORIENTED PROBLEMS

*CASE 16–1*

*A mother consulted her pediatrician after noticing that when her 11-month-old daughter began to stand independently, her legs seemed to be of different lengths. The pediatrician diagnosed congenital hip dysplasia.*

- ✱ Are the hip joints of these infants usually dislocated at birth?
- ✱ What are the probable causes of congenital dislocation of the hip?

## CASE 16–2

*A male infant was born with limb defects (see Fig. 16-12). His mother said that one of her relatives had similar defects.*

* Are limb defects similar to those caused by the drug thalidomide common?
* What was the characteristic syndrome produced by thalidomide?
* Name the limb and other defects commonly associated with the thalidomide syndrome.

## CASE 16–3

*A neonate presented with clubfeet. The physician explained that this is a common birth defect.*

* What is the most common type of clubfoot?
* How common is it?
* Describe the feet of infants born with this birth defect and the treatment.

## CASE 16–4

*A baby was born with syndactyly (webbing between her fingers). The doctor stated that this minor defect can be easily corrected surgically.*

* Is syndactyly common?
* Does it occur more often in the hands than in the feet?
* What is the embryologic basis of syndactyly?
* What is the difference between simple and complex (osseous) syndactyly?

Discussion of these problems appears in the Appendix at the back of the book.

## BIBLIOGRAPHY AND SUGGESTED READING

Ambler CA, Nowicki JL, Burke AC, et al: Assembly of trunk and limb blood vessels involves extensive migration and vasculogenesis of somite-derived angioblasts, *Dev Biol* 234:352, 2001.

Butterfield NC, McGlinn E, Wicking C: The molecular regulation of vertebrate limb patterning, *Curr Top Dev Biol* 90:319, 2010.

Cole P, Kaufman Y, Hatef DA, et al: Embryology of the hand and upper extremity, *J Craniofac Surg* 20:992, 2009.

Cooperman DR, Thompson GH: Congenital abnormalities of the upper and lower extremities and spine. In Martin RJ, Fanaroff AA, Walsh MC, editors: *Fanaroff and Martin's neonatal-perinatal medicine: diseases of the fetus and infant*, ed 8, Philadelphia, 2006, Mosby.

Dahn RD, Fallon JF: Limiting outgrowth: BMPs as negative regulators in limb development, *Bioessays* 21:721, 1999.

Elliott AM, Evans JA, Chudley AE: Split hand foot malformation (SHFM), *Clin Genet* 68:501, 2005.

Gold NB, Westgate MN, Holmes LB: Anatomic and etiological classification of congenital limb deficiencies, *Am J Med Genet A* 155:1225, 2011.

Goncalves LF, Kusanovic JP, Gotsch F, et al: The fetal musculoskeletal system. In Callen PW, editor: *Ultrasonography in obstetrics and gynecology*, ed 5, Philadelphia, 2008, Elsevier.

Grzeschik K-H: Human limb malformations: an approach to the molecular basis of development, *Int J Dev Biol* 46:983, 2002.

Hall BK: *Bones and cartilage: developmental skeletal biology*, Philadelphia, 2005, Elsevier.

Hinrichsen KV, Jacob HJ, Jacob M, et al: Principles of ontogenesis of leg and foot in man, *Ann Anat* 176:121, 1994.

Kabak S, Boizow L: Organogenese des extremitätenskeletts und der extremitätengelenke beim menschenembryo, *Anat Anz* 170:349, 1990.

Logan M: Finger or toe: the molecular basis of limb identity, *Development* 130:6401, 2003.

Manske PR, Oberg KC: Classification and developmental biology of congenital anomalies of the hand and upper extremity, *J Bone Joint Surg Am* 91:3, 2009.

Marini JC, Gerber NL: Osteogenesis imperfecta, *JAMA* 277:746, 1997.

Moore KL, Dalley AF, Agur AMR: *Clinically oriented anatomy*, ed 7, Baltimore, 2014, Lippincott Williams & Wilkins.

Muragaki Y, Mundlos S, Upton J, et al: Altered growth and branching patterns in synpolydactyly caused by mutations in HoxD13, *Science* 272:548, 1996.

O'Rahilly R, Müller F: *Developmental stages in human embryos*, Washington, DC, 1987, Carnegie Institution of Washington.

Robertson WW Jr, Corbett D: Congenital clubfoot, *Clin Orthop* 338:14, 1997.

Sammer DM, Chung KC: Congenital hand differences: embryology and classification, *Hand Clin* 25:151, 2009.

Talamillo A, Delgado I, Nakamura T, et al: Role of epiprofin, a zinc-finger transcription factor in limb development, *Dev Biol* 337:363, 2010.

Towers M, Tickle C: Generation of pattern and form in the developing limb, *Int J Dev Biol* 53:805, 2009.

Van Allen MI: Structural anomalies resulting from vascular disruption, *Pediatr Clin North Am* 39:255, 1992.

Van Heest AE: Congenital disorders of the hand and upper extremity, *Pediatr Clin North Am* 43:1113, 1996.

Zuniga A: Globalisation reaches gene regulation: the case for vertebrate limb development, *Curr Opin Genet Dev* 15:403, 2005.

# Nervous System

*T*he nervous system consists of three main regions:

- The **central nervous system (CNS)** consists of the brain and spinal cord and is protected by the cranium and vertebral column.
- The **peripheral nervous system (PNS)** includes the neurons outside the CNS as well as the cranial nerves and spinal nerves (and their associated ganglia), which connect the brain and spinal cord with peripheral structures.
- The **autonomic nervous system (ANS)** has parts in the CNS and PNS and consists of the neurons that innervate smooth muscle, cardiac muscle, glandular epithelium, and combinations of these tissues.

## DEVELOPMENT OF NERVOUS SYSTEM

The first indications of the developing nervous system appear during the third week as the **neural plate** and **neural groove** develop on the posterior aspect of the trilaminar embryo (Fig. 17-1*A*). The notochord and paraxial mesenchyme induce the overlying ectoderm to differentiate into the neural plate. *Signaling molecules involve members of the transforming growth factor β family, Sonic hedgehog (SHH), and bone morphogenic proteins (BMPs).*

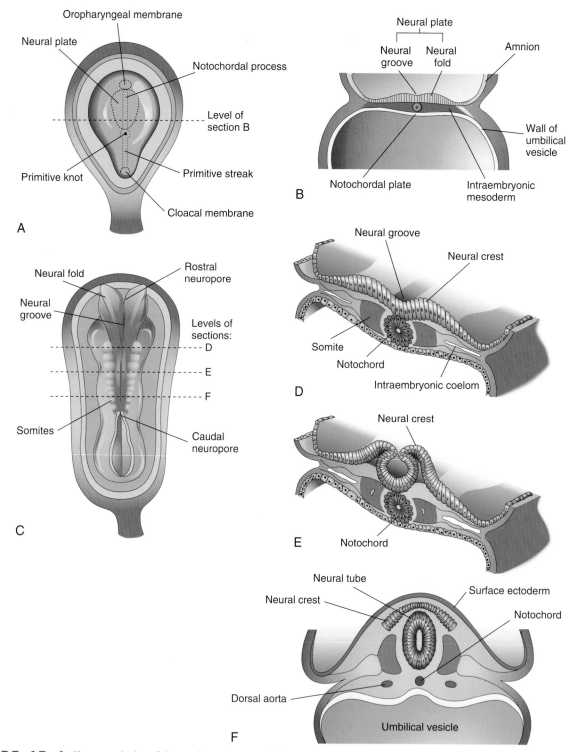

**FIGURE 17–1** The neural plate folds to form the neural tube. **A,** Dorsal view shows an embryo of approximately 17 days that was exposed by removing the amnion. **B,** Transverse section of the embryo shows the neural plate and early development of the neural groove and neural folds. **C,** Dorsal view of an embryo of approximately 22 days shows that the neural folds have fused opposite the fourth to sixth somites but are spread apart at both ends. **D** to **F,** Transverse sections of the embryo at the levels shown in **C** illustrate formation of the neural tube and its detachment from the surface ectoderm. Some neuroectodermal cells are not included in the neural tube but remain between it and the surface ectoderm as the neural crest.

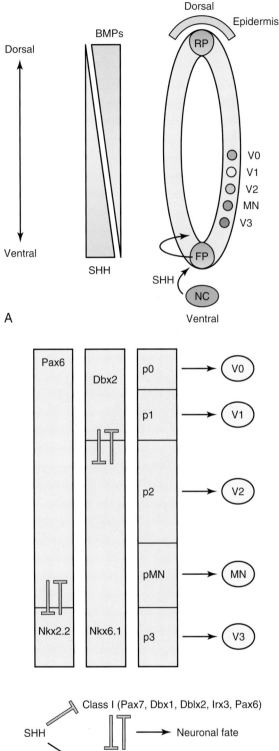

A

B

**FIGURE 17–2** Morphogens and transcription factors specify the fate of progenitors in the ventral neural tube. **A,** Sonic hedgehog *(SHH)* is secreted by the notochord *(NC)* and the floor plate *(FP)* of the neural tube in a ventral to dorsal gradient. Similarly, bone morphogenetic proteins *(BMPs),* members of the transforming growth factor-β superfamily, are secreted by the roof plate *(RP)* of the neural tube and the overlying epidermis in a dorsal to ventral gradient. These opposing morphogen gradients determine dorsal-ventral cell fates. **B,** SHH concentration gradients define the ventral expression domains of class I (repressed) and class II (activated) homeobox transcription factors. Reciprocal negative interactions assist to establish boundaries of gene expression in the embryonic ventral spinal cord. *p,* Progenitor; *MN,* motor neuron; *V,* ventral interneuron. *(Modified from Jessel TM: Neuronal specification in the spinal cord: inductive signals and transcription codes,* Nat Rev Genet *1:20, 2000.)*

region of the fourth to sixth pairs of somites (see Fig. 17-1C and D). At this stage, the cranial two thirds of the neural plate and tube as far caudal as the fourth pair of somites represent the future brain, and the caudal one third of the plate and tube represents the future spinal cord.

**Fusion of the neural folds** and formation of the **neural tube** begins at the fifth somite and proceeds in cranial and caudal directions until only small areas of the tube remain open at both ends (Fig. 17-3A and B). The lumen of the neural tube becomes the **neural canal**, which communicates freely with the amniotic cavity (see Fig. 17-3C). The cranial opening (**rostral neuropore**) closes at approximately the 25th day, and the **caudal neuropore** closes at approximately the 27th day (see Fig. 17-3D).

*Closure of the neuropores* coincides with the establishment of a vascular circulation for the neural tube. *Syndecan 4 (SDC4) and van gogh–like 2 (VANGL2) proteins appear to be involved with neural tube closure.* The neuroprogenitor cells of the wall of the neural tube thicken to form the brain and spinal cord (Fig. 17-4). The neural canal forms the ventricular system of the brain and the central canal of the spinal cord.

## NONCLOSURE OF NEURAL TUBE

The current hypothesis is that there are multiple (possibly five) closure sites involved in the formation of the neural tube. Failure of closure of site 1 results in spina bifida cystica (see Fig. 17-15). **Meroencephaly** (anencephaly) results from failure of closure of site 2 (see Fig. 17-13). **Craniorachischisis** results from failure of sites 2, 4, and 1 to close. Site 3 nonfusion is rare.

The **neural tube defects (NTDs)** are described later (see Fig. 17-17). It has been suggested that the most caudal region may have a fifth closure site from the second lumbar vertebra to the second sacral vertebra and that closure inferior to the second sacral vertebra occurs by secondary neurulation. Epidemiologic analysis of neonates with NTD supports the concept that there are multiple closures of the neural tube in humans.

Formation of the neural folds, neural crest, and neural tube is illustrated in Figures 17-1B to F and 17-2.

- The neural tube differentiates into the CNS.
- The neural crest gives rise to cells that form most of the PNS and ANS.

**Neurulation** (formation of the neural plate and neural tube) begins during the fourth week (22–23 days) in the

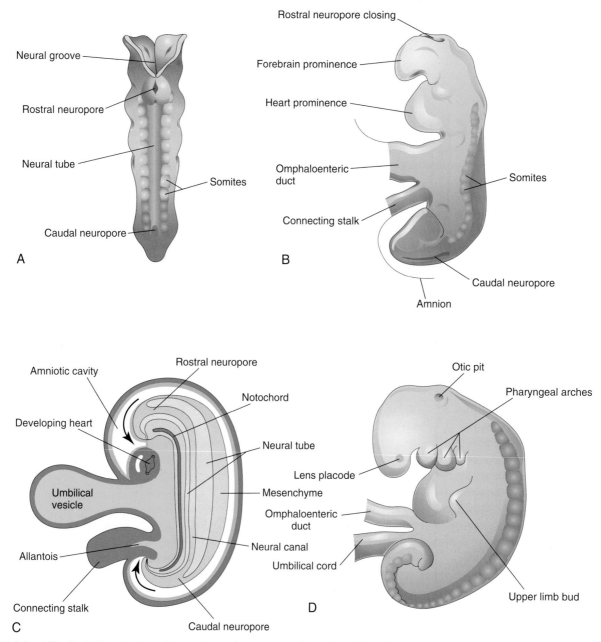

**FIGURE 17–3** A, Dorsal view of an embryo of approximately 23 days shows fusion of the neural folds, which forms the neural tube. B, Lateral view of an embryo of approximately 24 days shows the forebrain prominence and closing of the rostral neuropore. C, Diagrammatic sagittal section of the embryo at 23 days shows the transitory communication of the neural canal with the amniotic cavity *(arrows)*. D, In the lateral view of an embryo of approximately 27 days, notice that the neuropores shown in B are closed.

## DEVELOPMENT OF SPINAL CORD

The primordial spinal cord develops from the caudal part of the neural plate and caudal eminence. The neural tube caudal to the fourth pair of somites develops into the spinal cord (Fig. 17-5; see Figs. 17-3 and 17-4). The lateral walls of the neural tube thicken, gradually reducing the size of the **neural canal** until only a minute **central canal of the spinal cord** exists at 9 to 10 weeks (see Fig. 17-5C). *Retinoic acid signaling is essential in the development of the spinal cord from early patterning to neurogenesis.*

Initially, the wall of the neural tube is composed of a thick, pseudostratified, columnar neuroepithelium (see

Fig. 17-5D). These neuroepithelial cells constitute the **ventricular zone** (ependymal layer), which gives rise to all neurons and macroglial cells (macroglia) in the spinal cord (Fig. 17-6; see Fig. 17-5E). Macroglial cells are the larger members of the neuroglial family of cells, which includes astrocytes and oligodendrocytes. Soon, a **marginal zone** composed of the outer parts of the neuroepithelial cells becomes recognizable (see Fig. 17-5E). This zone gradually becomes the **white matter of the spinal cord** as axons grow into it from nerve cell bodies in the spinal cord, spinal ganglia, and brain.

Some dividing neuroepithelial cells in the ventricular zone differentiate into primordial neurons (**neuroblasts**).

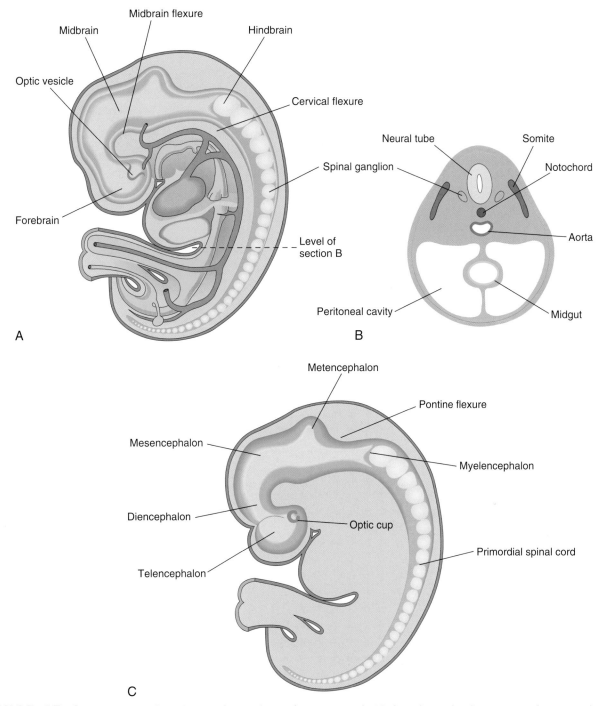

**FIGURE 17-4** A, Schematic lateral view of an embryo of approximately 28 days shows the three primary brain vesicles: forebrain, midbrain, and hindbrain. Two flexures demarcate the primary divisions of the brain. B, Transverse section of the embryo shows the neural tube that will develop into the spinal cord in this region. The spinal ganglia derived from the neural crest are also shown. C, Schematic lateral view of the central nervous system of a 6-week embryo shows the secondary brain vesicles and the pontine flexure that occurs as the brain grows rapidly.

These embryonic cells form an **intermediate zone** (mantle layer) between the ventricular and marginal zones. *Neuroblasts become neurons* as they develop cytoplasmic processes (see Fig. 17-6).

The supporting cells of the CNS, called **glioblasts** (spongioblasts), differentiate from neuroepithelial cells, mainly after neuroblast formation has ceased. The **glioblasts** migrate from the ventricular zone into the intermediate and marginal zones. Some glioblasts become **astroblasts** and later **astrocytes**, whereas others become **oligodendroblasts** and eventually **oligodendrocytes** (see Fig. 17-6). When the neuroepithelial cells cease producing neuroblasts and glioblasts, they differentiate into ependymal cells, which form the **ependyma** (ependymal epithelium)

**FIGURE 17–5** Development of the spinal cord. **A**, Transverse section of the neural tube of an embryo of approximately 23 days. **B** and **C**, Similar sections at 6 and 9 weeks, respectively. **D**, Section of the wall of the neural tube shown in **A**. **E**, Section of the wall of the developing spinal cord shows its three zones. Notice that the neural canal of the neural tube is converted into the central canal of the spinal cord (**A** to **C**).

lining the central canal of the spinal cord. *SHH signaling controls the proliferation, survival, and patterning of neuroepithelial progenitor cells by regulating GLI transcription factors* (see Fig. 17-2).

**Microglia** (microglial cells), which are scattered throughout the gray and white matter of the spinal cord, are small cells that are derived from **mesenchymal cells** (see Fig. 17-6). Microglia invade the CNS rather late in the fetal period after it has been penetrated by blood vessels. *Microglia originate in the bone marrow* and are part of the mononuclear phagocytic cell population.

Proliferation and differentiation of neuroepithelial cells in the developing spinal cord produce thick walls and thin roof plates and floor plates (see Fig. 17-5B). Differential thickening of the lateral walls of the spinal cord soon produces a shallow *longitudinal groove* on each side, the **sulcus limitans** (Fig. 17-7; see Fig. 17-5B). This groove separates the dorsal part (**alar plate**) from the ventral part (**basal plate**). The alar and basal plates produce longitudinal bulges extending through most of the length of the developing spinal cord. *This regional separation is of fundamental importance* because the alar and basal plates are later associated with afferent and efferent functions, respectively.

Cell bodies in the alar plates form the **dorsal gray columns**, which extend the length of the spinal cord. In transverse sections of the cord, these columns are the **dorsal gray horns** (see Fig. 17-7). Neurons in these columns constitute afferent nuclei and groups of them form the dorsal gray columns. As the alar plates enlarge, the **dorsal median septum** forms. Cell bodies in the basal plates form the ventral and lateral gray columns.

In transverse sections of the spinal cord, these columns are the **ventral gray horns** and **lateral gray horns**, respectively (see Fig. 17-5C). Axons of ventral horn cells grow out of the spinal cord and form the **ventral roots of the spinal nerves**. As the basal plates enlarge, they bulge ventrally on each side of the median plane. As this occurs, the **ventral median septum** forms, and a deep longitudinal groove (**ventral median fissure**) develops on the ventral surface of the spinal cord (see Fig. 17-5C).

## Development of Spinal Ganglia

The **unipolar neurons in the spinal ganglia** (dorsal root ganglia) are derived from **neural crest cells** (Figs. 17-8 and 17-9). The axons of cells in the spinal ganglia are at first bipolar, but the two processes soon unite in a T-shaped

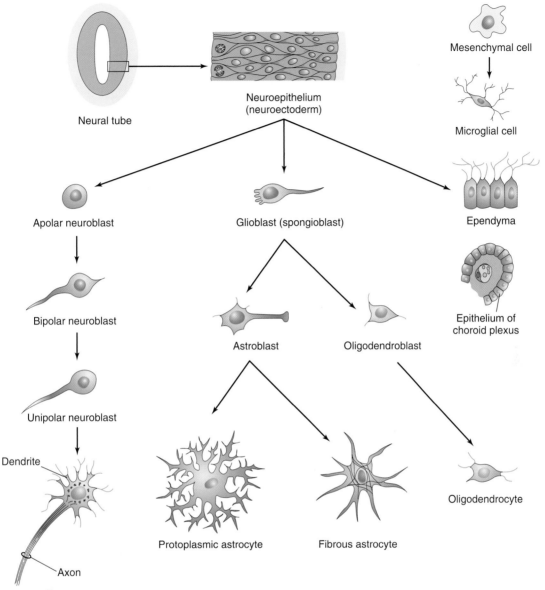

Neural tube

Neuroepithelium
(neuroectoderm)

Mesenchymal cell

Microglial cell

Apolar neuroblast

Glioblast (spongioblast)

Ependyma

Bipolar neuroblast

Unipolar neuroblast

Astroblast

Oligodendroblast

Epithelium of
choroid plexus

Dendrite

Protoplasmic astrocyte

Fibrous astrocyte

Oligodendrocyte

Axon

Neuron

**FIGURE 17–6** Histogenesis of cells in the central nervous system. After further development, the multipolar neuroblast *(lower left)* becomes a nerve cell or neuron. Neuroepithelial cells give rise to all neurons and macroglial cells. Microglial cells are derived from mesenchymal cells that invade the developing nervous system with the blood vessels.

fashion. Both processes of spinal ganglion cells have the structural characteristics of **axons**, but the peripheral process is a dendrite in that there is conduction toward the cell body. The peripheral processes of **spinal ganglion cells** pass in the spinal nerves to sensory endings in somatic or visceral structures (see Fig. 17-8). The central processes enter the spinal cord and constitute the **dorsal roots of spinal nerves.**

## Development of Spinal Meninges

The meninges (membranes covering the spinal cord) develop from cells of the neural crest and mesenchyme between 20 and 35 days. The cells migrate to surround the neural tube (primordium of the brain and spinal cord) and form the primordial meninges (see Fig. 17-1F).

The external layer of these membranes thickens to form the **dura mater** (Fig. 17-10A and B), and the internal layer, the *pia arachnoid,* is composed of **pia mater** and **arachnoid mater (leptomeninges)**. Fluid-filled spaces appear within the *leptomeninges* that soon coalesce to form the **subarachnoid space** (see Fig. 17-12A). The origin of the pia mater and arachnoid from a single layer is indicated in the adult by **arachnoid trabeculae,** which are numerous, delicate strands of connective tissue that pass between the pia and arachnoid. **Cerebrospinal fluid (CSF)** begins to form during the fifth week (see Fig. 17-12A).

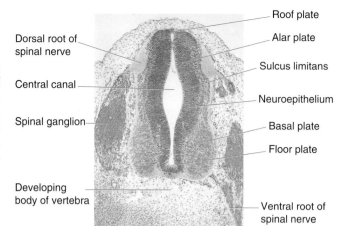

**FIGURE 17–7** Transverse section of an embryo (×100) at Carnegie stage 16 at approximately 40 days. The ventral root of the spinal nerve is composed of nerve fibers arising from neuroblasts in the basal plate (developing ventral horn of spinal cord), whereas the dorsal root is formed by nerve processes arising from neuroblasts in the spinal ganglion. *(From Moore KL, Persaud TVN, Shiota K: Color atlas of clinical embryology, ed 2, Philadelphia, 2000, Saunders.)*

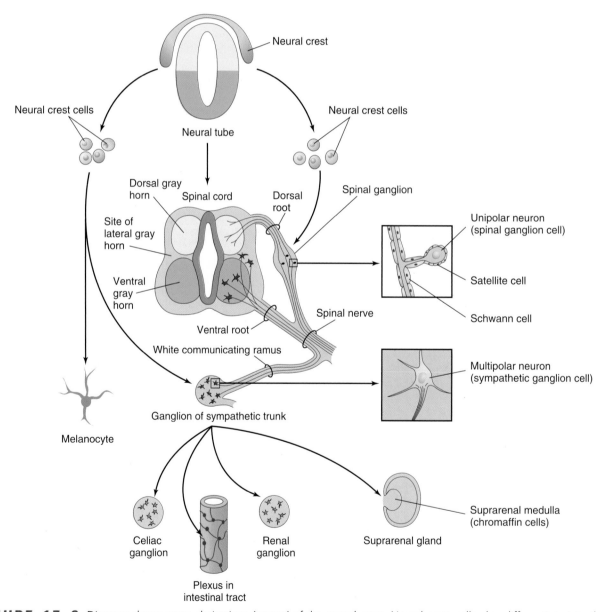

**FIGURE 17–8** Diagram shows some derivatives *(arrows)* of the neural crest. Neural crest cells also differentiate into the cells in the afferent ganglia of cranial nerves and many other structures (see Chapter 5, Fig. 5-5). Formation of a spinal nerve is also illustrated.

## Positional Changes of Spinal Cord

The spinal cord in the embryo extends the entire length of the vertebral canal (see Fig. 17-10A). The spinal nerves pass through the **intervertebral foramina** opposite their levels of origin. Because the vertebral column and dura mater grow more rapidly than the spinal cord, this positional relationship of the spinal nerves does not persist. The caudal end of the **spinal cord in fetuses** gradually comes to lie at relatively higher levels. In a 24-week-old fetus, it lies at the level of the first sacral vertebra (see Fig. 17-10B).

The **spinal cord in neonates** terminates at the level of the second or third lumbar vertebra (see Fig. 17-10C). In adults, the cord usually terminates at the inferior border of the first lumbar vertebra (see Fig. 17-10D). This is an average level because the caudal end of the spinal cord in adults may be as superior as the 12th thoracic vertebra or as inferior as the third lumbar vertebra. The **spinal nerve roots**, especially those of the lumbar and sacral segments, run obliquely from the spinal cord to the corresponding level of the vertebral column (see Fig. 17-10D). The nerve roots inferior to the end of the cord (**medullary cone**) form a bundle of spinal nerve roots called the **cauda equina** (Latin *horse tail*), which arises from the lumbosacral enlargement (swelling) and medullary cone of the spinal cord (see Fig. 17-10D).

Although the dura mater and arachnoid mater usually end at the S2 vertebra in adults, the pia mater does not. Distal to the caudal end of the spinal cord, the pia mater forms a long fibrous thread, the **filum terminale** (terminal filum), which indicates the original level of the caudal end of the embryonic spinal cord (see Fig. 17-10C). The **filum** (Latin *thread*) extends from the medullary cone and attaches to the periosteum of the first coccygeal vertebra (see Fig. 17-10D).

**A** Neural crest cell **B** Bipolar neuroblasts **C** **D** Unipolar afferent neuron

**FIGURE 17–9** A to D, Diagrams show successive stages in the differentiation of a neural crest cell into a unipolar afferent neuron in a spinal ganglion. *Arrows* indicate how a unipolar neuron is formed.

## Myelination of Nerve Fibers

**Myelin sheaths** around the nerve fibers within the spinal cord begin to form during the late fetal period and continue to form during the first postnatal year (Fig. 17-11E). Myelin basic proteins, a family of related polypeptide isoforms, are essential in myelination; $\beta_1$-integrins

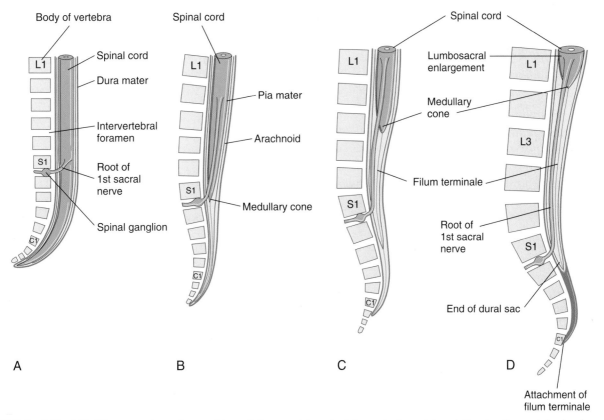

**FIGURE 17–10** Diagrams show the position of the caudal end of the spinal cord in relation to the vertebral column and meninges at various stages of development. The increasing inclination of the root of the first sacral nerve is also illustrated. **A,** At 8 weeks. **B,** At 24 weeks. **C,** Neonate. **D,** Adult.

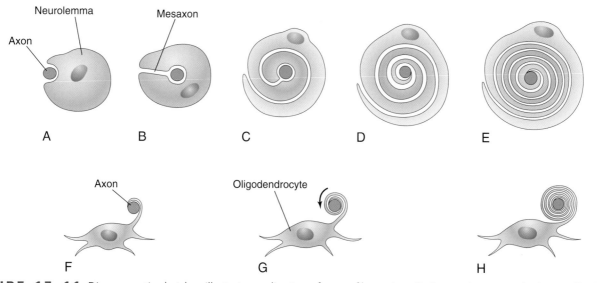

**FIGURE 17–11** Diagrammatic sketches illustrate myelination of nerve fibers. **A** to **E**, Successive stages in the myelination of an axon of a peripheral nerve fiber by the neurilemma (sheath of Schwann). The axon first indents the cell, and the cell then rotates around the axon as the mesaxon (site of invagination) elongates. The cytoplasm between the layers of the cell membrane gradually condenses. Cytoplasm remains on the inside of the sheath between the myelin and the axon. **F** to **H**, Successive stages in the myelination of a nerve fiber in the central nervous system by an oligodendrocyte. A process of the neuroglial cell wraps itself around an axon, and the intervening layers of cytoplasm move to the body of the cell.

regulate this process. Fiber tracts become functional at approximately the time they become myelinated. *Motor roots are myelinated before sensory roots.* The myelin sheaths around the nerve fibers in the spinal cord are formed by **oligodendrocytes (oligodendroglial cells)** are **types of glial cells** that originate from the neuroepithelium. The plasma membranes of these cells wrap around the axon, forming several layers (see Fig. 17-11*F* to *H*). *Profilin 1 (PFN1) protein is essential in the microfilament polymerization that promotes changes to the oligodendrocyte cytoskeleton.*

The **myelin sheaths** around the axons of peripheral nerve fibers are formed by the plasma membranes of the neurilemma (sheath of Schwann cells), which are analogous to oligodendrocytes. Neurilemma cells are derived from neural crest cells that migrate peripherally and wrap themselves around the **axons** of somatic motor neurons and **preganglionic autonomic motor neurons** as they pass out of the CNS (see Figs. 17-8 and 17-11*A* to *E*). These cells also wrap themselves around the central and peripheral processes of somatic and visceral sensory neurons and around the axons of postsynaptic autonomic motor neurons. Beginning at approximately 20 weeks, peripheral nerve fibers have a whitish appearance resulting from the deposition of myelin (layers of lipid and protein substances).

## BIRTH DEFECTS OF SPINAL CORD

Most defects result from **failure of fusion of one or more neural arches** of the developing vertebrae during the fourth week. NTDs affect the tissues overlying the spinal cord: meninges, neural arches, muscles, and skin (Fig. 17-12). Defects involving the embryonic **neural arches** are referred to as **spina bifida**; subtypes of this defect are based on the degree and pattern of the NTD. The term *spina bifida* denotes nonfusion of the halves of the embryonic **neural arches**, which is common to all types of spina bifida (see Fig. 17-12A). Severe defects also involve the spinal cord, meninges, and neurocranium (bones of cranium enclosing the brain) (Fig. 17-13). Spina bifida ranges from clinically significant types to minor defects that are functionally unimportant (Fig. 17-14).

## DERMAL SINUS

A dermal sinus is lined with epidermis and skin appendages extending from the skin to a deeper-lying structure, usually the spinal cord. The sinus (channel) is associated with closure of the neural tube and formation of the meninges in the lumbosacral region of the spinal cord. The birth defect is caused by *failure of the surface ectoderm (future skin) to detach from the neuroectoderm* and meninges that envelop it. As a result, the meninges are continuous with a narrow channel that extends to a dimple in the skin of the sacral region of the back (see Fig. 17-13). The dimple indicates the region of closure of the **caudal neuropore** at the end of the fourth week and therefore represents the last place of separation between the surface ectoderm and the neural tube.

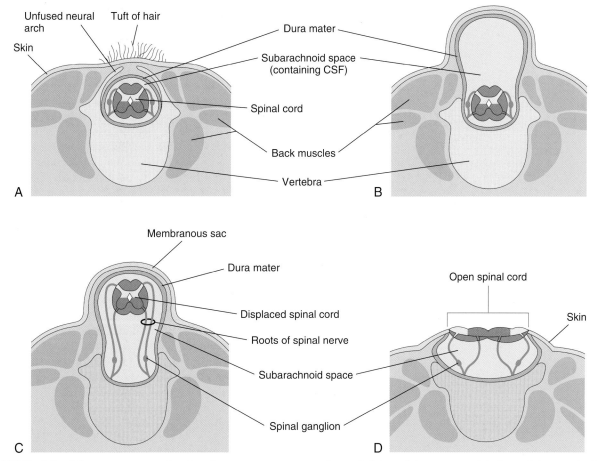

**FIGURE 17–12** Diagrammatic sketches illustrate various types of spina bifida and the associated defects of the vertebral arches (one or more), spinal cord, and meninges. **A,** Spina bifida occulta. Observe the unfused neural arch. **B,** Spina bifida with meningocele. **C,** Spina bifida with meningomyelocele. **D,** Spina bifida with myeloschisis. The defects illustrated in **B** to **D** are referred to collectively as *spina bifida cystica* because of the cyst-like sac or cyst associated with them. *CSF,* Cerebrospinal fluid.

**FIGURE 17–13** A fetus at 20 weeks with severe neural tube defects, including acrania, cerebral regression (meroencephaly), iniencephaly (enlargement of foramen magnum), and a sacral dimple *(arrow).*

**FIGURE 17–14** A female child with a tuft of hair in the lumbosacral region indicating the site of a spina bifida occulta.

## SPINA BIFIDA OCCULTA

Spina bifida occulta is an **NTD** resulting from failure of the halves of one or more **neural arches** to fuse in the median plane (see Fig. 17-12A). This NTD occurs in the L5 or S1 vertebra in approximately 10% of otherwise normal people. In the minor form, the only evidence of its presence may be a small dimple with a tuft of hair arising from it (see Figs. 17-12A and 17-14). An overlying lipoma dermal sinus or other birthmark may also occur. Spina bifida occulta usually produces no symptoms. A few affected infants have functionally significant defects of the underlying spinal cord and dorsal roots.

## SPINA BIFIDA CYSTICA

Severe types of spina bifida, which involve protrusion of the spinal cord and/or meninges through defects in the vertebral arches, are referred to collectively as **spina bifida cystica** because of the **meningeal cyst** (sac-like structure) that is associated with these defects (Fig. 17-15; see Fig. 17-12B to D). This NTD occurs in approximately 1 of 5000 births and shows considerable geographic variation in incidence. When the cyst contains meninges and CSF, the defect is **spinal bifida with meningocele** (see Fig. 17-12B). The spinal cord and spinal roots are in the normal position, but there may be spinal cord defects. Protrusion of the meninges and CSF of the spinal cord occurs through a defect in the vertebral column.

If the spinal cord or nerve roots are contained within the meningeal cyst, the defect is **spina bifida with meningomyelocele** (see Figs. 17-12C and 17-15A). Severe cases involving several vertebrae are associated with absence of the calvaria (skullcap), absence of most of the brain, and facial abnormalities; these severe defects are called **meroencephaly** (see Figs. 17-13 and 17-17). The defects entail drastic effects in some brain areas and lesser or no effects in others. For these neonates, death is inevitable. The term *anencephaly* for these severe defects is inappropriate because it indicates that no part of the brain exists.

Spina bifida cystica shows various degrees of neurologic deficit, depending on the position and extent of the lesion. Dermatomal loss of sensation along with complete or partial skeletal muscle paralysis occurs with the lesion (see Fig. 17-15B). The level of the lesion determines the area of **anesthesia** (area of skin without sensation) and the muscles affected. **Sphincter paralysis** (bladder or anal sphincters) is common with **lumbosacral meningomyelocele** (see Figs. 17-12C and 17-15A). A **saddle block anesthesia** typically occurs when the sphincters are involved; loss of sensation occurs in the body region that would contact a saddle.

**Meroencephaly** is strongly suspected in utero when there is a high level of **alpha fetoprotein (AFP)** in the amniotic fluid (see Chapter 6, box titled "Alpha-Fetoprotein and Fetal Anomalies"). The level of AFP may also be elevated in maternal blood serum. **Amniocentesis** is usually performed on pregnant women with high levels of serum AFP for the determination of the AFP level in the amniotic fluid (see Chapter 6, Fig. 6-13). An ultrasound scan may reveal an NTD that has resulted in spina bifida cystica. The fetal vertebral column can be detected by ultrasound at 10 to 12 weeks, and if there is a defect in the vertebral arch, a meningeal cyst may be detected in the affected area (see Figs. 17-12C and 17-15A).

**FIGURE 17–15** Infants with spina bifida cystica. **A,** Spina bifida with meningomyelocele in the lumbar region. **B,** Spina bifida with myeloschisis in the lumbar region. Notice that the nerve involvement has affected the lower limbs of the infant.

## MENINGOMYELOCELE

Meningomyelocele is a more common and a more severe defect than spina bifida with meningocele (see Figs. 17-15A and 17-12B). This NTD may occur anywhere along the vertebral column; however, they are most common in the lumbar and sacral region (see Fig. 17-17). More than 90% of cases have associated hydrocephalus due to coexistence of an Arnold-Chiari malformation. Most patients require surgical diversion of CSF to avoid high intracranial pressure–related complications. Some cases of meningomyelocele are associated with **craniolacunia** (defective development of the calvaria), which results in depressed, nonossified areas on the inner surfaces of the flat bones of the calvaria.

## MYELOSCHISIS

*Myeloschisis is the most severe type of spina bifida* (Fig. 17-16; see Figs. 17-12D and 17-15B). In this defect, the spinal cord in the affected area is open because the neural folds failed to fuse. As a result, the spinal cord is represented by a flattened mass of nervous tissue. Myeloschisis usually results in permanent paralysis or weakness of the lower limbs.

**FIGURE 17–16** A 19-week female fetus showing an open spinal defect in the lumbosacral region (spina bifida with myeloschisis).

## CAUSES OF NEURAL TUBE DEFECTS

Nutritional and environmental factors undoubtedly play a role in the production of NTDs. Gene-gene and gene-environment interactions are likely involved in most cases. Food fortification with folic acid and folic acid supplements taken before conception and continued for at least 3 months during pregnancy reduce the incidence of NTDs. In 2015, the Centers for Disease Control and Prevention urged "all women of childbearing age who can become pregnant to get 0.4 mg of folic acid every day to help reduce the risk of neural tube defects" (for more information, go to http://www.cdc.gov/folicacid). Epidemiologic studies have also shown that low maternal $B_{12}$ levels may significantly increase the risk of NTDs. Certain drugs (e.g., valproic acid) increase the risk of meningomyelocele. This anticonvulsant drug causes NTDs in 1% to 2% of pregnancies if taken during early pregnancy, when the neural folds are fusing (Fig. 17-17).

## DEVELOPMENT OF BRAIN

16   The brain begins to develop during the third week, when the neural plate and tube are developing from the neuroectoderm (see Fig. 17-1). The **neural tube**, cranial to the fourth pair of somites, develops into the brain. Neuroprogenitor cells proliferate, migrate, and differentiate to form specific areas of the brain. Fusion of the neural folds in the cranial region and closure of the rostral neuropore form **three primary brain vesicles** from which the brain develops (Fig. 17-18):

- **Forebrain** (prosencephalon)
- **Midbrain** (mesencephalon)
- **Hindbrain** (rhombencephalon)

During the fifth week, the forebrain partly divides into two **secondary brain vesicles**, the *telencephalon* and *diencephalon*; the midbrain does not divide. The hindbrain partly divides into two vesicles, the *metencephalon* and *myelencephalon*. Consequently, there are five secondary brain vesicles.

### Brain Flexures

16   During the fifth week, the embryonic brain grows rapidly and bends ventrally with the head fold. The bending produces the **midbrain flexure** in the midbrain region and the **cervical flexure** at the junction of the hindbrain and spinal cord (Fig. 17-19A). Later, unequal growth of the brain between these flexures produces the **pontine flexure** in the opposite direction. This flexure results in thinning of the roof of the hindbrain (see Fig. 17-19C).

Initially, the primordial brain has the same basic structure as the developing spinal cord; however, the brain flexures produce considerable variation in the outline of transverse sections at different levels of the brain and in the position of the gray and white matter. The **sulcus limitans** extends cranially to the junction of the midbrain and forebrain, and the alar and basal plates are recognizable only in the midbrain and hindbrain (see Figs. 17-5C and 17-19C).

### Hindbrain

The *cervical flexure* demarcates the hindbrain from the spinal cord (see Fig. 17-19A). Later, this junction is arbitrarily defined as the level of the superior rootlet of the first cervical nerve, which is located roughly at the foramen magnum. The *pontine flexure*, located in the future pontine region, divides the hindbrain into caudal (myelencephalon) and rostral (metencephalon) parts. The **myelencephalon** becomes the **medulla oblongata** (commonly called the *medulla*), and the **metencephalon** becomes the **pons** and **cerebellum**. The cavity of the hindbrain becomes the **fourth ventricle** and the **central canal** in the medulla (see Fig. 17-19B and C).

### Myelencephalon

The caudal part of the myelencephalon (closed part of the medulla) resembles the spinal cord developmentally and structurally (see Fig. 17-19B). The **neural canal** of the neural tube forms the small *central canal* of the myelencephalon. Unlike those of the spinal cord, **neuroblasts** from the alar plates in the myelencephalon migrate into the marginal zone and form isolated areas of gray matter: the **gracile nuclei** medially and the **cuneate nuclei** laterally (see Fig. 17-19B). These nuclei are associated with correspondingly named nerve tracts that enter the medulla from the spinal cord. The ventral area of the medulla contains a pair of fiber bundles (**pyramids**) that consist of corticospinal fibers descending from the developing cerebral cortex (see Fig. 17-19B).

The rostral part of the **myelencephalon** (open part of the medulla) is wide and rather flat, especially opposite the **pontine flexure** (see Fig. 17-19C and D). The pontine flexure causes the lateral walls of the medulla to move laterally like the pages of an open book. As a result, its **roof plate** is stretched and greatly thinned (see Fig. 17-19C). The cavity of this part of the myelencephalon (part of the future fourth ventricle) becomes somewhat rhomboidal (diamond shaped). As the walls of the medulla move laterally, the **alar plates** become lateral to the basal plates. As the positions of the plates change, the motor nuclei usually develop medial to the sensory nuclei (see Fig. 17-19C).

**Neuroblasts in the basal plates of the medulla**, like those in the spinal cord, develop into motor neurons. The neuroblasts form nuclei (groups of nerve cells) and organize into three cell columns on each side (see Fig. 17-19D). From medial to lateral, the columns are named as follows:

- **General somatic efferent**, represented by neurons of the hypoglossal nerve
- **Special visceral efferent**, represented by neurons innervating muscles derived from the pharyngeal arches (see Chapter 9, Fig. 9-6)
- **General visceral efferent**, represented by some neurons of the vagus and glossopharyngeal nerves (see Chapter 9, Fig. 9-6)

**Neuroblasts in the alar plates of the medulla** form neurons that are arranged in four columns on each side.

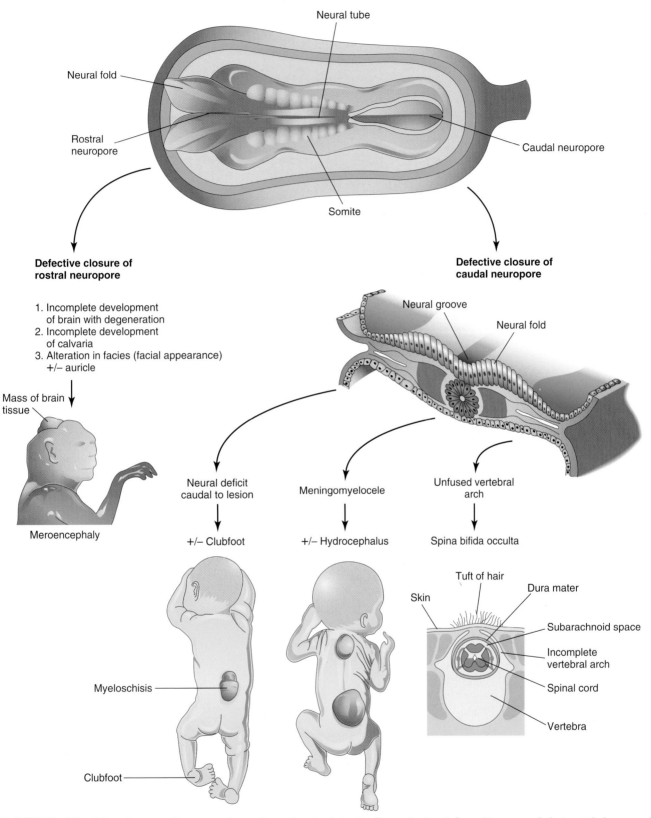

Neural tube

Neural fold

Rostral neuropore

Caudal neuropore

Somite

**Defective closure of rostral neuropore**

1. Incomplete development of brain with degeneration
2. Incomplete development of calvaria
3. Alteration in facies (facial appearance) +/− auricle

Mass of brain tissue

Meroencephaly

**Defective closure of caudal neuropore**

Neural groove

Neural fold

Neural deficit caudal to lesion

Meningomyelocele

Unfused vertebral arch

+/− Clubfoot

+/− Hydrocephalus

Spina bifida occulta

Tuft of hair

Skin

Dura mater

Subarachnoid space

Incomplete vertebral arch

Spinal cord

Vertebra

Myeloschisis

Clubfoot

**FIGURE 17–17** Schematic illustration shows the embryologic basis of neural tube defects. Meroencephaly (partial absence of brain) results from defective closure of the rostral neuropore, and meningomyelocele results from defective closure of the caudal neuropore. *(Modified from Jones KL: Smith's recognizable patterns of human malformations, ed 4, Philadelphia, 1988, Saunders.)*

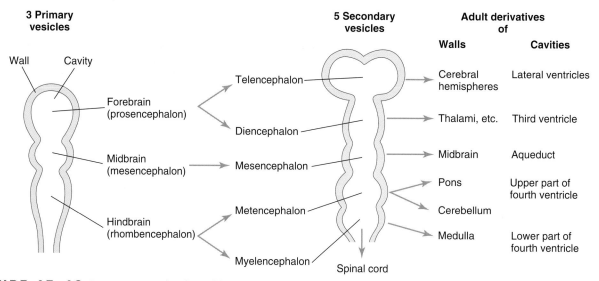

**FIGURE 17–18** Diagrammatic sketches of the brain vesicles indicate the adult derivatives of their walls and cavities. The rostral part of the third ventricle forms from the cavity of the telencephalon. Most of this ventricle is derived from the cavity of the diencephalon.

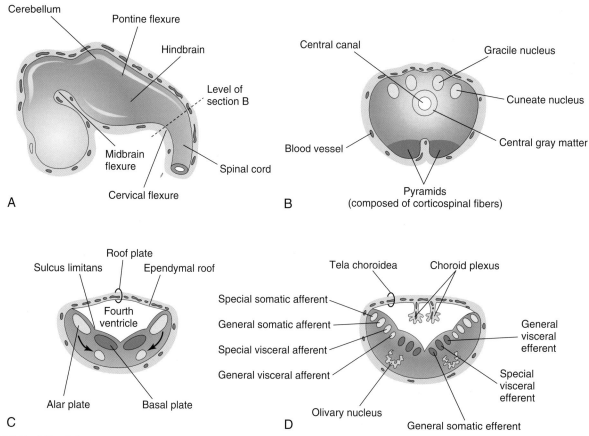

**FIGURE 17–19** A, Sketch of the developing brain at the end of the fifth week of gestation shows the three primary divisions of the brain and brain flexures. B, Transverse section of the caudal part of the myelencephalon (developing closed part of medulla). C and D, Similar sections of the rostral part of the myelencephalon (developing open part of medulla) show the position and successive stages of differentiation of the alar and basal plates. The *arrows* in C show the pathway taken by neuroblasts from the alar plates to form the olivary nuclei.

From medial to lateral, the columns are designated as follows:

- **General visceral afferent,** which receives impulses from the viscera
- **Special visceral afferent,** which receives taste fibers
- **General somatic afferent,** which receives impulses from the surface of the head
- **Special somatic afferent,** which receives impulses from the ear

Some neuroblasts from the alar plates migrate ventrally and form the neurons in the **olivary nuclei** (see Fig. 17-19C and *D*).

## Metencephalon

The walls of the metencephalon form the **pons** and **cerebellum,** and the cavity of the metencephalon forms the *superior part of the fourth ventricle* (Fig. 17-20A). As in the rostral part of the myelencephalon, the **pontine flexure** causes divergence of the **lateral walls of the pons,** which spreads the gray matter in the floor of the fourth ventricle (see Fig. 17-20B). As in the myelencephalon, neuroblasts

in each basal plate develop into motor nuclei and organize into three columns on each side.

The **cerebellum** develops from thickenings of **dorsal parts of the alar plates.** Initially, the **cerebellar swellings** project into the fourth ventricle (see Fig. 17-20B). As the swellings enlarge and fuse in the median plane, they overgrow the rostral half of the fourth ventricle and overlap the pons and medulla (see Fig. 17-20D).

Some neuroblasts in the intermediate zone of the alar plates migrate to the marginal zone and differentiate into the neurons of the **cerebellar cortex.** Other neuroblasts from these plates give rise to the *central nuclei,* the largest of which is the **dentate nucleus** (see Fig. 17-20D). Cells from the alar plates also give rise to the **pontine nuclei, cochlear and vestibular nuclei,** and the **sensory nuclei of the trigeminal nerve.**

The structure of the cerebellum reflects its phylogenetic (evolutionary) development (see Fig. 17-20C and *D*):

- The *archicerebellum* (**flocculonodular lobe**), the oldest part phylogenetically, has connections with the vestibular apparatus, especially the vestibule of the ear.

**FIGURE 17–20** **A,** Sketch of the developing brain at the end of the fifth week. **B,** Transverse section of the metencephalon (developing pons and cerebellum) shows the derivatives of the alar and basal plates. **C** and **D,** Sagittal sections of the hindbrain at 6 and 17 weeks, respectively, show successive stages in the development of the pons and cerebellum.

- The *paleocerebellum* (**vermis and anterior lobe**), of more recent development, is associated with sensory data from the limbs.
- The *neocerebellum* (**posterior lobe**), the newest part phylogenetically, is concerned with selective control of limb movements.

Nerve fibers connecting the cerebral and cerebellar cortices with the spinal cord pass through the marginal layer of the ventral region of the metencephalon. This region of the **brainstem** is the **pons** (Latin *bridge*) because of the robust band of nerve fibers that crosses the median plane and forms a bulky ridge on its anterior and lateral aspects (see Fig. 17-20C and D).

## Choroid Plexuses and Cerebrospinal Fluid

The thin ependymal roof of the fourth ventricle is covered externally by **pia mater**, which is derived from mesenchyme associated with the hindbrain (see Fig. 17-20B to D). This vascular membrane, together with the ependymal roof, forms the **tela choroidea**, the sheet of pia covering the lower part of the fourth ventricle (see Fig. 17-19D). Because of the active proliferation of the pia, the tela choroidea invaginates the fourth ventricle, where it differentiates into the **choroid plexus**, infoldings of choroidal arteries of the pia (see Figs. 17-19C and D and 17-20C and D). Similar plexuses develop in the roof of the third ventricle and the medial walls of the lateral ventricles.

*The choroid plexuses secrete ventricular fluid*, which becomes CSF as additions are made to it from the surfaces of the brain, spinal cord, and the pia-arachnoid layer of the meninges. Various signaling morphogens are found in CSF and the choroid plexus that are necessary for brain development. The thin roof of the fourth ventricle evaginates in three locations. These outpouchings rupture to form openings, the **median** and **lateral apertures** (foramen of Magendie and foramina of Luschka, respectively), which permit the CSF to enter the subarachnoid space from the fourth ventricle. Specific neurogenic molecules (e.g., retinoic acid) control the proliferation and differentiation of neuroprogenitor cells. The epithelial lining of the choroid plexus is derived from neuroepithelium, whereas the stroma develops from mesenchymal cells.

The main site of absorption of CSF into the venous system is through the **arachnoid villi**, which are protrusions of arachnoid mater into the **dural venous sinuses** (large venous channels between the layers of the **dura mater**). The arachnoid villi consist of a thin cellular layer derived from the epithelium of the arachnoid and the endothelium of the sinus.

## Midbrain

The midbrain (**mesencephalon**) undergoes less change than other parts of the developing brain (Fig. 17-21A), except for the caudal part of the hindbrain. The **neural canal** narrows and becomes the **cerebral aqueduct** (see Figs. 17-20D and 17-21D), a channel that connects the third and fourth ventricles.

**Neuroblasts** (Greek *blastos*, germ) are embryonic nerve cells that migrate from the **alar plates of the midbrain** into the **tectum** (roof-like covering) and aggregate to form *four large groups of neurons*, the paired **superior and inferior colliculi** (see Fig. 17-21C to E), which are concerned with visual and auditory reflexes, respectively. Neuroblasts from the **basal plates** may give rise to groups of neurons in the **tegmentum of the midbrain** (red nuclei, nuclei of third and fourth cranial nerves, and reticular nuclei). The **substantia nigra**, a broad layer of gray matter adjacent to the **crus cerebri** (cerebral peduncles) may also differentiate from the basal plate (see Fig. 17-21B, D, and E); however, some authorities think the substantia nigra is derived from cells in the alar plate that migrate ventrally.

Fibers growing from the **cerebrum** (principal part of brain, including the diencephalon and cerebral hemispheres) form the **crus cerebri** (cerebral peduncles) anteriorly (see Fig. 17-21B). The peduncles become progressively more prominent as more descending fiber groups (*corticopontine, corticobulbar,* and *corticospinal*) pass through the developing midbrain on their way to the **brainstem** (the medulla is the caudal subdivision of the brainstem that is continuous with the spinal cord) and **spinal cord** (see Fig. 17-21C).

## Forebrain

As closure of the **rostral neuropore** occurs (see Fig. 17-3B), two lateral outgrowths (**optic vesicles**) appear (see Fig. 17-4A), one on each side of the forebrain. These vesicles are the *primordia of the retinae and optic nerves* (see Chapter 18, Figs. 18-1C, F, and H and 18-11). A second pair of diverticula, the **telencephalic vesicles**, soon arise more dorsally and rostrally (see Fig. 17-21C). They are the *primordia of the cerebral hemispheres*, and their cavities become the **lateral ventricles** (see Fig. 17-26B).

The rostral (anterior) part of the forebrain, including the primordia of the **cerebral hemispheres**, is the **telencephalon**; the caudal (posterior) part of the forebrain is the **diencephalon**. The cavities of the telencephalon and diencephalon contribute to the formation of the **third ventricle**, although the cavity of the diencephalon contributes more (Fig. 17-22E).

### Diencephalon

Three swellings develop in the lateral walls of the third ventricle, which later become the *thalamus, hypothalamus,* and *epithalamus* (see Fig. 17-22C to E). The **thalamus** is separated from the **epithalamus** by the **epithalamic sulcus** and from the hypothalamus by the **hypothalamic sulcus** (see Fig. 17-22E). The latter sulcus is not a continuation of the **sulcus limitans** into the forebrain, and it does not, like the sulcus limitans, divide sensory and motor areas (see Fig. 17-22C).

The **thalamus** (large, ovoid mass of gray matter) develops rapidly on each side of the third ventricle and bulges into its cavity (see Fig. 17-22E). The thalami meet and fuse in the midline in approximately 70% of brains, forming a bridge of gray matter across the third ventricle, which is the interthalamic adhesion (variable connection

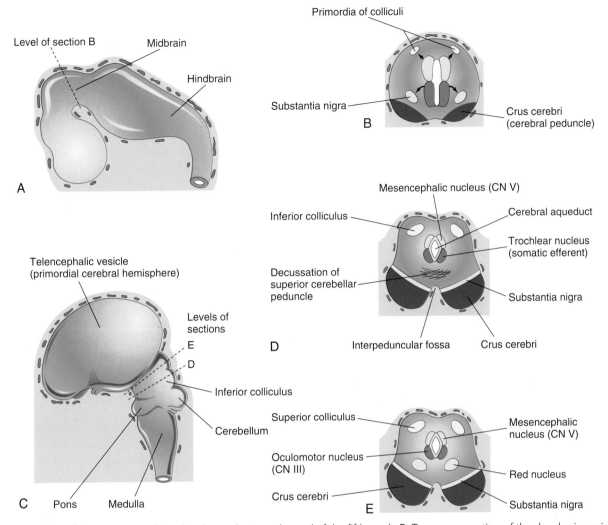

**FIGURE 17–21** A, Sketch of the developing brain at the end of the fifth week. B, Transverse section of the developing midbrain shows the early migration of cells from the basal and alar plates. C, Sketch of the developing brain at 11 weeks. D and E, Transverse sections of the developing midbrain at the level of the inferior and superior colliculi, respectively.

between the two thalamic masses across the third ventricle); the bridge is absent in about 20% of brains.

The **hypothalamus** arises by proliferation of neuroblasts in the intermediate zone of the diencephalic walls, ventral to the **hypothalamic sulci** (see Fig. 17-22E). *Differential expression of Wnt/β-catenin signaling is involved in the patterning of the hypothalamus.* Later, a number of nuclei concerned with endocrine activities and homeostasis develop. A pair of nuclei forms pea-sized swellings (**mammillary bodies**) on the ventral surface of the hypothalamus (see Fig. 17-22C).

The **epithalamus** develops from the roof and dorsal portion of the lateral wall of the diencephalons (see Fig. 17-22C to E). Initially, the **epithalamic swellings** are large, but later they become relatively small.

The **pineal gland** (pineal body) develops as a median diverticulum of the caudal part of the roof of the diencephalon (see Fig. 17-22D). Proliferation of cells in its walls soon converts it into a solid, cone-shaped gland.

The **pituitary gland** *(hypophysis)* is ectodermal in origin (Fig. 17-23 and Table 17-1). The Notch signaling

pathway has been implicated in the proliferation and differentiation of pituitary progenitor cells. The pituitary develops from two sources:

- An upgrowth from the ectodermal roof of the stomodeum, the **hypophyseal diverticulum** (Rathke pouch)
- A downgrowth from the neuroectoderm of the diencephalon, the **neurohypophyseal diverticulum**

This double origin explains why the pituitary gland is composed of two different types of tissue:

- The **adenohypophysis** (glandular tissue), or anterior lobe, arises from oral ectoderm
- The **neurohypophysis** (nervous tissue), or posterior lobe, arises from neuroectoderm

By the third week, the **hypophyseal diverticulum** projects from the roof of the stomodeum and lies adjacent to the floor (ventral wall) of the diencephalon (see Fig. 17-23C). By the fifth week, the diverticulum has elongated and constricted at its attachment to the oral epithelium. By this stage, it has come into contact with the

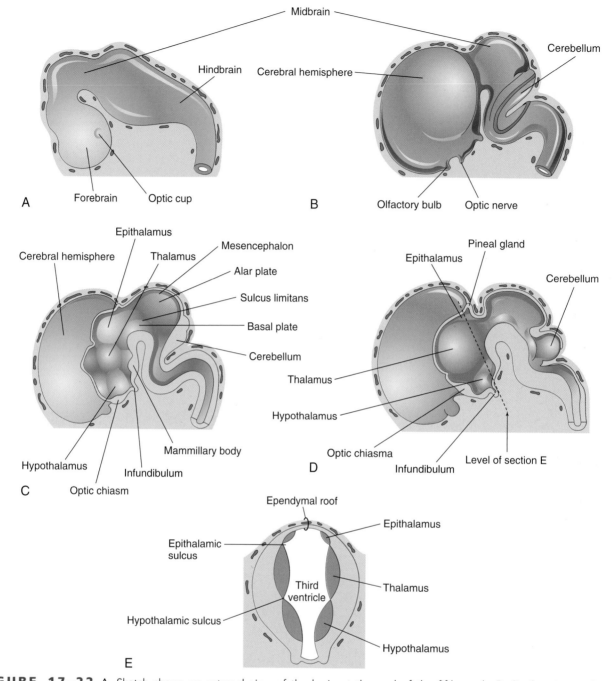

**FIGURE 17-22** A, Sketch shows an external view of the brain at the end of the fifth week. B, Similar view at 7 weeks. C, Median section of the brain at 7 weeks shows the medial surface of the forebrain and midbrain. D, Similar section at 8 weeks. E, Transverse section of the diencephalon shows the epithalamus dorsally, the thalamus laterally, and the hypothalamus ventrally.

**infundibulum** (derived from the neurohypophyseal diverticulum), a ventral downgrowth of the diencephalon (see Figs. 17-22C and D and 17-23).

The *stalk of the hypophyseal diverticulum* passes between the chondrification centers of the developing presphenoid and basisphenoid bones of the cranium (see Fig. 17-23E). During the sixth week, the connection of the diverticulum with the oral cavity degenerates (see Fig. 17-23D and E). Cells of the anterior wall of the hypophyseal diverticulum proliferate and give rise to the **pars anterior of the pituitary gland** (see Table 17-1). Later, an

extension, the **pars tuberalis,** grows around the **infundibular stem** (see Fig. 17-23E). The extensive proliferation of the anterior wall of the hypophyseal diverticulum reduces its lumen to a narrow cleft (see Fig. 17-23E). The **residual cleft** is usually not recognizable in the adult pituitary gland; however, it may be represented by a zone of cysts. Cells in the posterior wall of the hypophyseal pouch do not proliferate; they give rise to the thin, poorly defined **pars intermedia** (see Fig. 17-23F).

The part of the pituitary gland that develops from the **neuroectoderm** (neurohypophyseal diverticulum) is the

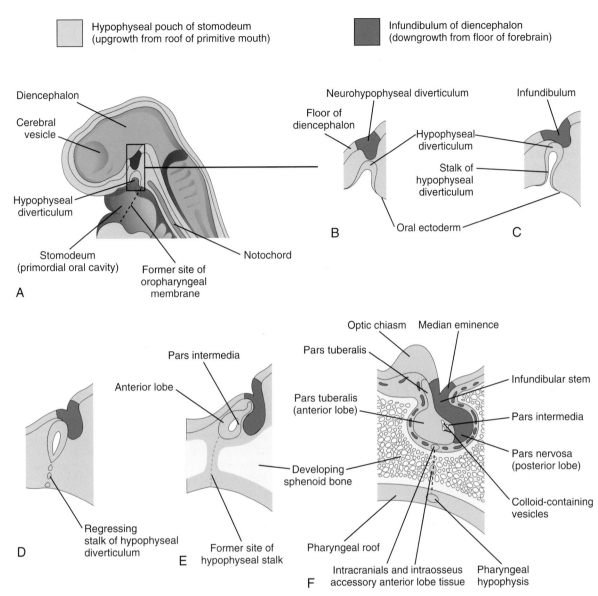

**FIGURE 17–23** Diagrammatic sketches illustrate development of the pituitary gland. **A,** Sagittal section of the cranial end of an embryo at approximately 36 days shows the hypophyseal diverticulum, an upgrowth from the stomodeum, and the neurohypophyseal diverticulum, a downgrowth from the forebrain. **B** to **D,** Successive stages of the developing pituitary gland. By 8 weeks, the diverticulum loses its connection with the oral cavity and is in close contact with the infundibulum and posterior lobe (neurohypophysis) of the pituitary gland. **E** and **F,** Sketches of later stages show proliferation of the anterior wall of the hypophyseal diverticulum to form the anterior lobe (adenohypophysis) of the pituitary gland.

| Table 17–1 | Pituitary Gland Derivation and Terminology | | |
|---|---|---|---|
| **DERIVATION** | **TISSUE TYPE** | **PART** | **LOBE** |
| **Oral ectoderm** | | | |
| Hypophyseal diverticulum from the roof of the stomodeum | Adenohypophysis (glandular tissue) | Pars anterior Pars tuberalis Pars intermedia | Anterior lobe |
| **Neuroectoderm** | | | |
| Neurohypophyseal diverticulum from the floor of the diencephalon | Neurohypophysis (nervous tissue) | Pars nervosa Infundibular stem Median eminence | Posterior lobe |

neurohypophysis (see Fig. 17-23B to F and Table 17-1). The **infundibulum** gives rise to the **median eminence, infundibular stem,** and **pars nervosa**. Initially, the walls of the infundibulum are thin, but the distal end of the infundibulum soon becomes solid as the neuroepithelial cells proliferate. These cells later differentiate into **pituicytes**, the primary cells of the posterior lobe of the pituitary gland, which are closely related to **neuroglial cells**. Nerve fibers grow into the pars nervosa from the hypothalamic area, to which the infundibular stem is attached (see Fig. 17-23F).

*Studies indicate that secreted inductive molecules (e.g., FGF8, BMP4, and WNT5A) from the diencephalon are involved in the formation of the anterior and intermediate lobes of the pituitary gland. The LIM homeobox gene LHX2 appears to control development of the posterior lobe.*

## PHARYNGEAL HYPOPHYSIS AND CRANIOPHARYNGIOMA

A remnant of the stalk of the hypophyseal diverticulum may persist and form a **pharyngeal hypophysis** in the roof of the oropharynx (see Fig. 17-23F). Rarely, masses of anterior lobe tissue develop outside the capsule of the pituitary gland, within the sella turcica of the sphenoid bone (Fig. 17-24). A remnant of the hypophyseal diverticulum, the **basipharyngeal canal**, is visible in sections of the neonate's sphenoid bone in approximately 1% of cases. It can also be identified in a small number of radiographs of crania of neonates (usually those with cranial defects).

Occasionally, a rare, benign tumor (**craniopharyngioma**) develops in or superior to the sella turcica. Less often, these tumors form in the pharynx or basisphenoid (posterior part of the sphenoid) from remnants of the stalk of the hypophyseal diverticulum (see Fig. 17-24). These tumors arise along the path of the hypophyseal diverticulum from epithelial remnants (see Fig. 17-23D to F).

## Telencephalon

The telencephalon consists of a median part and two lateral diverticula, the **cerebral vesicles** (see Fig. 17-23A). These vesicles are the primordia of the **cerebral hemispheres** (see Figs. 17-22B and 17-23A). The cavity of the median portion of the telencephalon forms the extreme anterior part of the **third ventricle** (Fig. 17-25). At first, the cerebral hemispheres are in wide communication with the cavity of the third ventricle through the **interventricular foramina** (Fig. 17-26B; see Fig. 17-25).

Along the **choroid fissure**, part of the medial wall of the developing **cerebral hemisphere** becomes very thin (see Figs. 17-25 and 17-26A and B). Initially, this ependymal portion lies in the roof of the hemisphere and is continuous with the ependymal roof of the third ventricle (see Fig. 17-26A). The **choroid plexus of the lateral ventricle** later forms at this site (Fig. 17-27; see Fig. 17-25).

As the **cerebral hemispheres** expand, they cover successively the diencephalon, midbrain, and hindbrain. The hemispheres eventually meet each other in the midline, and their medial surfaces become flattened. The mesenchyme trapped in the longitudinal fissure between them gives rise to the **cerebral falx** *(falx cerebri)*, a median fold of dura mater.

The **corpus striatum** appears during the sixth week as a prominent swelling in the floor of each cerebral hemisphere (see Fig. 17-27B). The floor of each hemisphere expands more slowly than its thin cortical walls because it contains the rather large **corpus striatum**, and the cerebral hemispheres become C shaped (Fig. 17-28A and B).

The growth and curvature of the cerebral hemispheres affect the shape of the lateral ventricles. They become

**FIGURE 17–24** Sagittal magnetic resonance image of the brain of a 4-year-old boy whose presenting symptoms were headaches and optic atrophy (vision loss). A large mass (4 cm) occupies an enlarged sella turcica, expanding inferiorly into the sphenoid bone and superiorly into the suprasellar cistern. A craniopharyngioma was confirmed by surgery. The inferior half of the mass is solid and appears dark, whereas the superior half is cystic and appears brighter.

Corpus callosum
Thalamus
Midbrain
Cerebellum
Craniopharyngioma
Pons

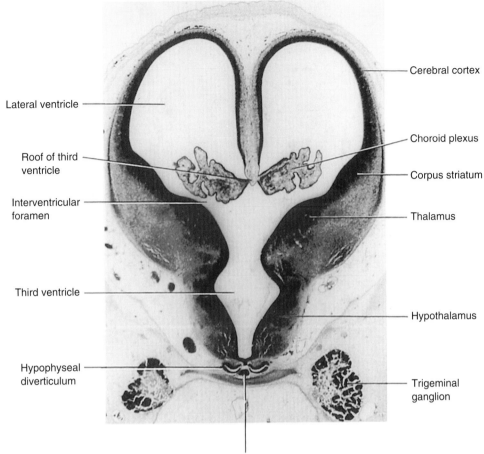

Labels (clockwise from top): Cerebral cortex, Choroid plexus, Corpus striatum, Thalamus, Hypothalamus, Trigeminal ganglion, Neurohypophyseal diverticulum, Hypophyseal diverticulum, Third ventricle, Interventricular foramen, Roof of third ventricle, Lateral ventricle

**FIGURE 17–25** Photomicrograph of a transverse section through the diencephalon and cerebral vesicles of a human embryo (approximately 50 days) at the level of the interventricular foramina (×20). The choroid fissure is located at the junction of the choroid plexus and the medial wall of the lateral ventricle.

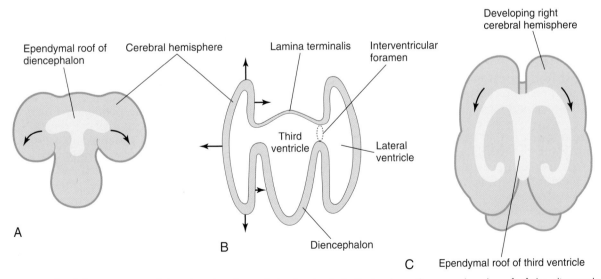

Labels: Ependymal roof of diencephalon, Cerebral hemisphere, Lamina terminalis, Interventricular foramen, Developing right cerebral hemisphere, Third ventricle, Lateral ventricle, Diencephalon, Ependymal roof of third ventricle

A          B          C

**FIGURE 17–26** A, Sketch of the dorsal surface of the forebrain indicates how the ependymal roof of the diencephalon is carried out to the dorsomedial surface of the cerebral hemispheres (*arrows*). B, Diagrammatic section of the forebrain shows how the developing cerebral hemispheres grow from the lateral walls of the forebrain and expand in all directions until they cover the diencephalon. The *arrows* indicate some directions in which the hemispheres expand. The rostral wall of the forebrain, the lamina terminalis, is very thin. C, Sketch of the forebrain shows how the ependymal roof is finally carried into the temporal lobes as a result of the C-shaped growth pattern of the cerebral hemispheres (*arrows*).

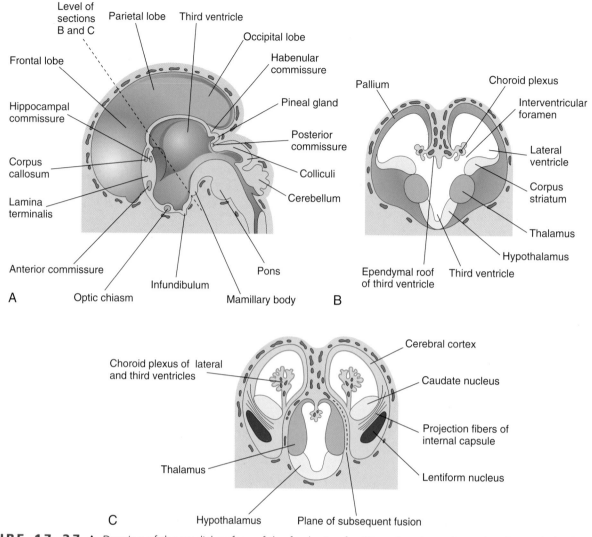

**FIGURE 17–27** A, Drawing of the medial surface of the forebrain of a 10-week embryo shows the diencephalic derivatives, the main commissures, and the expanding cerebral hemispheres. B, Transverse section of the forebrain at the level of the interventricular foramina shows the corpus striatum and choroid plexuses of the lateral ventricles. C, Similar section at approximately 11 weeks shows division of the corpus striatum into the caudate and lentiform nuclei by the internal capsule. The developing relationship of the cerebral hemispheres to the diencephalon is also illustrated.

roughly C-shaped cavities filled with CSF. The caudal end of each hemisphere turns ventrally and then rostrally, forming the **temporal lobe** (Fig. 17-29C); in so doing, it carries the lateral ventricle (forming its **temporal horn**) and choroid fissure with it (see Fig. 17-28B and C). The thin medial wall of the hemisphere is invaginated along the choroid fissure by vascular pia mater to form the *choroid plexus of the temporal horn* (see Fig. 17-27B).

As the **cerebral cortex** differentiates, fibers coursing to and from it pass through the **corpus striatum** and divide it into **caudate and lentiform nuclei**. This fiber pathway (**internal capsule**) (see Fig. 17-27C) becomes C shaped as the hemisphere assumes this form. The **caudate nucleus** becomes elongated and C shaped, conforming to the outline of the lateral ventricle (see Fig. 17-28C). Its pear-shaped head and elongated body lie in the floor of the frontal horn and body of the **lateral ventricle**, whereas its tail makes a U-shaped turn to gain the roof of the temporal or inferior horn.

## Cerebral Commissures

As the cerebral cortex develops, groups of nerve fibers (commissures) connect corresponding areas of the **cerebral hemispheres** with one another (see Fig. 17-27). The most important of these commissures crosses in the **lamina terminalis**, which is the rostral (anterior) end of the forebrain (see Fig. 17-26A and B and 17-27A). This lamina extends from the roof plate of the diencephalon to the **optic chiasm** (decussation or crossing of the optic nerve fibers). The lamina terminalis is the natural pathway from one hemisphere to the other.

The first commissures to form are the *anterior commissure* and *hippocampal commissure*. They are small fiber bundles that connect phylogenetically older parts of the brain (see Fig. 17-27A). The anterior commissure connects the **olfactory bulb** (rostral extremity of the olfactory tract) and related areas of one hemisphere with those of the opposite side. The hippocampal commissure connects the hippocampal formations.

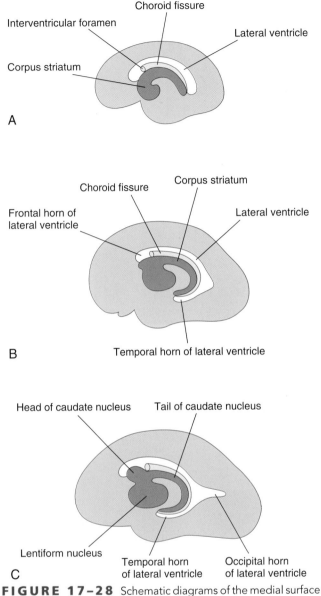

**FIGURE 17–28** Schematic diagrams of the medial surface of the developing right cerebral hemisphere show development of the lateral ventricle, choroid fissure, and corpus striatum. A, At 13 weeks. B, At 21 weeks. C, At 32 weeks.

The largest cerebral commissure is the corpus callosum (see Figs. 17-27A and 17-28A), which connects neocortical areas. The corpus callosum initially lies in the lamina terminalis, but fibers are added to it as the cortex enlarges, and it gradually extends beyond the lamina terminalis. The rest of the **lamina terminalis** lies between the corpus callosum and the fornix. It becomes stretched to form the *septum pellucidum*, a thin plate of brain tissue containing nerve cells and fibers.

At birth, the **corpus callosum** extends over the roof of the diencephalon. The **optic chiasm**, which develops in the ventral part of the lamina terminalis (see Fig. 17-27A), consists of fibers from the medial halves of the retinae (layer at back of the eyeball that is sensitive to light) that cross to join the optic tract of the opposite side.

The walls of the developing cerebral hemispheres initially show three typical zones of the neural tube:

*ventricular, intermediate,* and *marginal*; later a fourth one, the *subventricular zone,* appears. Cells of the intermediate zone migrate into the marginal zone and give rise to the cortical layers. The gray matter is located peripherally, and axons from its cell bodies pass centrally to form the large volume of white matter (**medullary center**).

Initially, the surface of the cerebral hemispheres is smooth (see Fig. 17-29A); however, as growth proceeds, **sulci** (grooves) between the gyri (tortuous convolutions) develop (Fig. 17-30A; see Fig. 17-29B and D). The gyri are caused by infolding of the **cerebral cortex**. The sulci and gyri permit a considerable increase in the surface area of the cerebral cortex without requiring an extensive increase in the size of the neurocranium (see Fig. 17-30B and C). As each cerebral hemisphere grows, the cortex covering the external surface of the corpus striatum grows relatively slowly and is soon overgrown (see Fig. 17-29D). This buried cortex, hidden from view in the depths of the **lateral sulcus** of the cerebral hemisphere (see Fig. 17-30A), is the **insula** (Latin *island*).

## BIRTH DEFECTS OF BRAIN

Because of the complexity of its embryologic history, abnormal development of the brain is common (approximately 3 of 1000 births). Most major birth defects, such as **meroencephaly** and **meningoencephalocele**, result from *defective closure of the rostral neuropore* (an NTD) during the fourth week (Fig. 17-31C) and involve the overlying tissues (meninges and calvaria). The factors causing NTDs are genetic, nutritional, and environmental. Birth defects of the brain can be caused by alterations in the morphogenesis or histogenesis of the nervous tissue, or they can result from developmental failures occurring in associated structures (notochord, somites, mesenchyme, and cranium).

**Abnormal histogenesis of the cerebral cortex** can result in **seizures** (Fig. 17-32) and various degrees of **mental deficiency**. Subnormal intellectual development may result from exposure of the embryo or fetus during the 8- to 16-week period to viruses such as **Rubella virus** and **high levels of radiation** (see Table 20-6). **Prenatal risk factors**, such as maternal infection or thyroid disorder, Rh factor incompatibility, and some hereditary and genetic conditions, cause most cases of **cerebral palsy**, but the central motor deficit may result from events during birth.

*Text continued on p. 412*

### ENCEPHALOCELE

Encephalocele is a herniation of intracranial contents resulting from a defect in the cranium (**cranium bifidum**). Encephaloceles are most common in the occipital region (Figs. 17-33 and 17-34; see Fig. 17-31A to D). The hernia may contain meninges (**meningocele**), meninges and part of the brain (**meningoencephalocele**), or meninges, part of the brain, and part of the ventricular system (**meningohydroencephalocele**). Encephalocele occurs in approximately 1 of 2000 births.

**FIGURE 17–29** Sketches of lateral views of the left cerebral hemisphere, diencephalon, and brainstem show successive stages in the development of the sulci and gyri in the cerebral cortex. Notice the gradual narrowing of the lateral sulcus and burying of the insula, an area of cerebral cortex that is concealed from surface view. The surface of the cerebral hemispheres grows rapidly during the fetal period, forming many gyri (convolutions), which are separated by many sulci (grooves). A, At 14 weeks. B, At 26 weeks. C, At 30 weeks. D, At 38 weeks. E, Magnetic resonance image of a pregnant woman shows a mature fetus. Observe the brain and spinal cord. *Inset at upper right,* The smooth lateral *(top)* and medial *(bottom)* surfaces of a human fetal brain (14 weeks).

**FIGURE 17–30** *A*, Lateral view of the brain of a fetus that died before delivery (25 weeks). *B*, The medial *(top)* and lateral *(bottom)* surfaces of the fetal brain (week 25). *C*, The lateral *(top)* and medial *(bottom)* surfaces of the fetal brain at week 38 (label on photo: 40 weeks from last normal menstrual period). As the brain enlarges, the gyral pattern of the cerebral hemispheres becomes more complex (compare with Figure 17-29). *(A, From Nishimura H, Semba R, Tanimura T, Tanaka O: Prenatal development of the human with special reference to craniofacial structures: an atlas, Bethesda, MD, 1977, U.S. Department of Health, Education, and Welfare, National Institutes of Health.)*

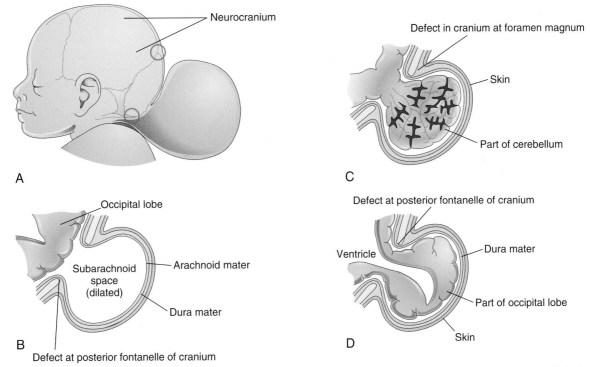

**FIGURE 17–31** Schematic drawings illustrate encephalocele (cranium bifidum) and various types of herniation of the brain and meninges. *A*, Sketch of the head of a neonate with a large protrusion from the occipital region of the cranium. The *upper red circle* indicates a cranial defect at the posterior fontanelle (membranous interval between cranial bones). The *lower red circle* indicates a cranial defect near the foramen magnum. *B*, *Meningocele* consists of a protrusion of the cranial meninges that is filled with cerebrospinal fluid. *C*, *Meningoencephalocele* consists of a protrusion of part of the cerebellum that is covered by meninges and skin. *D*, *Meningohydroencephalocele* consists of a protrusion of part of the occipital lobe that contains part of the posterior horn of a lateral ventricle.

**FIGURE 17–32** A, Focal heterotopic cerebral cortex. Magnetic resonance image of the brain of a 19-year-old woman with seizures shows a focal heterotopic cortex of the right parietal lobe, indenting the right lateral ventricle. Notice the lack of organized cortex at the overlying surface of the brain. Heterotopic cortex is the result of an arrest of centrifugal migration of neuroblasts along the radial processes of glial cells. B, Coronal section of an adult brain with periventricular heterotopia (arrow) in the parietal cerebrum. The lobulated gray matter structures along the ventricle represent cells that failed to migrate but nevertheless differentiated into neurons.

**FIGURE 17–33** A neonate with a large meningoencephalocele in the occipital area.

## MEROENCEPHALY

**Meroencephaly** is a severe defect of the calvaria and brain that results from *failure of the rostral neuropore to close* during the fourth week. The forebrain, midbrain, and most of the hindbrain and calvaria are absent (Fig. 17-35; see Figs. 17-13 and 17-17). Most of the embryo's brain is exposed or extruding from the cranium (**exencephaly**). Because of the abnormal structure and **vascularization** (formation of new blood vessels) of the **embryonic exencephalic brain**, the nervous tissue undergoes degeneration. The remains of the brain appear as a spongy, vascular mass consisting mostly of hindbrain structures.

**Meroencephaly is a common lethal defect**, occurring in at least 1 of 1000 births. It is two to four times more common among girls than boys, and it is always associated with **acrania** (complete or partial absence of neurocranium). It may be associated with **rachischisis** (failure of fusion of neural arches) when defective neural tube closure is extensive (see Figs. 17-13 and 17-35). Meroencephaly is the most common serious defect seen in stillborn fetuses. Neonates with this severe NTD may survive briefly. *Meroencephaly can be easily diagnosed by ultrasonography, magnetic resonance imaging (MRI) fetoscopy, and radiography* because extensive parts of the brain and calvaria are absent (see Fig. 17-35).

**Meroencephaly usually has a multifactorial mode of inheritance** (see Chapter 20, Figs. 20-1 and 20-23). An excess of amniotic fluid (*polyhydramnios*) is often associated with meroencephaly, possibly because the fetus lacks the neural control for swallowing amniotic fluid. The fluid does not pass into the intestines for absorption and subsequent transfer to the placenta for disposal.

**FIGURE 17–34** Magnetic resonance images (MRIs) of a 1-day-old neonate show a meningocele. **A,** Sagittal MRI taken so that the cerebrospinal fluid (CSF) appears bright. The image is blurred because of movement of the neonate. **B,** Axial image located at the cranial defect near the foramen magnum and taken so that CSF appears dark. Compare with Figure 17-31C.

**FIGURE 17–35** **A,** Sonogram of a normal fetus at 12 weeks *(left)* and a fetus at 14 weeks with acrania and meroencephaly *(right)*. **B,** Magnetic resonance image of diamniotic-monochorionic twins, one with meroencephaly. Notice the absent calvaria *(white arrow)* of the abnormal twin and the amnion of the normal twin *(black arrow)*. (**A,** *From Pooh RK, Pooh KH: Transvaginal 3D and Doppler ultrasonography of the fetal brain,* Semin Perinatol *25:38, 2001.)*

## MICROCEPHALY

*Microcephaly is a neurodevelopmental disorder.* The calvaria and brain are small, but the face is normal sized (Fig. 17-36). These infants are **grossly mentally deficient** because the brain is underdeveloped. *Microcephaly is the result of a reduction in brain growth.* Inadequate pressure from the growing brain leads to the small size of the **neurocranium (bones of cranium)**. In the United States, about 25,000 infants are diagnosed annually.

Some cases appear to be genetic in origin. In autosomal recessive primary microcephaly, embryonic brain growth is reduced without affecting the structure of the brain. Exposure to large amounts of ionizing radiation, infectious agents (e.g., cytomegalovirus, rubella virus, *Toxoplasma gondii*), and certain drugs (e.g., maternal alcohol abuse) during the fetal period are contributing factors in some cases (see Chapter 20, Table 20-6).

Microcephaly can be detected in utero by ultrasound scans carried out over the period of gestation. A small head may result from **premature synostosis** (osseous union) of all the cranial sutures (see Chapter 14, Fig. 14-12D); however, the neurocranium is thin with exaggerated convolutional markings.

**FIGURE 17–36** An infant with microcephaly showing the typical normal-sized face and small neurocranium. This defect is usually associated with mental deficiency.

## AGENESIS OF CORPUS CALLOSUM

In agenesis of corpus callosum, there is a complete or partial **absence of the corpus callosum**, which is the main neocortical commissure of the cerebral hemispheres (Fig. 17-37A and B). The condition may be asymptomatic, but seizures and mental deficiency are common. Agenesis of the corpus callosum is associated with more than 50 human congenital syndromes.

**FIGURE 17–37** **A,** Sagittal magnetic resonance image of the brain of a 22-year-old, normal-functioning man. There is complete absence of the corpus callosum. **B,** A coronal slice through a child's brain shows agenesis of the corpus callosum, which would normally cross the midline to connect the two cerebral hemispheres. Notice the thalamus (*T*) and the downward displacement of the cingulum (well-marked fiber bundle) into the lateral and third ventricles (*arrow*).

# HYDROCEPHALUS

Significant **enlargement of the head** results from an imbalance between the production and absorption of CSF; as a result, there is an *excess of CSF in the ventricular system of the brain* (Fig. 17-38). Hydrocephalus results from impaired circulation and absorption of CSF and, in rare cases, from increased production of CSF by a **choroid plexus adenoma** (benign tumor). A premature infant may develop intraventricular hemorrhage leading to hydrocephalus through the obstruction of the lateral aperture (foramen of Luschka) and median aperture (foramen of Magendie). Rarely, impaired CSF circulation results from **congenital aqueductal stenosis** (Fig. 17-39; see Fig. 17-38); the **cerebral aqueduct** is narrow or consists of several minute channels. In a few cases, stenosis results from transmission of an **X-linked recessive trait**, but most cases appear to result from a fetal **viral infection** (e.g., cytomegalovirus) or *Toxoplasma gondii* (see Chapter 20, Table 20-6). Blood in the **subarachnoid space** may cause obliteration of the cisterns or arachnoid villi (thin, limiting membrane).

**Blockage of CSF circulation** results in dilation of the ventricles proximal to the obstruction, internal **accumulation of CSF**, and pressure on the cerebral hemispheres (see Fig. 17-39). This squeezes the brain between the ventricular fluid and the neurocranium. In infants, the internal pressure results in an accelerated rate of expansion of the brain and neurocranium because most of the fibrous sutures are not fused. Hydrocephalus usually refers to **obstructive or noncommunicating hydrocephalus**, in which all or part of the ventricular system is enlarged. All ventricles are enlarged if the apertures of the fourth ventricle or the subarachnoid spaces are blocked, whereas the lateral and third ventricles are dilated when only the **cerebral aqueduct** is obstructed (see Fig. 17-39). **Obstruction of an interventricular foramen** can produce dilation of one ventricle.

Hydrocephalus resulting from obliteration of the subarachnoid cisterns or malfunction of the arachnoid villi is called **nonobstructive or communicating hydrocephalus**. Although hydrocephalus may be associated with spina bifida cystica, enlargement of the head may not be obvious at birth. Hydrocephalus often produces thinning of the bones of the calvaria, prominence of the forehead, atrophy of the cerebral cortex and white matter (see Fig. 17-38*B* and *C*), and compression of the basal ganglia and diencephalon.

**FIGURE 17–38** A, An infant with hydrocephalus and bilateral cleft palate. B and C, The brain of a 10-year-old child who developed hydrocephalus in utero as a result of aqueductal stenosis. The thin white matter is well myelinated. Notice that the shunt tube in B, which was meant to treat the hydrocephalus, lies in the frontal horn of the ventricle.

**FIGURE 17–39** Congenital stenosis of the cerebral aqueduct. Sagittal magnetic resonance image shows large lateral and third ventricles. The cerebrospinal fluid appears bright in this image. There is also a marked flow void within the cerebral aqueduct. *(From Dr. Frank Gaillard, Radiopaedia.org.)*

**FIGURE 17–40** Frontal view of an intact (**A**) and coronally sectioned (**B**) fetal brain with holoprosencephaly at 21 weeks. This defect results from failure of cleavage of the prosencephalon (rostral neural tube) into right and left cerebral hemispheres, telencephalon and diencephalon, and olfactory bulbs and optic tracts.

## HOLOPROSENCEPHALY

Holoprosencephaly (HPE) results from *incomplete separation of the cerebral hemispheres* and most are associated with facial abnormalities. Genetic and environmental factors have been implicated in this severe and relatively common defect (1 in 250 fetuses and 1 in 15,000 neonates) (Fig. 17-40). **Maternal diabetes** and teratogens (e.g., alcohol) can destroy embryonic cells in the median plane of the embryonic disc during the third week, producing a wide range of birth defects resulting from **defective formation of the forebrain**. In familial alobar holoprosencephaly, the forebrain is small, and the lateral ventricles often merge to form one large ventricle.

Defects in forebrain development often cause facial anomalies resulting from a reduction in tissue in the frontonasal prominence (see Chapter 9, Figs. 9-26 and 9-27). HPE is often indicated when the eyes are abnormally close together (**hypotelorism**). *Molecular studies have identified several holoprosencephaly-related genes, including SHH.*

**FIGURE 17–41** Magnetic resonance image of a fetus with massive hydrocephalus or hydrocephaly *(asterisk)* shows excessive accumulation of cerebrospinal fluid. Notice the greatly reduced and displaced cerebral hemispheres and cerebellum.

## HYDRANENCEPHALY

Hydranencephaly is a rare anomaly. The **cerebral hemispheres are absent** or represented by membranous sacs with remnants of the cerebral cortex dispersed over the membranes (Fig. 17-41). The brainstem (midbrain, pons, and medulla) is relatively intact. These infants appear normal at birth, but the head grows excessively after birth because of **CSF accumulation**. A **ventriculoperitoneal shunt** is usually made to prevent further enlargement of the neurocranium. Mental development fails to occur, and there is little or no cognitive development. The cause of this unusual, severe anomaly is uncertain, but evidence indicates that it may result from an early obstruction of blood flow to the areas supplied by the internal carotid arteries.

## CHIARI MALFORMATION

Chiari malformation (Fig. 17-42) is a structural defect of the cerebellum. It is characterized by a tongue-like projection of the medulla and inferior displacement of the cerebral tonsil through the foramen magnum into the vertebral canal. The posterior cranial fossa is usually abnormally small, causing pressure on the cerebellum and brainstem. The condition may lead to a type of non-communicating hydrocephalus that obstructs the absorption and flow of CSF; as a result, the entire ventricular system is distended. Magnetic resonance imaging is now used to diagnose Chiari malformation, and as a result, more cases have been detected than before.

Several types of Chiari malformations have been described. In **type I**, the inferior part of the cerebellum herniates through the foramen magnum. This is the most common form. It is usually asymptomatic and detected in adolescence. In **type II**, also known as **Arnold-Chiari malformation**, cerebellar tissue and the brainstem herniate through the foramen magnum, often accompanied by occipital encephalocele and lumbar myelomeningocele. In **type III**, the most severe form, there is herniation of the cerebellum and brainstem through the foramen magnum into the vertebral canal, which has serious neurologic consequences. In **type IV**, the cerebellum is absent or underdeveloped; these infants do not survive.

## MENTAL DEFICIENCY

Impairment of intelligence may result from various genetically determined conditions (e.g., Down syndrome [trisomy 21], trisomy 18 syndrome) (see Chapter 20, Table 20-1). **Mental deficiency** may also result from the action of a mutant gene or a chromosomal abnormality (e.g., extra chromosome 13, 17, or 21). **Chromosomal aberrations** and mental deficiency are discussed later (see Chapter 20, Figs. 20-1 and 20-2). Approximately 25% of cases have a demonstrable cause.

**Maternal alcohol abuse** is a common identifiable cause of mental deficiency. The 8th to 16th week of development is also the period of greatest sensitivity for fetal brain damage resulting from **large doses of radiation**. By the end of the 16th week, most neuronal proliferation and cell migration to the cerebral cortex are completed.

Cell depletion of sufficient degree in the cerebral cortex results in severe mental deficiency. Disorders of protein, carbohydrate, or fat metabolism may also cause mental deficiency. **Maternal and fetal infections** (e.g., syphilis, rubella virus, toxoplasmosis, cytomegalovirus) and congenital **hypothyroidism** are commonly associated

**FIGURE 17–42** A, An Arnold-Chiari type II malformation in a 23-week fetus. In situ exposure of the hindbrain reveals cerebellar tissue (*arrow*) well below the foramen magnum. B, Magnetic resonance image of a child with Arnold-Chiari type I malformation. The cerebellar tonsils lie inferior to the foramen magnum (*red arrow*).

## MENTAL DEFICIENCY—cont'd

with mental deficiency. *Deficient mental development* throughout the postnatal growth period can result from birth injuries, toxins (e.g., lead), cerebral infections (e.g., meningitis), cerebral trauma from head injuries, and poisoning.

# DEVELOPMENT OF PERIPHERAL NERVOUS SYSTEM

The peripheral nervous system (PNS) consists of cranial, spinal, and visceral nerves and cranial, spinal, and autonomic ganglia. The PNS develops from various sources but mostly from the neural crest. All sensory cells (somatic and visceral) of the PNS are derived from neural crest cells. The cell bodies of these sensory cells are located outside the CNS.

With the exception of the cells in the spiral ganglion of the cochlea and the vestibular ganglion of CN VIII (vestibulocochlear nerve), all peripheral sensory cells are at first bipolar. Later, the two processes unite to form a single process with peripheral and central components, resulting in a unipolar type of neuron (see Fig. 17-9D). The peripheral process terminates in a sensory ending, whereas the central process enters the spinal cord or brain (see Fig. 17-8). The sensory cells in the ganglion of CN VIII remain bipolar.

The cell body of each afferent neuron is closely invested by a capsule of modified Schwann cell (satellite cells) (see Fig. 17-8), which are derived from neural crest cells. This capsule is continuous with the neurilemma (sheath of Schwann) that surrounds the axons of afferent neurons. External to the satellite cells is a layer of connective tissue that is continuous with the endoneurial sheath of the nerve fibers. This connective tissue and the endoneurial sheath are derived from mesenchyme.

Neural crest cells in the developing brain migrate to form sensory ganglia only in relation to the trigeminal (CN V), facial (CN VII), vestibulocochlear (CN VIII), glossopharyngeal (CN IX), and vagus (CN X) nerves. Neural crest cells also differentiate into multipolar neurons of the autonomic ganglia (see Fig. 17-8), including ganglia of the sympathetic trunks that lie along the sides of the vertebral bodies; collateral (prevertebral) ganglia in plexuses of the thorax and abdomen (e.g., cardiac, celiac, and mesenteric plexuses); and parasympathetic (terminal) ganglia in or near the viscera (e.g., submucosal or Meissner plexus).

Cells of the paraganglia (chromaffin cells) are also derived from the neural crest The term *paraganglia* includes several widely scattered groups of cells that are similar in many ways to medullary cells of the suprarenal glands. The cell groups largely lie retroperitoneally, often in association with sympathetic ganglia. The carotid and aortic bodies also have small islands of chromaffin cells associated with them. These widely scattered groups of cells constitute the chromaffin system. Neural crest cells also give rise to melanoblasts (precursors of melanocytes) and cells of the medulla of the suprarenal gland.

## Spinal Nerves

Motor nerve fibers arising from the spinal cord begin to appear at the end of the fourth week (see Figs. 17-4, 17-7, and 17-8). The nerve fibers arise from cells in the basal plates of the developing spinal cord and emerge as a continuous series of rootlets along its ventrolateral surface. The fibers destined for a particular developing muscle group become arranged in a bundle, forming a ventral nerve root. The nerve fibers of the dorsal nerve root are formed from neural crest cells that migrate to the dorsolateral aspect of the spinal cord, where they differentiate into the cells of the spinal ganglion (see Figs. 17-8 and 17-9).

The central processes of neurons in the spinal ganglion form a single bundle that grows into the spinal cord opposite the apex of the dorsal horn of gray matter (see Fig. 17-5B and C). The distal processes of spinal ganglion cells grow toward the ventral nerve root and eventually join it to form a spinal nerve.

Immediately after being formed, a mixed spinal nerve divides into dorsal and ventral primary *rami* (Latin *branches*). The dorsal primary ramus, the smaller division, innervates the dorsal axial musculature (see Chapter 15, Fig. 15-1), vertebrae, posterior intervertebral joints, and part of the skin of the back. The ventral primary ramus, the major division of each spinal nerve, contributes to the innervation of the limbs and ventrolateral parts of the body wall. The major nerve plexuses (cervical, brachial, and lumbosacral) are formed by ventral primary rami.

As the limb buds develop, the nerves from the spinal cord segments opposite to the bud elongate and grow into the limb. The nerve fibers are distributed to its muscles, which differentiate from myogenic cells that originate from the somites (see Chapter 15, Fig. 15-1).

The skin of the developing limbs is also innervated in a segmental manner. Early in development, successive ventral primary rami are joined by connecting loops of nerve fibers, especially those supplying the limbs (e.g., brachial plexus). The dorsal division of the trunks of these plexuses supplies the extensor muscles and the extensor surface of the limbs. The ventral divisions of the trunks supply the flexor muscles and the flexor surface. The dermatomes and cutaneous innervation of the limbs were described earlier (see Chapter 16, Fig. 16-10).

## Cranial Nerves

Twelve pairs of cranial nerves form during the fifth and sixth weeks. They are classified into three groups, according to their embryologic origins.

### Somatic Efferent Cranial Nerves

The trochlear (CN IV), abducent (CN VI), hypoglossal (CN XII), and greater part of the oculomotor (CN III) nerves are homologous with the ventral roots of spinal nerves (Fig. 17-43). The cells of origin of these nerves are located in the *somatic efferent column*, which is derived from the basal plates of the brainstem. Their axons are distributed to muscles derived from the head myotomes (preotic and occipital) (see Chapter 15, Fig. 15-4).

The hypoglossal nerve (CN XII) resembles a spinal nerve more than do the other somatic efferent cranial nerves. CN XII develops by the fusion of the ventral root fibers of three or four occipital nerves (see Fig. 17-43A). Sensory roots, which correspond to the dorsal roots of spinal nerves, are absent. The somatic motor fibers originate from the hypoglossal nucleus, consisting of motor cells resembling those of the ventral horn of the spinal cord. These fibers leave the ventrolateral wall of the

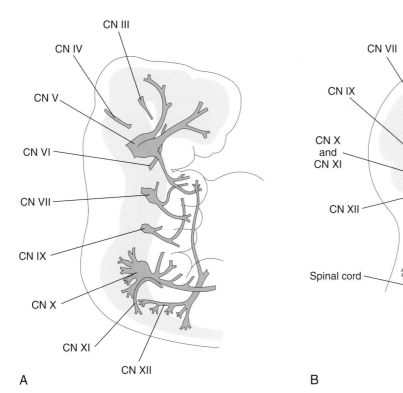

A

B

**FIGURE 17–43** A, Schematic drawing of a 5-week embryo shows distribution of most of the cranial nerves, especially those supplying the pharyngeal arches. B, Schematic drawing of the head and neck of an adult shows the general distribution of most of the cranial nerves.

medulla in several groups, the hypoglossal nerve roots, which converge to form the common trunk of CN XII (see Fig. 17-43B). They grow rostrally and eventually innervate the muscles of the tongue, which are thought to be derived from occipital myotomes (see Chapter 15, Fig. 15-4). With development of the neck, the hypoglossal nerve comes to lie at a progressively higher level.

The **abducent nerve** (CN VI) arises from nerve cells in the basal plates of the metencephalon. It passes from its ventral surface to the posterior of the three preotic myotomes from which the lateral rectus muscle of the eye is thought to originate.

The **trochlear nerve** (CN IV) arises from nerve cells in the somatic efferent column in the posterior part of the midbrain. Although it is a motor nerve, it emerges from the brainstem dorsally and passes ventrally to supply the superior oblique muscle of the eye.

The **oculomotor nerve** (CN III) supplies most muscles of the eye, including the superior, inferior, and medial recti and the inferior oblique muscles. They are derived from the first preotic myotomes.

### Nerves of Pharyngeal Arches

**CN V, VII, IX, and X** supply the embryonic pharyngeal arches. The structures that develop from these arches are therefore innervated by these cranial nerves (see Fig. 17-43A and see Chapter 9, Table 9-1).

The **trigeminal nerve** (CN V) is the nerve of the first arch, but it has an ophthalmic division that is not a pharyngeal arch component. *CN V is chiefly sensory and is the principal sensory nerve for the head.* The large **trigeminal ganglion** lies beside the rostral end of the pons, and its cells are derived from the most anterior part of the neural crest. The central processes of cells in this ganglion form the large sensory root of CN V, which enters the lateral portion of the pons. The peripheral processes of cells in this ganglion separate into three large divisions (ophthalmic, maxillary, and mandibular nerves). Their sensory fibers supply the skin of the face and the lining of the mouth and nose (see Chapter 9, Fig. 9-6).

The **motor fibers of CN V** arise from cells in the most anterior part of the special visceral efferent column in the metencephalon. The **motor nucleus of CN V** lies at the midlevel of the pons. The fibers leave the pons at the site of the entering sensory fibers and pass to the **muscles of mastication** and other muscles that develop in the **mandibular prominence** of the first pharyngeal arch (see Chapter 9, Table 9-1). The mesencephalic nucleus of CN V differentiates from cells in the midbrain that extend rostrally from the metencephalon.

The **facial nerve** (CN VII) is the nerve of the second pharyngeal arch. It consists mostly of motor fibers that arise principally from a nuclear group in the special visceral efferent column in the caudal part of the pons. These fibers are distributed to the **muscles of facial expression** and to other muscles that develop in the mesenchyme of the second arch (see Chapter 9, Table 9-1). The small general visceral efferent component of CN VII terminates in the peripheral autonomic ganglia of the head. The sensory fibers of CN VII arise from the cells of the geniculate ganglion. The central processes of these cells enter the pons, and the peripheral processes pass to the greater superficial petrosal nerve and, through the **chorda tympani nerve**, to the taste buds in the anterior two thirds of the tongue.

The **glossopharyngeal nerve** (CN IX) is the nerve of the third pharyngeal arch. Its motor fibers arise from the special and, to a lesser extent, general visceral efferent columns of the anterior part of the myelencephalon. CN IX forms from several rootlets that arise from the medulla just caudal to the developing internal ear. All fibers from the special visceral efferent column are distributed to the **stylopharyngeus muscle**, which is derived from mesenchyme in the third arch (see Chapter 9, Table 9-1). The general efferent fibers are distributed to the **otic ganglion**, from which postganglionic fibers pass to the **parotid and posterior lingual glands**. The sensory fibers of CN IX are distributed as general sensory and special visceral afferent fibers (taste fibers) to the posterior part of the tongue.

The **vagus nerve** (CN X) is formed by fusion of the nerves of the fourth and sixth pharyngeal arches (see Chapter 9, Table 9-1). It has large visceral efferent and visceral afferent components that are distributed to the heart, foregut and its derivatives, and a large part of the midgut. The nerve of the fourth arch becomes the **superior laryngeal nerve**, which supplies the cricothyroid muscle and constrictor muscles of the pharynx. The nerve of the sixth arch becomes the recurrent laryngeal nerve, which supplies various **laryngeal muscles**.

The **spinal accessory nerve** (CN XI) emerges as a series of rootlets from the cranial five or six cervical segments of the spinal cord (see Fig. 17-43). The fibers of the traditional cranial root are now considered to be part of CN X. The fibers of the CN X supply the sternocleidomastoid and trapezius muscles.

### Special Sensory Nerves

The **olfactory nerve** (CN I) arises from the olfactory organ. The olfactory receptor neurons differentiate from cells in the epithelial lining of the primordial nasal sac. The central processes of the **bipolar olfactory neurons** are collected into bundles to form approximately 20 **olfactory nerves** around which the cribriform plate of the ethmoid bone develops. These unmyelinated nerve fibers end in the **olfactory bulb**.

The **optic nerve** (CN II) is formed by more than a million nerve fibers that grow into the brain from neuroblasts in the primordial retina. Because the retina develops from the evaginated wall of the forebrain, the optic nerve represents a fiber tract of the brain.

The **vestibulocochlear nerve** (CN VIII) consists of two kinds of sensory fiber in two bundles; these fibers are known as the *vestibular* and *cochlear nerves*. The **vestibular nerve** originates in the semicircular ducts, and the **cochlear nerve** proceeds from the cochlear duct, in which the **spiral organ** (of Corti) develops. The bipolar neurons of the vestibular nerve have their cell bodies in the **vestibular ganglion**. The central processes of these cells terminate in the **vestibular nuclei** in the floor of the fourth ventricle. The bipolar neurons of the cochlear nerve have their cell bodies in the **spiral ganglion**. The central processes of these cells end in the ventral and dorsal cochlear nuclei in the medulla.

## DEVELOPMENT OF AUTONOMIC NERVOUS SYSTEM

16

Functionally, the autonomic nervous system (**ANS**) can be divided into sympathetic (thoracolumbar) and parasympathetic (craniosacral) parts.

### Sympathetic Nervous System

During the fifth week, **neural crest cells** in the thoracic region migrate along each side of the spinal cord, where they form paired cellular masses (ganglia) dorsolateral to the aorta (see Fig. 17-8). All of these segmentally arranged **sympathetic ganglia** are connected in a bilateral chain by longitudinal nerve fibers. The ganglionated cords (**sympathetic trunks**) are located on each side of the vertebral bodies. Some neural crest cells migrate ventral to the aorta and form neurons in the **preaortic ganglia**, such as the *celiac* and *mesenteric ganglia* (see Fig. 17-8). Other neural crest cells migrate to the area of the heart, lungs, and gastrointestinal tract, where they form terminal ganglia in **sympathetic organ plexuses**, located near or within these organs.

After the sympathetic trunks have formed, axons of sympathetic neurons, which are located in the **intermediolateral cell column** (lateral horn) of the thoracolumbar segments of the spinal cord, pass through the ventral root of a spinal nerve and a **white ramus communicans** (communicating branch) to a paravertebral ganglion (see Fig. 17-8). They may synapse there with neurons or ascend or descend in the sympathetic trunk to synapse at other levels. Other presynaptic fibers pass through the **paravertebral ganglia** without synapsing, forming splanchnic nerves to the viscera. The postsynaptic fibers course through a **gray communicating branch** (gray ramus communicans), passing from a sympathetic ganglion into a spinal nerve; the sympathetic trunks are composed of ascending and descending fibers. *BMP signaling regulates the development of the sympathetic system through SMAD4 pathways.*

### Parasympathetic Nervous System

The **presynaptic parasympathetic fibers** arise from neurons in nuclei of the brainstem and in the sacral region of the spinal cord. The fibers from the brainstem leave through the oculomotor (CN III), facial (CN VII), glossopharyngeal (CN IX), and vagus (CN X) nerves. The **postsynaptic neurons** are located in peripheral ganglia or in plexuses near or within the structure being innervated (e.g., pupil of the eye, salivary glands).

## SUMMARY OF NERVOUS SYSTEM

- The central nervous system (**CNS**) develops from a dorsal thickening of ectoderm (**neural plate**), which appears around the middle of the third week. The neural plate is induced by the underlying notochord and paraxial mesenchyme.

● The neural plate bends to form a **neural groove** that has neural folds on each side. When the **neural folds** start to fuse to form the neural tube beginning during the fourth week, some neuroectodermal cells are not included in it but remain between the neural tube and surface ectoderm as the **neural crest**. As the neural folds are fusing to form the **neural tube**, its ends are open. The openings at each end, the **rostral** and **caudal neuropores**, communicate with the overlying amniotic cavity. Closure of the rostral neuropore occurs by the 25th day, and the caudal neuropore closes 2 days later.

● *The cranial end of the neural tube forms the brain*, the primordia of which are the forebrain, midbrain, and hindbrain. The **forebrain** gives rise to the **cerebral hemispheres** and **diencephalon**. The **midbrain** becomes the adult midbrain, and the **hindbrain** gives rise to the **pons, cerebellum**, and **medulla**. The remainder of the neural tube forms the spinal cord.

● The **neural canal**, which is the lumen of the neural tube, becomes the **ventricles of the brain** and the **central canal of the medulla and spinal cord**. The walls of the neural tube thicken by proliferation of its neuroepithelial cells. These cells give rise to all nerve and **macroglial cells** in the CNS. The microglia differentiate from mesenchymal cells that enter the CNS with the blood vessels.

● The **pituitary gland** develops from two completely different parts (see Table 17-1): an *ectodermal upgrowth* from the stomodeum, the **hypophyseal diverticulum** that forms the **adenohypophysis**, and a *neuroectodermal downgrowth* from the diencephalon, the **neurohypophyseal diverticulum** that forms the **neurohypophysis**.

● Cells in the cranial, spinal, and autonomic ganglia are derived from **neural crest cells** that originate in the neural crest. **Schwann cells**, which myelinate the axons external to the spinal cord, also arise from neural crest cells. Similarly, most of the ANS and all chromaffin tissue, including the suprarenal medulla, develop from neural crest cells.

● **Birth defects of the CNS** are common (approximately 3 per 1000 births). **Neural tube defects (NTDs)** in the closure of the neural tube account for most severe defects (e.g., spinal bifida cystica). Some birth defects are caused by genetic factors (e.g., numeric chromosomal abnormalities such as trisomy 21 [Down syndrome]). Others result from **environmental factors** such as infectious agents, drugs, and metabolic disease. Other CNS defects are caused by a combination of genetic and environmental factors (**multifactorial inheritance**).

● **Major birth defects** (e.g., meroencephaly) are incompatible with life. Severe birth defects (e.g., spina bifida with meningomyelocele) cause functional disability (e.g., muscle paralysis in the lower limbs).

● The two main types of **hydrocephalus** are **obstructive or noncommunicating hydrocephalus** (blockage of CSF flow in the ventricular system) and **nonobstructive or communicating hydrocephalus** (blockage of CSF flow in the subarachnoid space). In most cases, *congenital hydrocephalus is associated with spina bifida with meningomyelocele.*

● **Mental deficiency** may result from chromosomal abnormalities occurring during gametogenesis, metabolic disorders, maternal alcohol abuse, or infections occurring during prenatal life.

## CLINICALLY ORIENTED PROBLEMS

### CASE 17–1

*A pregnant woman developed acute polyhydramnios. After an ultrasound examination, a radiologist reported that the fetus had acrania and meroencephaly.*

* How soon can meroencephaly be detected by ultrasound scanning?
* Why is polyhydramnios associated with meroencephaly?
* What other techniques can confirm the diagnosis of meroencephaly?

### CASE 17–2

*A male infant had a large lumbar meningomyelocele that was covered with a thin membranous sac. Within a few days, the sac ulcerated and began to leak. A marked neurologic deficit was detected inferior to the level of the sac.*

* What is the embryologic basis of this defect?
* What is the basis of the neurologic deficit?
* What structures are likely to be affected?

### CASE 17–3

*An MRI scan of an infant with an enlarged head showed dilation of the lateral and third ventricles.*

* What is this condition called?
* Where is the blockage most likely located to produce dilation of the ventricles?
* Is this condition usually recognizable before birth?
* How should this condition be treated surgically?

### CASE 17–4

*An infant had an abnormally small head.*

* What condition is usually associated with an abnormally small head?
* Does growth of the cranium depend on growth of the brain?
* What environmental factors cause microencephaly?

---

**CASE 17–5**

*A radiologist reported that a child's cerebral ventricles were dilated posteriorly and that the lateral ventricles were widely separated by a dilated third ventricle. Agenesis of the corpus callosum was diagnosed.*

* ❋ What is the common symptom associated with agenesis of the corpus callosum?
* ❋ Are some patients asymptomatic?
* ❋ What is the basis of the dilated third ventricle?

Discussion of these problems appears in the Appendix at the back of the book.

## BIBLIOGRAPHY AND SUGGESTED READING

Amron D, Walsh CA: Genetic malformations of the human frontal lobe, *Epilepsia* 51(Suppl 1):13, 2010.

Barros CS, Nguyen T, Spencer KS, et al: Beta1 integrins are required for normal CNS myelination and promote AKT-dependent myelin outgrowth, *Development* 136:2717, 2009.

Bekiesinska-Figatowska M, Herman-Sucharska I, Romaniuk-Doroszewska A, et al: Brain development of the human fetus in magnetic resonance imaging, *Med Wieku Rozwoj* 14:5, 2010.

Bell JE: The pathology of central nervous system defects in human fetuses of different gestational ages. In Persaud TVN, editor: *Advances in the study of birth defects: central nervous system and craniofacial malformations*, vol 7, New York, 1982, Alan R Liss.

Biencowe H, Cousens S, Modell B, et al: Folic acid to reduce neonatal mortality from neural tube disorders, *Int J Epidemiol* 39(Suppl 1): i110, 2010.

Cau E, Blader P: Notch activity in the nervous system: to switch or not switch, *Neural Dev* 4:36, 2009.

Copp AJ, Greene ND: Genetics and development of neural tube defects, *J Pathol* 220:217, 2010.

Cordero A, Mulinare J, Berry RJ, et al: CDC grand rounds: additional opportunities to prevent neural tube defects with folic acid fortification, *MMWR Morb Mortal Wkly Rep* 59:980, 2010.

Davis SW, Castinetti F, Carvalho LR, et al: Molecular mechanisms of pituitary organogenesis: in search of novel regulatory genes, *Mol Cell Endocrinol* 323:4, 2010.

De Wals P, Tairou F, Van Allen MI, et al: Reduction in neural-tube defects after folic acid fortification in Canada, *N Engl J Med* 357:135, 2007.

Diaz AL, Gleeson JG: The molecular and genetic mechanisms of neocortex development, *Clin Perinatol* 36:503, 2009.

Evans OB, Hutchins JB: Development of the nervous system. In Haines DE, editor: *Fundamental neuroscience*, ed 3, New York, 2006, Churchill Livingstone.

Gressens P, Hüppi PS: Normal and abnormal brain development. In Martin RJ, Fanaroff AA, Walsh MC, editors: *Fanaroff and Martin's neonatal-perinatal medicine: diseases of the fetus and infant*, ed 8, Philadelphia, 2006, Mosby.

Guillemont F, Molnar Z, Tarabykin V, et al: Molecular mechanisms of cortical differentiation, *Eur J Neurosci* 23:857, 2006.

Haines DE: *Neuroanatomy: an atlas of structures, sections, and systems*, ed 8, Baltimore, 2012, Lippincott Williams & Wilkins.

Howard B, Chen Y, Zecevic N: Cortical progenitor cells in the developing human telencephalon, *Glia* 53:57, 2006.

Johnston MV, Kinsman S: Congenital anomalies of the central nervous system. In Behrman RE, Kliegman RM, Jenson HB, editors: *Nelson textbook of pediatrics*, ed 17, Philadelphia, 2004, Saunders.

Liu W, Komiya Y, Mezzacappa C, et al: MIM regulates vertebrate neural tube closure, *Development* 138:2035, 2011.

Lowery LA, Sive H: Totally tubular: the mystery behind function and origin of the brain ventricular system, *Bioessays* 31:446, 2009.

Moore KL, Dalley AF, Agur AMR: *Clinically oriented anatomy*, ed 7, Baltimore, 2014, Lippincott Williams & Wilkins.

Nakatsu T, Uwabe C, Shiota K: Neural tube closure in humans initiates at multiple sites: evidence from human embryos and implications for the pathogenesis of neural tube defects, *Anat Embryol (Berl)* 201:455, 2000.

Noden DM: Spatial integration among cells forming the cranial peripheral neurons, *J Neurobiol* 24:248, 1993.

O'Rahilly R, Müller F: *Embryonic human brain: an atlas of developmental stages*, ed 2, New York, 1999, Wiley-Liss.

ten Donkelaar HT, Lammens M: Development of the human cerebellum and its disorders, *Clin Perinatol* 36:513, 2009.

Thomaidou D, Politis PK, Matsas R: Neurogenesis in the central nervous system: cell cycle progression/exit and differentiation of neuronal progenitors. In Giordano A, Galderisi U, editors: *Cell cycle regulation and differentiation in cardiovascular and neural systems*, New York, 2010, Springer.

# Development of Eyes and Ears

## DEVELOPMENT OF EYES AND RELATED STRUCTURES

The eyes begin to develop in 22-day embryos when **optic grooves** appear (Fig. 18-1*A* 17 and *B*). The eyes are derived from four sources:

- **Neuroectoderm** of the forebrain
- **Surface ectoderm** of the head
- **Mesoderm** between the previous two layers
- **Neural crest cells**

The **neuroectoderm** differentiates into the retina, posterior layers of iris, and optic nerve. The **surface ectoderm** forms the lens of the eye and the corneal epithelium. The **mesoderm** between the neuroectoderm and surface ectoderm gives rise to the fibrous and vascular coats of the eye. **Neural crest cells** migrate into the mesenchyme and differentiate into the choroid, sclera, and corneal endothelium.

Early eye development results from a series of inductive signals. *Homeobox-containing genes, including the transcription regulator PAX6, fibroblast growth factors, and other inducing factors play important roles in the molecular development of the eye.*

The first evidence of eye development is the appearance of **optic grooves** in the neural folds at the cranial end of the embryo (see Fig. 18-1*A* and *B*). As the **neural folds** fuse to

**417**

**FIGURE 18-1** Early stages of eye development. A, Dorsal view of the cranial end of an embryo at approximately 22 days shows the optic grooves, which are the first indication of eye development. B, Transverse section of a neural fold shows the optic groove in it. C, Schematic drawing of the forebrain of an embryo at approximately 28 days shows its covering layers of mesenchyme and surface ectoderm. D, F, and H, Schematic sections of the developing eye show the successive stages in the development of the optic cup and lens vesicle. E, Lateral view of the brain of an embryo at approximately 32 days shows the external appearance of the optic cup. G, Transverse section of the optic stalk shows the retinal fissure and its contents. The edges of the retinal fissure are growing together, thereby completing the optic cup and enclosing the central artery and vein of the retina in the optic stalk and cup.

form the forebrain, the optic grooves evaginated (protruded) from the future diencephalon to form hollow diverticula (outpocketings) called **optic vesicles,** which project from the wall of the forebrain into the adjacent mesenchyme. The vesicles soon come in contact with the surface ectoderm (Fig. 18-1*C* and *D*). The cavities of the optic vesicles are continuous with the cavity of the forebrain. Formation of the optic vesicles is induced by the mesenchyme adjacent to the developing brain.

As the optic vesicles grow, their distal ends expand, and their connections with the forebrain constrict to form hollow **optic stalks** (see Fig. 18-1*D*). Concurrently, the surface ectoderm adjacent to the vesicles thickens to form **lens placodes,** which are the primordia of the lenses (see Fig. 18-1*C* and *D*). Formation of placodes in a precursor field (preplacodal region) is induced by the **optic vesicles** after the surface ectoderm has been conditioned by the underlying mesenchyme. An inductive message passes from the vesicles, stimulating the surface ectodermal cells to form the **primordia of the lens.** The lens placodes invaginated as they sink deep to the surface ectoderm, forming **lens pits** (Fig. 18-2; see 18-1*D*). The edges of the lens pits approach each other and fuse to form spherical **lens vesicles** (see Figs. 18-1*F* and *H*), which gradually lose their connection with the surface ectoderm.

As the lens vesicles are developing, the optic vesicles invaginate to form double-walled **optic cups,** which consist of two layers that are connected to the developing brain by optic stalks (see Figs. 18-1*E* and *F* and 18-2). *The optic cup becomes the retina, and the optic stalk becomes the optic nerve.* The lens and part of the cornea develop from the ectoderm and mesoderm. The opening of each optic cup is large at first, but the rim of the cup infolds around the lens (Fig. 18-3*A*). By this time, the lens vesicles have lost their connection with the surface ectoderm and have entered the cavities of the optic cups (Fig. 18-4).

Linear grooves (**retinal fissures**) develop on the ventral surface of the optic cups and along the optic stalks (see Figs. 18-1*E* to *H* and 18-3*A* to *D*). The center of the optic cup, where the retinal fissure is deepest, forms the **optic disc,** where the neural retina is continuous with the optic stalk (see Figs. 18-2 and 18-3*C* and *D*). The developing **axons of the ganglion cells** pass directly into the optic stalk and convert it into the optic nerve (see Fig. 18-3*B* and *C*). **Myelination of nerve fibers** (forming a sheath around the fibers) begins during the latter part of fetal development and during the first postnatal year.

The *retinal fissures contain vascular mesenchyme* from which **hyaloid blood vessels** develop (see Fig. 18-3*C* and *D*). The **hyaloid artery,** a branch of the ophthalmic artery, supplies the inner layer of the optic cup, the lens vesicle, and the mesenchyme in the **cavity of the optic cup** (see Figs. 18-1*H* and 18-3*C*). The **hyaloid vein** returns blood from these structures. As the edges of the retinal fissure fuse, the **hyaloid vessels** are enclosed within the **primordial optic nerve** (see Fig. 18-3*C* to *F*). Distal parts of the hyaloid vessels eventually degenerate, but proximal parts of them persist as the **central artery** and **vein of retina** (see Fig. 18-3*E* and 18-9*D*). *Bone morphogenic protein (BMP), sonic hedgehog (SHH), and fibroblast growth factor (FGF) are essential for signaling of the optical vesicle and closure of the retinal fissure.*

## Retina

The retina develops from the walls of the optic cup, an outgrowth of the forebrain (see Figs. 18-1*C* to *F*

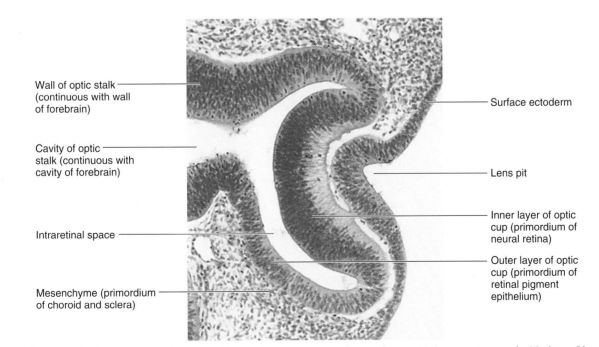

Wall of optic stalk (continuous with wall of forebrain)

Cavity of optic stalk (continuous with cavity of forebrain)

Intraretinal space

Mesenchyme (primordium of choroid and sclera)

Surface ectoderm

Lens pit

Inner layer of optic cup (primordium of neural retina)

Outer layer of optic cup (primordium of retinal pigment epithelium)

**FIGURE 18–2** Photomicrograph of a sagittal section of the eye of an embryo (×200) at approximately 32 days. Observe the primordium of the lens (invaginated lens placode), the walls of the optic cup (primordium of retina), and the optic stalk (primordium of optic nerve). *(From Moore KL, Persaud TVN, Shiota K: Color atlas of clinical embryology, ed 2, Philadelphia, 2000, Saunders.)*

**FIGURE 18–3** Closure of the retinal fissure and formation of the optic nerve. A, C, and E, Views of the inferior surface of the optic cup and stalk show progressive stages in the closure of the retinal fissure. C₁, Schematic drawing of a longitudinal section of a part of the optic cup and stalk shows the optic disc and axons of ganglion cells of the retina growing through the optic stalk to the brain. B, D, and F, Transverse sections of the optic stalk show successive stages in the closure of the retinal fissure and formation of the optic nerve. The lumen of the optic stalk is gradually obliterated as axons of ganglion cells accumulate in the inner layer of the optic stalk as the optic nerve forms.

- Retinal pigment epithelium
- Neuroepithelium
- Anterior lens epithelium
- Lens fibers
- Iris
- Vitreous body
- Surface ectoderm
- Sclera

Optic nerve
Branches of hyaloid artery
Intraretinal space
Choroid

**FIGURE 18–4** Photomicrograph of a sagittal section of the eye of an embryo (×100) at approximately 44 days. The posterior wall of the lens vesicle forms the lens fibers. The anterior wall does not change appreciably as it becomes the anterior lens epithelium. *(From Nishimura H, editor:* Atlas of human prenatal histology, *Tokyo, 1983, Igaku-Shoin.)*

and 18-2). The walls of the cup develop into the two layers of the retina: the *outer, thin layer of the cup* becomes the **pigment layer of retina**, and the *inner, thick (neural) layer* differentiates into the **neural retina** (see Figs. 18-1*H*, 18-4, and 18-9*A*). *The proliferation and differentiation of retinal precursor cells are regulated by forkhead transcription factors.* By the sixth week, **melanin** appears in the retinal pigment epithelium (see Fig. 18-9*A*).

During the embryonic and early fetal periods, the two layers of the retina are separated by an **intraretinal space** (see Figs. 18-4 and 18-9*A* and *B*), which is derived from the cavity of the optic cup. This space gradually disappears as the two layers of the retina fuse (see Figs. 18-8 and 18-9*D*), but the fusion is not firm. Because the optic cup is an outgrowth of the forebrain, the layers of the optic cup are continuous with the wall of the brain (see Fig. 18-1*H*).

Under the influence of the developing lens, the inner layer of the optic cup proliferates to form a thick **neuroepithelium** (see Figs. 18-2 and 18-4). Subsequently, the cells of this layer differentiate into the neural retina, the light-sensitive region of the retina. This region contains **photoreceptors** (rods and cones) and the **cell bodies of neurons** (e.g., bipolar cells, ganglion cells). *FGF signaling regulates retinal ganglion cell differentiation.*

Because the optic vesicle invaginates as it forms the optic cup, the neural retina is inverted; light-sensitive parts of the photoreceptor cells are adjacent to the outer retinal pigment epithelium. As a result, light traverses the thickest part of the retina before reaching the photoreceptors. However, because the neural retina is

transparent, it does not form a barrier to light. The axons of ganglion cells in the superficial layer of the neural retina grow proximally in the wall of the **optic stalk** (see Figs. 18-3*B* to *D* and 18-4). As a result, the cavity of the optic stalk is gradually obliterated as the axons of the many ganglion cells form the **optic nerve** (see Fig. 18-3*E* and *F*).

*The optic nerve is surrounded by three sheaths* that evaginate with the optic vesicle and stalk. Consequently, they are continuous with the meninges of the brain (see Fig. 18-3*F*).

- The **outer dural sheath** from the dura mater is thick and fibrous and blends with the sclera.
- The **intermediate sheath** from the arachnoid mater is thin.
- The **inner sheath** from the pia mater is vascular and closely invests the optic nerve and central arterial and venous vessels of the retina as far as the optic disc.

**Cerebrospinal fluid** is found in the subarachnoid space between the intermediate and inner sheaths of the optic nerve.

*Myelination of the axons within the optic nerves begins in the late fetal period.* After the eyes have been exposed to light for approximately 10 weeks, myelination is complete, but the process normally stops short of the **optic disc,** where the optic nerves leave the eyeballs. Normal neonates can see but not too well because they are farsighted. They respond to changes in illumination and are able to fixate points of contrast. Visual acuity improves rapidly over the first year of infancy to almost normal adult levels.

# BIRTH DEFECTS OF EYES

## Coloboma

Coloboma results when there is incomplete closure of the retinal fissure, creating a gap in the eye structure. These defects can occur in any ocular structure from the cornea to the optic nerve. The eyelid may be involved, but it is caused by other mechanisms. **Retinochoroidal coloboma** is characterized by a localized gap in the retina, usually inferior to the optic disc. The defect is bilateral in most cases.

**Coloboma of the iris** is a defect in the inferior sector of the iris or a notch in the pupillary margin, giving the pupil a keyhole appearance (Fig. 18-5). The defect may be limited to the iris, or it may extend deeper and involve the ciliary body and retina. The coloboma may be caused by environmental factors, but a simple coloboma often is hereditary and is transmitted as an autosomal dominant characteristic.

## Detachment of Retina

Retinal detachment occurs when the inner and outer layers of the optic cup fail to fuse during the fetal period to form the retina and obliterate the **intraretinal space** (see Figs. 18-3 and 18-9A and B). It occurs in conjunction with **Down syndrome** and **Marfan syndrome** (connective tissue multisystemic disorder). The separation of the neural and pigment layers of the retina may be partial or complete. **Retinal detachment** may result from unequal rates of growth of the two retinal layers; as a result, the layers of the optic cup are not in perfect apposition. Sometimes, the layers of the optic cup appear to have fused and separated later; secondary detachments usually are associated with other defects of the eye and head or trauma.

When there is a detached retina, it is not detachment of the entire retina; the retinal pigment layer remains firmly attached to the **choroid** (vascular layer of eyeball) (see Fig. 18-9D). The detachment is at the site of adherence of the outer and inner layers of the optic cup. Although separated from the pigment layer of the retina, the neural retina retains its blood supply (**central artery of retina**), which is derived from the embryonic hyaloid artery (see Fig. 18-9A and D).

Postnatally, the pigment layer normally becomes fixed to the choroid, however, because its attachment to the neural retina is not firm, a detached retina may follow a blow to the eye or occur spontaneously. Fluid accumulates between the pigment and neural layers, and vision is impaired.

## Cyclopia

Cyclopia is a rare defect. The eyes are partially or completely fused, forming a single **median eye** enclosed in a single orbit (Fig. 18-6). There is usually a tubular nose (**proboscis**) superior to the eye. **Cyclopia** (single midline eye) and **synophthalmia** (fusion of the eyes) represent a spectrum of ocular defects. These severe defects are associated with other craniocerebral defects that are incompatible with life. Cyclopia appears to result from severe suppression of midline cerebral structures (**holoprosencephaly**) (see Chapter 17, Fig. 17-40) that develop from the cranial part of the neural plate. Cyclopia is a hereditary condition transmitted by a recessive trait.

## Microphthalmia

Congenital microphthalmia is a heterogeneous group of eye defects. The eye may be very small and associated with other ocular defects, such as a facial cleft (see Chapter 9, Fig. 9-44A) and trisomy 13 (see Chapter 20, Fig. 20-8 and Table 20-1), or it may be normal-appearing. The affected side of the face is underdeveloped, and the orbit is small.

Severe microphthalmia results from **arrested development of the eye** before or shortly after the optic vesicles have formed in the fourth week. The eye is essentially underdeveloped, and the lens does not form. If the interference with development occurs before the retinal fissure closes in the sixth week, the eye is larger, but the microphthalmos is associated with gross ocular defects. When eye development is arrested in the eighth week or during the early fetal period, simple microphthalmos results (small eye with minor ocular abnormalities). Some cases of microphthalmos are inherited. The hereditary pattern may be autosomal dominant, autosomal recessive, or X-linked. Most cases of simple microphthalmia are caused by **infectious agents** (e.g., rubella virus, *Toxoplasma gondii*, herpes simplex virus) that cross the placental membrane during the late embryonic and early fetal periods (see Chapter 20, Table 20-6).

## Anophthalmia

Unilateral or bilateral anophthalmia denotes absence of the eye, which is rare. The eyelids form, but no eyeball develops (Fig. 18-7). Because formation of the orbit relies on stimulation from the developing eye, orbital defects are always present. This severe defect is usually accompanied by other severe craniocerebral defects. In **primary anophthalmos**, eye development is arrested early in the fourth week and results from failure of the optic vesicle to form. In **secondary anophthalmos**, development of the forebrain is suppressed, and absence of the eye or eyes is one of several associated defects.

**FIGURE 18–5** Coloboma of the left iris. Observe the defect in the inferior part of the iris. *(From Guercio J, Martyn L: Congenital malformations of the eye and orbit, Otolaryngol Clin North Am 40:113, 2007.)*

**FIGURE 18–7** Photograph of an infant with anophthalmia (congenital absence of most eye tissues) and a single nostril. The eyelids are formed but are mostly fused.

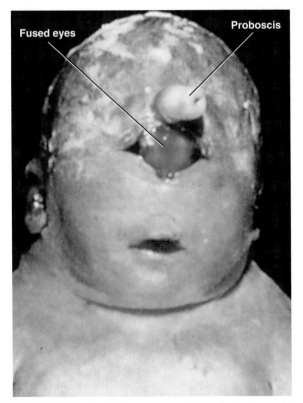

**FIGURE 18–6** Male neonate with cyclopia (synophthalmia). Cyclopia (fusion of the eyes) is a severe, uncommon birth defect of the face and eyes that is associated with a proboscis that represents the nose. The white substance covering his head is vernix caseosa, a normal fatty protective covering.

## Ciliary Body

The ciliary body is a wedge-shaped extension of the choroid (see Fig. 18-4). Its medial surface projects toward the lens, forming **ciliary processes** (see Fig. 18-9C and D). The pigmented portion of the ciliary epithelium is derived from the outer layer of the optic cup, which is continuous with the pigment layer of the retina (Figs. 18-8 and 18-9D). The **nonvisual retina** is the nonpigmented **ciliary epithelium**, which represents the anterior prolongation of the neural retina in which no neural elements develop (Fig. 18-10).

The **ciliary muscle** (smooth muscle of the ciliary body) is responsible for focusing the lens. The connective tissue in the ciliary body develops from mesenchyme located at the edge of the optic cup in the region between the anterior scleral condensation and the ciliary pigment epithelium.

## Iris

The iris develops from the **rim of the optic cup** (see Fig. 18-3A), which grows inward and partially covers the lens (see Figs. 18-7 and 18-9). The two layers of the optic cup remain thin in this area. The epithelium of the iris represents both layers of the optic cup; it is continuous with the double-layered epithelium of the **ciliary body** and with the retinal pigment epithelium and neural retina. The connective tissue framework (stroma) of the iris is derived from neural crest cells that migrate into the iris.

The **dilator pupillae** and **sphincter pupillae muscles** of the iris are derived from *neuroectoderm of the optic cup*. They appear to arise from the anterior epithelial cells of the iris. These smooth muscles result from a transformation of epithelial cells into smooth muscle cells.

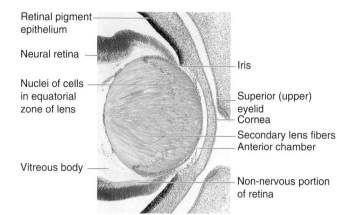

Retinal pigment epithelium

Neural retina

Nuclei of cells in equatorial zone of lens

Vitreous body

Iris

Superior (upper) eyelid

Cornea

Secondary lens fibers

Anterior chamber

Non-nervous portion of retina

**FIGURE 18-8** Sagittal section of part of the developing eye of an embryo (×280) at approximately 56 days. The lens fibers have elongated and obliterated the cavity of the lens vesicle. The inner layer of the optic cup has thickened to form the primordial neural retina. The outer layer is heavily pigmented and is the primordium of the pigment layer of the retina. *(From Moore KL, Persaud TVN, Shiota K: Color atlas of clinical embryology, ed 2, Philadelphia, 2000, Saunders.)*

## COLOR OF THE IRIS

The iris color is typically light blue or gray in most neonates. The iris acquires its definitive color as pigmentation occurs during the first 6 to 10 months. The concentration and distribution of pigment-containing cells (**chromatophores**) in the loose vascular connective tissue of the iris determine eye color. If the **melanin pigment** is confined to the pigmented epithelium on the posterior surface of the iris, the iris appears blue. If melanin is also distributed throughout the **stroma** (supporting tissue) of the iris, the eye appears brown. Iris heterochromia can also result from changes to the sympathetic innervations to the eye.

**FIGURE 18-9** Diagrams of sagittal sections of the eye show successive developmental stages of the lens, retina, iris, and cornea. **A,** At 5 weeks. **B,** At 6 weeks. **C,** At 20 weeks. **D,** Neonate. The retina and optic nerve are formed from the optic cup and optic stalk (see Fig. 18-1D).

Retinal pigment epithelium

Intraretinal space

Lateral rectus muscle

Vitreous body

Neural retina

Choroid

Sclera

Iris

Superior (upper) eyelid

Lens

Cornea

Inferior (lower) eyelid

Inferior rectus muscle

**FIGURE 18–10** Photomicrograph of a sagittal section of the eye of an embryo (×50) at approximately 56 days. Observe the developing neural retina and pigment layer of the retina. The large intraretinal space disappears when these two layers of the retina fuse. *(From Moore KL, Persaud TVN, Shiota K: Color atlas of clinical embryology, ed 2, Philadelphia, 2000, Saunders.)*

**FIGURE 18–11** Clouding of the cornea caused by congenital glaucoma. Clouding may also result from infection, trauma, or metabolic disorders. *(From Guercio J, Martyn L: Congenital malformations of the eye and orbit, Otolaryngol Clin North Am 40:113, 2007.)*

**FIGURE 18–12** Typical appearance of a congenital cataract that may have been caused by rubella virus infection,. Cardiac defects and deafness are other birth defects commonly attributed to this infection. *(From Guercio J, Martyn L: Congenital malformations of the eye and orbit, Otolaryngol Clin North Am 40:113, 2007.)*

## CONGENITAL ANIRIDIA

Congenital aniridia is a rare anomaly. There is a lack of iris tissue or almost complete **absence of the iris**. This defect results from an *arrest of development at the rim of the optic cup* during the eighth week (see Fig. 18-3A). The defect may be associated with glaucoma, cataracts, and other eye abnormalities (Figs. 18-11 and 18-12). Aniridia may be **familial** (occurring in members of a family); the trait may be transmitted in a dominant or sporadic pattern. Mutation of the *PAX6* gene results in aniridia.

## Lens

The lens develops from the **lens vesicle**, a derivative of the surface ectoderm (see Fig. 18-1*F* and *H*). The anterior wall of the vesicle, which is composed of cuboidal epithelium, becomes the subcapsular **lens epithelium** (see Fig. 18-9*C*). The nuclei of the tall columnar cells forming the posterior wall of the **lens vesicle** undergo dissolution (see Fig. 18-4). These cells lengthen considerably to form highly transparent epithelial cells, the **primary lens fibers**. As these fibers grow, they gradually obliterate the cavity of the lens vesicle (see Figs. 18-9*A* to *C* and 18-10). *Expression of PAX6 and SOX2 is required for the induction of the lens. The transcription factors PITX3, GATA3, and FOXE3, regulate formation and differentiation of the lens fibers.*

The rim of the lens is called the *equatorial zone* because it is located midway between the anterior and posterior poles of the lens (see Figs. 18-9C and 18-10). The cells in the equatorial zone are cuboidal. As they elongate, they lose their nuclei and become **secondary lens fibers**. These new lens fibers are added to the external sides of the primary lens fibers. Although secondary lens fibers continue to form during adulthood and the lens increases in diameter, the **primary lens fibers** must last a lifetime.

The developing lens is supplied with blood by the distal part of the **hyaloid artery** (see Figs. 18-4 and 18-9). However, it becomes avascular in the fetal period, when this part of the hyaloid artery degenerates. Thereafter, the lens depends on diffusion from the **aqueous humor** (watery fluid) in the **anterior chamber of the eye** (see Fig. 18-9C), which bathes its anterior surface, and from the **vitreous humor** (fluid component of vitreous body) in other parts. The developing lens is invested by a vascular mesenchymal layer, the **tunica vasculosa lentis** (see Fig. 18-9C). The anterior part of this capsule is the **pupillary membrane** (see Fig. 18-9B).

The pupillary membrane develops from the mesenchyme posterior to the cornea in continuity with the mesenchyme developing in the sclera. The part of the hyaloid artery that supplies the tunica vasculosa lentis disappears during the late fetal period (see Fig. 18-9A and D). *The tunica vasculosa lentis and pupillary membrane degenerate* (see Fig. 18-9C and D), but the **lens capsule** produced by the anterior lens epithelium and the lens fibers persists. This capsule represents a greatly thickened basement membrane and has a lamellar structure because of its development. The former site of the hyaloid artery is indicated by the **hyaloid canal** in the vitreous body (see Fig. 18-9D), which is usually inconspicuous in the living eye.

The **vitreous body** forms within the cavity of the optic cup (see Figs. 18-4 and 18-9C). It is composed of **vitreous humor**, which is the fluid component of the vitreous body. The **primary vitreous humor** is derived from mesenchymal cells of neural crest origin, which secrete a **gelatinous matrix**; this surrounding substance is called the **primary vitreous body**. The primary humor is surrounded later by a gelatinous **secondary vitreous humor**, which is thought to arise from the inner layer of the optic cup. The secondary humor consists of primitive **hyalocytes** (vitreous cells), collagenous material, and traces of hyaluronic acid.

## PERSISTENT PUPILLARY MEMBRANE

Remnants of the pupillary membrane, which cover the anterior surface of the lens during the embryonic period and most of the fetal period (see Fig. 18-9B), may persist as web-like strands of connective tissue or vascular arcades over the pupil in neonates, especially in premature newborns. This tissue seldom interferes with vision and tends to atrophy. Rarely, the entire pupillary membrane persists, giving rise to **congenital atresia of pupil** (absence of a pupil opening). Surgery or laser treatment is needed in some cases to provide an adequate pupil.

## PERSISTENCE OF HYALOID ARTERY

The distal part of the hyaloid artery normally degenerates as its proximal part becomes the central artery of the retina (see Fig. 18-9C and D). If the distal part of the hyaloid artery persists, it may appear as a freely moving, nonfunctional vessel or as a worm-like structure projecting from the optic disc (see Fig. 18-3C). The hyaloid artery remnant sometimes may appear as a fine strand traversing the vitreous body. A remnant of the artery may also form a cyst. In unusual cases, the entire distal part of the artery persists and extends from the optic disc through the vitreous body to the lens. In most of these unusual cases, the eye is **microphthalmic**.

## CONGENITAL APHAKIA

Absence of the lens is rare and results from failure of the lens placode to form during the fourth week. Aphakia may also result from failure of lens induction by the optic vesicle.

## Aqueous Chambers

The **anterior chamber of the eye** develops from a cleft-like space that forms in the mesenchyme located between the developing lens and cornea (see Figs. 18-9A to C and 18-10). The mesenchyme superficial to this space forms the **substantia propria** (transparent connective tissue) of the cornea and the mesothelium of the anterior chamber. After the lens is established, it induces the surface ectoderm to develop into the epithelium of the cornea and conjunctiva.

The **posterior chamber of the eye** develops from a space that forms in the mesenchyme posterior to the developing iris and anterior to the developing lens. When the pupillary membrane disappears and the pupil forms

## CONGENITAL GLAUCOMA

Abnormal elevation of intraocular pressure in neonates usually results from abnormal development of the drainage mechanism of the aqueous humor during the fetal period (see Fig. 18-11). *Intraocular tension* rises because of an imbalance between the production of aqueous humor and its outflow. This imbalance may result from abnormal development of the *scleral venous sinus* (see Fig. 18-9D). Congenital glaucoma is genetically **heterogeneous** (includes several phenotypes that appear similar but are determined by different genotypes), but the condition may also result from a rubella infection during early pregnancy (see Chapter 20, Table 20-6). *Mutations in the CYP1B1 gene are associated with approximately 85% of cases of congenital glaucoma.*

(see Fig. 18-9C and D), the anterior and posterior chambers of the eye are able to communicate with each other through the **scleral venous sinus** (see Fig. 18-9D). This vascular structure encircling the anterior chamber of the eye is the outflow site of aqueous humor from the anterior chamber to the venous system.

## CONGENITAL CATARACTS

In cases of congenital cataracts, the lens is opaque and frequently appears grayish white. Without treatment, blindness results. Many lens opacities are inherited; dominant transmission is more common than recessive or sex-linked transmission. Some cataracts are caused by teratogenic agents, particularly the **rubella virus** (see Fig. 18-12 and Chapter 20, Table 20-6), that affect early development of the lenses. The lenses are vulnerable to rubella virus between the fourth and seventh weeks, when primary lens fibers are forming. Cataract and other ocular defects caused by the rubella virus can be completely prevented in all women of reproductive age by ensuring immunity through rubella virus vaccination.

Physical agents such as **radiation** can damage the lens and produce cataracts. Another cause of cataracts is an enzymatic deficiency (**congenital galactosemia**). These cataracts are not present at birth, but they may appear in the neonatal period. Because of the enzyme deficiency, large amounts of **galactose** from milk accumulate in the infant's blood and tissues, causing injury to the lens and resulting in cataract formation.

## Cornea

The cornea is induced by the lens vesicle. The inductive influence results in transformation of the surface ectoderm into the transparent, multilayered, avascular cornea. The cornea is formed from three sources:

- **External corneal epithelium**, derived from surface ectoderm
- **Mesenchyme**, derived from mesoderm that is continuous with the developing sclera
- **Neural crest cells** that migrate from the optic cup, corneal epithelium, and middle stromal layer of collagen-rich extracellular matrix

## EDEMA OF THE OPTIC DISC

The relationship of the sheaths of the optic nerve to the meninges of the brain and the subarachnoid space is important clinically. An increase in cerebrospinal fluid pressure (often resulting from increased intracranial pressure) slows venous return from the retina, causing **papilledema** (fluid accumulation) of the optic disc. This edema occurs because the retinal vessels are covered by pia mater and lie in the extension of the subarachnoid space that surrounds the optic nerve.

## Choroid and Sclera

The mesenchyme surrounding the optic cup (largely of neural crest origin) reacts to the inductive influence of the retinal pigment epithelium by differentiating into an inner vascular layer, the **choroid**, and an outer fibrous layer, the **sclera** (see Fig. 18-9C and D). The **sclera** develops from a condensation of mesenchyme external to the choroid and is continuous with the **stroma** (supporting tissue) of the cornea. Toward the rim of the optic cup, the choroid becomes modified to form the **cores** (central masses) of the **ciliary processes** (see Fig. 18-9D), consisting chiefly of capillaries supported by delicate connective tissue. The first **choroidal blood vessels** appear during the 15th week; by the 23rd week, arteries and veins can be easily distinguished.

## Eyelids

The eyelids develop during the sixth week from mesenchyme derived from neural crest cells and from two cutaneous folds of the surface ectoderm that grow over the cornea (see Fig. 18-9B and C). The eyelids begin to adhere to one another during the eighth week and remain adherent until the 26th to 28th week (see Fig. 18-9C). While the eyelids are adherent, there is a closed **conjunctival sac** anterior to the cornea. As the eyelids open, the **bulbar conjunctiva** is reflected over the anterior part of the sclera and the surface epithelium of the cornea (see Fig. 18-9D). The **palpebral conjunctiva** lines the inner surface of the eyelids.

The **eyelashes** and **glands** in the eyelids are derived from the surface ectoderm in a manner similar to that described for other parts of the integument (see Chapter 9, Fig. 19-1). The connective tissue and **tarsal plates** (fibrous plates in the eyelids) develop from mesenchyme in the developing eyelids. The **orbicularis oculi muscle** is derived from mesenchyme in the second pharyngeal arch (see Chapter 9, Fig. 9-6B) and is supplied by the facial nerve (CN VII).

## CONGENITAL PTOSIS OF EYELID

Drooping of the superior (upper) eyelids is relatively common in neonates (Fig. 18-13). **Ptosis** (blepharoptosis) may result from failure of normal development of the **levator palpebrae superioris muscle**. Congenital ptosis may also result from prenatal injury or **dystrophy** (defective nutrition) of the superior division of the **oculomotor nerve** (CN III), which supplies this muscle. If ptosis is associated with an inability to move the eyeball superiorly, there is also failure of the **superior rectus muscle** of the eyeball to develop normally. Congenital ptosis may be transmitted as an autosomal dominant trait. Ptosis also is commonly associated on the affected side with absence of sweat (anhidrosis) and a small pupil (miosis), which is known as Horner syndrome. Vision can be affected if the margin of the eyelid partially or completely covers the pupil; early surgical correction is indicated.

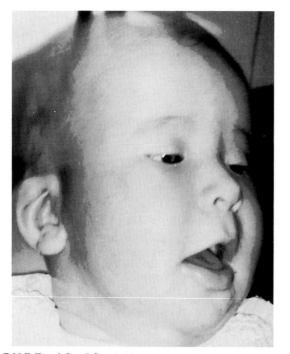

**FIGURE 18-13** Child with congenital bilateral ptosis. Drooping of the superior eyelids usually results from abnormal development or failure of development of the levator palpebrae superioris, the muscle that elevates the eyelids. The infant is contracting the frontalis muscle of the forehead in an attempt to raise the eyelids. *(From Avery ME, Taeusch HW Jr: Schaffer's diseases of the newborn, ed 5, Philadelphia, 1984, Saunders.)*

## COLOBOMA OF THE EYELID

Large defects of the eyelid (**palpebral colobomas**) are uncommon. A coloboma is usually characterized by a small notch in the superior eyelid, but the defect may involve almost the entire lid. Palpebral colobomas appear to result from local developmental disturbances in the formation and growth of the eyelids. Drying and ulceration of the cornea can result from a lower eyelid coloboma.

## CRYPTOPHTHALMOS

Cryptophthalmos is a rare disorder that results from congenital absence of the eyelids; as a result, skin covers the eyes. The eyeball is small and defective, and the cornea and conjunctiva usually do not develop. Fundamentally, the defect means an absence of the **palpebral fissure** (slit) between eyelids. There is usually some degree of eyelash and eyebrow absence, and there are other eye defects. Cryptophthalmos is an autosomal recessive condition that is usually part of the *cryptophthalmos syndrome, which includes urogenital anomalies.*

## Lacrimal Glands

At the superolateral angles of the orbits, the lacrimal glands develop from a number of solid buds from the surface ectoderm. The lacrimal ducts drain into the lacrimal sac and eventually into **nasolacrimal duct**. The glands are small at birth and do not function fully until approximately 6 weeks; neonates therefore do not produce tears when they cry. Tears are often not produced when crying until 1 to 3 months.

## DEVELOPMENT OF EARS

The ears are composed of three parts:

- **External ear,** consisting of the auricle (pinna), external acoustic meatus (passage), and external layer of the tympanic membrane (eardrum)
- **Middle ear,** consisting of three small auditory ossicles (ear bones) and the internal layer of the tympanic membranes, which are connected to the oval windows of the internal ears by the ossicles
- **Internal ear,** consisting of the vestibulocochlear organ, which functions in hearing and balance

The external and middle parts are concerned with the transference of sound waves to the internal ears, which convert the waves into nerve impulses and registers changes in equilibrium.

### Internal Ears

The internal ears are the first of the three parts of the ears to develop. Early in the fourth week, a thickening of surface ectoderm, the **otic placode**, appears in a preplacodal field of precursor neurons on each side of the myelencephalon, which is the caudal part of the hindbrain (Fig. 18-14*A*, *B*, and *D*). *Inductive signals, including those of FGF3 and FGF10 from the paraxial mesoderm and notochord, stimulate the surface ectoderm to form the placodes* (see Chapter 4, Fig. 4-9). Each otic placode soon invaginates and sinks deep to the surface ectoderm into the underlying mesenchyme. In so doing, it forms an **otic pit** (see Fig. 18-14*C* and *D*). The edges of the pit come together and fuse to form an **otic vesicle**, which is the *primordium of the membranous labyrinth* (Fig. 18-15; see Fig. 18-14*E* to *G*). The vesicle soon loses its connection with the surface ectoderm, and a diverticulum grows from the vesicle and elongates to form the **endolymphatic duct** and **sac** (Fig. 18-16*A* to *E*).

Two regions of the otic vesicles are recognizable (see Fig. 18-16*A*):

- **Dorsal utricular parts**, from which the small endolymphatic ducts, utricles, and semicircular ducts arise
- **Ventral saccular parts**, which give rise to the saccules and cochlear ducts

Three disc-like diverticula grow out from the utricular parts of the **primordial membranous labyrinths**. Soon the central parts of these diverticula fuse and disappear (see Fig. 18-16*B* to *E*). The peripheral unfused parts of the diverticula become **semicircular ducts**, which are attached

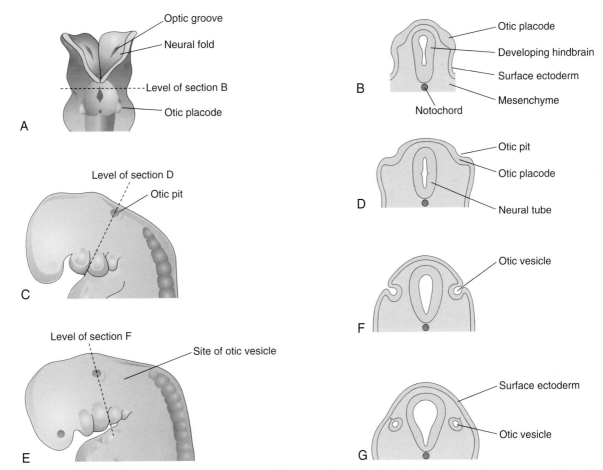

**FIGURE 18–14** Drawings of early development of the internal ear. **A,** Dorsal view of an embryo at approximately 22 days shows the otic placodes. **B, D, F,** and **G,** Schematic coronal sections show successive stages in the development of otic vesicles. **C** and **E,** Lateral views of the cranial region of embryos at approximately 24 and 28 days, respectively.

**FIGURE 18–15** Photomicrograph **(A)** of a transverse section of an embryo (×55) at approximately 26 days. The otic vesicles (primordia of the membranous labyrinths) give rise to the internal ears. Photomicrograph **(B)** at higher magnification of the right otic vesicle (×120). The ectodermal stalk is still attached to the remnant of the otic placode. The otic vesicle will soon lose its connection with the surface ectoderm. *(From Nishimura H, editor:* Atlas of human prenatal histology, *Tokyo, 1983, Igaku-Shoin.)*

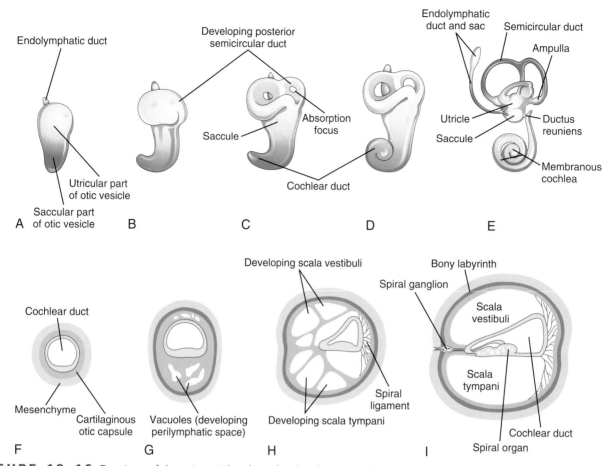

**FIGURE 18-16** Drawings of the otic vesicles show the development of the membranous and bony labyrinths of the internal ear. A to E, Lateral views show successive stages in the development of the otic vesicle into the membranous labyrinth from the fifth to eighth weeks and the development of a semicircular duct. F to I, Sections through the cochlear duct show successive stages in the development of the spiral organ and the perilymphatic space from the 8th to the 20th weeks.

to the utricle and are later enclosed in the **semicircular canals of the bony labyrinth** (see Fig. 18-16*I*). Localized dilatations, the **ampullae**, develop at one end of each semicircular duct (see Fig. 18-16*E*). Specialized receptor areas (**cristae ampullares**) differentiate in the ampullae and the utricle and saccule (maculae utriculi and sacculi).

From the saccular part of the otic vesicle, a tubular diverticulum (**cochlear duct**) grows and coils to form the **membranous cochlea** (see Fig. 18-16*A* and *C* to *E*). *TBX1 expression in the mesenchyme surrounding the otic vesicle regulates the formation of the cochlear duct by controlling retinoic acid activity.* A connection of the cochlea with the saccule (**ductus reuniens**) soon forms (see Fig. 18-16*E*). The **spiral organ** differentiates from cells in the wall of the cochlear duct (see Fig. 18-16*F* to *I*). Ganglion cells of the **vestibulocochlear nerve** (CN VIII) migrate along the coils of the membranous cochlea and form the **spiral ganglion** (see Fig. 18-16*I*). Nerve processes extend from this ganglion to the **spiral organ**, where they terminate on the **hair cells**. The cells in the spiral ganglion retain their embryonic bipolar condition.

Inductive influences from the otic vesicle stimulate the mesenchyme around the otic vesicle to condense and differentiate into a **cartilaginous otic capsule** (see Fig. 18-16*F*). *Studies indicate that the PAX2 gene is*

*required for formation of the spiral organ of Corti and the spiral ganglion. Retinoic acid and transforming growth factor β₁ play a role in modulating epithelial-mesenchymal interaction in the internal ear and in directing the formation of the otic capsule or bony labyrinth.*

As the **membranous labyrinth** enlarges, vacuoles appear in the cartilaginous otic capsule and soon coalesce to form the **perilymphatic space** (see Fig. 18-16*G*). The membranous labyrinth is now suspended in **perilymph** (fluid in perilymphatic space). The perilymphatic space, which is related to the cochlear duct, develops two divisions, the **scala tympani** and **scala vestibuli** (see Fig. 18-16*H* and *I*). The cartilaginous otic capsule later ossifies to form the **bony labyrinth** of the internal ear (see Fig. 18-16*I*). The internal ear reaches its adult size and shape by the middle of the fetal period (20–22 weeks).

## Middle Ears

Development of the **tubotympanic recess** (Fig. 18-17*B*) from the first pharyngeal pouch is described in Chapter 9. The proximal part of the tubotympanic recess forms the **pharyngotympanic tube** (auditory tube). The distal part of the recess expands and becomes the **tympanic cavity** (Fig. 18-17*C*), which gradually envelops the small

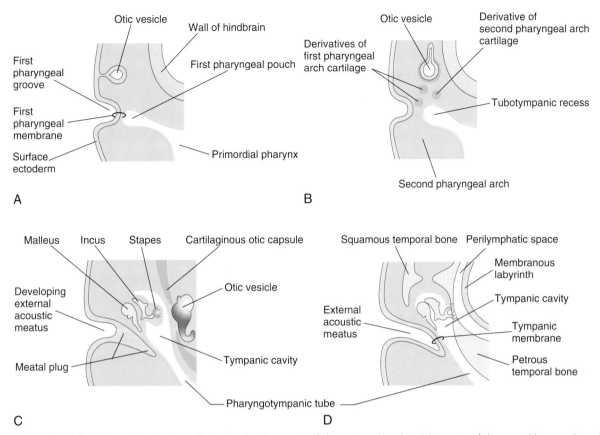

**FIGURE 18-17** Schematic drawings illustrate development of the external and middle parts of the ear. Observe the relationship of these parts to the otic vesicle, the primordium of the internal ear. **A**, At 4 weeks, the drawing shows the relationship of the otic vesicle to the pharyngeal apparatus. **B**, At 5 weeks, the drawing shows the tubotympanic recess and pharyngeal arch cartilages. **C**, Drawing of a later stage shows the tubotympanic recess (future tympanic cavity and mastoid antrum) beginning to envelop the ossicles. **D**, Drawing of the final stage of ear development shows the relationship of the middle ear to the perilymphatic space and the external acoustic meatus. The tympanic membrane develops from three germ layers: surface ectoderm, mesenchyme, and endoderm of the tubotympanic recess.

bones of the middle ear (**auditory ossicles** [malleus, incus, and stapes]), their tendons and ligaments, and the chorda tympani nerve. The malleus and incus are derived from the cartilage of the first pharyngeal arch. The crus, base of the foot plate, and the head of the stapes appear to be formed from neural crest, whereas the outer rim of the foot plate is derived from mesodermal cells. These structures receive a more or less complete epithelial investment derived from neural crest cells of the endoderm. The neural crest cells undergo an epithelial-mesenchymal transformation. In addition to apoptosis in the middle ear, an epithelium-type organizer located at the tip of the tubotympanic recess probably plays a role in the early development of the middle ear cavity and tympanic membrane.

During the late fetal period, expansion of the **tympanic cavity** gives rise to the **mastoid antrum**, which is located in the petromastoid part of the temporal bone. The mastoid antrum is almost adult size at birth, but no mastoid cells are present in neonates. By 2 years of age, the mastoid cells are well developed and produce conical projections of the temporal bones, the **mastoid processes**. The middle ear continues to grow through puberty. The **tensor tympani muscle**, which is attached to the malleus,

is derived from mesenchyme in the first pharyngeal arch and is innervated by trigeminal nerve (CN V), the nerve of this arch. The **stapedius muscle** is derived from the second pharyngeal arch and is supplied by the facial nerve (CN VII), the nerve of this arch. *The signaling molecules fibroblast growth factor 8 (FGF8), endothelin 1 (EDN1), and T-box 1 (TBX1) are involved in middle ear development.*

## External Ears

The **external acoustic meatus**, which is the passage of the external ear leading to the **tympanic membrane**, develops from the dorsal part of the *first pharyngeal groove* (see Fig. 18-17A; see Chapter 9, Fig 9-7C). The ectodermal cells at the bottom of this funnel-shaped tube proliferate to form a solid epithelial plate, the **meatal plug** (see Fig. 18-17C). Late in the fetal period, the central cells of this plug degenerate, forming a cavity that becomes the internal part of the external acoustic meatus (see Fig. 18-17D). The meatus, which is relatively short at birth, attains its adult length in approximately the ninth year.

The primordium of the **tympanic membrane** is the first pharyngeal membrane, which forms the external surface of the tympanic membrane. In the embryo, the pharyngeal membrane separates the first pharyngeal groove from the first pharyngeal pouch (see Fig. 18-17A). As development proceeds, mesenchyme grows between the two parts of the pharyngeal membrane and differentiates into the collagenic fibers in the tympanic membrane.

The tympanic membrane develops from three sources:

- **Ectoderm** of the first pharyngeal groove
- **Endoderm** of the tubotympanic recess, a derivative of the first pharyngeal pouch
- **Mesenchyme** of the first and second pharyngeal arches

The **auricle** (pinna), which projects from the side of the head, develops from mesenchymal proliferations in the first and second pharyngeal arches (**auricular hillocks**) surrounding the first pharyngeal groove (Fig. 18-18A). As the auricle grows, the contribution from the first arch is reduced. The **lobule** (earlobe) of the auricle is the last part of the auricle to develop. The auricles begin to develop at the base of the neck (Fig. 18-18A and B). As the mandible develops, the auricles assume their normal position at the side of the head (see Fig. 18-22).

The parts of the auricle derived from the first pharyngeal arch are supplied by the mandibular branch of the **trigeminal nerve (CN V)**; the parts derived from the second arch are supplied by cutaneous branches of the

Auricular hillocks derived from the first and second pharyngeal arches

A — First pharyngeal groove

B 1 mm

**FIGURE 18–18** Development of the auricle, which is the part of the external ear that is not within the head. **A**, At 6 weeks, three of the auricular hillocks are located on the first pharyngeal arch and three on the second arch. **B**, Photograph of a 7-week embryo shows the developing external ear.

cervical plexus, especially the **lesser occipital and greater auricular nerves.** The nerve of the second pharyngeal arch, the **facial nerve,** has few cutaneous branches; some of its fibers contribute to the sensory innervation of the skin in the mastoid region and probably in small areas on both aspects of the auricle.

## CONGENITAL DEAFNESS

Because formation of the internal ear is independent of development of the middle and external ears, congenital impairment of hearing may be the result of maldevelopment of the sound-conducting apparatus of the middle and external ears or of the neurosensory structures of the internal ear. Approximately 3 in 1000 neonates have significant hearing loss, of which there are many subtypes.

Most types of congenital deafness are caused by genetic factors, and many of the genes responsible have been identified. Mutations in the *GJB2* gene are responsible for approximately 50% of nonsyndromic recessive hearing loss. Congenital deafness may be associated with several other head and neck defects as a part of the **first arch syndrome** (see Chapter 9, Fig. 9-14). Abnormalities of the malleus and incus are often associated with this syndrome (see Chapter 14, Fig. 14-8D). A **rubella infection** during the critical period of development of the internal ear, particularly the seventh and eighth weeks, can cause defects of the spiral organ and deafness (see Chapter 20, Table 20-6). **Congenital fixation of the stapes** results in conductive deafness in an otherwise normal ear. Failure of differentiation of the anular ligament, which attaches the base of the stapes to the oval window (*fenestra vestibuli*), results in fixation of the stapes to the bony labyrinth.

## AURICULAR ABNORMALITIES

Severe defects of the external ear are rare, but minor deformities are common. There is a wide variation in the shape of the auricle. Almost any minor auricular defect may occasionally be found as a usual feature in a particular family. Minor defects of the auricles may serve as indicators of a specific pattern of congenital defects. For example, the auricles are often abnormal in shape and low set in infants with **chromosomal syndromes** (Fig. 18-19) such as trisomy 18 (see Chapter 20, Fig. 20-7 and Table 20-1) and in infants affected by maternal ingestion of certain drugs (e.g., trimethadione) (see Chapter 20, Table 20-6).

### Auricular Appendages

Auricular appendages (skin tags) are common and may result from the development of **accessory auricular hillocks** (Fig. 18-20). The appendages usually appear anterior to the auricle, more often unilaterally than bilaterally. The appendages, which often have narrow pedicles, consist of skin, but they may contain some cartilage.

### Absence of Auricle

Anotia (absence of the auricle) is rare but is commonly associated with the first pharyngeal arch syndrome. This defect results from failure of mesenchymal proliferation.

## AURICULAR ABNORMALITIES—cont'd

### Microtia

Microtia (small or rudimentary auricle) results from suppressed mesenchymal proliferation (Fig. 18-21). This defect often serves as an indicator of associated birth defects, such as atresia of the external acoustic meatus (80% of cases) and middle ear anomalies. The cause can be both genetic and environmental.

### Preauricular Sinuses and Fistulas

Pit-like cutaneous depressions or shallow sinuses are occasionally located in a triangular area anterior to the auricle (Fig 18-22; see Chapter 9, Fig. 9-9F). The sinuses are usually narrow tubes or shallow pits that have pinpoint external openings. Some sinuses contain a vestigial cartilaginous mass. Preauricular sinuses may be associated with internal anomalies such as deafness and kidney malformations. The embryologic basis of auricular sinuses is uncertain, but it may relate to incomplete fusion of the auricular hillocks or to abnormal mesenchymal proliferation and defective closure of the dorsal part of the first pharyngeal groove. Most of this pharyngeal groove normally disappears as the external acoustic meatus forms.

Other auricular sinuses appear to represent ectodermal folds that are sequestered during formation of the auricle. The preauricular sinus usually is unilateral and involves the right side, and bilateral preauricular sinuses are typically familial. Most sinuses are asymptomatic and have only minor cosmetic importance; however, they can become infected. **Auricular fistulas** (narrow canals) connecting the preauricular skin with the tympanic cavity or the tonsillar fossa (see Chapter 9, Fig. 9-9F) are rare.

### Atresia of the External Acoustic Meatus

Atresia (blockage) of the external acoustic meatus results from failure of the meatal plug to canalize (Figs. 18-23 and 18-24; see Fig. 18-17C). The deep part of the meatus is usually open, but the superficial part is blocked by bone or fibrous tissue. Most cases are associated with the *first arch syndrome* (see Chapter 9, Fig. 9-14). Abnormal development of the first and second pharyngeal arches often is involved. The auricle is also severely affected, and middle and internal ear defects sometimes occur. Atresia of the external acoustic meatus can occur bilaterally or unilaterally and usually results from inheritance of an autosomal dominant trait.

### Absence of External Acoustic Meatus

Absence of the external acoustic meatus is rare; usually, the auricle is normal (see Fig. 18-23). This defect results from failure of inward expansion of the first pharyngeal groove and failure of the meatal plug to disappear (see Fig. 18-17C).

### Congenital Cholesteatoma

A congenital cholesteatoma is a fragment of keratinized epithelial cells that is retained after birth. The embryonic rest remnants form epithelial tissue that appears as a white, cyst-like structure medial to and behind the tympanic membrane. The rest may consist of cells from the meatal plug that was displaced during its canalization (see Fig. 18-17C). It has been suggested that congenital cholesteatoma may originate from an epidermoid formation that normally involutes by 33 weeks' gestation. Cholesteatomas can exhibit growth and invasion of neighboring bone.

**FIGURE 18–19** Potter facies consists of low-set ears and a small, hooked nose associated with renal agenesis and pulmonary hypoplasia.

**FIGURE 18–20** Child with a preauricular tag or skin tag.

**FIGURE 18–21** Child with a rudimentary auricle (microtia). She also has several other birth defects.

**FIGURE 18–23** This child has no external acoustic meatus, but the auricle is normal. There is no opening of the external acoustic meatus, but computed tomography revealed normal middle and internal ear structures.

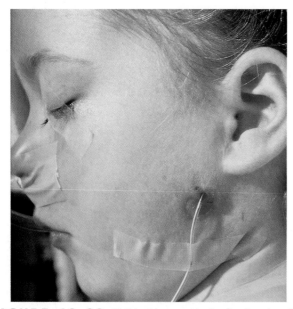

**FIGURE 18–22** Child with an auricular fistula related to the first pharyngeal arch. Notice the external orifice of the fistula below the auricle, the upward direction of the catheter (in the sinus tract) toward the external acoustic meatus, and the normal position of the auricle.

**FIGURE 18–24** Computed tomogram of a 9-month-old infant with atresia of the external acoustic meatus (external auditory canal) (asterisk) shows the osseous atresia plate (black arrow) and the middle ear cavity (white arrow).

## SUMMARY OF EYE DEVELOPMENT

- The first indication of the eyes is the **optic grooves** in the neural folds at the cranial end of the embryo. The grooves form at the beginning of the fourth week and deepen to form hollow optic vesicles that project from the forebrain.

- The **optic vesicles** contact the surface ectoderm and induce development of the **lens placodes**.
- As the lens placode thickens to form a **lens pit** and **lens vesicle**, the optic vesicle invaginates to form the **optic cup**. The retina forms from the two layers of the optic cup.
- The retina, optic nerve fibers, muscles of the iris, and epithelium of the iris and ciliary body are derived from

the **neuroectoderm of the forebrain**. The sphincter and dilator muscles of the iris develop from the ectoderm at the rim of the optic cup. The surface ectoderm gives rise to the **lens** and the epithelium of the lacrimal glands, eyelids, conjunctiva, and cornea. The mesenchyme gives rise to the eye muscles, except those of the iris, and to all connective and vascular tissues of the cornea, iris, ciliary body, choroid, and sclera.

- The eyes are sensitive to the teratogenic effects of **infectious agents** (e.g., cytomegalovirus). Defects of sight may result from infection of tissues and organs by certain microorganisms during the fetal period (e.g., rubella virus, *Treponema pallidum* [causes syphilis]).
- Most ocular defects are caused by defective closure of the retinal fissure during the sixth week (e.g., coloboma of the iris).
- Congenital cataract and glaucoma may result from intrauterine infections, but most congenital cataracts are inherited.

## SUMMARY OF EAR DEVELOPMENT

- The **otic vesicle** develops from the surface ectoderm during the fourth week. The vesicle develops into the **membranous labyrinth** of the internal ear.
- The otic vesicle divides into a *dorsal utricular part*, which gives rise to the **utricle, semicircular ducts**, and **endolymphatic duct**, and a *ventral saccular part*, which gives rise to the **saccule** and **cochlear duct**. The cochlear duct gives rise to the **spiral organ**.
- The **bony labyrinth** develops from the mesenchyme adjacent to the membranous labyrinth. The epithelium lining the tympanic cavity, mastoid antrum, and pharyngotympanic tube is derived from the endoderm of the **tubotympanic recess**, which develops from the first pharyngeal pouch.
- The auditory ossicles develop from the dorsal ends of the cartilages in the first two pharyngeal arches. The epithelium of the **external acoustic meatus** develops from the ectoderm of the first pharyngeal groove.
- The **tympanic membrane** is derived from three sources: endoderm of the first pharyngeal pouch, ectoderm of the first pharyngeal groove, and mesenchyme between the previous two layers.
- The **auricle** develops from the fusion of six **auricular hillocks**, which form from mesenchymal prominences around the margins of the first pharyngeal groove.
- **Congenital deafness** may result from abnormal development of the membranous labyrinth, bony labyrinth, or auditory ossicles. Inheritance of a recessive trait is the most common cause of congenital deafness, but a **rubella virus infection** near the end of the embryonic period is a major cause of abnormal development of the spiral organ and defective hearing.
- There are many minor anomalies of the auricle; however, some of them may alert clinicians to the possible presence of associated major anomalies (e.g., defects of middle ear). Low-set, severely malformed ears are often associated with **chromosomal abnormalities**, particularly trisomy 13 and trisomy 18.

## CLINICALLY ORIENTED PROBLEMS

### CASE 18–1

A fetus was born blind and deaf with congenital heart disease. The mother had a severe viral infection early in her pregnancy.

- Name the virus that was probably responsible for the birth defects.
- What is the common congenital cardiovascular lesion found in infants whose mothers have this infection early in pregnancy?
- Is the history of a rash during the first trimester an essential factor in the development of embryonic disease (embryopathy)?

### CASE 18–2

An infant was born with bilateral ptosis.

- What is the probable embryologic basis of this condition?
- Are hereditary factors involved?
- Injury to what nerve can cause congenital ptosis?

### CASE 18–3

An infant had small, multiple calcifications in the brain, microcephaly, and microphthalmia. The mother was known to consume rare meat.

- What protozoon is likely involved?
- What is the embryologic basis of the infant's birth defects?
- What advice should the doctor give the mother concerning future pregnancies?

### CASE 18–4

A mentally deficient female infant had low-set, malformed ears; a prominent occiput; and rocker-bottom feet. A chromosomal abnormality was suspected.

- What is the type of chromosomal aberration?
- What is the usual cause of this abnormality?
- How long is the infant likely to survive?

### CASE 18–5

An infant had partial detachment of the retina in one eye. The eye was microphthalmic, and *there was persistence of the distal end of the hyaloid artery.*

* What is the embryologic basis of congenital detachment of the retina?
* What is the usual fate of the hyaloid artery?

Discussion of problems appears in the Appendix at the back of the book.

## BIBLIOGRAPHY AND SUGGESTED READING

Barishak YR: *Embryology of the eye and its adnexa*, ed 2, Basel, Switzerland, 2001, Karger.

Bauer PW, MacDonald CB, Melhem ER: Congenital inner ear malformation, *Am J Otol* 19:669, 1998.

Box J, Chang W, Wu DK: Patterning and morphogenesis of the vertebrate ear, *Int J Dev Biol* 51:521, 2007.

Carlson BM: *Human embryology and developmental biology*, ed 5, St. Louis, 2014, Mosby.

Chung HA, Medina-Ruiz S, Harland RM: Sp8 regulates inner ear development, *Proc Natl Acad Sci U S A* 111:632, 2014.

Graw J: Eye development, *Curr Top Dev Biol* 90:343, 2010.

Haddad J Jr: The ear. congenital malformations. In Kliegman RM, Stanton BF, St. Geme JW III, et al, editors: *Nelson textbook of pediatrics*, ed 19, Philadelphia, 2011, Saunders.

Jason R, Guercio BS, Martyn LJ: Congenital malformations of the eye and orbit, *Otolaryngol Clin North Am* 40:113, 2007.

Jones KL, Jones MC, Campo MD, editors: *Smith's recognizable patterns of human malformation*, ed 7, Philadelphia, 2013, Saunders.

Moore KL, Dalley AF, Agur AMR: *Clinically oriented anatomy*, ed 7, Baltimore, 2014, Lippincott Williams & Wilkins.

Munnamalai V, Fekete DM: Wnt signaling during cochlear development, *Semin Cell Dev Biol* 24:480, 2013.

Olitsky SE, Hug D, Plummer LS, et al: Disorders of the eye: growth and development. In Kliegman RM, Stanton BF, St. Geme JW III, et al, editors: *Nelson textbook of pediatrics*, ed 19, Philadelphia, 2011, Saunders.

O'Rahilly R: The early development of the otic vesicle in staged human embryos, *J Embryol Exp Morphol* 11:741, 1963.

O'Rahilly R: The prenatal development of the human eye, *Exp Eye Res* 21:93, 1975.

Porter CJW, Tan SW: Congenital auricular anomalies: topographic anatomy, embryology, classification, and treatment strategies, *Plast Reconstr Surg* 115:1701, 2005.

Rodriguez-Vázquez JF: Development of the stapes and associated structures in human embryos, *J Anat* 207:165, 2005.

Sellheyer K: Development of the choroid and related structures, *Eye* 4:255, 1990.

Smith AN, Radice G, Lang RA: Which FGF ligands are involved in lens induction? *Dev Biol* 337:195, 2010.

Thompson H, Ohazama A, Sharpe PT, et al: The origin of the stapes and relationship to the otic capsule and oval window, *Dev Dynam* 241:1396, 2012.

Wilson E, Saunders R, Trivedi R: *Pediatric ophthalmology: current thought and a practical guide*, New York, 2008, Springer.

# 19

# Integumentary System

The integumentary system consists of skin and its appendages: sweat glands, nails, hairs, sebaceous glands, arrector muscles of hairs (arrector pili muscles), mammary glands, and teeth.

## DEVELOPMENT OF SKIN AND APPENDAGES

The skin, which is the outer protective covering of the body, is a complex organ system, and it is the body's largest organ. The skin consists of two layers (Fig. 19-1):

- The **epidermis** is a superficial epithelial tissue that is derived from surface embryonic ectoderm.
- The **dermis,** which underlies the epidermis, is a deep layer composed of dense, irregularly arranged connective tissue that is derived from **mesenchyme.**

**Ectodermal** (epidermal) and **mesenchymal** (dermal) interactions involve mutual inductive mechanisms that are mediated by a conserved set of signaling molecules, including WNT, fibroblast growth factor (FGF), transforming growth factor-β (TGF-β), and sonic hedgehog (SHH). Skin structures vary from one part of the body to another. For example, the skin of the eyelids is thin and soft and has fine hairs, whereas the skin of the eyebrows is thick and has coarse hairs. The **embryonic skin** at 4 to 5 weeks consists of a single layer of **surface ectoderm** overlying the mesoderm (see Fig. 19-1A).

### Epidermis

Epidermal growth occurs in stages and increases epidermal thickness. The primordium of the epidermis is a single layer of surface ectodermal cells (see Fig. 19-1A). These cells

**437**

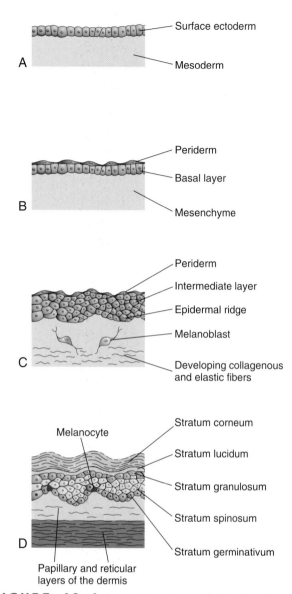

**FIGURE 19-1** Successive stages of skin development. A, At 4 weeks. B, At 7 weeks. C, At 11 weeks. D, Neonate. Observe the melanocytes in the basal layer of the epidermis; their processes extend between the epidermal cells to supply them with melanin.

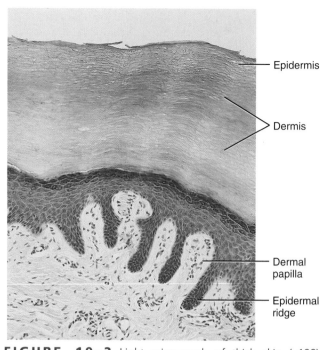

**FIGURE 19-2** Light micrograph of thick skin (×132). Observe the epidermis, the dermis, and the dermal papillae interdigitating with the epidermal ridges. *(From Gartner LP, Hiatt JL: Color textbook of histology, ed 2nd, Philadelphia, 2001, Saunders.)*

proliferate and form a layer of squamous epithelium, the **periderm**, and a basal layer (see Fig. 19-1*B* and *C*). The **cells of the periderm** continually undergo **keratinization** (keratin formation or development of a horny layer) and **desquamation** (shedding of **cuticle**, the outer, thin layer), and they are replaced by cells arising from the basal layer. The **exfoliated peridermal cells** form part of a white, greasy substance (**vernix caseosa**) that covers the fetal skin (see Fig. 19-3). During the fetal period, the vernix protects the developing skin from constant exposure to amniotic fluid with its high content of urine, bile salts, and sloughed cells. The greasy vernix also facilitates birth of the fetus.

The basal layer of the epidermis becomes the **stratum germinativum** (see Fig. 19-1*B* and *D*), which produces new cells that are displaced into the more superficial layers. By 11 weeks, cells from the stratum germinativum have formed an **intermediate layer** (see Fig. 19-1*C*). Replacement of peridermal cells continues until approximately the 21st week; thereafter, the *periderm disappears* and the **stratum corneum** forms from the **stratum lucidum** (see Fig. 19-1*D*).

Proliferation of cells in the stratum germinativum also forms *epidermal ridges* that extend into the developing dermis (Fig. 19-2). These ridges begin to appear in embryos at 10 weeks and are permanently established by 19 weeks. Those of the hand appear approximately 1 week earlier than ridges in the feet.

The *epidermal ridges produce grooves* on the surface of the palms and soles, including the digits (fingers and toes). The type of pattern that develops is determined genetically and constitutes the basis for examining fingerprints in criminal investigations and medical genetics. Abnormal chromosome complements can affect the development of ridge patterns. For instance, approximately 50% of infants with Down syndrome have distinctive patterns on their hands and feet that have diagnostic value.

Late in the embryonic period, **neural crest cells** migrate into the mesenchyme of the developing dermis and differentiate into **melanoblasts** (cells derived from the neural crest) (see Fig. 19-1*C*). These cells migrate to the **dermo-epidermal junction** and differentiate into **melanocytes** (pigment-producing cells) (see Fig. 19-1*D*). Differentiation of melanoblasts into melanocytes involves the formation **of pigment granules (grain-like particles).** *Signaling by WNT molecules regulates this process.*

Melanocytes appear in the developing skin at 40 to 50 days, immediately after the migration of neural crest cells. In Caucasians, the cell bodies of melanocytes are usually confined to basal layers of the epidermis (see Fig. 19-1*B*); however, the **dendritic processes of the melanocytes** extend between the epidermal cells (see Fig. 19-1*C*).

Only a few melanin-containing cells are normally present in the dermis (see Fig. 19-1*D*). The melanocytes begin producing melanin before birth and distribute it to the epidermal cells. Pigment formation can be observed prenatally in the epidermis of dark-skinned races; however, there is little evidence of such activity in light-skinned fetuses. The relative content of melanin inside the melanocytes accounts for the different colors of skin.

The transformation of the surface ectoderm into the multilayered **definitive epidermis** results from continuing inductive interactions with the dermis. Skin is classified as thick or thin based on the thickness of the epidermis.

- **Thick skin** covers the palms of the hands and soles of the feet; it lacks hair follicles, arrector muscles of hairs, and sebaceous glands, but it has sweat glands.
- **Thin skin** covers most of the rest of the body; it contains hair follicles, arrector muscles of hairs, sebaceous glands, and sweat glands (Fig. 19-3).

## Dermis

The dermis develops from mesenchyme, which is derived from the mesoderm underlying the surface ectoderm (see Fig. 19-1*A* and *B*). Most of the mesenchyme that differentiates into the connective tissue of the dermis originates from the somatic layer of lateral mesoderm; however, some of it is derived from the dermatomes of the somites (see Fig. 14-1*C* and *E*). By 11 weeks, the mesenchymal cells have begun to produce collagenous and elastic connective tissue fibers (see Figs. 19-1*D* and 19-3).

As the **epidermal ridges** form, the dermis projects into the epidermis, forming **dermal papillae,** which interdigitate with the epidermal ridges (see Fig. 19-2). **Capillary loops of blood vessels** develop in some of the papillae and provide nourishment for the epidermis (see Fig. 19-3); sensory nerve endings form in other papillae. The **developing afferent nerve fibers** apparently play an important role in the spatial and temporal sequence of dermal ridge formation. The development of the **dermatomal pattern** of innervation of the skin of the limbs is described elsewhere (see Chapter 16, Fig. 16-10).

The **blood vessels in the dermis** begin as simple, endothelium-lined structures that differentiate from mesenchyme (vasculogenesis). As the skin grows, new

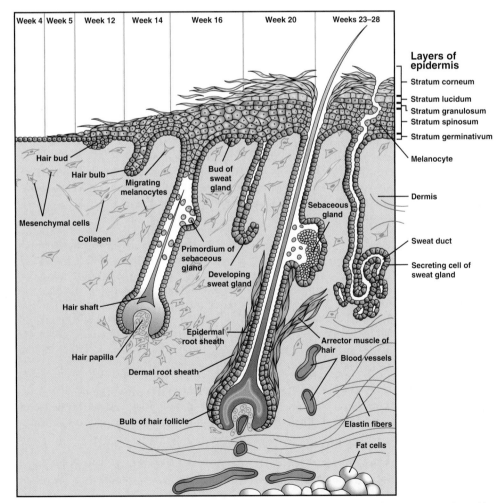

**FIGURE 19–3** Successive stages in the development of hairs, sebaceous glands, and arrector muscles of hair. The sebaceous gland develops as an outgrowth from the side of the hair follicle.

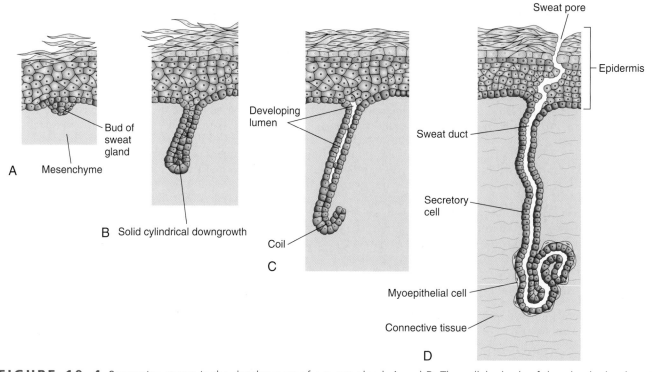

**FIGURE 19–4** Successive stages in the development of a sweat gland. A and B, The cellular buds of the glands develop at approximately 20 weeks as a solid growth of epidermal cells into the mesenchyme. C, Its terminal part coils and forms the body of the gland. The central cells degenerate to form the lumen of the gland. D, The peripheral cells differentiate into secretory cells and contractile myoepithelial cells.

capillaries grow out from the primordial vessels (**angiogenesis**). These capillary-like vessels have been observed in the dermis at the end of the fifth week. Some capillaries acquire muscular coats through differentiation of myoblasts developing in the surrounding mesenchyme and become arterioles and arteries. Other capillaries, through which a return flow of blood is established, acquire muscular coats and become venules and veins. As new blood vessels form, some transitory ones disappear. By the end of the first trimester, the major vascular organization of the fetal dermis is established.

## Glands

The glands of the skin include eccrine and apocrine sweat glands, sebaceous glands, and mammary glands. They are derived from the epidermis and grow into the dermis.

### Sebaceous Glands

Sebaceous glands are derived from the epidermis. Cellular buds develop from the sides of the developing **epidermal root sheaths of hair follicles** (see Fig. 19-3). The buds invade the surrounding dermal connective tissue and branch to form the primordia of several alveoli (hollow sacs) and their associated ducts. The central cells of the alveoli break down, forming an oily substance (**sebum**), which is a secretion from sebaceous glands that protects the fetal skin against friction and dehydration. The secretion is released into **hair follicles** and passes to the surface of the skin, where it mixes with desquamated peridermal cells (see Fig. 19-3).

Sebaceous glands, independent of hair follicles, such as those of the glans penis and labia minora, develop as **cellular buds** from the epidermis that invade the dermis.

### Sweat Glands

Coiled, tubular **eccrine sweat glands** are located in the skin throughout most of the body. They develop as cellular buds from the epidermis that grow into the underlying mesenchyme (see Fig. 19-3). As the buds elongate, their ends coil to form the bodies of the secretory parts of the glands (Fig. 19-4). The epithelial attachments of the developing glands to the epidermis form the **primordia of the sweat ducts**. The central cells of these ducts degenerate, forming **lumina** (canals of tubular eccrine glands). The peripheral cells of the secretory parts of the glands differentiate into myoepithelial and secretory cells (see Fig. 19-4D). The **myoepithelial cells** are thought to be specialized smooth muscle cells that assist in expelling sweat from the glands. Eccrine sweat glands begin to function soon after birth.

Distribution of the large sudoriferous (producing sweat) **apocrine sweat glands** is mostly confined to the axillary, pubic, and perineal regions and to the areolae (circular pigmented areas) surrounding the nipples. The glands develop from downgrowths of the stratum germinativum of the epidermis (see Fig. 19-3). As a result, the ducts of these glands do not open onto the skin surface, as do eccrine sweat glands, but into the canals of the hair follicles superficial to the entry of the sebaceous gland ducts. Secretion by apocrine sweat glands is influenced by hormones and does not begin until puberty.

**FIGURE 19–5** *A,* Child with congenital hypertrichosis and hyperpigmentation. Notice the excessive hairiness on the shoulders and back. *B,* Child with severe keratinization of the skin (ichthyosis) from the time of birth.

## DISORDERS OF KERATINIZATION

**Ichthyosis** is a general term that is applied to a group of skin disorders resulting from excessive **keratinization of skin** (Fig. 19-5*B*). The skin is characterized by dryness and scaling, which may involve the entire surface of the body.

**Harlequin ichthyosis** results from a rare keratinizing disorder that is transmitted as an autosomal recessive trait with a mutation in the *ABCA12* gene. The skin is markedly thickened, ridged, and cracked. Affected neonates require intensive care, and even so, more than 50% die early.

A **collodion infant** is covered by a thick, taut membrane that resembles collodion (a protective film) or parchment. The membranous skin cracks with the first respiratory efforts and begins to fall off in large sheets. Deficiency of transglutaminase 1 (TGM1) is the most common cause. Complete shedding may take several weeks, occasionally leaving normal-appearing skin.

**Lamellar ichthyosis** is an autosomal recessive disorder. A neonate with this condition may appear to be a collodion baby at first; however, the scaling persists. Growth of hair may be curtailed, and development of sweat glands is often impeded. Affected infants usually suffer severely in hot weather because of their inability to sweat.

## CONGENITAL ECTODERMAL DYSPLASIA

Congenital ectodermal dysplasia represents a group of rare **hereditary disorders** involving tissues derived from ectoderm. The teeth are completely or partially absent, and the hairs and nails often are affected. **Ectrodactyly–ectodermal dysplasia–clefting syndrome** is a congenital skin condition that is transmitted as an autosomal dominant trait. It involves ectodermal and mesodermal tissues and consists of **ectodermal dysplasia** (incomplete development of epidermis and skin appendages; the skin is smooth and hairless). The **dysplasia** is associated with **hypopigmentation of skin**, scanty hair and eyebrows, absence of eyelashes, nail dystrophy, hypodontia and microdontia, **ectrodactyly** (absence of all or part of one or more fingers or toes), and cleft lip and palate. *This appears to be caused by a defect in the* TP63 *gene, which codes for a transcription factor.*

## ANGIOMAS OF THE SKIN

Angiomas are **vascular anomalies**. Transitory or surplus primitive blood or lymphatic vessels persist in these developmental defects. Those composed of blood vessels may be mainly arterial, venous, or **cavernous** angiomas, but they are often a mixed type. Angiomas composed of lymphatics are called **cystic lymphangiomas** or **cystic hygromas** (see Chapter 13, Fig. 13-55). True angiomas are benign tumors of endothelial cells that usually are composed of solid or hollow cords; the hollow cords contain blood.

**Nevus flammeus** denotes a flat, pink or red, flame-like blotch that often appears on the posterior surface of the neck. A **port-wine stain (hemangioma)** is a larger and darker angioma than a nevus flammeus and is typically anterior or lateral on the face or neck (Fig. 19-6). It is sharply demarcated when it is near the median plane, whereas the **common angioma** (pinkish red blotch) may cross the median plane. A port-wine stain in the area of distribution of the trigeminal nerve is sometimes associated with a similar type of angioma of the meninges of the brain and seizures at birth (**Sturge-Weber syndrome**). Hemangiomas are among the most common benign neoplasms found in infants and children. When multiple, they may be associated with internal hemangiomas that affect the airways, or if in the liver, they may cause hematologic disturbances such as platelet consumption (Kasabach-Merritt syndrome).

## ALBINISM

In **generalized albinism**, which is an autosomal recessive condition, the skin, hairs, and retina lack pigment; however, the iris usually shows some pigmentation. Albinism occurs when the **melanocytes fail to produce melanin** because of the lack of the enzyme tyrosinase or other pigment enzymes. In *localized albinism* (piebaldism), which is transmitted as an autosomal dominant trait, patches of skin and hair lack melanin.

## Mammary Glands

Mammary glands are modified and highly specialized types of sweat glands. Gland development is similar in male and female embryos. The first evidence of mammary development appears in the fourth week when **mammary crests** (ridges) develop along each side of the ventral surface of the embryo. These crests extend from the axillary region (armpit) to the inguinal region (Fig. 19-7A). The crests usually disappear except for the parts at the site of the future breasts (see Fig. 19-7B).

**FIGURE 19–6** Hemangioma (port-wine stain) in an infant. *(From Dorland's Illustrated Medical Dictionary, ed 30, Philadelphia, 2003, Saunders.)*

Involution of the remaining mammary crests in the fifth week produces the **primary mammary buds** (see Fig. 19-7C). These buds are downgrowths of the epidermis into the underlying mesenchyme. The changes occur in response to an inductive influence from the mesenchyme. Each primary mammary bud soon gives rise to several **secondary mammary buds**, which develop into **lactiferous ducts** and their branches (see Fig. 19-7D to E). **Canalization** (formation of canals) of these buds is induced by **placental sex hormones** entering the fetal circulation. This process continues until the late fetal period, and by term, 15 to 19 lactiferous ducts are formed. The fibrous connective tissue and fat of the mammary glands develop from the surrounding mesenchyme.

During the late fetal period, the epidermis at the site of origin of the mammary glands become depressed, forming shallow **mammary pits** (see Fig. 19-7E). The nipples are poorly formed and depressed in neonates. Soon after birth, the **nipples** usually rise from the mammary pits because of proliferation of the surrounding connective tissue of the **areola**, the circular area of pigmented skin around the nipples. The smooth muscle fibers of the nipples and areolae differentiate from surrounding mesenchymal cells.

The **rudimentary mammary glands** of male and female neonates are identical and are often enlarged. Some secretion (galactorrhea) may be produced. These transitory changes are caused by maternal hormones that pass through the placental membrane into the fetal circulation (see Chapter 7, Fig. 7-7). The breasts of neonates contain **lactiferous ducts** but no **alveoli** that are arranged in grape-clusters; these will be the sites of milk secretion.

In girls, the breasts enlarge rapidly during puberty (Fig. 19-8), mainly because of development of the mammary glands and the accumulation of the fibrous **stroma** (connective tissue) and fat associated with them. Full development occurs at approximately 19 years (see Fig. 19-8F). Normally, the **lactiferous ducts** of boys remain rudimentary throughout life.

*Several transcription factors, including the MYC protein, which is a basic helix-loop-helix transcription factor, are essential for the formation of the lactiferous ducts and function of the female breast.*

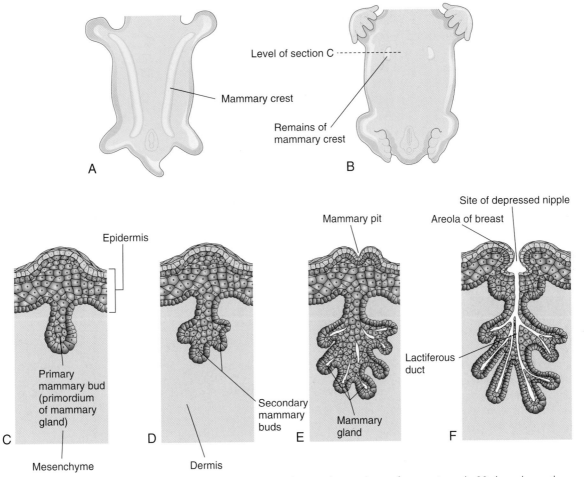

**FIGURE 19-7** Development of mammary glands. **A,** Ventral view of an embryo of approximately 28 days shows the mammary crests. **B,** Similar view at 6 weeks shows the remains of these crests. **C,** Transverse section of a mammary crest at the site of a developing mammary gland. **D** to **F,** Similar sections show successive stages of breast development between the 12th week and birth.

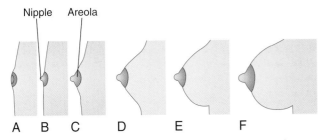

**FIGURE 19-8** Sketches of progressive stages in the postnatal development of female breasts. **A,** Neonate. **B,** Child. **C,** Early puberty. **D,** Late puberty. **E,** Young adult. **F,** Pregnant female. Notice that the nipple is inverted at birth (**A**). At puberty (12–15 years), female breasts enlarge because of development of the mammary glands and the increased deposition of fat.

## GYNECOMASTIA

The rudimentary lactiferous ducts in boys normally undergo no postnatal development. **Gynecomastia** refers to the development of the rudimentary lactiferous ducts in the male mammary tissue. During midpuberty, approximately two thirds of boys develop various degrees of **hyperplasia** (enlargement) of the breasts. This subareolar hyperplasia may persist for a few months to 2 years. A decreased ratio of testosterone to estradiol is found in boys with gynecomastia. Approximately 40% of boys with **Klinefelter syndrome** have gynecomastia (see Chapter 20, Fig. 20-9), which is associated with an XXY chromosome complement.

## ABSENCE OF NIPPLES OR BREASTS

Absence of nipples (athelia) or breasts (amastia) may occur bilaterally or unilaterally. These rare birth defects result from failure of development or disappearance of the mammary crests. They may also result from failure of mammary buds to form. More common is enlargement (**hypoplasia of breast**), which often is associated with **gonadal agenesis** (absence or failure gonads to form) and **Turner syndrome** (see Chapter 20, Fig. 20-4). **Poland syndrome** is associated with hypoplasia or absence of the breast or nipple (see Chapter 15, Fig. 15-5).

**FIGURE 19–9** Female infant with an extra nipple (polythelia) on the left side.

## APLASIA OF BREAST

Postpubertal female breasts often are somewhat different in size. Marked differences are regarded as anomalies because both glands are exposed to the same hormones at puberty. In these cases, there is often associated rudimentary development of muscles of the thoracic wall, usually the **pectoralis major** (see Chapter 15, Fig. 15-5).

**FIGURE 19–10** Man with polythelia (extra nipples) in the axillary and thigh regions. *Insets* are enlargements of the nipples (*arrowheads*). The *broken line* indicates the original position of the left mammary crest.

## SUPERNUMERARY BREASTS AND NIPPLES

An extra breast (**polymastia**) or nipple (**polythelia**) occurs in approximately 0.2% to 5.6% of the female population (Fig. 19-9); it is an inheritable condition. An extra breast or nipple usually develops just inferior to the normal breast. **Supernumerary nipples** are also relatively common in boys; often they are mistaken for moles (Fig. 19-10). Polythelia is often associated with other congenital defects such as renal and urinary tract anomalies. Less commonly, **supernumerary breasts or nipples** appear in the axillary or abdominal regions of girls. In these positions, the nipples or breasts develop from extramammary buds that develop from remnants of the mammary crests. They usually become more obvious in women when they are pregnant. Approximately one third of affected persons have two extra nipples or breasts. **Supernumerary mammary tissue** rarely occurs in a location other than along the course of the mammary crests (milk lines). It probably develops from tissue that was displaced from these crests.

## INVERTED NIPPLES

The nipples sometimes fail to elevate above the skin surface after birth or during puberty, and they remain in their prenatal location (see Figs. 19-7F and 19-8A). Inverted nipples may make breast-feeding of a neonate or infant difficult, but several breast-feeding techniques may be used to reduce this difficulty.

## Hairs

Hairs begin to develop early in the fetal period (weeks 9–12), but they do not become easily recognizable until approximately the 20th week (see Fig. 19-3). Hairs are first recognizable on the eyebrows, upper lip, and chin. The **hair follicles** begin as proliferations of the *stratum germinativum of the epidermis* and extend into the underlying dermis. The **hair buds** become club shaped in the 12th week, forming **hair bulbs** in the 14th week (see Fig. 19-3). The epithelial cells of the hair bulbs constitute the **germinal matrix**, which later produces the hair shafts.

The hair bulbs (**primordia of hair roots**) are soon invaginated by small mesenchymal **hair papillae** (Fig. 19-11; see Fig. 19-3). The peripheral cells of the developing hair follicles form **epithelial root sheaths**, and the surrounding mesenchymal cells differentiate into the **dermal root sheaths.** As cells in the **germinal matrix** (substance of tissue) proliferate, they are pushed toward the surface, where they become keratinized to form **hair shafts** (see Fig. 19-3). The hairs grow through the epidermis on the eyebrows and upper lip by the end of the 12th week.

The first hairs to appear are called **lanugo** (downy hair). They are fine, soft, and lightly pigmented. Lanugo begins to appear toward the end of the 12th week and is plentiful by 17 to 20 weeks (see Fig. 19-3). These hairs help to hold the **vernix caseosa**, which covers and protects the skin of the fetus. Lanugo is replaced by coarser hairs during the perinatal period. This hair persists over most of the body, except in the axillary and pubic regions, where it is replaced at puberty by even coarser terminal hairs. In boys, similar coarse hairs also appear on the face and often on the chest and back.

**Melanoblasts** migrate into the hair bulbs and differentiate into **melanocytes** (pigment-producing cells) (see Fig. 19-3). The **melanin** produced by these cells is transferred to the hair-forming cells in the germinal matrix several weeks before birth. The relative content of melanin accounts for different hair colors.

**Arrector muscles of hairs**, small bundles of smooth muscle fibers, differentiate from the mesenchyme surrounding the hair follicles and attach to the **dermal root sheaths of hair follicles** and the **papillary layer of the dermis**, which interdigitates with the epidermis (see Figs. 19-1D and 19-3). Contractions of the arrector muscles depress the skin over their attachment and elevate the skin around the hair shafts, causing the hairs to stand up ("goose bumps"). The arrector muscles are poorly developed in the hairs of the axillary region and in certain parts of the face. The hairs forming the eyebrows and cilia forming the eyelashes have no arrector muscles.

### ALOPECIA

Absence or loss of scalp hairs may occur alone or with other defects of the skin and its derivatives. **Congenital alopecia** (hair loss) may be caused by failure of hair follicles to develop, or it may result from follicles producing poor-quality hairs. Up to 70% of men and 40% of women have a scalp that is wholly or partly hairless sometime during their lives. Genetic and environmental factors play a role in baldness.

### HYPERTRICHOSIS

**Excessive hairiness** results from the development of **supernumerary hair follicles** or from the **persistence of lanugo hairs** that normally disappear during the perinatal period. It may be localized (e.g., on the shoulders and back) or diffuse (see Fig. 19-5A). **Localized hypertrichosis** is often associated with spina bifida occulta (see Chapter 17, Fig. 17-14).

### PILI TORTI

Pili torti is a familial disorder in which the hairs are twisted and bent. Other ectodermal defects (e.g., distorted fingernails) may be associated with this condition. Pili torti is usually recognized at 2 to 3 years of age.

**FIGURE 19–11** Light micrograph of a longitudinal section of a hair follicle with its hair root *(R)* and papilla *(P)* (×132). *(From Gartner LP, Hiatt JL: Color textbook of histology, ed 2, Philadelphia, 2001, Saunders.)*

## Nails

Toenails and fingernails begin to develop at the tips of the digits at approximately 10 weeks (Fig. 19-12). Development of **fingernails** precedes that of **toenails** by approximately 4 weeks (see Chapter 6, Table 6-1). The primordia of nails appear as thickened areas or **nail fields** of the epidermis at the tip of each digit (see Fig. 19-12A). Later, these **fields** migrate onto the dorsal surfaces of the nails, carrying their innervation from the ventral surface. The **nail fields** are surrounded laterally and proximally by folds of epidermis, the **nail folds** (see Fig. 19-12B). Cells from the proximal nail fold grow over the nail field and become keratinized to form the **nail plate** (see Fig. 19-12C).

At first, the developing nail is covered by a narrow band of epidermis, the **eponychium** (corneal layer of epidermis). It later degenerates, exposing the nail except at its base, where it persists as the **cuticle**. The cuticle of the nail is a thin layer of the deep surface of the **proximal nail fold** (eponychium). The skin under the free margin of the nail is the **hyponychium** (see Fig. 19-12C). The fingernails reach the fingertips by approximately 32 weeks; the toenails reach the toe tips by approximately 36 weeks. Nails that have not reached the tips of the digits at birth indicate prematurity.

### APLASTIC ANONYCHIA

**Congenital absence of fingernails or toenails** is rare. Anonychia results from failure of nail fields to form or from failure of the proximal nail folds to form nail plates. This birth defect is permanent. **Aplastic anonychia** (defective development or absence of nails) may be associated with extremely poor development of hairs and with defects of the teeth. Anonychia may be restricted to one or more nails of the digits of the hands and feet.

## Teeth

Two sets of teeth develop: the primary dentition (**deciduous teeth**) and the secondary dentition (**permanent teeth**). Teeth develop from the oral ectoderm, mesenchyme, and neural crest cells (Fig. 19-13B). The **enamel of teeth** is derived from ectoderm of the oral cavity; all other tissues differentiate from the surrounding mesenchyme and neural crest cells (Fig. 19-14G and H). Neural crest cells are imprinted with morphogenetic information before or shortly after they migrate from the neural crest. *The molecular mechanisms and signaling pathways involve*

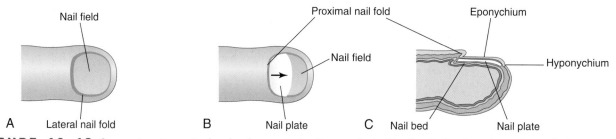

**FIGURE 19–12** Successive stages in the development of a fingernail. A, The first indication of a nail is a thickening of the epidermis, the nail field, at the tip of the finger. B, As the nail plate develops, it slowly grows toward the tip of the finger. C, The fingernail reaches the end of the finger by 32 weeks.

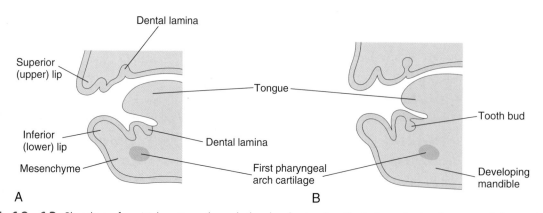

**FIGURE 19–13** Sketches of sagittal sections through the developing jaw illustrate early development of the teeth. A, Early in the sixth week, the dental laminae are present. B, Later in the sixth week, tooth buds arise from the laminae.

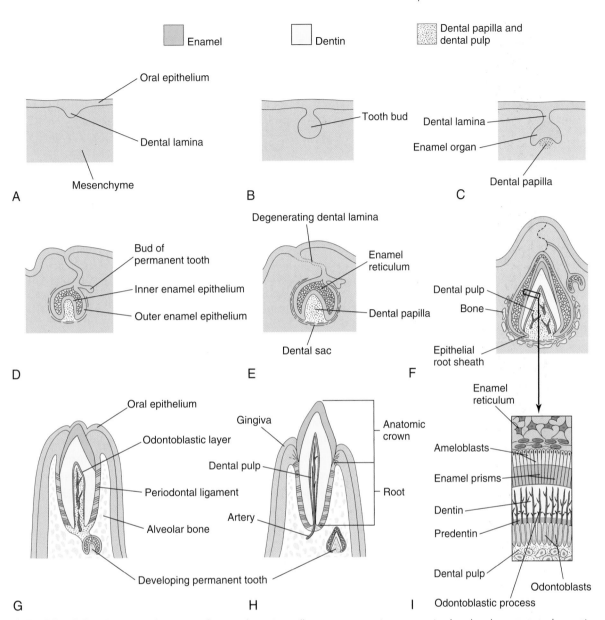

**FIGURE 19-14** Schematic drawings of sagittal sections illustrate successive stages in the development and eruption of an incisor tooth. **A,** At 6 weeks, the dental lamina is present. **B,** At 7 weeks, the tooth bud is developing from the dental lamina. **C,** The cap stage of tooth development occurs at 8 weeks. **D,** The early bell stage of a deciduous tooth and the bud stage of a permanent tooth are shown at 10 weeks. **E,** At 14 weeks, the drawing shows the advanced bell stage of tooth development. The connection (dental lamina) of the tooth to the oral epithelium is degenerating. **F,** At 28 weeks, the enamel and dentin layers can be seen. **G,** At 6 months postnatally, the early stage of tooth eruption is shown. **H,** At 18 months postnatally, the deciduous incisor tooth is fully erupted. The permanent incisor tooth has a well-developed crown. **I,** Section through a developing tooth shows ameloblasts (enamel producers) and odontoblasts (dentin producers).

*the expression and effects of FGF, BMP, SHH, TNF, and WNT.* As the mandible and maxilla grow to accommodate the developing teeth, the shape of the face changes.

**Odontogenesis** (tooth development) is a property of the oral epithelium (see Fig. 19-14G). Development is a continuous process involving reciprocal induction between neural crest–induced mesenchyme and the overlying oral epithelium (see Fig. 19-14A). It is usually divided into stages for descriptive purposes based on the appearance of the developing teeth. The first tooth buds appear in the anterior mandibular region (see Figs. 19-13B and 19-14B); later, tooth development occurs in the anterior maxillary region and then progresses posteriorly in both jaws.

**Tooth development continues for years after birth** (Table 19-1). The first indication of tooth development occurs early in the sixth week as a thickening of the oral epithelium (see Fig. 19-13A). These U-shaped bands **(dental laminae)** follow the curves of the primitive jaws (see Fig. 19-14A).

| Table 19–1 | Eruption and Shedding of Teeth | |
| --- | --- | --- |
| **TOOTH** | **ERUPTION TIME** | **SHEDDING TIME** |
| **Deciduous** | | |
| Medial incisor | 6–8 mo | 6–7 yr |
| Lateral incisor | 8–10 mo | 7–8 yr |
| Canine | 16–20 mo | 10–12 yr |
| First molar | 12–16 mo | 9–11 yr |
| Second molar | 20–24 mo | 10–12 yr |
| **Permanent\*** | | |
| Medial incisor | 7–8 yr | |
| Lateral incisor | 8–9 yr | |
| Canine | 10–12 yr | |
| First premolar | 10–11 yr | |
| Second premolar | 11–12 yr | |
| First molar | 6–7 yr | |
| Second molar | 12 yr | |
| Third molar | 13–25 yr | |

Data from Moore KL, Dalley AF, Agur AMR: *Clinically oriented anatomy*, ed 7, Baltimore, 2014, Lippincott Williams & Wilkins, 2014.
\*The permanent teeth are not shed.

## Bud Stage of Tooth Development

**Each dental lamina** (see Fig. 19-13A) develops 10 centers of proliferation from which swellings (**tooth buds**) grow into the underlying mesenchyme (see Figs. 19-13B and 19-14A to C). These buds develop into **deciduous teeth** (see Table 19-1). The tooth buds for permanent teeth that have deciduous predecessors begin to appear at approximately 10 weeks from deep continuations of the dental lamina (see Fig. 19-14D). They develop *lingual* (next to the tongue) to the **deciduous tooth buds**.

The permanent molars have no deciduous predecessors and develop as buds from posterior extensions of the **dental laminae** (horizontal bands). The tooth buds for the permanent teeth appear at different times, mostly during the fetal period (see Fig. 19-1D). *The buds for the second and third permanent molars develop after birth.* The deciduous teeth have well-developed crowns at birth (see Fig. 19-14H), whereas the permanent teeth remain as tooth buds (see Table 19-1).

## Cap Stage of Tooth Development

As each tooth bud is invaginated by mesenchyme (primordium of the dental papilla and dental follicle), the buds become cap shaped (Fig. 19-15; see Fig. 19-14C). The ectodermal part of the developing tooth, which is the **enamel organ** (mass of ectodermal cells budded from the dental lamina), eventually produces enamel (see Fig. 19-14E and G). The internal part of each cap-shaped

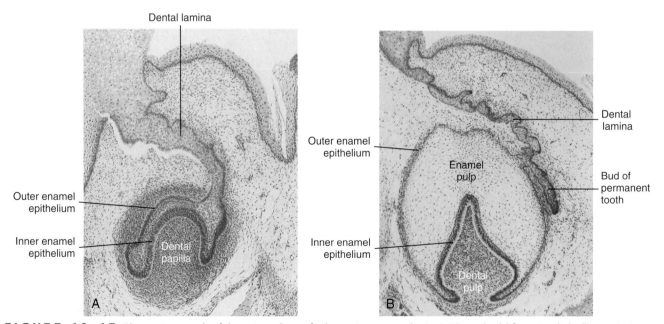

**FIGURE 19–15** Photomicrograph of the primordium of a lower incisor tooth. *A*, A 12-week-old fetus (early bell stage). A cap-like enamel organ has formed, and the dental papilla is developing beneath it. *B*, Primordium of a lower incisor tooth in a 15-week-old fetus (late bell stage). Observe the inner and outer enamel layers, the dental papilla, and the bud of the permanent tooth. *(From Moore KL, Persaud TVN, Shiota K: Color atlas of clinical embryology, ed 2, Philadelphia, 2000, Saunders, 2000.)*

tooth (**dental papilla**) is the primordium of dentin and dental pulp (see Fig. 19-14*E*). Together, the dental papilla and enamel organ form the tooth bud. The *outer cell layer* of the enamel organ is the **outer enamel epithelium**, and the *inner cell layer* lining the papilla is the **inner enamel epithelium** (see Fig. 19-14*D*).

The central core of loosely arranged cells between the layers of enamel epithelium is the **enamel reticulum** or stellate reticulum (see Fig. 19-14*E*). As the enamel organ and dental papilla develop, the mesenchyme surrounding the developing tooth condenses to form the **dental sac** (dental follicle), a vascularized capsular structure (see Fig. 19-14*E*). The dental sac is the primordium of the *cement* and *periodontal ligament* (see Fig. 19-14*G*). The cement is the bone-like, mineralized connective tissue covering the root of the tooth. The **periodontal ligament**, which is derived from neural crest cells, is a specialized vascular connective tissue that surrounds the root of the tooth, attaching it to the alveolar bone (see Fig. 19-14*G*).

## Bell Stage of Tooth Development

As the **enamel organ** differentiates, the developing tooth assumes the shape of a bell (Fig. 19-15; see Fig. 19-14*D* and *E*). The mesenchymal cells in the **dental papilla** adjacent to the internal enamel epithelium differentiate into **odontoblasts** (dentin-forming cells), which produce predentin and deposit it adjacent to the epithelium (see Fig. 19-14*G*). Later, the **predentin** calcifies and becomes **dentin**, the second hardest tissue in the body. As the dentin thickens, the odontoblasts regress toward the center of the dental papilla; however, their finger-like cytoplasmic processes (**odontoblastic processes**) remain embedded in the dentin (Fig. 19-16; see Fig. 19-14*F* and *I*).

Cells of the inner enamel epithelium differentiate into **ameloblasts** (cells of the inner layer of the enamel organ) under the influence of the odontoblasts, which produce enamel in the form of prisms (rods) over the dentin (see Fig. 19-14*I*). As the enamel increases, the ameloblasts migrate toward the outer enamel epithelium (see Fig. 19-15*A* and *B*). Enamel is the hardest tissue in the body; it overlies and protects the dentin from being fractured (see Fig. 19-16). The color of the translucent enamel is based on the thickness and color of the underlying dentin. Enamel and dentin formation begins at the cusp (tip) of the tooth and progresses toward the future root.

The **root of the tooth** begins to develop after dentin and enamel formations are well advanced (Fig. 19-17; see Fig. 19-14*H*). The inner and outer enamel epithelia come together at the **neck of the tooth** (cementoenamel junction), where they form a fold, the **epithelial root sheath** (see Figs. 19-14*F* and 19-15). This sheath grows into the mesenchyme and initiates root formation.

The **odontoblasts** adjacent to the epithelial root sheath form dentin that is continuous with that of the crown of the tooth. As the dentin increases, it reduces the **pulp cavity** to a narrow **root canal** through which the vessels and nerves pass (see Fig. 19-14*H*). The inner cells of the dental sac differentiate into **cementoblasts**, which produce cement that is restricted to the root. Cement is deposited over the dentin of the root and meets the enamel at the

**FIGURE 19–16** Photomicrograph of a section of the crown and neck of a tooth (×17). Observe the enamel (*E*), dentin (*D*), dental pulp (*P*), and odontoblasts (*O*). (*From Gartner LR, Hiatt JL: Color textbook of histology, ed 2, Philadelphia, 2001, Saunders.*)

**neck of the tooth**, the constricted part of the tooth, between the crown and the root (see Fig. 19-14*H*).

As the teeth develop and the jaws ossify, the outer cells of the **dental sac** also become active in bone formation see (Fig. 19-14*E*). Each tooth soon becomes surrounded by bone, except over the crown (see Fig. 19-14*G* and *H*). The tooth is held in its **alveolus** (tooth socket) by the strong **periodontal ligament**, a derivative of the dental sac (see Fig. 19-14*G* and *H*). Some fibers of this ligament are embedded in the cement of the root; other fibers are embedded in the bony wall of the alveolus.

## Tooth Eruption

As the **deciduous teeth** develop, they begin a continuous, slow movement toward the **oral cavity**, which is the narrow cleft between the teeth and gingiva (see Fig. 19-14*G*). This process (**eruption**) results in the emergence of the tooth from the dental follicle in the jaw to its functional position in the mouth. The **mandibular teeth** usually erupt before the **maxillary teeth**, and girls' teeth usually erupt sooner than boys' teeth. The child's dentition contains **20 deciduous teeth**. As the root of the tooth grows, its crown gradually erupts through the **oral epithelium** (see Fig. 19-14*G*). The part of the oral mucosa around the erupted crown becomes the **gingiva** (see Fig. 19-14*H*).

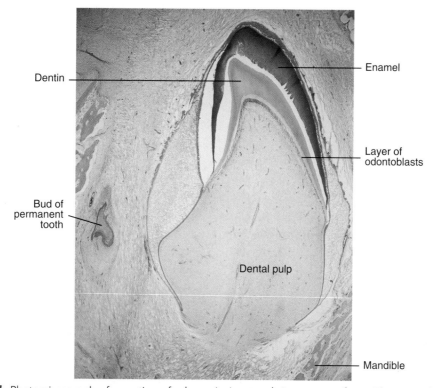

Dentin

Enamel

Layer of
odontoblasts

Bud of
permanent
tooth

Dental pulp

Mandible

**FIGURE 19–17** Photomicrograph of a section of a lower incisor tooth in a mature fetus. The enamel and dentin layers and the pulp are clearly demarcated. *(From Moore KL, Persaud TVN, Shiota K: Color atlas of clinical embryology, ed 2, Philadelphia, 2000, Saunders.)*

The usual eruption time of the deciduous teeth is between 6 and 24 months (see Table 19-1). The mandibular medial (**central incisor teeth**) typically erupt from 6 to 8 months, but this process may not begin until 12 or 13 months in some children. Despite this, all 20 deciduous teeth are usually present by the end of the second year in healthy children. Delayed eruption of all teeth may indicate a systemic or nutritional disturbance such as **hypopituitarism** (diminished activity of the anterior lobe of the hypophysis) or **hypothyroidism** (diminished production of thyroid hormone).

The **permanent dentition** consists of 32 teeth. The permanent teeth develop in a manner similar to that described for deciduous teeth. As a permanent tooth grows, the root of the corresponding deciduous tooth is gradually resorbed by **osteoclasts** (odontoclasts). Consequently, when the deciduous tooth is shed, it consists only of the crown and uppermost part of the root. The permanent teeth usually begin to erupt during the sixth year and continue to appear until early adulthood (Fig. 19-18; see Table 19-1).

The shape of the face is affected by the development of the **paranasal sinuses** (air-filled cavities in the bones of the face) and the growth of the maxilla and mandible to accommodate the teeth (see Chapter 9, Fig. 9-26). Lengthening of the **alveolar processes** (tooth sockets supporting the teeth) increases the length of the face during childhood.

**FIGURE 19–18** Cranium of a 4-year-old child. Bone has been removed from the mandible and maxilla to expose the relationship of the developing permanent teeth to the erupted deciduous teeth.

## NATAL TEETH

Neonates may have one or more **erupted teeth at birth** (**natal teeth**). These teeth are usually the lower incisors. One or more teeth may also erupt later in the neonatal period (up to 4 weeks); they are called **neonatal teeth**. Natal teeth are observed in 1 in 2000 neonates. This anomaly is often transmitted as an autosomal dominant trait. Only the crowns of the teeth are calcified, and their roots are usually loose. These teeth may produce maternal discomfort during breast-feeding, and the neonate's tongue may be lacerated, or the teeth may detach and be aspirated; for these reasons, natal teeth are usually extracted. Because they are prematurely erupting decidual teeth, spacers may be required to prevent overcrowding of the other teeth.

## ENAMEL HYPOPLASIA

**Defective enamel formation** causes pits and fissures in the enamel of teeth (Figs. 19-19 and 19-20A). These defects result from temporary disturbances of enamel formation. Various factors (e.g., nutritional deficiency, tetracycline therapy, infectious diseases such as measles) may injure ameloblasts, which are the **enamel builders**. **Rickets** occurring during the critical period of tooth development (6–12 weeks) is a common cause of enamel hypoplasia. Rickets, a disease in children who are deficient in vitamin D, is characterized by *disturbance of ossification of the epiphysial cartilage* plates and disorientation of cells at the metaphysis (see Fig. 14-4E).

**FIGURE 19–19** Common anomalies of teeth. **A**, Enamel pearl (with furcation [forking] of a permanent maxillary third molar). **B**, Gemination and tetracycline staining (maxillary third molar). **C**, Fusion of permanent mandibular central and lateral incisors. **D**, Abnormally short root (microdont permanent maxillary central incisor). **E**, Dens invaginatus (talon cusps on the lingual surface of the permanent maxillary central incisor). **F**, Taurodont tooth (radiograph of the mesial surface of the permanent maxillary second molar). **G**, Fusion (primary mandibular central and lateral incisors).

**FIGURE 19–20** Additional common anomalies of teeth. **A,** Amelogenesis imperfecta. **B,** Extra root (mandibular molar). **C,** Extra root (mandibular canine). **D,** Accessory root (maxillary lateral incisor). Extra roots present challenges for root canal therapy and extraction. **E,** Tetracycline staining (root of maxillary third molar). **F,** A midline supernumerary tooth (mesiodens [M]) located near the apex of the central incisor. The prevalence of supernumerary teeth is 1% to 3% in the general population.

## Variations of Tooth Shape

Abnormally shaped teeth are relatively common (see Figs. 19-19 and 19-20A to E). Occasionally, there is a spherical mass of enamel (**enamel pearl**) on the root of a tooth that is separate from the enamel of the crown (see Fig. 19-19A). The pearl is formed by **aberrant groups of ameloblasts**. In other cases, the maxillary lateral incisor teeth may have a slender, tapering shape (peg-shaped incisors).

**Congenital syphilis** affects differentiation of the permanent teeth, resulting in incisors with central notches in their incisive edges. The molars are also affected and are called **mulberry molars** because of their characteristic features.

## NUMERIC ABNORMALITIES OF TEETH

One or more **supernumerary teeth** (mesiodens) may develop, or the normal number of teeth may fail to form (see Fig. 19-20F). Many studies report a higher prevalence among girls. Supernumerary teeth usually develop in the area of the maxillary incisors and can disrupt the position and eruption of normal teeth. The extra teeth commonly erupt posterior to the normal ones (or remain unerupted) and are asymptomatic in most cases.

In **partial anodontia**, one or more teeth are absent; this is often a familial trait. In **total anodontia**, no teeth develop; this is an extremely rare condition. It is usually associated with **ectodermal dysplasia** (congenital defect of ectodermal tissues). Occasionally, a tooth bud partially or completely divides into two separate teeth.

A partially divided tooth germ is called **gemination**. The result is a **macrodontia** (large teeth) with a common root canal system; small teeth (**microdontia**) also occur. If the tooth germ completely divides into two separate teeth, the result is twinning, with one additional tooth in the dentition. Fusion of two teeth results in one fewer tooth in the dentition. This condition can be differentiated radiographically from gemination by **two separate root canal systems** found with fusion.

## DENTIGEROUS CYST

A cyst may develop in a mandible, maxilla, or a maxillary sinus that contains an unerupted tooth. The **dentigerous** (*tooth-bearing*) **cyst** develops because of cystic degeneration of the enamel reticulum of the enamel organ of an unerupted tooth. Most cysts are deeply situated in the jaw and are associated with misplaced or malformed secondary teeth that have failed to erupt.

## AMELOGENESIS IMPERFECTA

Amelogenesis imperfecta is a complex group of at least 14 clinical entities that involve **aberrations in enamel formation** in the absence of any systemic disorder. This is an **inherited ectodermal birth defect** that primarily affects the enamel only. The enamel may be **hypoplastic**, **hypocalcified**, or **hypomature** (not fully developed). Depending on the type of amelogenesis imperfecta, the enamel may be hard or soft, pitted or smooth, and thin or normal in thickness. The incidence of amelogenesis imperfecta ranges from 1 in 700 to 8000 people, depending on the population studied. Multiple modes of inheritance patterns are involved. Mutational defects of the genes that encode for enamel, dentin, and mineralization are likely involved. Classification of this condition is based on clinical and radiographic findings and on the mode of inheritance.

## DENTINOGENESIS IMPERFECTA

This autosomal dominant disorder of the teeth is characterized clinically by translucent gray to yellow-brown teeth involving primary and permanent dentition. The teeth have an opalescent sheen because the *odontoblasts fail to differentiate normally*, and poorly calcified dentin results. The enamel tends to wear down rapidly, exposing the dentin. This disorder in most cases is localized on chromosome 4q, and this condition is relatively common among white children (Fig. 19-21).

**FIGURE 19–21** Teeth of a child with dentinogenesis imperfecta. (*From Thompson MW: Genetics in medicine, ed 4, Philadelphia, 1986, Saunders.*)

## DISCOLORED TEETH

Foreign substances incorporated into the developing enamel and dentin discolor the teeth. The hemolysis associated with **erythroblastosis fetalis** or hemolytic disease of the neonate may produce blue to black discoloration of the teeth. All **tetracyclines** are extensively incorporated into the teeth. The critical period at risk for this disease is from approximately 14 weeks of fetal life to the 10th postnatal month for deciduous teeth and from approximately 14 weeks of fetal life to the eighth postnatal year for permanent teeth.

**Tetracycline staining** affects enamel and dentin because it binds to **hydroxyapatite** (modified natural mineral structure that forms the crystal lattice of bones and teeth). The brownish yellow discoloration (mottling) of teeth produced by tetracycline is caused by the conversion of tetracycline to a colored by-product under the action of light. The dentin is probably affected more than the enamel because it is more permeable than enamel after tooth mineralization is complete. The enamel is completely formed on all but the third molars by approximately 8 years of age. For this reason, **tetracyclines** (broad-spectrum antibiotics) should not be administered to pregnant women or children younger than 8 years of age.

## SUMMARY OF INTEGUMENTARY SYSTEM

- The skin and its appendages develop from ectoderm, mesenchyme, and neural crest cells. The epidermis is derived from surface ectoderm, and the dermis is derived from mesenchyme. **Melanocytes** are derived from **neural crest cells** that migrate into the epidermis.
- Cast-off cells from the epidermis mix with secretions of sebaceous glands to form the **vernix caseosa**, a whitish, greasy coating of the skin that protects the epidermis of the fetuses.
- **Hairs** develop from downgrowths of the epidermis into the dermis. By approximately 20 weeks, the fetus is completely covered with fine, downy hairs (**lanugo**). These fetal hairs are shed before birth or shortly thereafter and are replaced by coarser hairs.
- Most **sebaceous glands** develop as outgrowths from the sides of hair follicles; however, some glands develop as downgrowths of the epidermis into the dermis. **Sweat glands** also develop from epidermal downgrowths into the dermis. **Mammary glands** develop in a similar manner.
- **Birth defects of the skin** are mainly disorders of keratinization (**ichthyosis**) and pigmentation (**albinism**). Abnormal blood vessel development results in various types of angioma.
- **Nails** may be absent or malformed. Hair may be absent or excessive.
- Absence of **mammary glands** is rare, but supernumerary breasts (**polymastia**) and nipples (**polythelia**) are relatively common.
- **Teeth** develop from ectoderm, mesoderm, and neural crest cells. The **enamel** is produced by **ameloblasts**, which are derived from the oral ectoderm; all other dental tissues develop from mesenchyme, which is derived from mesoderm and neural crest cells.
- **Common birth defects of teeth** are defective formation of enamel and dentin, abnormalities in shape, and variations in number and position.
- **Tetracyclines** are extensively incorporated into the enamel and dentin of developing teeth, producing brownish yellow discoloration and hypoplasia of the enamel. *They should not be prescribed for pregnant women or children younger than 8 years of age.*

## CLINICALLY ORIENTED PROBLEMS

### CASE 19–1

*A neonate had two erupted mandibular incisor teeth.*

- What are these teeth called?
- How common is this anomaly?
- Are they supernumerary teeth?
- What problems or danger is associated with the presence of teeth at birth?

### CASE 19–2

*The deciduous teeth of an infant had a brownish yellow color and some hypoplasia of the enamel. The mother recalled that she had been given antibiotics during the second trimester of her pregnancy.*

- What is the probable cause of the infant's tooth discoloration?
- Dysfunction of what cells causes enamel hypoplasia?
- Will the secondary dentition be discolored?

### CASE 19–3

*An infant had a small, irregularly shaped, light red blotch on the posterior surface of the neck. It was level with the surrounding skin and blanched when light pressure was applied.*

- What is this birth defect called?
- What do these observations indicate?
- Is this condition common?
- Are there other names for this skin defect?

### CASE 19–4

*A female neonate had a tuft of hair in the lumbosacral region of her back.*

- What does this tuft of hair indicate?
- Is this condition common?
- Is this birth defect clinically important?

### CASE 19–5

*The skin of a male neonate had a collodion type of covering that fissured and exfoliated shortly after birth. Later, lamellar ichthyosis developed.*

- Briefly describe this condition.
- Is it a common defect?
- How is it inherited?

Discussion of these problems appears in the Appendix at the back of the book.

## BIBLIOGRAPHY AND SUGGESTED READING

Caton J, Tucker AS: Current knowledge of tooth development: patterning and mineralization of the murine dentition, *J Anat* 214:407, 2009.

Chiu YE: Dermatology. In Marcdante KJ, Kliegman KJ, editors: *Nelson essentials of pediatrics*, ed 7, Philadelphia, 2015, Saunders.

Coletta RD, McCoy EL, Burns V, et al: Characterization of the Six 1 homeobox gene in normal mammary gland morphogenesis, *BMC Dev Biol* 10:4, 2010.

Crawford PJM, Aldred MJ: Anomalies of tooth formation and eruption. In Welbury RR, Duggal MS, Hosey MT, editors: *Paediatric dentistry*, ed 4, Oxford, UK, 2012, Oxford University Press.

Felipe AF, Abazari A, Hammersmith KM, et al: Corneal changes in ectrodactyly-ectodermal dysplasia-cleft lip and palate syndrome: case series and literature review, *Int Ophthalmol* 32:475, 2012.

Galli-Tsinopoulou A, Stergidou D: Polythelia: simple atavistic remnant or a suspicious clinical sign for investigation?, *Pediatr Endocrinol Rev* 11:290, 2014.

Harryparsad A, Rahman L, Bunn BK: Amelogenesis imperfecta: a diagnostic and pathological review with case illustration, *SADJ* 68:404, 2013.

Kliegman RM, Stanton B, St Geme J, et al, editors: *Nelson textbook of pediatrics*, ed 19, Philadelphia, 2011, Saunders.

Lee K, Gjorevski N, Boghaert E, et al: Snail1, Snail2, and E47 promote mammary epithelial branching morphogenesis, *EMBO J* 30:2662, 2011.

Marwaha M, Nanda KD: Ectrodactyly, ectodermal dysplasia, cleft lip, and palate (EEC syndrome), *Contemp Clin Dent* 3:205, 2012.

McDermottt KM, Liu BY, Tisty TD, et al: Primary cilia regulate branching morphogenesis during mammary gland development, *Curr Biol* 20:731, 2010.

Moore KL, Dalley AF, Agur AMR: *Clinically oriented anatomy*, ed 7, Baltimore, 2014, Lippincott Williams & Wilkins.

Müller M, Jasmin JR, Monteil RA, et al: Embryology of the hair follicle, *Early Hum Dev* 26:59, 1999.

Nanci A: *Ten Cate's oral histology: development, structure, and function*, ed 8, St Louis, 2013, Mosby.

Osborne MP, Boolbol SK: Breast anatomy and development. In Harris JR, Lippman ME, Morrow M, et al, editors: *Diseases of the breast*, ed 4, Philadelphia, 2010, Lippincott Williams & Wilkins.

Paller AS, Mancini AJ: *Hurwitz clinical pediatric dermatology: a textbook of skin disorders of childhood and adolescence*, ed 4, Philadelphia, 2011, Saunders.

Papagerakis P, Mitsiadis T: Development and structure of teeth and periodontal tissues. In Rosen CJ, editor: *Primer on the metabolic bone diseases and disorders of mineral metabolism*, ed 8, New Jersey, 2013, John Wiley & Sons.

Patil S, Doni B, Kaswan S, et al: Prevalence of dental anomalies in Indian population, *J Clin Exp Dent* 5:e183, 2013.

Rudel RA, Fenton SE, Ackerman JM, et al: Environmental exposures and mammary gland development: state of the science, public health implications, and research recommendations, *Environ Health Perspect* 119:1053, 2011.

Smolinski KN: Hemangiomas of infancy: clinical and biological characteristics, *Clin Pediatr* 44:747, 2005.

Watts A, Addy MA: Tooth discolouration and staining: a review of the literature, *Br Dent J* 190:309, 2001.

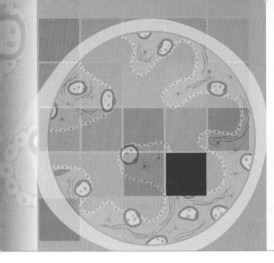

# Human Birth Defects

*T*he Humane Foetus tho no bigger then a Green Pea, yet is furnifhed with all its parts.
        —Antonj van Leeuwenhoek, 1683

*We ought not to set them aside with idle thoughts or idle words about "curiosities" or "chances." Not one of them is without meaning; not one that might not become the beginning of excellent knowledge, if only we could answer the question—why is it rare, or being rare, why did it in this instance happen?*

        —James Paget, Lancet 2:1017, 1882

Birth defects (anomalies) are developmental disorders present at birth. Defects are the leading cause of infant mortality (fetal outcome). They may be structural, functional, metabolic, behavioral, or hereditary. Birth defects are a global problem; close to 8 million children worldwide have a serious birth defect.

## CLASSIFICATION OF BIRTH DEFECTS

The most widely used reference guide for classifying birth defects is the *International Classification of Diseases*, but no single classification has universal appeal. Each is limited by being designed for a particular purpose. Attempts to classify human birth defects, especially those that result from **errors of morphogenesis** (development of form), reveal the frustration and obvious difficulties in the formulation of concrete proposals for use in medical practice. A practical classification system for birth defects that takes into consideration the time of onset of the injury, possible cause, and pathogenesis is now widely accepted among clinicians.

# TERATOLOGY: STUDY OF ABNORMAL DEVELOPMENT

*Teratology* is the branch of embryology and pathology concerned with the production, developmental anatomy, and the classification of malformed embryos and fetuses. *A fundamental concept in teratology is that certain stages of embryonic development are more vulnerable to disruption than others* (see Fig. 20-15). Until the 1940s, it was thought that embryos were protected from environmental agents such as drugs, viruses, and chemicals by their extraembryonic or fetal membranes (amnion and chorion) and their mothers' uterine and abdominal walls.

In 1941, the first well-documented cases reported that an environmental agent (**rubella virus**) could produce severe birth defects such as cataracts (see Chapter 18, Fig. 18-13), cardiac defects, and deafness if the rubella infection occurred during the critical period of development of the eyes, heart, and ears. In the 1950s, severe limb defects and other developmental disorders were found in infants of mothers who had consumed a sedative (**thalidomide**) during early pregnancy (see Fig. 20-20). These discoveries, made more than seven decades ago, focused worldwide attention on the role of drugs and viruses as *causes of human birth defects.* An estimated 7% to 10% of birth defects result from the disruptive actions of drugs, viruses, and environmental toxins.

*More than 20% of infant deaths in North America are attributed to birth defects.* Major structural defects, such as **spina bifida cystica**, a severe type of vertebral defect in which part of the neural tube fails to fuse (see Chapter 17, Fig. 17-15), are observed in approximately 3% of neonates. Additional defects can be detected during infancy, and the incidence reaches approximately 6% among 2-year-old children and 8% among 5-year-old children.

The **causes of birth defects** are divided into three broad categories:

- **Genetic factors** such as chromosomal abnormalities
- **Environmental factors** such as drugs and viruses
- **Multifactorial inheritance** (genetic and environmental factors acting together)

*For 50% to 60% of birth defects, the cause is unknown* (Fig. 20-1). The defects may be single or multiple and may have major or minor clinical significance. **Single minor defects** occur in approximately 14% of neonates. Defects of the external ears, for example, are of no serious medical significance, but they may indicate the presence of associated major defects. For instance, the finding of a single umbilical artery alerts the clinician to possible cardiovascular and renal anomalies (see Chapter 7, Fig. 7-18).

*Ninety percent of infants with three or more minor defects also have one or more major defects.* Of the 3% born with clinically significant defects, **multiple major defects** are found in 0.7%, and most of these infants die. **Major developmental defects** are much more common in young embryos (10%–15%), but *most of them abort spontaneously* during the first 6 weeks. **Chromosomal abnormalities** are detected in 50% to 60% of spontaneously aborted embryos.

## BIRTH DEFECTS CAUSED BY GENETIC FACTORS

*Numerically, genetic factors are the most important causes of birth defects.* Mutant genes cause approximately one third of all defects (see Fig. 20-1). Any mechanism as complex as **mitosis** or **meiosis** may occasionally malfunction (see Fig. 20-1; see Chapter 2, Figs. 2-1 and 2-2). Chromosomal aberrations occur in 6% to 7% of zygotes (single-cell embryos).

Most early abnormal embryos never undergo normal cleavage and become blastocysts (see Chapter 2, Figs. 2-16 and 2-17). In vitro studies of cleaving zygotes less than 5 days old have revealed a high incidence of abnormalities. More than 60% of day 2 cleaving zygotes were found to be abnormal. Many defective zygotes, blastocysts, and 3-week-old embryos abort spontaneously, and the overall frequency of chromosomal aberrations in these embryos is at least 50%.

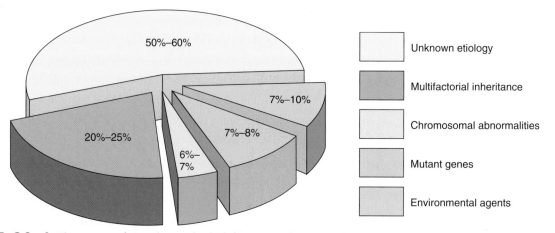

**FIGURE 20–1** The causes of most human birth defects are unknown, and 20% to 25% of them are caused by a combination of genetic and environmental factors (multifactorial inheritance).

*Two kinds of changes occur in chromosome comple-
ments:* numeric and structural. The changes may affect
the **sex chromosomes** or the **autosomes** (chromosomes
other than sex chromosomes). In some instances, both
kinds of chromosomes are affected. Persons with chromosomal aberrations usually have characteristic **phenotypes** (morphologic characteristics), such as the physical
characteristics of infants with Down syndrome (see Fig.
20-6). They often look more like other persons with the
same chromosomal abnormality than their own siblings.
*This characteristic appearance results from a genetic
imbalance.* Genetic factors initiate defects by biochemical
or other means at the subcellular, cellular, or tissue level.
The abnormal mechanisms initiated by the genetic factors
may be identical or similar to the causal mechanisms
initiated by **teratogens,** such as drugs and infections (see
Table 20-6).

## Numeric Chromosomal Abnormalities

In the United States, approximately 1 in 120 neonates has
a chromosomal abnormality. Numeric aberrations of
chromosomes usually result from **nondisjunction,** an
error in cell division in which there is failure of a chromosomal pair or two chromatids of a chromosome to
disjoin during mitosis or meiosis (see Chapter 2, Figs. 2-2
and 2-3). As a result, the chromosomal pair or chromatids pass to one daughter cell and the other daughter cell
receives neither (Fig. 20-2). Nondisjunction may occur
during maternal or paternal gametogenesis. The chromosomes in somatic cells are normally paired and called
**homologous chromosomes** (homologs). Normal human
females have 22 pairs of autosomes plus two X chromosomes, whereas normal males have 22 pairs of autosomes
plus one X and one Y chromosome.

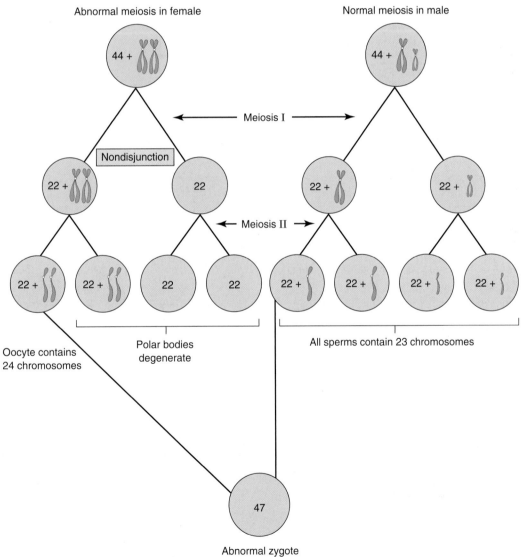

**FIGURE 20–2** Nondisjunction of chromosomes during the first meiotic division of a primary oocyte results in an abnormal
oocyte with 24 chromosomes. Subsequent fertilization by a normal sperm produces a zygote with 47 chromosomes (aneuploidy), which
is a deviation from the human diploid number of 46.

## GLOSSARY OF TERATOLOGIC TERMS

A birth defect is a structural abnormality of any type, but *not all variations of development are defects or anomalies (marked deviation from the average or norm)*. **Anatomical variations are common**; for example, bones vary in their basic shape and in lesser details of surface structure. The four *clinically significant types of birth defects* are malformation, disruption, deformation, and dysplasia.

- **Malformation** is a morphologic defect of an organ, part of an organ, or larger region of the body that results from an *intrinsically abnormal developmental process*. *Intrinsic* implies that the developmental potential of the primordium of an organ is abnormal from the beginning, such as a chromosomal abnormality of a gamete (oocyte or sperm) at fertilization. Most malformations are considered to be a defect of a *morphogenetic or developmental field* that responds as a coordinated unit to embryonic interaction and results in complex or multiple malformations.
- **Disruption** is a morphologic defect of an organ, part of an organ, or a larger region of the body that *results from the extrinsic breakdown of or an interference with an originally normal developmental process*. Morphologic alterations after exposure to **teratogens** (e.g., drugs, viruses) should be considered as disruptions. *A disruption cannot be inherited*, but inherited factors can predispose to and influence the development of a disruption.
- **Deformation** is an abnormal form, shape, or position of a part of the body that *results from mechanical forces*. **Intrauterine compression in utero** that results from **oligohydramnios** (insufficient amount of amniotic fluid) may produce an *equinovarus foot* or *clubfoot* (see Chapter 16, Fig. 16-15). Some central nervous system (CNS) neural tube defects, such as *meningomyelocele* (severe type of spina bifida), produce intrinsic functional disturbances, which cause fetal deformation (see Chapter 17, Figs. 17-12C and 17-15A).
- **Dysplasia** is an abnormal organization of cells in tissues and its morphologic results. Dysplasia is the process and the consequence of **dyshistogenesis** (abnormal tissue formation). All abnormalities relating to histogenesis are therefore classified as dysplasias, such as *congenital ectodermal dysplasia* (see Chapter 19, box titled "Congenital Ectodermal Dysplasia"). Dysplasia is causally nonspecific and often affects several organs because of the nature of the underlying cellular disturbances.

Other descriptive terms are used to describe infants with multiple defects, and the terms have evolved to express causation and pathogenesis:

- A *polytopic field defect* is a pattern of defects derived from the disturbance of a single developmental field.
- A *sequence* is a pattern of multiple defects derived from a single known or presumed structural defect or mechanical factor.
- A *syndrome* is a pattern of multiple defects thought to be pathogenetically related and not known to represent a single sequence or a polytopic field defect.
- An *association* is a nonrandom occurrence in two or more individuals of multiple defects not known to be a polytopic field defect, sequence, or syndrome.

Whereas a sequence is a **pathogenetic** (causing disease or abnormality) and not a causal concept, a syndrome often implies a single cause, such as **trisomy 21 (Down syndrome)**. In both cases, the pattern of defects is known or considered to be pathogenetically related. In the case of a sequence, the *primary initiating factor and cascade of secondary developmental complications are known*. For example, the *Potter syndrome* (*sequence*), which is attributed to **oligohydramnios** (insufficient amount of amniotic fluid), results from renal agenesis or leakage of amniotic fluid (see Chapter 12, Fig. 12-12C). An association, in contrast, refers to statistically, not pathogenetically or causally, related defects. One or more sequences, syndromes, or field defects may constitute an association.

**Dysmorphology** is an area of clinical genetics that is concerned with the diagnosis and interpretation of patterns of structural defects. *Recurrent patterns of birth defects enable syndrome recognition*. Identifying these patterns in individuals has improved understanding of the causes and pathogenesis of these conditions.

## INACTIVATION OF GENES

During embryogenesis, one of the two X chromosomes in female somatic cells is randomly inactivated and appears as a mass of **sex chromatin. Inactivation of genes** on one X chromosome in somatic cells of female embryos occurs during implantation. X inactivation is important clinically because it means that each cell from a carrier of an X-linked disease has the mutant gene causing the disease on the active X chromosome or on the inactivated X chromosome that is represented by sex chromatin. Uneven X inactivation in monozygotic (identical) twins is one reason given for discordance in a variety of birth defects. The genetic basis for discordance is that one twin preferentially expresses the paternal X and the other the maternal X.

## ANEUPLOIDY AND POLYPLOIDY

Changes in chromosome number result in aneuploidy or polyploidy. **Aneuploidy** is any deviation from the diploid number of 46 chromosomes. *In humans, this disorder is the most common and clinically significant of numeric chromosomal abnormalities.* It occurs in 3% to 4% of clinically recognized pregnancies. An **aneuploid** is an individual who has a chromosome number that is not an exact multiple of the haploid number of 23 (e.g., 45, 47). A **polyploid** is a person who has a chromosome number that is a multiple of the haploid number of 23 other than the diploid number (e.g., 69) (see Fig. 20-10).

The principal cause of aneuploidy is nondisjunction during cell division (see Fig. 20-2), which results in an unequal distribution of one pair of homologous chromosomes to the daughter cells. One cell has two chromosomes, and the other has neither chromosome of the pair. As a result, the embryo's cells may be hypodiploid (45,X as in Turner syndrome) (Figs. 20-3 to 20-5) or **hyperdiploid** (usually 47, as in trisomy 21 [Down syndrome]) (Fig. 20-6). Embryos with **monosomy** (missing a chromosome) usually die. *Approximately 99% of embryos lacking a sex chromosome (e.g., 45,X) abort spontaneously* (see Fig. 20-5).

**FIGURE 20–3** Female infant with Turner syndrome (45,X). **A,** Face of the infant. **B,** Lateral view of the infant's head and neck shows a short, webbed neck and prominent ears. Infants with this syndrome have defective gonadal development (gonadal dysgenesis). **C,** The infant's feet show the characteristic lymphedema (puffiness and swelling), which is a useful diagnostic sign. **D,** Lymphedema of the toes is a condition that usually leads to nail underdevelopment (hypoplasia).

**FIGURE 20-4** Turner syndrome (45,X) in a 14-year-old girl. Features of the syndrome include short stature; a webbed neck; absence of sexual maturation; a broad chest with widely spaced nipples; and lymphedema swelling of the hands and feet.

**FIGURE 20-5** Female fetus with Turner syndrome (45,X) at 16 weeks. Notice the excessive accumulation of watery fluid (hydrops) and the large cystic hygroma (lymphangioma) in the posterior head and cervical region. The hygroma causes the loose neck skin and webbing seen postnatally (see Fig. 20-3B).

## Turner Syndrome

*Approximately 1% of monosomy X female embryos survives;* the incidence of 45,X (Turner syndrome) in female neonates is approximately 1 in 8000 live births. One half of affected individuals have 45,X; the others have a variety of abnormalities of a sex chromosome. *The phenotype of Turner syndrome is female* (see Figs. 20-3 to 20-5). Secondary sexual characteristics do not develop in 90% of affected females, and hormone replacement is required.

**Phenotype** refers to the morphologic characteristics of a person as determined by the genotype and environment in which it is expressed. The **monosomy X chromosome abnormality** is the most common cytogenetic abnormality observed in fetuses that abort spontaneously (see Fig. 20-5); it accounts for approximately 18% of all abortions caused by chromosomal abnormalities. The error in gametogenesis (**nondisjunction**) that causes monosomy X (Turner syndrome), when it can be traced, is in the paternal gamete (sperm) in approximately 75% of cases; it is the paternal X chromosome that is usually missing. The most frequent chromosome constitution in **Turner syndrome** is 45,X; however, almost 50% of these people have other **karyotypes** (chromosomal characteristics of an individual cell or cell line).

## Trisomy of Autosomes

Three chromosome copies in a given chromosome pair is called **trisomy**. *Trisomies are the most common abnormalities of chromosome number.* The usual cause of this numeric error is **meiotic nondisjunction of chromosomes** (see Fig. 20-2), which results in a gamete with 24 instead of 23 chromosomes and subsequently in a zygote with 47 chromosomes. Trisomy of autosomes is mainly associated with three syndromes (Table 20-1):

- Trisomy 21 or Down syndrome (see Fig. 20-6)
- Trisomy 18 or Edwards syndrome (Fig. 20-7)
- Trisomy 13 or Patau syndrome (Fig. 20-8)

**FIGURE 20–6** A, Anterior view of a female fetus with Down syndrome (trisomy 21) at 16.5 weeks. B, Hand of the fetus shows the single, transverse palmar flexion crease (simian crease, *arrow*) and the clinodactyly (incurving) of the fifth digit. C, Anterior view of the faces of dizygotic male twins that are discordant for Down syndrome (trisomy 21). The smaller twin has Down syndrome and developed from a zygote that contained an extra chromosome 21. The characteristic facial features of the syndrome in this infant include upslanting palpebral fissures, epicanthal folds, and a flat nasal bridge. D, A girl aged 2 years 6 months has Down syndrome.

*Infants with trisomy 13 and trisomy 18 are severely malformed and mentally deficient;* they usually die early in infancy. More than one half of **trisomic embryos** spontaneously abort early. *Trisomy of the autosomes occurs with increasing frequency as maternal age increases.* For example, trisomy 21 occurs once in approximately 1400 births among mothers between the ages of 20 and 24 years but once in approximately 25 births among mothers 45 years and older (Table 20-2). Trisomy 13 syndrome is the most common chromosomal abnormality in neonates (1 in 12,000).

*Errors in meiosis occur with increasing maternal age,* and the most common aneuploidy seen in older mothers is trisomy 21 (**Down syndrome**) (see Fig. 20-6).

| Table 20–1 | Trisomy of Autosomes | |
|---|---|---|

| CHROMOSOMAL ABERRATION AND SYNDROME | INCIDENCE | USUAL CLINICAL MANIFESTATIONS |
|---|---|---|
| Trisomy 21 (Down syndrome)* (see Fig. 20-6) | 1 in 800 | Mental deficiency; brachycephaly, flat nasal bridge; upward slant to palpebral fissures; protruding tongue; transverse palmar flexion crease; clinodactyly of the fifth digit; congenital heart defects; gastrointestinal tract abnormalities |
| Trisomy 18 syndrome (Edwards syndrome)† (see Fig. 20-7) | 1 in 8000 | Mental deficiency; growth retardation; prominent occiput; short sternum; ventricular septal defect; micrognathia; low-set, malformed ears, flexed digits, hypoplastic nails; rocker-bottom feet |
| Trisomy 13 syndrome (Patau syndrome)† (see Fig. 20-8) | 1 in 12,000 | Mental deficiency; severe central nervous system malformations; sloping forehead; malformed ears, scalp defects; microphthalmia; bilateral cleft lip and/or palate; polydactyly; posterior prominence of the heels |

*The importance of this disorder in the overall problem of mental deficiency is indicated by the fact that persons with Down syndrome represent 10% to 15% of institutionalized individuals with severe mental retardation. The incidence of trisomy 21 at fertilization is greater than at birth; however, 75% of embryos are spontaneously aborted, and at least 20% are stillborn.
†Infants with this syndrome rarely survive beyond 6 months.

**FIGURE 20–7** A female neonate with the trisomy 18 syndrome has growth retardation, clenched fists with characteristic positioning of the fingers (second and fifth ones overlapping the third and fourth ones), short sternum, and narrow pelvis.

| Table 20–2 | Incidence of Down Syndrome among Neonates |
|---|---|

| MATERNAL AGE (YEARS) | INCIDENCE |
|---|---|
| 20–24 | 1 in 1400 |
| 25–29 | 1 in 1100 |
| 30–34 | 1 in 700 |
| 35 | 1 in 350 |
| 37 | 1 in 225 |
| 39 | 1 in 140 |
| 41 | 1 in 85 |
| 43 | 1 in 50 |
| 45+ | 1 in 30 |

**FIGURE 20–8** A female neonate with trisomy 13 syndrome has a bilateral cleft lip, low-set and malformed left ear, and polydactyly (extra digits). A small omphalocele (herniation of viscera into umbilical cord) can be seen.

Because of the current trend of increasing maternal age, it has been estimated that by the end of this decade, children born to women older than 34 years will account for 39% of infants with trisomy 21. Translocation or mosaicism occurs in approximately 5% of the affected children. **Mosaicism**, which is a condition in which two or more cell types contain different numbers of chromosomes (normal and abnormal), leads to a less severe phenotype, and the IQ of the child may be almost normal.

**Table 20–3** Trisomy of Chromosomes

| CHROMOSOME COMPLEMENT* | SEX | INCIDENCE† | USUAL CHARACTERISTICS |
|---|---|---|---|
| 47,XXX | Female | 1 in 1000 | Normal in appearance; usually fertile; 15% to 25% are mildly mentally deficient |
| 47,XXY | Male | 1 in 1000 | Klinefelter syndrome: small testes, hyalinization of seminiferous tubules; aspermatogenesis; often tall with disproportionately long lower limbs. Intelligence of siblings is less than normal. Approximately 40% of these males have gynecomastia (see Fig. 20-9). |
| 47,XYY | Male | 1 in 1000 | Normal in appearance, usually tall, and often exhibit aggressive behavior |

*The numbers designate the total number of chromosomes, including the sex chromosomes shown after the comma.
†Data from Hook EB, Hamerton JL: The frequency of chromosome abnormalities detected in consecutive newborn studies; differences between studies; results by sex and by severity of phenotypic involvement. In Hook EB, Porter IH, editors: *Population cytogenetics: studies in humans*, New York, 1977, Academic Press. More information is provided by Nussbaum RL, McInnes RR, Willard HF: *Thompson and Thompson genetics in medicine*, ed 7, Philadelphia, 2007, Saunders.

**FIGURE 20–9** A male adolescent with Klinefelter syndrome (XXY trisomy) has breasts. Approximately 40% of males with this syndrome have gynecomastia (development of breasts) and small testes.

## Trisomy of Sex Chromosomes

Trisomy of the sex chromosomes is a common disorder (Table 20-3). However, because there are no characteristic physical findings in infants or children, the disorder is not usually detected until puberty (Fig. 20-9). **Sex chromatin studies** have detected some types of trisomy because two masses of sex chromatin are found in the nuclei of **XXX females** (trisomy X), and the nuclei of **XXY males** (Klinefelter syndrome) contain a mass of sex chromatin (see Table 20-3 and Fig. 20-9). Diagnosis is best achieved by **chromosome analysis** or other molecular cytogenetic techniques.

## TETRASOMY AND PENTASOMY

Persons with tetrasomy or pentasomy have cell nuclei with four or five sex chromosomes, respectively. Several chromosome complexes have been reported in females (48,XXXX and 49,XXXXX) and in males (48,XXXY, 48,XXYY, 49,XXXYY, and 49,XXXXY). The extra sex chromosomes do not accentuate sexual characteristics. However, the greater the number of sex chromosomes in males, the greater the severity of mental deficiency and physical impairment. The **tetrasomy X syndrome** (48,XXXX) is associated with serious mental deficiency and physical development. The **pentasomy X syndrome** (49,XXXXX) usually includes severe metal deficiency and multiple physical defects.

## MOSAICISM

A person with at least two cell lines with two or more **genotypes** (genetic constitutions) is a **mosaic**. The autosomes or sex chromosomes may be involved. The defects usually are less serious than in persons with monosomy or trisomy. For instance, the features of Turner syndrome are not as evident in 45,X/46,XX **mosaic females** as in the usual 45,X females. Mosaicism usually results from nondisjunction during early cleavage of the zygote (see Chapter 2, Fig. 2-16). Mosaicism resulting from **loss of a chromosome by anaphase lagging** also occurs. The chromosomes separate normally, but one of them is delayed in its migration and is eventually lost.

## TRIPLOIDY

The most common type of **polyploidy** (cell nucleus containing three or more haploid sets) (see Chapter 2, Fig. 2-1) is **triploid fetus** (69 chromosomes). **Triploid fetuses** have severe **intrauterine growth retardation** with severe head-body disproportion (Fig. 20-10). Although triploid fetuses are born, they do not survive very long.

**Triploidy** most frequently results from fertilization of an oocyte by two sperms (**dispermy**). Failure of one of the meiotic divisions (see Chapter 2, Fig. 2-1), resulting in a **diploid oocyte or sperm**, may account for some cases. **Triploid fetuses** account for approximately 20% of chromosomally abnormal spontaneous abortions.

## TETRAPLOIDY

Doubling of the diploid chromosome number from 46 to 92 (**tetraploidy**) probably occurs during the first cleavage division of the zygote (see Chapter 2, Fig. 2-17A). Division of this abnormal zygote subsequently results in an embryo with cells containing 92 chromosomes. *Tetraploid embryos abort very early*, and often all that is recovered is an empty chorionic sac (*blighted embryo*).

## Structural Chromosomal Abnormalities

Most structural chromosomal abnormalities result from **chromosome breakage**, followed by reconstitution in an abnormal combination (Fig. 20-11). The breakage may be **induced by environmental factors** such as ionizing radiation, viral infections, drugs, and chemicals. The type of structural abnormality depends on what happens to the broken chromosome pieces. The only two aberrations of chromosome structure that are likely to be transmitted from a parent to an embryo are **structural rearrangements**, such as inversion and translocation. Overall, structural abnormalities of chromosomes occur in about 1 in 375 neonates.

### Translocation

**Translocation** is the transfer of a piece of one chromosome to a nonhomologous chromosome. If two nonhomologous chromosomes exchange pieces, it is called a **reciprocal translocation** (see Fig. 20-11A and G). *Translocation does not necessarily cause abnormal development.* For example, persons with a translocation between a number 21 chromosome and a number 14 chromosome (see Fig. 20-11G) are phenotypically normal. They are called **balanced translocation carriers**. They have a tendency, independent of age, to produce germ cells with an **abnormal translocation chromosome**. Between 3% and 4% of infants with Down syndrome have **translocation trisomies;** the extra chromosome 21 is attached to another chromosome.

### Deletion

When a chromosome breaks, part of it may be lost (see Fig. 20-11B). A partial terminal deletion from the short arm of chromosome 5 causes the **cri du chat syndrome** (Fig. 20-12). Affected infants have a weak cat-like cry, microcephaly (small neurocranium), severe mental deficiency, and congenital heart disease.

A **ring chromosome** is a type of deletion chromosome from which both ends have been lost, and the broken ends have rejoined to form a **ring-shaped chromosome** (see Fig. 20-11C). *Ring chromosomes are rare, but they have been found for all chromosomes.* These abnormal chromosomes have been described in persons with **45,X** (Turner syndrome), **trisomy 18** (Edwards syndrome), and other structural chromosomal abnormalities.

**FIGURE 20-10** Triploid fetus (69 chromosomes) illustrates severe head-to-body disproportion. Triploid fetuses account for almost 20% of chromosomally abnormal miscarriages. *(From Crane JP: Ultrasound evaluation of fetal chromosome disorders. In Callen PW, editor: Ultrasonography in obstetrics and gynecology, ed 3, Philadelphia, 1994, Saunders.)*

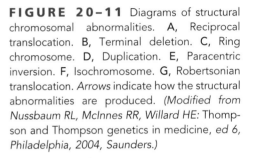

**FIGURE 20–11** Diagrams of structural chromosomal abnormalities. **A**, Reciprocal translocation. **B**, Terminal deletion. **C**, Ring chromosome. **D**, Duplication. **E**, Paracentric inversion. **F**, Isochromosome. **G**, Robertsonian translocation. *Arrows* indicate how the structural abnormalities are produced. *(Modified from Nussbaum RL, McInnes RR, Willard HE: Thompson and Thompson genetics in medicine, ed 6, Philadelphia, 2004, Saunders.)*

**FIGURE 20–12** A, Male child with cri du chat syndrome (cat-like cry) has microcephaly and hypertelorism (increased distance between orbits). B, Partial karyotype of the child shows a terminal deletion of the short arm (end) of chromosome 5. The *arrow* indicates the site of the deletion. *(A, From Gardner EJ: Principles of genetics, ed 5, New York, 1975, John Wiley & Sons.)*

## MICRODELETION AND MICRODUPLICATION

With **high-resolution banding techniques**, very small interstitial and terminal **deletions in several chromosomal disorders** have been detected. An acceptable resolution of chromosome banding on routine analysis reveals 550 bands per haploid set, whereas high-resolution chromosome banding reveals up to 1300 bands per haploid set. Because the deletions span several contiguous genes, these disorders and those with microduplications are referred to as **contiguous gene syndromes** (Table 20-4), as in these examples:

- **Prader-Willi syndrome** (PWS) is a sporadically occurring disorder associated with short stature, mild mental deficiency, obesity, **hyperphagia** (overeating), and hypogonadism.
- **Angelman syndrome** (AS) is characterized by severe mental deficiency, **microcephaly, brachycephaly,** seizures, and **ataxic (jerky) movements** of the limbs and trunk.

PWS and AS are often associated with a visible deletion of band q12 on chromosome 15. The clinical phenotype is determined by the parental origin of the deleted chromosome 15. If the deletion is in the mother, AS occurs; if passed on by the father, the child exhibits the PWS phenotype. This suggests the phenomenon of **genetic imprinting**, in which differential expression of genetic material depends on the sex of the transmitting parent. One of the two parental alleles is active and the other inactive because of epigenetic factors. Loss of expression of the active allele leads to neurodevelopmental disorders.

## MOLECULAR CYTOGENETICS

Methods for merging classic cytogenetics with **DNA technology** have facilitated precise definitions of chromosome abnormalities, location, and origins, including unbalanced translocations, accessory or marker chromosomes, and **gene mapping**. One approach to chromosome identification is based on **fluorescent in situ hybridization (FISH)**, in which chromosome-specific **DNA probes** adhere to complementary regions located on specific chromosomes. This allows improved identification of chromosome location and number in metaphase spreads or interphase cells. **FISH techniques** applied to interphase cells may soon obviate the need to culture cells for specific chromosome analysis, as in the case of **prenatal diagnosis of fetal trisomies**.

Studies using **subtelomeric FISH probes** in individuals with mental deficiency of unknown origin, with or without birth defects, have identified **submicroscopic chromosome deletions** or duplications in 5% to 10% of these individuals. Alterations in DNA sequence copy number are identified in solid tumors and are associated with developmental abnormalities and mental deficiency.

**Comparative genomic hybridization (CGH)** can detect and map changes in specific regions of the genome. **Microarray-based CGH** (array comparative genomic hybridization) is being used to identify genomic rearrangements in individuals who were previously considered to have mental deficiency or multiple birth defects of unknown origin despite normal test results from traditional chromosome or gene analysis. These investigations have become important in the routine evaluation of patients with previously unexplained mental deficiency, autism, and multiple congenital anomalies.

## DUPLICATIONS

Some abnormalities are represented as a duplicated part of a chromosome within a chromosome (see Fig. 20-11D), attached to a chromosome, or as a separate fragment. *Duplications are more common than deletions and are less harmful because there is no loss of genetic material.* However, the resulting phenotype often includes mental impairment or birth defects. Duplication may involve part of a gene, a whole gene, or a series of genes.

## INVERSION

Inversion is a chromosomal aberration in which a segment of a chromosome is reversed. **Paracentric inversion** is confined to a single arm of the chromosome (see Fig. 20-11E), whereas **pericentric inversion** involves both arms and includes the centromere. **Carriers of pericentric inversions** risk having offspring with birth defects because of unequal crossing over and malsegregation at meiosis (see Chapter 2, Fig. 2-2).

| Table 20–4 | Contiguous Gene Syndromes | | |
| --- | --- | --- | --- |
| SYNDROME | CLINICAL FEATURES | CHROMOSOME FINDINGS | PARENTAL ORIGIN |
| Prader-Willi | Hypotonia, hypogonadism, extreme obesity with hyperphagia, distinct face, short stature, small hands and feet, mild developmental delay, learning disability | del 15 q12 (most cases) | Paternal |
| Angelman | Microcephaly, macrosomia, ataxia, excessive laughter, seizures, severe mental deficiency | del 15 q12 (most cases) | Maternal |
| Miller-Dieker | Type 1 lissencephaly, dysmorphic face, seizures, severe developmental delay, cardiac defects | del 17 p13.3 (most cases) | Either parent |
| DiGeorge | Thymic hypoplasia, parathyroid hypoplasia, conotruncal cardiac defects, facial dysmorphism | del 22 q11 (some cases) | Either parent |
| Velocardiofacial (Shprintzen) | Palatal defects, hypoplastic alae nasi, long nose, conotruncal cardiac defects, speech delay, learning disorder, schizophrenia-like disorder | del 22 q11 (most cases) | Either parent |
| Smith-Magenis | Brachycephaly, broad nasal bridge, prominent jaw, short and broad hands, speech delay, mental deficiency | del 17 p11.2 | Either parent |
| Williams | Short stature; hypercalcemia; cardiac defects, especially supravalvular aortic stenosis; characteristic elfin-like face; mental deficiency | del 17 q11.23 (most cases) | Either parent |
| Beckwith-Wiedemann | Macrosomia, macroglossia, omphalocele (some cases), hypoglycemia, hemihypertrophy, transverse ear lobes | dup 11 p15 (some cases) | Paternal |

## ISOCHROMOSOMES

An **isochromosome** results when the centromere divides transversely instead of longitudinally (see Fig. 20-11E), creating a chromosome in which one arm is missing and the other is duplicated. *This chromosome appears to be the most common structural abnormality of the X chromosome.* Persons with this aberration often have short stature and the other **stigmata** (visible evidence of disease) of **Turner syndrome** (see Figs. 20-3 to 20-5). These characteristics are related to the loss of an arm of an X chromosome.

## Birth Defects Caused by Mutant Genes

*Between 7% and 8% of birth defects are caused by gene defects* (see Fig. 20-1). A **mutation**, usually involving a loss or change in the function of a gene, is any permanent, heritable change in the sequence of genomic DNA. Because a random change is unlikely to lead to an improvement in development, *most mutations are deleterious, and some are lethal.*

The **mutation rate** can be increased by a number of environmental agents, such as *large doses of ionizing radiation.* Defects resulting from gene mutations are inherited according to mendelian laws (laws of inheritance of single-gene traits that form the basis of the science of genetics); consequently, predictions can be made about the probability of their *occurrence in the affected person's children and other relatives.* An example

of a dominantly inherited birth defect is **achondroplasia** (Fig. 20-13), which results from a G-to-A transition mutation at nucleotide 1138 of the cDNA in the fibroblast growth factor receptor 3 gene on chromosome 4p. Other defects, such as **congenital suprarenal hyperplasia** (see Fig. 20-18) and **microcephaly** (see Chapter 17, Fig. 17-36), are attributed to autosomal recessive inheritance. *Autosomal recessive genes manifest only when homozygous*; as a consequence, many carriers of these genes (heterozygotes) remain undetected.

**Fragile X syndrome** is the second most commonly inherited cause of moderate intellectual disability after Down syndrome (Fig. 20-14). It is one of more than 200 X-linked disorders associated with mental impairment. Fragile X syndrome occurs in 1 of 4000 male births. Autism spectrum disorders are prevalent in this condition. Diagnosis of this syndrome can be confirmed by chromosome analysis demonstrating the fragile X chromosome at Xq27.3 or by DNA studies showing an expansion of CGG nucleotides in a specific region of the *FMR1* gene.

Several genetic disorders are caused by **expansion of trinucleotides** (combination of three adjacent nucleotides) in specific genes. Other examples include *myotonic dystrophy, Huntington chorea, spinobulbar atrophy* (Kennedy syndrome), *Friedreich ataxia,* and others. X-linked recessive genes usually manifest in affected (hemizygous) males and occasionally in carrier (heterozygous) females, as in Fragile X syndrome (see Fig. 20-14).

The *human genome comprises an estimated 20,000 to 25,000 genes per haploid set* or 3 billion base pairs. Because of the **Human Genome Project** and international research collaboration, many disease- and birth defect–causing mutations in genes have been and will continue

**FIGURE 20-13** A young boy with achondroplasia has short stature, short limbs and fingers, normal length of trunk, bowed legs, a relatively large head, a prominent forehead, and a depressed nasal bridge.

to be identified. Most genes will be sequenced and their specific function determined.

Determining the causes of birth defects requires a better understanding of gene expression during early development. Most genes are expressed in a wide variety of cells and are involved in basic cellular metabolic functions, such as nucleic acid and protein synthesis, cytoskeleton and organelle biogenesis, and nutrient transport and other cellular mechanisms. These genes are referred to as **housekeeping genes.** The specialty genes are expressed at specific times in specific cells and define the hundreds of cell types that make up the human organism. *An essential aspect of developmental biology is **regulation of gene expression.*** Regulation is often achieved by transcription factors that bind to regulatory or promoter elements of specific genes.

**Epigenetic regulation** refers to changes in phenotype (appearance) or gene expression caused by mechanisms other than changes in the underlying DNA sequence. The mechanisms of epigenetic change are not entirely clear, but modifying transcriptional factors, DNA methylation, and histone modification may be key in altering developmental events. Several birth defects, including neurodevelopmental problems (e.g., autism spectrum disorder), may be the result of altered gene expression due to environmental chemicals, drugs, and maternal stress or altered nutrition rather than changes in DNA sequences.

**Genomic imprinting** is an epigenetic process in which the allele inherited from the mother or father is marked by methylation (imprinted), silencing the gene and allowing expression of the nonimprinted gene from the other parent. Only the **paternal or maternal allele** (any one of a series of two or more different genes) of a gene is active in the offspring. The sex of the transmitting parent therefore influences expression or nonexpression of certain genes (see Table 20-4).

In Prader-Willi syndrome (**PWS**) and Angelman syndrome (**AS**) the phenotype is determined by whether the

**FIGURE 20-14** Siblings with fragile X syndrome. A, An 8-year-old mentally deficient boy has a relatively normal appearance with a long face and prominent ears. B, His 6-year-old sister, who also has this syndrome, has a mild learning disability and similar features of a long face and prominent ears. Notice the strabismus (crossed right eye). Although it is an X-linked disorder, female carriers sometimes express the disease.

microdeletion is transmitted by the father (PWS) or the mother (AS). In a substantial number of cases of PWS and AS and in several other genetic disorders, the condition arises from a phenomenon referred to as **uniparental disomy**. In PWS and AS, both copies of chromosome 15 originate from only one parent. PWS occurs when both are derived from the mother, and AS occurs when both are paternally derived. The mechanism is thought to begin with a trisomic conceptus, followed by a loss of the extra chromosome in an early postzygotic cell division. This results in a "rescued" cell in which both chromosomes have been derived from one parent.

Uniparental disomy has involved several chromosome pairs. Some are associated with adverse clinical outcomes involving pairs of chromosome 6 (transient neonatal diabetes mellitus), 7 (Silver-Russell syndrome), and 15 (PWS and AS), whereas others (1 and 22) are not associated with abnormal phenotypic effects.

**Homeobox genes are found in all vertebrates.** They have highly conserved sequences and order. They are involved in early embryonic development and specify identity and spatial arrangements of body segments. Protein products of these genes bind to DNA and form transcriptional factors that regulate gene expression. Disorders associated with some homeobox gene mutations are described in Table 20-5.

## Developmental Signaling Pathways

Normal embryogenesis is regulated by several complex signaling cascades (see Chapter 21). *Mutations or alterations in any of these signaling pathways can lead to birth defects.* Many pathways are cell autonomous and alter the differentiation of only that particular cell, as seen in proteins produced by *HOXA* and *HOXD* gene clusters (in which mutations lead to a variety of limb defects). Other **transcriptional factors** act by influencing the pattern of gene expression of adjacent cells. These short-range signal controls can act as simple on-off switches *(paracrine signals)*; those called **morphogens** elicit many responses in target cells depending on their level of expression (concentration).

One developmental signaling pathway is initiated by the secreted protein called **sonic hedgehog** (SHH) that sets off a chain of events resulting in activation and repression of target cells by transcription factors in the GLI family. Perturbations (disturbances) in the regulation of the Shh-Patched-Gli (SHH-PTCH-GLI) signaling pathway lead to several human diseases, including some cancers and birth defects.

SHH is expressed in the notochord, the floor plate of the neural tube, the brain, and other regions, such as the zone of polarizing activity of the developing limbs and the gut. Sporadic and inherited mutations in the human *SHH* gene leads to **holoprosencephaly** (see Chapter 17, Fig. 17-40), a midline defect of variable severity involving abnormal CNS septation, facial clefting, single central incisor, hypotelorism, or a single cyclopic eye (see Chapter 18, Fig. 18-6). The SHH protein needs to be processed to an active form and is modified by the addition of a cholesterol moiety. Defects in cholesterol biosynthesis, such as in the autosomal recessive disorder **Smith-Lemli-Opitz syndrome** (mental deficiency, small stature, ptosis, and male genital defects), share many features, particularly brain and limb defects reminiscent of SHH-related diseases. This suggests that signaling through SHH may play a key role in several genetic disorders.

Three transcriptional factors encoded by *GLI* genes are in the SHH-PTCH-GLI pathway. Mutations in the *GLI3* gene have been implicated in several autosomal dominant disorders, including **Greig cephalopolysyndactyly syndrome** (deletions or point mutations); **Pallister-Hall syndrome** with hypothalamic hamartomas, central or postaxial polydactyly, and other defects of the face, brain, and limbs (frameshift or nonsense mutations); simple familial postaxial polydactyly type A and B; and preaxial polydactyly type IV (nonsense, missense, and frameshift mutations).

A comprehensive, authoritative, and daily updated listing of all known human genetic disorders and gene loci can be found at the Online Mendelian Inheritance in Man (OMIM) website (www.ncbi.nlm.nih.gov/omim). The OMIM is maintained by the McKusick-Nathans Institute for Genetic Medicine at Johns Hopkins University

| Table 20–5 | Human Disorders Associated with Homeobox Mutations | |
| --- | --- | --- |
| **SYNDROME** | **CLINICAL FEATURES** | **GENE** |
| Waardenburg syndrome (type I) | White forelock, lateral displacement of medial canthi of the eyes, cochlear deafness, heterochromia, tendency to facial clefting, autosomal dominant inheritance | *PAX3* (formerly *HUP2*) gene, homologous to mouse *Pax3* gene |
| Synpolydactyly (type II syndactyly) | Webbing and duplication of fingers, supernumerary metacarpals, autosomal dominant inheritance | *HOXD13* mutation |
| Holoprosencephaly (one form) | Incomplete separation of lateral cerebral ventricles, anophthalmia or cyclopia, midline facial hypoplasia or clefts, single maxillary central incisors, hypotelorism, autosomal dominant inheritance with widely variable expression | *SHH* (formerly *HPE3*) mutation, homologous to the *Drosophila* sonic hedgehog gene for segment polarity |
| Schizencephaly (type II) | Full-thickness cleft within the cerebral ventricles often leading to seizures, spasticity, and mental deficiency | Germline mutation in the *EMX2* homeobox gene, homologous to the mouse *Emx2* |

and by the National Center for Biotechnology Information at the National Library of Medicine.

# BIRTH DEFECTS CAUSED BY ENVIRONMENTAL FACTORS

Although the human embryo is well protected in the uterus, many environmental agents (**teratogens**) may cause developmental disruptions after maternal exposure to them (Table 20-6). *A teratogen is any agent that can produce a birth defect (congenital anomaly) or increase the incidence of a defect in the population.* **Environmental factors** (e.g., infections, drugs) may simulate genetic conditions, as when two or more children of normal parents are affected. *An important principle is that not everything that is familial is genetic.*

The organs and parts of an embryo are most sensitive to teratogenic agents during periods of rapid differentiation (Fig. 20-15). Environmental factors cause 7% to 10% of birth defects (see Fig. 20-1). Because biochemical differentiation precedes morphologic differentiation, the period during which structures are sensitive to interference by teratogens often precedes the stage of their visible development by a few days.

*Teratogens do not appear to cause defects until cellular differentiation has begun*; however, their early actions (e.g., during the first 2 weeks) may cause death of the embryo. The exact mechanisms by which drugs, chemicals, and other environmental factors disrupt embryonic development and induce abnormalities remain obscure. Even thalidomide's mechanisms of action on the embryo are a mystery, and more than 20 hypotheses have been postulated to explain how this **hypnotic agent** disrupts embryonic development.

Many studies have shown that certain hereditary and environmental influences may adversely affect embryonic development by altering fundamental processes such as the intracellular compartment, surface of the cell, extracellular matrix, and fetal environment. It has been suggested that the initial cellular response may take more than one form (genetic, molecular, biochemical, or biophysical), resulting in different sequences of cellular changes (cell death, faulty cellular interaction or induction, reduced biosynthesis of substrates, impaired morphogenetic movements, and mechanical disruption). Eventually, these different types of pathologic lesion may lead to the final defect (intrauterine death, developmental defects, fetal growth retardation, or functional disturbances) through a common pathway.

Rapid progress in molecular biology is providing more information about the genetic control of differentiation and the cascade of events involved in the expression of homeobox genes and pattern formation. It is reasonable to speculate that disruption of gene activity at any critical stage could lead to a developmental defect. This view is supported by studies that showed that exposure of mouse and amphibian embryos to the teratogen **retinoic acid** (metabolite of vitamin A) altered gene expression domains and disrupted normal morphogenesis. **Retinoic acid is highly teratogenic.** Researchers are focusing on the molecular mechanisms of abnormal development in an attempt to understand better the pathogenesis of birth defects.

## Principles of Teratogenesis

When considering the possible teratogenicity of a drug or chemical, *three important principles must be considered:*

- Critical periods of development
- Dose of the drug or chemical
- Genotype (genetic constitution) of the embryo

## Critical Periods of Human Development

The embryo's stage of development when it encounters a drug or virus determines its susceptibility to the teratogen (see Fig. 20-15). The most critical period of development is when cell division, cell differentiation, and morphogenesis are at their peak. Table 20-7 indicates the relative frequencies of birth defects for certain organs.

The **critical period for brain development is from 3 to 16 weeks,** but development may be disrupted after this because the brain is differentiating and growing rapidly at birth. Teratogens may produce mental deficiency during the embryonic and fetal periods (see Fig. 20-15).

**Tooth development** continues long after birth (see Chapter 19, Table 19-1). Development of permanent teeth may be disrupted by **tetracyclines** from 14 weeks of fetal life up to 8 years after birth (see Chapter 19, Fig. 19-20E). The **skeletal system** also has a prolonged critical period of development extending into childhood, and the growth of skeletal tissues provides a good gauge of general growth.

**Environmental disturbances** during the first 2 weeks after fertilization may interfere with cleavage of the zygote and implantation of the blastocyst and may cause early death and **spontaneous abortion of an embryo.** However, disturbances during the first 2 weeks are not known to cause birth defects (see Fig. 20-15). *Teratogens acting during the first 2 weeks kill the embryo or their disruptive effects are compensated for by powerful regulatory properties of the early embryo.* Most development during the first 4 weeks is concerned with the formation of extraembryonic structures such as the amnion, umbilical vesicle, and chorionic sac (see Chapter 3, Fig. 3-8 and Chapter 5, Figs. 5-1 and 5-18).

*Development of the embryo is most easily disrupted when the tissues and organs are forming* (Fig. 20-16, see Fig. 20-15). During this **organogenetic period** (4 to 8 weeks; see Chapter 1, Fig. 1-1), teratogens may induce major birth defects. **Physiologic defects** such as minor morphologic defects of the external ears and functional disturbances such as mental deficiency are likely to result from *disruption of development during the fetal period (ninth week to birth).* Some **microorganisms,** such as *Toxoplasma gondii,* cause serious birth defects, particularly of the brain and eyes, when they infect the fetus (see Figs. 20-22 and 20-23 and Table 20-6).

Each tissue, organ, and system of an embryo has a critical period during which its development may be disrupted (see Fig. 20-15). The type of birth defect produced

| Table 20–6 | Teratogens That Cause Human Birth Defects |
|---|---|

| AGENTS | MOST COMMON BIRTH DEFECTS |
|---|---|
| **Drugs** | |
| Alcohol | Fetal alcohol syndrome: IUGR, mental deficiency, microcephaly, ocular anomalies, joint abnormalities, short palpebral fissures |
| Androgens and high doses of progestogens | Various degrees of masculinization of female fetuses: ambiguous external genitalia resulting in labial fusion and clitoral hypertrophy |
| Aminopterin | IUGR; skeletal defects; CNS malformations, notably meroencephaly (most of the brain is absent) |
| Carbamazepine | NTD, craniofacial defects, developmental retardation |
| Cocaine | IUGR, prematurity, microcephaly, cerebral infarction, urogenital defects, neurobehavioral disturbances |
| Diethylstilbestrol | Abnormalities of uterus and vagina, cervical erosion and ridges |
| Isotretinoin (13-*cis*-retinoic acid) | Craniofacial abnormalities; NTDs such as spina bifida cystica; cardiovascular defects; cleft palate; thymic aplasia |
| Lithium carbonate | Various defects, usually involving the heart and great vessels |
| Methotrexate | Multiple defects, especially skeletal, involving the face, cranium, limbs, and vertebral column |
| Misoprostol | Limb abnormalities, ocular and cranial nerve defects, autism spectrum disorder |
| Phenytoin | Fetal hydantoin syndrome: IUGR, microcephaly, mental deficiency, ridged frontal suture, inner epicanthal folds, eyelid ptosis, broad and depressed nasal bridge, phalangeal hypoplasia |
| Tetracycline | Stained teeth, hypoplasia of enamel |
| Thalidomide | Abnormal development of limbs such as meromelia (partial absence) and amelia (complete absence); facial defects; systemic anomalies such as cardiac, kidney, and ocular defects |
| Trimethadione | Development delay, V-shaped eyebrows, low-set ears, cleft lip and/or palate |
| Valproic acid | Craniofacial anomalies, NTDs, cognitive abnormalities, often hydrocephalus, heart and skeletal defects |
| Warfarin | Nasal hypoplasia, stippled epiphyses, hypoplastic phalanges, eye anomalies, mental deficiency |
| **Chemicals** | |
| Methylmercury | Cerebral atrophy, spasticity, seizures, mental deficiency |
| Polychlorinated biphenyls | IUGR, skin discoloration |
| **Infections** | |
| Cytomegalovirus | Microcephaly, chorioretinitis, sensorineural hearing loss, delayed psychomotor/mental development, hepatosplenomegaly, hydrocephaly, cerebral palsy, brain (periventricular) calcification |
| Hepatitis B virus | Preterm birth, low birth weight, fetal macrosomia |
| Herpes simplex virus | Skin vesicles and scarring, chorioretinitis, hepatomegaly, thrombocytopenia, petechiae, hemolytic anemia, hydranencephaly |
| Human parvovirus B19 | Fetal anemia, nonimmune hydrops fetalis, fetal death |
| Rubella virus | IUGR, postnatal growth retardation, cardiac and great vessel abnormalities, microcephaly, sensorineural deafness, cataract, microphthalmos, glaucoma, pigmented retinopathy, mental deficiency, neonate bleeding, hepatosplenomegaly, osteopathy, tooth defects |
| *Toxoplasma gondii* | Microcephaly, mental deficiency, microphthalmia, hydrocephaly, chorioretinitis, cerebral calcifications, hearing loss, neurologic disturbance |
| *Treponema pallidum* | Hydrocephalus, congenital deafness, mental deficiency, abnormal teeth and bones |
| Venezuelan equine encephalitis virus | Microcephaly, microphthalmia, cerebral agenesis, CNS necrosis, hydrocephalus |
| Varicella virus | Cutaneous scars (dermatome distribution), neurologic defects (e.g., limb paresis [incomplete paralysis]), hydrocephaly, seizures, cataracts, microphthalmia, Horner syndrome, optic atrophy, nystagmus, chorioretinitis, microcephaly, mental deficiency, skeletal anomalies (e.g., hypoplasia of limbs, fingers, toes), urogenital anomalies |
| **Radiation** | |
| High levels of ionizing radiation | Microcephaly, mental deficiency, skeletal anomalies, growth retardation, cataracts |

*CNS,* Central nervous system; *IUGR,* intrauterine growth restriction; *NTD,* neural tube defect.

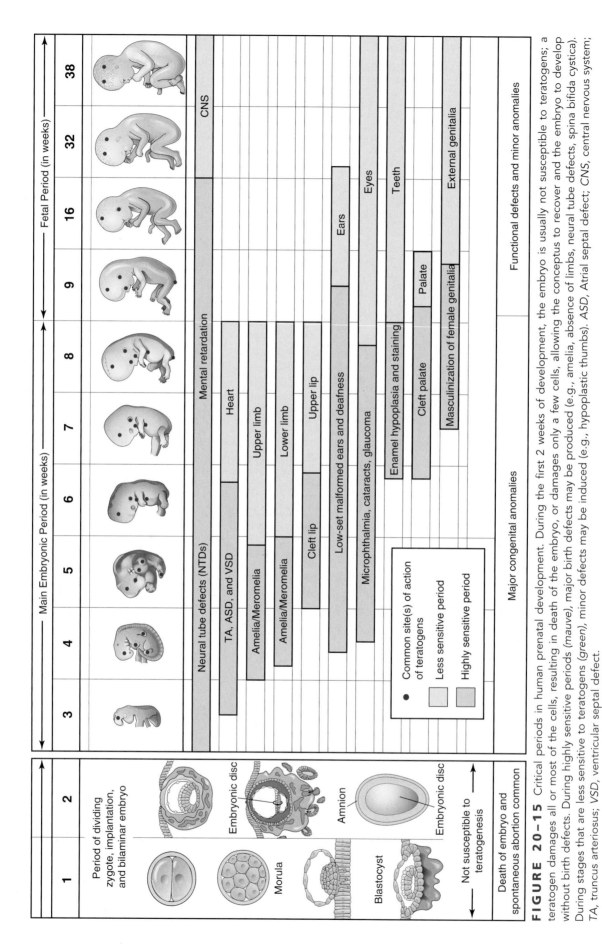

**FIGURE 20–15**  Critical periods in human prenatal development. During the first 2 weeks of development, the embryo is usually not susceptible to teratogens; a teratogen damages all or most of the cells, resulting in death of the cells, allowing the conceptus to recover and the embryo to develop without birth defects. During highly sensitive periods (*mauve*), major birth defects may be produced (e.g., amelia, absence of limbs, neural tube defects, spina bifida cystica). During stages that are less sensitive to teratogens (*green*), minor defects may be induced (e.g., hypoplastic thumbs). *ASD*, Atrial septal defect; *CNS*, central nervous system; *TA*, truncus arteriosus; *VSD*, ventricular septal defect.

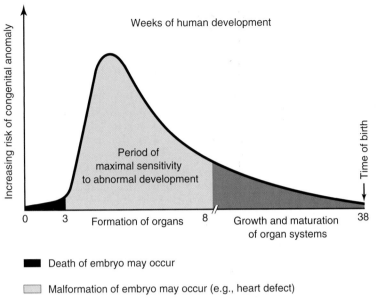

Weeks of human development

Increasing risk of congenital anomaly

Period of maximal sensitivity to abnormal development

Time of birth

0    3    Formation of organs    8    Growth and maturation of organ systems    38

**FIGURE 20–16** The risk of birth defects increases during organogenesis.

■ Death of embryo may occur

▨ Malformation of embryo may occur (e.g., heart defect)

■ Functional disturbance of fetus may occur (e.g., mental deficiency)

| Table 20–7 | Major Defects in Human Organs at Birth |
| --- | --- |
| **ORGAN** | **INCIDENCE** |
| Brain | 10 in 1000 |
| Heart | 8 in 1000 |
| Kidneys | 4 in 1000 |
| Limbs | 2 in 1000 |
| All other | 6 in 1000 |
| Total | 30 in 1000 |

Data from Connor JM, Ferguson-Smith MA: *Essential medical genetics,* ed 2, Oxford, UK, 1987, Blackwell Scientific Publications.

depends on which parts, tissues, and organs are most susceptible at the time the teratogen is encountered. Several examples show how teratogens may affect different organ systems that are developing at the same time:

- **High levels of ionizing radiation** produce defects of the CNS (brain and spinal cord) and eyes.
- **Rubella virus infection** causes eye defects (glaucoma and cataracts), deafness, and cardiac defects.
- **Drugs such as thalidomide** induce limb defects and other anomalies such as cardiac and kidney defects.

Early in the critical period of limb development, thalidomide causes severe defects such as meromelia, which is an absence of parts of the upper and lower limbs (see Fig. 20-20). Later in the sensitive period, thalidomide causes mild to moderate limb defects such as hypoplasia of the radius and ulna.

**Embryologic timetables** (see Fig. 20-15) are helpful when considering the cause of a human birth defect, but

it is wrong to assume that defects always result from a single event occurring during the critical period or that it is possible to determine from these tables the exact day the defect was produced. It can only be stated that the teratogen would have had to disrupt development before the end of the critical period for the tissue, part, or organ. For example, the critical period for limb development is 24 to 36 days after fertilization (see Chapter 1, Fig. 1-1).

## Dose of Drugs or Chemicals

Animal research has shown that there is a dose-response relationship for teratogens, but the dose used in animals to produce defects is often at levels much higher than human exposures. Consequently, *animal studies are not readily applicable to human pregnancies.* For a drug to be considered a **human teratogen**, a dose-response relationship has to be observed, and the greater the exposure during pregnancy, the more severe the phenotypic effect.

## Genotype of Embryo

Numerous examples in experimental animals and several suspected cases in humans show that there are genetic differences in response to a teratogen. **Phenytoin**, for example, is a well-known human teratogen (see Table 20-6). Between 5% and 10% of embryos exposed to this anticonvulsant medication develop the **fetal hydantoin syndrome** (see Fig. 20-19). Approximately one third of exposed embryos, however, have only some of the birth defects, and more than one half of the embryos are unaffected. It appears that the genotype of the embryo determines whether a teratogenic agent will disrupt its development.

## Human Teratogens

Awareness that certain agents can disrupt prenatal development offers the opportunity to prevent some birth defects. For example, if women are aware of the **harmful** effects of drugs such as alcohol, environmental chemicals (e.g., polychlorinated biphenyls), and some viruses, most will not expose their embryos to these teratogenic agents.

The objective of **teratogenicity testing** of drugs, chemicals, food additives, and pesticides is to identify agents that may cause malformations during human development and to alert pregnant women about the dangers to their embryos or fetuses.

## PROOF OF TERATOGENICITY

To prove that agents are teratogens, it must be shown that the frequency of defects is increased above the spontaneous rate in pregnancies in which the mother is exposed to the agent (**prospective approach**), or that *malformed infants* have a history of maternal exposure to the agent more often than normal children (**retrospective approach**). Both types of data are difficult to obtain in an unbiased form. *Case reports are not convincing unless both the agent and type of defect are so uncommon that their association in several cases can be judged not coincidental.*

## DRUG TESTING IN ANIMALS

Although testing of drugs in pregnant animals is important, the results are of limited value for predicting drug effects in human embryos. Animal experiments can suggest only that similar effects may occur in humans. If a drug or chemical produces teratogenic effects in two or more species, the probability of potential human hazard must be considered to be high, but the dose of the drug also must be considered.

### Drugs as Teratogens

*The teratogenicity of drugs varies considerably.* Some teratogens (e.g., **thalidomide**) cause severe disruption of development if administered during the organogenetic period from the fourth to eighth weeks (see Figs. 20-15 and 20-20). Other teratogens cause mental deficiency, growth restriction, and other defects if used excessively throughout development. In the case of alcohol, there is no safe amount during pregnancy.

*The use of prescription and nonprescription drugs during pregnancy is surprisingly high.* Between 40% and 90% of women consume at least one nonprescription drug during pregnancy. A report that was based on a database of prescribed drugs showed that pregnant women might be prescribed as many as 10 drugs. Several studies have indicated that some pregnant women take an average of four drugs, excluding nutritional supplements, and that approximately one half of these women take them during the highly sensitive period (see Fig. 20-15).

*Drug consumption tends to be higher during the critical period of development among heavy smokers and drinkers.* Despite this, less than 2% of birth defects are caused by drugs and chemicals. Only a few drugs have been positively implicated as human teratogenic agents (see Table 20-6).

Although only 7% to 10% of birth defects are caused by recognizable teratogens (environmental agents) (see Fig. 20-1), new agents continue to be identified. *Women should avoid all medications during the first trimester unless there is a strong medical reason for their use* and then only if the drugs are recognized as reasonably safe for the embryo. Even though well-controlled studies of certain drugs (e.g., marijuana) have failed to demonstrate a teratogenic risk to embryos, they affect development of the embryo (e.g., fetal decreased growth, birth weight).

***Cigarette smoking*** Maternal smoking during pregnancy is a well-established cause of **intrauterine growth restriction (IUGR)**. Despite warnings that cigarette smoking is harmful to the embryo or fetus, some women continue to smoke during their pregnancies. Among heavy cigarette smokers, premature delivery is twice as frequent as among mothers who do not smoke (see Chapter 6, Fig. 6-11). **Low birth weight** (<2000 g) is the chief predictor of infant death.

In a population-based case-control study, there was a modest increase in the incidence of **conotruncal and atrioventricular septal heart defects** associated with maternal smoking in the first trimester. There is some evidence that maternal smoking may cause urinary tract anomalies, behavioral problems, and IUGR.

**Nicotine** constricts uterine blood vessels, *decreasing uterine blood flow* and lowering the supply of oxygen and nutrients available to the embryo or fetus from the maternal blood in the intervillous space of the placenta (see Chapter 7, Figs. 7-5 and 7-7) The resulting deficiency impairs cell growth and may have an adverse effect on mental development. High levels of carboxyhemoglobin resulting from cigarette smoking appear in the maternal and fetal blood and may alter the capacity of the blood to transport oxygen. **Chronic fetal hypoxia** (low oxygen levels) may occur and affect fetal growth and development. *Maternal smoking is also associated with smaller brain volumes in preterm infants.*

***Alcohol*** Alcoholism affects 1% to 2% of women of childbearing age. Moderate and high levels of alcohol intake during early pregnancy may alter growth and morphogenesis of the embryo or fetus. Neonates born to **chronic alcoholic mothers** exhibit a specific pattern of defects, including prenatal and postnatal growth deficiency, mental deficiency, and other defects (Fig. 20-17; see Table 20-6).

**Microcephaly (small neurocranium)** (see Chapter 17, Fig. 17-36), short palpebral fissures, epicanthal folds, maxillary hypoplasia, short nose, thin upper lip, abnormal palmar creases, joint defects, and **congenital heart disease** are also seen in most infants. The pattern of defects produced by **fetal alcohol syndrome (FAS)** is detected in 1 to 2 infants per 1000 live births (see Fig. 20-17).

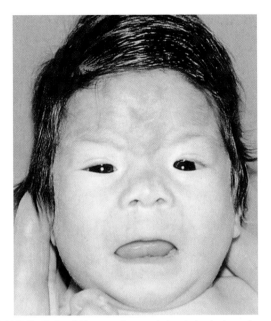

**FIGURE 20–17** An infant with fetal alcohol syndrome has a thin upper lip, elongated and poorly formed philtrum (vertical groove in medial part of upper lip), short palpebral fissures, flat nasal bridge, and short nose.

**FIGURE 20–18** Masculinized external genitalia of a 46,XX female infant. Observe the enlarged clitoris and fused labia majora. Virilization was caused by excessive androgens produced by the suprarenal glands during the fetal period (congenital adrenal hyperplasia). The *arrow* indicates the opening of the urogenital sinus.

*The incidence of FAS is related to the population studied.* Clinical experience is often necessary to make an accurate diagnosis of FAS because the physical defects in affected children are nonspecific. Nonetheless, the overall pattern of clinical features is unique but may vary from subtle to severe.

*Maternal alcohol abuse is thought to be the most common cause of mental deficiency.* Moderate maternal alcohol consumption (1–2 oz of alcohol per day) can result in cognitive impairment and behavioral problems. The term *fetal alcohol effects* (FAEs) was introduced after recognition that many children exposed to alcohol in utero had no external dysmorphic features but they had neurodevelopmental impairments.

The preferred term for the range of prenatal alcohol effects is **fetal alcohol spectrum disorder (FASD).** The prevalence of fetal alcohol spectrum in the general population disorder may be as high as 1%. Because the susceptible period of brain development spans the major part of gestation (see Fig. 20-15), *the safest advice is total abstinence from alcohol during pregnancy.*

**Androgens and progestogens** The terms *progestogens* and *progestins* are used for natural or synthetic substances that induce some or all of the biologic changes produced by **progesterone,** a hormone secreted by the *corpus luteum of the ovaries* that promotes and maintains a gravid endometrium (see Chapter 2, Figs. 2-7 and 2-10D). Some of these substances have **androgenic (masculinizing)** properties that may affect the female fetus, producing masculinization of the external genitalia (Fig. 20-18). The incidence of birth defects varies with the hormone and the dose. *Preparations that should be avoided are* the *progestins* ethisterone and norethisterone.

From a practical standpoint, the teratogenic risk of these hormones is low. Progestin exposure during the critical period of development is also associated with an increased prevalence of **cardiovascular defects,** and exposure of male fetuses during this period may double the incidence of **glanular hypospadias** (see Chapter 12, Fig. 12-42).

Many women use **contraceptive hormones** (birth control pills). **Oral contraceptives** containing progestogens and estrogens taken during the early stages of an unrecognized pregnancy are suspected of being **teratogenic agents,** but the results of several epidemiologic studies are inconsistent. One study found that the infants of 13 of 19 mothers who had taken progestogen-estrogen birth control pills during the critical period of development exhibited the **VACTERL syndrome** (*v*ertebral, *a*nal, *c*ardiac, *t*racheal, *e*sophageal, *r*enal, and *l*imb anomalies). Use of oral contraceptives should be stopped as soon as pregnancy is suspected or detected because of these possible teratogenic effects.

**Diethylstilbestrol (DES),** which is a synthetic nonsteroidal estrogenic compound, is **a human teratogen.** Gross and microscopic congenital abnormalities of the uterus and vagina have been detected in women who were exposed to DES in utero. Three types of lesions were observed: vaginal adenosis (generalized glandular diseases), cervical erosions, and transverse vaginal ridges. Some young women between the ages 16 and 22 years have developed **clear cell adenocarcinoma of the vagina** after a common history of exposure to this synthetic estrogen in utero. However, the probability of cancers developing at this early age in females exposed to DES in utero appears to be relatively low. The risk of cancer from DES exposure in utero is estimated to be about 1 in 1000.

Male fetuses who were exposed to DES in utero after maternal treatment before the 11th week of gestation had a higher incidence of **genital tract anomalies**, including epididymal cysts and hypoplastic (underdeveloped) testes. However, fertility in the men exposed to DES in utero seems to be unaffected. *Expression of the homeobox gene HOXA10 is altered after in utero exposure to DES.*

**Antibiotics** Tetracyclines (broad-spectrum antibiotics) cross the placental membrane and are deposited in the embryo's bones and teeth at sites of active calcification (see Chapter 7, Fig. 7-7). Relatively small doses of **tetracycline** during the third trimester can produce yellow staining of the deciduous and permanent teeth (see Chapter 19, Fig. 19-20E). **Tetracycline therapy** during the fourth to ninth months of pregnancy may also cause tooth defects (e.g., **enamel hypoplasia;** see Chapter 19, Figs. 19-19 and 19-20A), yellow to brown discoloration of the teeth, and diminished growth of long bones. Calcification of the permanent teeth begins at birth and, except for the third molars, is complete by 7 to 8 years of age. Long-term tetracycline therapy during childhood can affect the permanent teeth.

**Deafness** has been reported in infants of mothers who have been treated with high doses of **streptomycin** and **dihydrostreptomycin** as antituberculosis agents. More than 30 cases of *hearing deficit* and vestibulocochlear nerve damage (CN VIII) have been reported in infants exposed to streptomycin derivatives in utero. *Penicillin has been used extensively during pregnancy and appears to be harmless to the embryo and fetus.*

**Anticoagulants** All anticoagulants except heparin cross the placental membrane and may cause hemorrhage in the embryo or fetus. *Warfarin and other coumarin derivatives are antagonists of vitamin K.* Warfarin is used for the treatment of **thromboembolitic disease** and in patients with atrial fibrillation or artificial heart valves. **Warfarin is a known teratogen.** There are reports of infants with hypoplasia of the nasal cartilage, stippled epiphyses, and various CNS defects whose mothers took this anticoagulant during the critical period of embryonic development. **The period of greatest sensitivity is between 6 and 12 weeks after fertilization.** Second- and third-trimester exposure may result in **mental deficiency,** optic nerve atrophy, and microcephaly. **Heparin is not a teratogen,** and it does not cross the placental membrane (see Chapter 7, Fig. 7-7).

**Anticonvulsants** *Approximately 1 in 200 pregnant women is epileptic and requires treatment with an anticonvulsant.* Of the anticonvulsant drugs available, there is strong evidence that **trimethadione is a teratogen.** The main features of the **fetal trimethadione syndrome** are prenatal and postnatal growth retardation, developmental delay, V-shaped eyebrows, low-set ears, cleft lip or palate, and cardiac, genitourinary, and limb defects. *Use of this drug is contraindicated during pregnancy.*

**Phenytoin is a teratogen** (Fig. 20-19). **Fetal hydantoin syndrome** occurs in 5% to 10% of children of mothers treated with *phenytoin* or *hydantoin anticonvulsants.* The usual pattern of defects consists of IUGR, **microcephaly** (see Chapter 17, Fig. 17-36), mental deficiency,

**FIGURE 20-19** Fetal hydantoin syndrome in a young girl. She has a learning disability due to microcephaly and mental deficiency. She has large ears, a wide space between the eyes (hypertelorism), epicanthal folds, and a short nose (**A**). Her mother has epilepsy and ingested phenytoin (Dilantin) throughout her pregnancy. **B,** Right hand of a girl with severe digital hypoplasia (short fingers) born to a mother who took phenytoin (Dilantin) throughout her pregnancy. (*B, From Chodirker BN, Chudley AE, Reed MH, Persaud TV: Possible prenatal hydantoin effect in a child born to a nonepileptic mother, Am J Med Genet 27:373, 1987.*)

ridged frontal suture, inner epicanthal folds, eyelid ptosis (see Chapter 18, Fig. 18-13), broad depressed nasal bridge, nail and distal phalangeal hypoplasias (underdevelopment), and hernias.

**Valproic acid** has been the drug of choice for the management of different types of epilepsy, but the *use of valproic acid in pregnant women has led to a pattern of birth defects* consisting of craniofacial, heart, and limb defects, and postnatal cognitive developmental delay. There is also an increased risk of **neural tube defects** (e.g., spina bifida cystica) (see Chapter 17, Fig. 17-15). *Phenobarbital is considered to be a safe antiepileptic drug for use during pregnancy.* Magnesium sulfate and diazepam are also widely used for seizure prophylaxis.

*Antineoplastic agents* With the exception of the folic acid antagonist **aminopterin**, few well-documented reports of teratogenic effects are available for assessment. Because the data available on the possible teratogenicity of antineoplastic drugs are inadequate, it is recommended that they should be avoided, especially during the first trimester of pregnancy.

**Tumor-inhibiting chemicals are highly teratogenic** because they inhibit mitosis in rapidly dividing cells (see Chapter 2, Fig. 2-2). The use of **aminopterin** during the embryonic period often results in intrauterine death of embryos, and 20% to 30% of those that survive are severely malformed. **Busulfan** and **6-mercaptopurine** administered in alternating courses throughout pregnancy have produced multiple severe abnormalities, but neither drug alone appears to cause major defects (see Table 20-6).

**Methotrexate**, a folic acid antagonist and a derivative of aminopterin, is a *potent teratogen* that produces major birth defects. It is most often used as a single agent or in combination therapy for **neoplastic diseases,** but it may also be indicated in patients with **severe rheumatic diseases,** including rheumatoid arthritis. Multiple skeletal and other birth defects were found in an infant of a mother who attempted to terminate her pregnancy by taking methotrexate.

*Corticosteroids* Low doses of corticosteroids, including cortisone and hydrocortisone, do not induce cleft palate or any other defect in human embryos. Because of the risks of fetal bleeding and **premature closure of the ductus arteriosus,** *nonsteroidal anti-inflammatory drugs should not be taken during the last few weeks of pregnancy.*

*Angiotensin-converting enzyme inhibitors* Exposure of the fetus to **angiotensin-converting enzyme inhibitors** used as antihypertensive agents causes oligohydramnios (insufficient amount of amniotic fluid), fetal death, hypoplasia of the bones of the calvaria, IUGR, cardiovascular abnormalities, and renal dysfunction. During early pregnancy, the risk to the embryo is apparently less, and there is no indication to terminate a pregnancy. *Because of the high incidence of serious perinatal complications, it is recommended that angiotensin-converting enzyme inhibitors not be prescribed during pregnancy.*

*Insulin and hypoglycemic drugs* Insulin is not teratogenic in human embryos *except possibly in maternal insulin coma therapy.* Hypoglycemic drugs (e.g., **tolbutamide**) have been implicated, but evidence of their teratogenicity is weak. There is no convincing evidence that oral hypoglycemic agents (particularly *sulfonylureas*) are teratogenic in embryos.

The incidence of birth defects (e.g., **sacral agenesis, absence of a part**) is increased two to three times among the offspring of **diabetic mothers.** Approximately 40% of perinatal deaths of diabetic infants are the result of birth defects. *Women with insulin-dependent diabetes mellitus may significantly decrease their risk of having infants with birth defects by achieving good control of their disease before conception.*

*Retinoic acid* Retinoic acid is a metabolite of vitamin A. **Isotretinoin** (13-*cis*-retinoic acid), which is used for treating severe cystic acne, is a **teratogen.** The critical period for exposure appears to be from the third to fifth week. *The risk of spontaneous abortion and birth defects after exposure is high.* The most common major defects observed are **craniofacial dysmorphism,** microtia (see Chapter 18, Fig. 18-21), micrognathia (small jaws), cleft palate, thymic aplasia, cardiovascular defects, and neural tube defects. Postnatal longitudinal follow-up of children exposed in utero to **isotretinoin** revealed significant **neuropsychological impairment.**

Vitamin A is a valuable and necessary nutrient during pregnancy, but *pregnant women should avoid high levels of vitamin A.* An increased risk of birth defects was reported for the offspring of women who took more than 10,000 IU of vitamin A daily.

*Analgesics* Aspirin (acetylsalicylic acid [ASA]) and acetaminophen (paracetamol) are commonly used during pregnancy for the relief of fever or pain. *Clinical trials suggest that large doses of analgesics are potentially harmful to the embryo or fetus.* Although epidemiologic studies indicate that aspirin is not a teratogenic agent, large doses should be avoided, especially during the first trimester. A large survey of women who consumed **acetaminophen** during early pregnancy showed an increased incidence of behavioral problems, including attention deficit hyperactivity disorder (ADHD), among their children.

*Thyroid drugs* *Potassium iodide in cough mixtures and large doses of radioactive iodine may cause* **congenital goiter.** Iodides readily cross the placental membrane and interfere with thyroxin production (see Chapter 7, Fig. 7-7). They may also cause thyroid enlargement and **cretinism** (arrested physical and mental development and dystrophy of bones and soft parts). **Maternal iodine deficiency may also cause congenital cretinism.**

Pregnant women have been advised to avoid douches or creams containing **povidone-iodine** because it is absorbed by the vagina, enters the maternal blood, and may be teratogenic. **Propylthiouracil** interferes with thyroxin formation in the fetus and may cause goiter. *Administration of antithyroid substances for the treatment of maternal thyroid disorders may cause congenital goiter if*

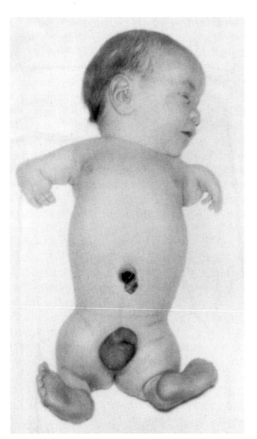

**FIGURE 20–20** Male neonate has typically malformed limbs (meromelia or limb reduction) resulting from thalidomide ingestion by his mother during the critical period of limb development (see Fig. 20-15). (*From Moore KL: The vulnerable embryo. Causes of malformation in man, Manit Med Rev 43:306, 1963.*)

*the mother is given the substances in excess of the amount required to control the disease.*

**Tranquilizers** Thalidomide is a potent teratogen, and it has been estimated that almost *12,000 neonates had defects caused by this drug.* The characteristic presenting feature is **meromelia** (absence of part of a limb), but the defects range from **amelia** (absence of limbs) through intermediate stages of development (*rudimentary limbs*) to **micromelia** (abnormally small or short limbs). **Phocomelia** ("seal limbs"), a type of meromelia, occurred in some of these individuals (Fig. 20-20).

Thalidomide also caused anomalies of other organs, such as absence of the external and internal ears, **hemangioma** on the face (see Chapter 19, Fig. 19-6), heart defects, and anomalies of the urinary and alimentary systems. *The period when thalidomide caused these congenital anomalies was 20 to 36 days after fertilization.* This sensitive period coincides with the critical periods for the development of the affected parts and organs (see Figs. 20-15 and 20-16).

Thalidomide is currently used for the treatment of leprosy, multiple myeloma, and several autoimmune diseases. *It is absolutely contraindicated in women of childbearing age.* The problem remains topical because of ongoing class action suits.

**Psychotropic drugs** Lithium is the drug of choice for the long-term maintenance of patients with bipolar disorders. However, *lithium has caused birth defects*, mainly of the heart and great vessels, in infants whose mothers were given the drug early in pregnancy. Although **lithium carbonate** is a known human teratogen, *the U.S. Food and Drug Administration has stated that the agent may be used during pregnancy if "in the opinion of the physician the potential benefits outweigh the possible hazards."*

**Benzodiazepines** such as **diazepam** and **oxazepam** are frequently prescribed for pregnant women. *These drugs readily cross the placental membrane* (see Chapter 7, Fig. 7-7) and their use during the first trimester of pregnancy is associated with craniofacial anomalies in neonates. **Selective serotonin reuptake inhibitors** (SSRIs) are used to treat depression during pregnancy. Several reports warn of an increased risk of atrial and ventricular septal defects (see Chapter 13, Figs. 13-28 and 13-29), persistent pulmonary hypertension, and neurobehavioral disturbances, including autism spectrum disorder, in infants exposed to SSRIs in utero. The mechanism is thought to be SSRIs blocking catecholamine transport, which affects placental blood flow.

**Illicit drugs** Several popular street drugs are used for their hallucinogenic properties. There is no evidence that marijuana is a human teratogen, but there is an indication that its use during the first 2 months of pregnancy affects fetal growth and birth weight. Sleep and electroencephalographic patterns in neonates exposed prenatally to marijuana were altered.

*Cocaine is the most widely used illicit drug among women of childbearing age.* Reports dealing with prenatal effects of cocaine include placental abruption, spontaneous abortion, prematurity, IUGR, microcephaly, cerebral infarction, urogenital anomalies, neurobehavioral disturbances, and neurologic abnormalities.

**Methadone** is used during withdrawal treatment of morphine and heroin addiction. Methadone is considered to be a *behavioral teratogen*, as is heroin. Infants of narcotic-dependent women maintained on methadone therapy were found to have **CNS dysfunction**, lower birth weights, and smaller head circumferences than nonexposed infants. *There is also concern about the long-term postnatal developmental effects of methadone.* The problem is difficult to resolve because other drugs are often used in combination with methadone, and heavy use of alcohol and cigarettes is prevalent among narcotic-dependent women. Maternal use of **methamphetamine**, a sympathetic nervous system stimulant, results in small-for-gestational-age fetuses with neurobehavioral changes.

## Environmental Chemicals as Teratogens

There is increasing concern about the possible *teratogenicity of environmental chemicals*, including industrial and agricultural chemicals, pollutants, and food additives. Most of these chemicals have not been positively implicated as teratogens in humans.

**Organic mercury** Infants of mothers whose main diet during pregnancy consists of fish containing abnormally high levels of organic mercury acquire fetal **Minamata**

disease, characterized by *neurologic and behavioral disturbances* resembling those of cerebral palsy. Severe brain damage, mental deficiency, and blindness have been detected in infants of mothers who received **methylmercury** in their food. This liquid metal is a teratogen that causes cerebral atrophy, spasticity, seizures, and mental deficiency. Similar observations have been made in infants whose mothers ate pork that became contaminated when the pigs ate corn grown from seeds sprayed with a **mercury-containing fungicide**.

**Lead** Abundantly present in the workplace and environment, *lead passes through the placental membrane* (see Chapter 7, Fig. 7-7) and accumulates in embryonic and fetal tissues. Prenatal exposure to lead is associated with increased abortions, fetal defects, IUGR, and functional deficits. Several reports have indicated that children of mothers who were exposed to subclinical levels of lead revealed neurobehavioral and psychomotor disturbances.

**Polychlorinated biphenyls** Polychlorinated biphenyls are teratogenic chemicals that produce IUGR and skin discoloration. The main dietary source of these chemicals in North America is probably *sport fish caught in contaminated waters*. In Japan and Taiwan, the teratogenic chemical was *detected in contaminated cooking oil*.

## Infectious Agents as Teratogens

Throughout prenatal life, embryos and fetuses are endangered by a variety of **microorganisms**. In most cases, the assault is resisted, but in some cases, spontaneous abortion or stillbirth occurs. If they survive, fetuses are born with **IUGR**, birth defects, or neonatal diseases (see Table 20-6). The microorganisms cross the **placental membrane** and enter the embryonic and fetal bloodstream (see Chapter 7, Fig. 7-7). There is a propensity for the CNS to be affected, and the **fetal blood-brain barrier** (BBB) offers little resistance to microorganisms. The BBB is a selective mechanism opposing the passage of most ions and high-molecular-weight compounds from the blood to brain tissue.

**Congenital rubella** A high incidence of birth defects in fetuses results from **maternal rubella virus infection** during the first trimester. *The fetus acquires the infection transplacentally; the virus crosses the placental membrane and infects the embryo or fetus* (see Chapter 7, Fig. 7-7). The virus that causes rubella is the prime example of an **infective teratogen**. The overall risk of embryonic or fetal infection is approximately 20%.

The clinical features of **congenital rubella syndrome** are cataracts (see Chapter 18, Fig. 18-12), cardiac defects, and deafness. However, other abnormalities are occasionally observed: mental deficiency, chorioretinitis (inflammation of the retina extending to the choroid), **glaucoma** (see Chapter 18, Fig. 18-11), microphthalmia (abnormal smallness of the eye), and tooth defects (see Table 20-6).

Most infants have birth defects when the disease occurs during the first 4 to 5 weeks after fertilization. This period includes the most susceptible organogenetic periods of the eyes, internal ears, heart, and brain (see Fig. 20-15). The risk of defects from a rubella infection during the second and third trimesters is approximately 10%; however, functional defects of the CNS (e.g., **mental deficiency**) and internal ears (**hearing loss**) may result. Because of widespread immunization against rubella virus, fewer infants are affected.

**Cytomegalovirus** Cytomegalovirus (**CMV**) is a member of the herpesvirus family. As with rubella, it is likely that the virus infects the placenta and then the fetus. Fetuses with this virus are often delivered prematurely. CMV is the most common viral infection of the fetus, occurring in approximately 1% of neonates. Most pregnancies end in spontaneous abortion when the infection occurs during the first trimester. *It is the leading cause of congenital infection with morbidity at birth.* Neonates infected during the **early fetal period** usually show no clinical signs and are identified through screening programs. CMV infection **later in pregnancy** may result in severe birth defects: IUGR, microphthalmia, chorioretinitis, blindness, microcephaly, cerebral calcification, mental deficiency, deafness, cerebral palsy, and *hepatosplenomegaly* (enlargement of the liver and spleen). Of particular concern are cases of asymptomatic CMV infection, which are often associated with audiologic, neurologic, and *neurobehavioral disturbances in infancy* (see Table 20-6).

**Herpes simplex virus** Maternal infection with herpes simplex virus in early pregnancy increases the abortion rate by threefold. Infection after the 20th week is associated with a higher rate of *prematurity* (fetus born at a gestational age of less than 37 weeks). Infection of the fetus with this virus usually occurs very late in pregnancy. It is likely that most infections are acquired from the mother shortly before or after delivery. The congenital defects that have been observed in neonates include cutaneous lesions, microcephaly, microphthalmia, spasticity, retinal dysplasia, and deficiency (see Table 20-6 and Chapter 17, Fig. 17-36).

**Varicella** Varicella (chickenpox) and **herpes zoster** (shingles) are caused by the same **varicella-zoster virus**, which is highly infectious. **Maternal varicella infection during the first two trimesters** causes the following birth defects: skin scarring, muscle atrophy, hypoplasia of limbs, rudimentary digits, eye and brain damage, and mental deficiency (see Chapter 20, Table 20-6). There is a 20% chance of these or other defects when the infection occurs during the **critical period of development** (see Fig. 20-15). After 20 weeks' gestation, there is no proven teratogenic risk.

**Human immunodeficiency virus** Human immunodeficiency virus (HIV) causes **acquired immunodeficiency syndrome (AIDS)**. There is conflicting information on the fetal effects of in utero infection with HIV. Reported birth defects include growth failure, microcephaly, and specific craniofacial features. Most cases of transmission of the virus from mother to fetus probably occur at the time of delivery. Breast-feeding increases the risk of transmitting the virus to the neonate. Preventing transmission of the virus to women and their infants is important because of the potential effects.

***Toxoplasmosis*** *Toxoplasma gondii* is an intracellular parasite named after *Ctenodactylus gundi*, a North African rodent in which the organism was first detected. This parasite may be found in the bloodstream, tissues, or reticuloendothelial cells, leukocytes, and epithelial cells.

Maternal infection is usually acquired by two routes:

- Eating raw or poorly cooked meat (usually pork or lamb) containing *Toxoplasma* cysts
- Close contact with infected domestic animals (e.g., cats) or infected soil

It is thought that the soil and garden vegetables may become contaminated with infected animal feces carrying **oocysts** (encapsulated zygotes in the life cycle of sporozoan protozoa). Oocysts can also be transported to food by flies and cockroaches.

The *T. gondii* organism crosses the placental membrane and infects the fetus (Figs. 20-21 and 20-22; see Chapter 7, Fig. 7-7), causing destructive changes in the brain (**intracranial calcifications**) and eyes (**chorioretinitis**) that result in mental deficiency, microcephaly, microphthalmia, and hydrocephaly. *Fetal death may follow infection,* especially during the early stages of pregnancy.

Mothers of congenitally defective infants are often unaware of having had **toxoplasmosis**, the disease caused by the parasitic organism. Because domestic and wild animals (e.g., cats, dogs, rabbits) may be infected with this parasite, *pregnant women should avoid them and eating raw or poorly cooked meat from them* (e.g., rabbits). Unpasteurized milk should also be avoided.

***Congenital syphilis*** The incidence of congenital syphilis is steadily increasing with more cases now than in any of the past 2 decades. One in 10,000 neonates in the United States is infected. *Treponema pallidum*, the small, spiral microorganism that causes syphilis, rapidly crosses the **placental membrane** as early as 6 to 8 weeks of development (see Chapter 7, Fig. 7-7). The fetus can become infected during any stage of the disease or any stage of pregnancy.

**Primary maternal infections** (acquired during pregnancy) usually cause *serious fetal infection* and *birth defects.* However, adequate treatment of the mother kills the microorganisms, preventing them from crossing the placental membrane and infecting the fetus.

**Secondary maternal infections** (acquired before pregnancy) seldom result in fetal disease and birth defects. If the mother is untreated, stillbirths occur in approximately one fourth of cases. Only 20% of untreated pregnant women will deliver a normal fetus.

**Early fetal manifestations** of *untreated maternal syphilis* are congenital deafness, abnormal teeth and bones, *hydrocephalus* (excessive accumulation of CSF) and mental deficiency (see Chapter 17, Fig. 17-38 and Chapter 19, Figs. 19-19 and 19-20). **Late fetal manifestations** of untreated congenital syphilis are destructive lesions of the palate and nasal septum, dental abnormalities (centrally notched, widely spaced peg-shaped upper central incisors [**Hutchinson teeth**], and facial defects (frontal bossing, including protuberance or swelling, saddle nose, and poorly developed maxilla).

**FIGURE 20–21** Chorioretinitis of congenital ocular toxoplasmosis induced by *Toxoplasma* infection. **A,** Necrotizing cicatricial lesion of the macula *(arrow).* **B,** Satellite lesion around and adjacent to the necrotizing cicatricial main lesion *(arrows).* **C,** Recrudescent lesion adjacent to a large necrotizing cicatricial main lesion *(arrows). (From Yokota K: Congenital anomalies and toxoplasmosis,* Congenit Anom (Kyoto) *35:151, 1995.)*

**FIGURE 20–22** Congenital cerebral defects induced by *Toxoplasma* infection. The diagnostic images were obtained at 2 years 9 months of age. **A,** Plain computed tomogram shows that the lateral ventricles are moderately dilated. Multiple calcified foci are apparent in the brain parenchyma *(arrows 1)* and along the ventricular wall *(arrow 2)*. **B,** T1-weighted magnetic resonance image (MRI) (400/22, 0.5 T) shows that the cortical gyri are widened on the left side, and the cortex is thickened in the left frontal lobe *(arrow)* compared with the corresponding structure on the right. **C,** T2-weighted MRI (2500/120, 0.5 T) shows abnormal hypointensity *(arrow)* of the left frontal lobe. *(From Yokota K: Congenital anomalies and toxoplasmosis, Congenit Anom (Kyoto) 35:151, 1995.)*

## Radiation as a Teratogen

**Exposure to high levels of ionizing radiation** may injure embryonic cells, resulting in cell death, chromosome injury, mental deficiency, and deficient physical growth. The severity of the embryonic damage is related to the absorbed dose of radiation, the dose rate, and the stage of embryonic or fetal development when the exposure to radiation occurs.

In the past, large amounts of ionizing radiation (hundreds to several thousand rads) were given inadvertently to embryos and fetuses of pregnant women who had cancer of the cervix. *In all cases, their embryos were severely malformed or killed.* Growth retardation, microcephaly, spina bifida cystica (see Chapter 17, Figs. 17-15 and 17-36 and Chapter 18, Fig. 18-12), pigment changes in the retina, cataracts, cleft palate, skeletal and visceral abnormalities, and mental deficiency have been observed in infants who survived after receiving high levels of ionizing radiation. Development of the CNS typically was affected.

Observations of Japanese **atomic bomb survivors** and their children suggest that 8 to 16 weeks after fertilization is the period of greatest sensitivity for *radiation damage to the brain*, resulting in severe mental deficiency. By the end of the 16th week, most neuronal proliferation is completed, after which the risk of mental deficiency decreases.

It is generally accepted that large doses of radiation (>25,000 mrad) are harmful to the developing CNS. *There is no conclusive proof that human birth defects have been caused by diagnostic levels of radiation (<10 rads).* Scattered radiation from a radiographic examination of a region of the body that is not near the uterus (e.g., thorax, sinuses, and teeth) produces a *dose of only a few millirads, which is not teratogenic to the embryo or fetus.* For example, pelvic computed tomography (CT) in the third trimester of pregnancy results in a wholebody dose to the fetus of approximately 1 to 5 rads. *The risk to the embryo is minuscule from a radiation exposure of 5 rads or less.* However, it is prudent to be cautious during diagnostic examinations of the pelvic region in pregnant women (radiographic examinations and medical diagnostic tests using radioisotopes) because they result in exposure of the embryo to 0.3 to 2 rads. *The recommended limit of maternal exposure of the whole body to radiation from all sources is 500 mrad (0.005 Gy) for the entire gestational period.*

### Ultrasonic Waves

Ultrasonography is widely used during pregnancy for embryonic or fetal diagnosis and prenatal care. A review of the safety of obstetric ultrasonography indicates that there are no confirmed harmful effects on the fetus from the use of routine diagnostic ultrasound examination.

### Maternal Factors as Teratogens

Approximately 4% of pregnant women have diabetes. Poorly controlled **diabetes mellitus** in the mother, particularly during embryonic development, is associated with an increased rate of spontaneous miscarriages and a twofold to threefold higher incidence of birth defects. **Neonates of diabetic mothers** are usually large (**macrosomia**), with prominent fat pads over the upper back and lower jaw. *These infants are at an increased risk for brain anomalies,* skeletal defects, sacral agenesis, and congenital heart defects. In addition to *neonatal metabolic complications,* respiratory distress syndrome and neurodevelopmental abnormalities may occur.

**Phenylketonuria** (autosomal recessive inborn error of metabolism) occurs in 1 of 10,000 infants born in the

United States. If untreated, women who are homozygous for **phenylalanine hydroxylase deficiency** (phenylketonuria) and those with **hyperphenylalaninemia** (abnormally high blood levels of phenylalanine) are at a higher risk for offspring with **microcephaly** (see Chapter 17, Fig. 17-36), cardiac defects, mental deficiency, and IUGR. *The brain damage and mental deficiency can be prevented if the phenylketonuric mother is placed on a phenylalanine-restricted diet before and during pregnancy.*

The risk of neural tube defects (see Chapter 17, Fig. 17-17) is greater in the offspring of mothers with low levels of **folic acid** and **vitamin B$_{12}$**.

### Mechanical Factors as Teratogens

*Amniotic fluid absorbs mechanical pressures, protecting the embryo from most external trauma.* A significantly reduced quantity of amniotic fluid (**oligohydramnios**) may result in mechanically induced deformation of the limbs, such as hyperextension of the knee. Congenital dislocation of the hip and clubfoot may be caused by mechanical forces, particularly in a malformed uterus. Deformations may be caused by any factor that restricts the mobility of the fetus and produces prolonged compression in an abnormal posture. Intrauterine amputations or other anomalies caused by local constriction during fetal growth may result from **amniotic bands**, which are thin strands or rings of tissue formed as a result of rupture of the amnion during early pregnancy (see Chapter 7, Fig. 7-21).

## BIRTH DEFECTS CAUSED BY MULTIFACTORIAL INHERITANCE

Multifactorial traits are often single major defects, such as cleft lip, isolated cleft palate, neural tube defects (e.g., meroencephaly, spina bifida cystica), pyloric stenosis, and congenital dislocation of the hips (see Chapter 11, Fig. 11-4C and Chapter 17, Figs. 17-12D, 17-15, and 17-17). Some of these defects may also occur as part of the phenotype in syndromes determined by single-gene inheritance, a chromosomal abnormality, or an environmental teratogen.

A central problem of *defining the cause of genetic abnormalities* such as cleft lip and cleft palate (CLP) is that the number of genes involved is unknown (multiple gene versus a single gene). Previously, a multifactorial threshold hypothesis for CLP was proposed. It stated that at least one genetic and one environmental factor were involved in the development of each case of CLP. However, this hypothesis left some unanswered questions regarding how genes interact to produce this anomaly and to what extent.

Identifying nonsyndromic orofacial clefts associated with well-known genetic markers has been an important step in understanding the contribution of genetic factors to CLP. Two types of approaches have been used to examine this contribution: large-scale family studies and linkage and association studies with specific genetic markers. *The multifactorial hypothesis has been replaced by the multiple genes of variable expression hypothesis,* supported by the strong statistical evidence from studies in humans and knockout mice showing that a few specific genes may explain the cause of facial clefts. Many reported cases of CLP have been attributed a single dominant gene of low penetration, contradicting the multifactorial hypothesis.

Based on clinical and experimental studies, the accepted hypothesis of multiple genes of variable expression involves a greater locus or relatively few loci (3–14 loci) that interact to cause facial clefts. There is strong evidence to support the fact that the genetic contribution to nonsyndromic orofacial clefts is higher than previously thought and is between 20% and 50%, with the remainder associated with environmental factors and genetic-environmental interactions. In the future, clinicians will have at hand these types of studies in diverse populations to have a complete map of the multiple loci involved in the generation of facial clefts (personal communication, Dr. David F. Gomez-Gill, 2012).

The recurrence risks used for **genetic counseling of families** having birth defects (determined by multifactorial inheritance) are empiric risks based on the frequency of the defect in the general population and in different categories of relatives. In individual families, these estimates may be inaccurate because they are usually averages for the population rather than precise probabilities for the individual family.

## SUMMARY OF BIRTH DEFECTS

- Birth defects are any type of structural abnormalities that are present at birth. The defect may be macroscopic or microscopic and on the surface or within the body. The **four clinically significant types of birth defect** are malformation, disruption, deformation, and dysplasia.
- Approximately 3% of neonates have an obvious major defect. Additional defects are detected after birth; the incidence is approximately 6% among 2-year-old children and 8% among 5-year-old children. Other defects (approximately 2%) are detected later (e.g., during surgery, dissection, autopsy).
- Birth defects may be single or multiple and have minor or major clinical significance. Single minor defects occur in approximately 14% of neonates. These defects have no serious medical consequences, but they alert clinicians to the possibility of an associated major defect.
- Ninety percent of infants with multiple minor defects have one or more associated major defects. Of the 3% of neonates with a major birth defect, multiple major anomalies are found in 0.7%. Major defects are more common in early embryos (up to 15%) than they are in neonates (up to 3%).
- Some birth defects are caused by genetic factors (e.g., chromosomal abnormalities, mutant genes), and a few defects are caused by environmental factors (e.g., infectious agents, environmental chemicals, drugs), but most common defects result from a complex interaction between genetic and environmental factors. The cause of most birth defects is unknown (see Fig. 20-1).

● During the **first 2 weeks of development**, teratogenic agents usually kill the embryo or have no effects. During the **organogenetic period**, teratogenic agents disrupt development and may cause major birth defects. During the **fetal period**, teratogens may produce morphologic and functional abnormalities, particularly of the brain and eyes.

## CLINICALLY ORIENTED PROBLEMS

### CASE 20–1

*A physician was concerned about the drugs a woman said she was taking when she first sought medical advice during her pregnancy.*

❋ What percentage of birth defects is caused by drugs, environmental chemicals, and infectious agents?

❋ Why may it be difficult for physicians to attribute specific birth defects to specific drugs?

❋ What should pregnant women know about the use of drugs during pregnancy?

### CASE 20–2

*During a pelvic examination, a 41-year-old woman learned that she was pregnant.*

❋ Do women this age have an increased risk of bearing fetuses with birth defects?

❋ If a 41-year-old woman becomes pregnant, what prenatal diagnostic tests will likely be performed?

❋ What genetic abnormality may be detected?

### CASE 20–3

*A pregnant woman asked her physician whether any drugs are considered safe during early pregnancy.*

❋ Name some commonly prescribed drugs that are safe to use.

❋ What commonly used drugs should be avoided during pregnancy?

### CASE 20–4

*A 10-year-old girl contracted a rubella infection (German measles), and her mother was worried that the child might develop cataracts and heart defects.*

❋ What did the physician tell the mother?

### CASE 20–5

*A pregnant woman who has two cats that often "spent the night out" was told by a friend that she should avoid close contact with her cats during her pregnancy. She was also told to avoid flies and cockroaches.*

❋ When she consulted her physician, what was she told?

Discussion of these problems appears in the Appendix at the back of the book.

## BIBLIOGRAPHY AND SUGGESTED READING

Adams Waldorf KM, McAdams RM: Influence of infection during pregnancy on fetal development, *Reproduction* 146:R151, 2013.

Bale JF Jr: Fetal infections and brain development, *Clin Perinatol* 36:639, 2009.

Berry RJ, Bailey L, Mulinarae J, et al: Fortification of flour with folic acid, *Food Nutr Bull* 31(Suppl 1):S22, 2010.

Biencowe H, Cousens S, Modell B, et al: Folic acid to reduce neonatal mortality from neural tube disorders, *Int J Epidemiol* 39(Suppl 1): i110, 2010.

Bober MB: Common multiple congenital anomaly syndromes. In Gomella TL, Cunningham M, editors: *Neonatology*, ed 7, New York, 2013, McGraw-Hill.

Briggs GG, Freeman RK, Yaffe SJ: *Drugs in pregnancy and lactation*, ed 9, Baltimore, 2011, Williams & Wilkins.

Burkey BW, Holmes AP: Evaluating medication use in pregnancy and lactation: what every pharmacist should know, *J Pediatr Pharmacol Ther* 18:247, 2013.

Callen PW, editor: *Ultrasonography in obstetrics and gynecology*, ed 5, Philadelphia, 2008, Saunders.

Carson G, Cox LV, Crane J, et al: for the Society of Obstetricians and Gynaecologists of Canada: Alcohol use and pregnancy consensus guidelines, *J Obstet Gynaecol Can* 32(Suppl 3):S1, 2010.

Chudley AE, Hagerman RJ: The fragile X syndrome, *J Pediatr* 110:821, 1987.

Correa C, Mallarinob C, Pena R, et al: Congenital malformations of pediatric surgical interest: prevalence, risk factors, and prenatal diagnosis between 2005 and 2012 in the capital city of a developing country: Bogotá, Colombia, *J Pediatr Surg* 49:1099, 2014.

Dior UP, Lawrence GM, Sitlani C, et al: Parental smoking during pregnancy and offspring cardio-metabolic risk factors at ages 17 and 32, *Atherosclerosis* 235:430, 2014.

Einfeld SL, Brown R: Down syndrome—new prospects for an ancient disorder, *JAMA* 303:2525, 2010.

Fonseca EB, Raskin S, Zugaib M: Folic acid for the prevention of neural tube defects, *Rev Bras Ginecol Obstet* 35:287, 2013.

Frey KA: Male reproductive health and infertility, *Prim Care* 37:643, 2010.

Gianicolo EA, Cresci M, Ait-Ait L, et al: Smoking and congenital heart disease: the epidemiological and biological link, *Curr Pharm Des* 16:2572, 2010.

Jones KL, Jones MC, Campo MD: *Smith's recognizable patterns of human malformation*, ed 7, Philadelphia, 2013, Saunders.

Kim MW, Ahn KH, Ryu KJ, et al: Preventive effects of folic acid supplementation on adverse maternal and fetal outcomes, *PLoS One* 19(9):e97273, 2014.

Levine DA: Growth and development. In Marcdante KJ, Kliegman KJ, editors: *Nelson essentials of pediatrics*, ed 7, Philadelphia, 2015, Saunders.

Levy PA, Marion RW: Human genetics and dysmorphology. In Marcdante KJ, Kliegman KJ, editors: *Nelson essentials of pediatrics*, ed 7, Philadelphia, 2015, Saunders.

Martin RJ, Fanaroff AA, Walsh MC, editors: *Fanaroff and Martin's neonatal-perinatal medicine: diseases of the fetus and infant*, ed 10, Philadelphia, 2014, Mosby.

Medicode, Inc: *Medicode's hospital and payer: international classification of diseases, ed 9 revised, clinical modification (ICD 9 CM)*, vol 1–3, Salt Lake City, 2010, Medicode.

Moore KL: *The sex chromatin*, Philadelphia, 1966, Saunders.

Moore KL, Barr ML: Smears from the oral mucosa in the determination of chromosomal sex, *Lancet* 2:57, 1955.

Nussbaum RL, McInnes RR, Willard HF: *Thompson & Thompson genetics in medicine*, ed 7 revised, Philadelphia, 2007, Saunders.

Persaud TVN: *Environmental causes of human birth defects*, Springfield, IL, 1990, Charles C Thomas.

Rasmussen SA: Human teratogens update 2011: can we ensure safety during pregnancy?, *Birth Defects Res A Clin Mol Teratol* 94(123):2012.

Reef SE, Strebel P, Dabbagh A, et al: Progress toward control of rubella and prevention of congenital rubella syndrome—worldwide, 2009, *J Infect Dis* 204(Suppl 1):S24, 2011.

Richardson GA, Goldschmidt L, Willford J: Continued effects of prenatal cocaine use: preschool development, *Neurotoxicol Teratol* 31:325, 2009.

Sackett C, Weller RA, Weller EB: Selective serotonin reuptake inhibitor use during pregnancy and possible neonatal complications, *Curr Psychiatry Rep* 11:253, 2009.

Shiota K, Uwabe C, Nishimura H: High prevalence of defective human embryos at the early postimplantation period, *Teratology* 35:309, 1987.

Simpson JL: Birth defects and assisted reproductive technologies, *Semin Fetal Neonatal Med* 19:177, 2014.

Slaughter SR, Hearns-Stokes R, van der Vlugt T, et al: FDA approval of doxylamine-pyridoxine therapy for use in pregnancy, *N Engl J Med* 370:1081, 2014.

Spranger J, Benirschke K, Hall JG, et al: Errors of morphogenesis, concepts and terms, *J Pediatr* 100:160, 1982.

Turnpenny P, Ellard S: *Emery's elements of medical genetics*, ed 14, Philadelphia, 2012, Churchill Livingstone.

Weiner CP, Buhimschi C: *Drugs for pregnant and lactating women*, ed 2, Philadelphia, 2009, Saunders.

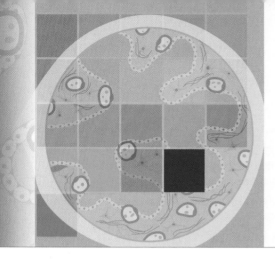

# Common Signaling Pathways Used During Development

*Jeffrey T. Wigle and David D. Eisenstat*

**D**uring the process of embryonic development, undifferentiated precursor cells differentiate and organize into the complex structures found in functional adult tissues. This intricate process requires cells to integrate many intrinsic and extrinsic cues for development to occur properly. These cues control the proliferation, differentiation, and migration of cells to determine the final size and shape of the developing organs. Disruption of these signaling pathways can result in human developmental disorders and birth defects. These key developmental signaling pathways are also frequently co-opted in the adult by diseases such as cancer.

Given the diverse changes that occur during embryogenesis, it may appear that a correspondingly diverse set of signaling pathways should regulate these processes. In contrast, the differentiation of many cell types is regulated through a relatively restricted set of molecular signaling pathways:

- **Intercellular communication:** Development involves the interaction of a cell with neighboring cell directly (gap junctions) or indirectly (cell adhesion molecules).
- **Morphogens:** These diffusible molecules specify which cell type is generated at a specific anatomic location and direct the migration of cells and their processes to their final

| Table 21–1 | | International Nomenclature Standards for Genes and Proteins | |
|---|---|---|---|
| Gene | Human | Italic, all letters capitalized | *PAX6* |
| | Mouse | Italic, first letter capitalized | *Pax6* |
| Protein | Human | Roman, all letters capitalized | PAX6 |
| | Mouse | Roman, all letters capitalized | PAX6 |

destinations. Morphogens include retinoic acid; the transforming growth factor-β (TGF-β) superfamily of proteins, including bone morphogenetic proteins (BMPs); and the hedgehog and WNT protein families. Table 21-1 explains gene and protein nomenclature.

- **Receptor tyrosine kinases (RTKs):** Many growth factors signal by binding to and activating membrane-bound RTKs. These kinases are essential for the regulation of cellular proliferation, apoptosis, and migration, as well as processes such as the growth of new blood vessels and axonal processes in the nervous system.
- **Notch-Delta:** This pathway often specifies which cell fate the precursor cells adopt.
- **Transcription factors:** These evolutionarily conserved proteins activate or repress downstream genes that are essential for many cellular processes. Many transcription factors are members of the homeobox (HOX) or helix-loop-helix (HLH) families. Their activity can be regulated by all of the other pathways described in this chapter.
- **Epigenetic effects:** These heritable changes in gene function do not result from a change in DNA sequence. Examples of epigenetic modifications are histone acetylation, histone methylation, and DNA methylation.
- **Stem cells:** Embryonic stem cells can give rise to all cells and tissues in the developing organism. Adult stem cells maintain tissues in the mature organism. These types of stem cells and induced pluripotent stem cells (iPS) are potential sources of cells for the regeneration and repair of injured or degenerating cells and organs.

## INTERCELLULAR COMMUNICATION

During embryonic development, cells receive signals from their external environment and communicate with neighboring cells. This communication directs the cell to undergo processes such as proliferation, differentiation, and migration. Two classes of proteins required for intercellular communication are discussed: gap junctions and cell adhesion molecules.

## Gap Junctions

**Gap junctions** are a means for cells to directly communicate with one another; this is known as *gap junction intercellular communication* (GJIC). Although the pore size of the channels vary, only small molecules (e.g.,

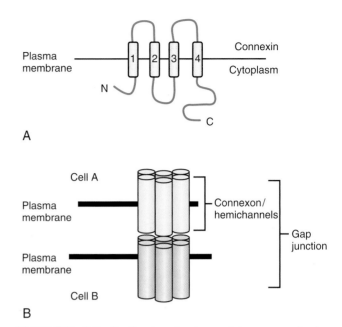

**FIGURE 21–1** Gap junction intercellular communication. *A,* The connexin molecule consists of four transmembrane domains and two extracellular domains, and its N- and C-termini are cytoplasmic. *B,* Connexons, or hemichannels, are hexameric structures consisting of six connexin subunits. A gap junction can be formed from two homophilic or heterophilic connexons. Small molecules (e.g., ions, adenosine triphosphate [ATP]) less than 1 kDa can pass through an open gap junction.

second messengers, ions such as calcium, adenosine triphosphate [ATP]) less than 1 kDa can pass through, which excludes most proteins and nucleic acids. In the nervous and cardiac systems, gap junctions help to establish electrical cell coupling ("electrical" synapse).

Although the function of gap junctions is quite straightforward, the structure of these intercellular channels is complex and highly regulated throughout development (Fig. 21-1). Each gap junction is composed of two hemichannels known as connexons. Each hexameric connexon consists of six individual connexin subunits. An individual connexin (Cx) molecule consists of four transmembrane domains. Vertebrates have more than 20 connexin molecules. Cellular and tissue functional diversity of gap junctions depends on whether individual connexons are the same (homotypic) or different (heterotypic) and whether each connexon is made from the same (homomeric) or different (heteromeric) connexin molecules.

Early in development, GJIC is important for the rapid distribution of ions and other molecules essential for regionalization before the establishment of distinct boundaries and compartments. The importance has been demonstrated in the developing chick hindbrain (rhombencephalon) by dye transfer and electrical coupling studies.

Some of the better-characterized connexins include Cx43 (heart, brain), Cx45 (heart, pancreas), Cx32 (myelin), and Cx36 (pancreas, brain). In this nomenclature system, the number following Cx refers to the molecular weight in kilodaltons (kDa) of the proteins. Mutations in Cx genes result in diseases such as the hereditary peripheral neuropathy X-linked Charcot-Marie-Tooth disease (*GJB1*, formerly *CX32*). It was previously thought that connexons had to bind to a connexon on an adjacent cell to functionally signal. However, it has since been shown that unbound connexons (hemichannels) enable the exchange of ions and small molecules between the cytoplasm and the extracellular space, especially during pathophysiologic conditions. Aberrant hemichannel activation through *GJB2* (formerly *CX26*) can result in keratitis-ichthyosis-deafness syndrome.

## Cell Adhesion Molecules

Cell adhesion molecules have large extracellular domains that interact with extracellular matrix (ECM) components or adhesion molecules on neighboring cells. These molecules often contain a transmembrane segment and a short cytoplasmic domain that regulate intracellular signaling cascades. Two classes of molecules that have important roles during embryonic development are cadherins and members of the immunoglobulin superfamily of cell adhesion molecules.

### Cadherins

**Cadherins** are critical for embryonic morphogenesis because they regulate the separation of cell layers (endothelial and epidermal), cell migration, cell sorting, establishment of well-defined boundaries, synaptic connections, and the growth cones of neurons. Cadherins mediate the interaction between the cell and its extracellular milieu (neighboring cells and ECM).

Cadherins were originally classified by their site of expression. E-cadherin (epithelial cadherin) is highly expressed in epithelial cells, whereas N-cadherin (neural cadherin) is highly expressed in neural cells.

Cadherins mediate homophilic, calcium-dependent binding. A typical cadherin molecule has a large extracellular domain, a transmembrane domain, and an intracellular tail (Fig. 21-2). The extracellular domain contains five extracellular repeats (EC repeats) and has four $Ca^{2+}$-binding sites. Cadherins form dimers that interact with cadherin dimers in adjacent cells. These complexes are found clustered in *adherens junctions*, which result in the formation of a tight barrier between epithelial or endothelial cells.

Through its intracellular domain, cadherins bind to p120 catenin, β-catenin, and α-catenin. These proteins connect cadherin to the cytoskeleton. E-cadherin expression is lost as epithelial cells transition to mesenchymal cells (**epithelial to mesenchymal transition [EMT]**). EMT is required for the formation of neural crest cells during development, and the same process can occur in tumors that develop from epithelial cell types.

### Immunoglobulin Superfamily

There are more than 700 members of the **immunoglobulin superfamily** of cell adhesion molecules in the human genome. This large family of proteins is involved in a wide variety of cellular processes. One member of this class, the neural cell adhesion molecule (NCAM), is an abundant protein in the brain and has three isoforms that

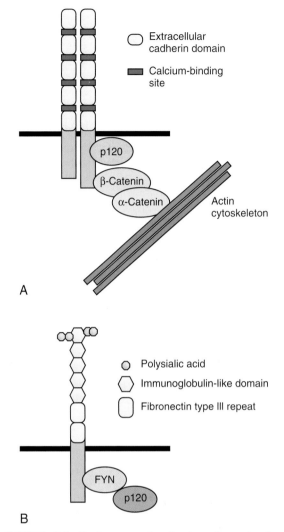

**FIGURE 21–2** Structure of cadherin and neural cell adhesion molecule (NCAM). **A**, The cadherin extracellular domain contains four calcium-binding sites and five repeated domains called extracellular cadherin domains. Each cadherin molecule forms a homodimer. On the intracellular domain, cadherin binds directly to p120 catenin and to β-catenin, which binds to α-catenin. This complex links the cadherin molecules to the actin cytoskeleton. **B**, Extracellularly, NCAM contains five immunoglobulin repeats and two fibronectin type III domains. The fifth immunoglobulin repeat is modified by polysialylation, which decreases the adhesiveness of the NCAM molecule. Intracellular signaling is transmitted by the FYN and FAK kinases.

result from alternative splicing. It has a large extracellular domain that contains five immunoglobulin (Ig) repeats and two fibronectin domains (see Fig. 21-2). This region mediates the calcium-independent homophilic binding of NCAM to itself and heterophilic binding to other cell adhesion molecules (L1 and TAG1), RTKs (fibroblast growth factor receptor [FGFR]), or the ECM. Ligand binding induces intracellular signaling through the FYN and FAK intracellular kinases.

NCAM undergoes polysialylation (PSA), a unique post-translational modification. PSA-NCAM is abundant early in neural development and becomes restricted to areas of neural plasticity and migration in the adult. It is thought that PSA decreases the adhesiveness of NCAM and facilitates migration. NCAM regulates neurite outgrowth, axonal path finding, survival, and plasticity.

## MORPHOGENS

Extrinsic signals guide the differentiation and migration of cells during development and thereby dictate the morphology and function of developing tissues (see Chapter 5). Many of these **morphogens** are found in concentration gradients in the embryo, and different morphogens can be expressed in opposing gradients in the dorsal-ventral, anterior-posterior, proximal-distal, and medial-lateral axes. The fate of a specific cell can be determined by its location along these gradients. Cells can be attracted or repelled by morphogens depending on the particular set of receptors expressed on the cell surface.

### Retinoic Acid

The anterior (rostral, head)–posterior (caudal, tail), or anteroposterior, axis of the embryo is crucial for determining the correct location for structures such as limbs and for the patterning of the nervous system. For decades, it has been clinically evident that alterations in the level of vitamin A (retinol) in the diet (excessive or insufficient amounts) can lead to the development of congenital malformations (see Chapters 17 and 20).

The bioactive form of vitamin A is **retinoic acid**, which is formed by the oxidation of retinol to retinal by retinol dehydrogenases and the subsequent oxidation of retinal by retinal aldehyde dehydrogenase. Free levels of retinoic acid can be further modulated by cellular retinoic acid–binding proteins that sequester retinoic acid. Retinoic acid also can be actively degraded into inactive metabolites by enzymes such as CYP26 (Fig. 21-3). Normally, retinoic acid posteriorizes the body plan. Excessive retinoic acid levels or inhibition of its degradation leads to a truncated body axis in which structures have a more posterior nature. Insufficient retinoic acid or defects in enzymes such as retinal aldehyde dehydrogenase lead to a more anteriorized structure.

At a molecular level, retinoic acid binds to its receptors inside the cell and activates them. Retinoic acid receptors are transcription factors, and their activation regulates the expression of downstream genes. Crucial targets of retinoic acid receptors in development are the *HOX* genes. Due to their profound influence on early development, retinoids are powerful teratogens, especially during the first trimester.

### Transforming Growth Factor-β and Bone Morphogenetic Proteins

Members of the TGF-β superfamily include TGF-β, BMPs, activin, and nodal. These molecules contribute to the establishment of dorsoventral patterning, cell fate decisions, and formation of specific organs, including the nervous system, kidneys, skeleton, and blood (see Chapters 5, 16, and 17).

**FIGURE 21–3** Regulation of retinoic acid metabolism and signaling. Dietary retinol (vitamin A) is converted to retinal by the action of retinol dehydrogenases. The concentration of free retinal is controlled by the action of cellular retinal-binding proteins. Similarly, retinal is converted to retinoic acid by retinal dehydrogenases, and its free level is modulated by sequestration by cellular retinoic acid–binding proteins and degradation by CYP26. The bioactive form of retinoic acid is all-*trans* retinoic acid.

In humans, there are three TGF-β isoforms (TGF-$\beta_1$, TGF-$\beta_2$, and TGF-$\beta_3$). Binding of these ligands to heterotetrameric (four-subunit) complexes, consisting of specific type I (inactive kinase domain) and type II TGF-β receptor subunit (TβR-II) (constitutively active) transmembrane serine-threonine kinase receptors results in intracellular signaling events (Fig. 21-4). When TGF-β ligands bind to their respective membrane-bound type II receptor, a type I receptor is recruited and transphosphorylated, and its kinase domain is activated, subsequently phosphorylating intracellular receptor-associated SMAD proteins (R-SMADs).

The SMADs are a large family of intercellular proteins that are divided into three classes: receptor-activated (R-SMADs 1–3, 5, and 8), common-partner (co-SMADs such as SMAD4), and inhibitory SMADs (I-SMADs such as SMAD6 and SMAD7). R-SMAD/SMAD4 complexes translocate to the nucleus and regulate target gene transcription by interacting with other proteins or function as transcription factors by directly binding to DNA.

Inhibitory SMAD proteins block the actions of I-SMAD by several mechanisms, such as preventing phosphorylation of R-SMADs by TβR-I, induction of R-SMAD degradation, and transcriptional repression. TβR-I activation is a highly regulated process that involves membrane-anchored coreceptors and other receptor-like molecules that can sequester ligands and prevent their binding to respective TβR-II receptors. Dominant negative forms of TβR-II have inactive kinase domains and cannot transphosphorylate TβR-I, thereby blocking downstream signaling events. The diversity of TGF-β ligand, TβR-I and

**FIGURE 21–4** Transforming growth factor-β *(TGF-β)/* SMAD signaling pathway. **A,** The type II TGF-β receptor subunit *(TβR-II)* is constitutively active. **B,** On binding of ligand to TβR-II, a type I receptor subunit is recruited to form a heterodimeric receptor complex, and the TβR-I kinase domain is transphosphorylated *(-P)*. Signaling from the activated receptor complex phosphorylates R-SMADs, which then bind to a co-SMAD, translocate from the cytoplasm to the nucleus, and activate gene transcription with cofactors *(X)*.

TβR-II, coreceptor, ligand trap, and R-SMAD combinations contributes to particular developmental and cell-specific processes, often in combination with other signaling pathways.

## Hedgehog

The **sonic hedgehog** gene *(SHH)* was the first identified mammalian ortholog of the *Drosophila* hedgehog gene *(Hh)*. SHH and other related proteins, including desert hedgehog and Indian hedgehog, are secreted morphogens critical to early patterning, cell migration, and differentiation of many cell types and organ systems (see Chapter 5).

In *Drosophila*, cells have various thresholds for response to the secreted Hh signal. The primary receptor for Shh is Patched (PTCH in humans, PTC family in mice), a 12-transmembrane domain protein that in the absence of Shh inhibits Smoothened (Smo), a seven-transmembrane domain G protein–linked protein, and downstream signaling to the nucleus. However, in the presence of Shh, Patched (Ptc) inhibition is blocked, and downstream events follow, including nuclear translocation of Gli (Gli1, Gli2, Gli3) with transcriptional

activation of target genes such as *Ptc1*, *Engrailed*, and others (Fig. 21-5).

Other membrane-bound SHH coreceptors have been identified with key roles in ventral neural patterning, including BOC and GAS1 (in mammals). Individually, these coreceptors bind the SHH ligand. BOC and GAS1 each interact with the SHH canonical receptor PTC/PTCH to form distinct receptor complexes essential for cell proliferation mediated by SHH. BOC's role is especially important for commissural axonal guidance during development and in medulloblastoma progression.

The SHH protein is modified post-translationally by the addition of cholesterol and palmitate moieties to the N- and C-termini, respectively. These lipid modifications affect SHH's association with the cell membrane, formation of SHH multimers, and movement of SHH, altering its tissue distribution and concentration gradients. One of the best explained activities of SHH in vertebrate development is its role in patterning the ventral neural tube (see Chapters 4 and 17). SHH is secreted at high levels by the *notochord*. The concentration of SHH is highest in the floor plate of the neural tube and lowest in the roof plate, where members of the TGF-β family are highly expressed. The cell fates of four ventral interneuron classes and motor neurons are determined by relative SHH concentrations and by a combinatorial code of homeobox and basic HLH (bHLH) genes.

The requirement of SHH signaling for many developmental processes is underscored by the discovery of human mutations of members of the Shh pathway and the corresponding phenotypes of genetically modified mice, in which members are inactivated (loss of function or knockout) or overexpressed (gain of function). Mutations of *SHH* and *PTCH* have been associated with holoprosencephaly, a congenital brain defect resulting in the fusion of the two cerebral hemispheres; anophthalmia or cyclopia (see Chapter 18); and dorsalization of forebrain structures. In sheep, this defect can also result from exposure to the teratogen cyclopamine, which disrupts SHH signaling (see Fig. 21-5). Some patients with severe forms of the inborn error of cholesterol synthesis, the autosomal recessive Smith-Lemli-Opitz syndrome, have holoprosencephaly (see Chapter 20).

*GLI3* mutations are associated with autosomal dominant polydactyly syndromes (see Chapter 16), such as the Greig and Pallister-Hall syndromes. Gorlin syndrome, which often is caused by germline *PTCH* mutations, is a constellation of congenital malformations mostly affecting the epidermis, craniofacial structures (see Chapter 9), and the nervous system. These patients are significantly predisposed to basal cell carcinomas, especially after radiation therapy, and a few develop malignant brain tumors (medulloblastomas) during childhood. Somatic mutations of *PTCH*, *SUFU*, and *SMO* have been identified in patients with sporadic medulloblastomas not associated with Gorlin syndrome.

In vertebrates, the Shh signaling pathway is linked to primary cilia (see Fig. 21-5, inset) and their constituent intraflagellar transport (IFT) and basal body proteins. IFT proteins act upstream of the GLI activator (GLI-A) and repressor (GLI-R) proteins and are necessary for their production. Mutations involving genes encoding basal

**FIGURE 21–5** Sonic hedgehog/Patched signaling pathway in vertebrates. **A,** The Patched *(Ptc)* receptor inhibits signaling from the Smoothened *(Smo)* receptor. In a complex with the kinesin-like protein Costal 2 *(Cos2)* and serine-threonine kinase Fused *(Fu)*, Gli is modified to become a transcriptional repressor *(Gli-R)*. **B,** Sonic hedgehog *(Shh)* is cleaved, and cholesterol *(Chol)* is added to its N-terminus. This modified Shh ligand inhibits the Ptc receptor, permitting Smo signaling, and activated Gli *(Gli-A)* ultimately translocates to the nucleus to activate target genes with cyclic AMP–binding protein *(CBP)*. In vertebrates, SHH signaling takes place in primary cilia *(inset)*. *CK1,* Casein kinase 1; *GSK3,* glycogen synthase kinase 3; *P,* phosphate group; *PKA,* protein kinase A; *SuFu,* suppressor of Fused.

body proteins, such as *KIAA0586* (formerly *TALPID3*) and oral-facial-digital syndrome 1 *(OFD1)*, affect SHH signaling in knockout mice. A group of human cilia-related diseases called *ciliopathies* includes rare genetic diseases and more common disorders such as autosomal recessive polycystic kidney disease.

## WNT/β-Catenin Pathway

The *WNT*-encoded glycoproteins are vertebrate orthologs of the *Drosophila* gene Wingless *(Wg/DWnt)*. Similar to the other morphogens previously discussed, the 19 WNT family members control several processes during development, including establishment of cell polarity, proliferation, apoptosis, cell fate specification, and migration. WNT signaling is very complex, and three signaling pathways have been elucidated. The classic or canonical β-catenin–dependent pathway is discussed here.

In mammals, specific WNTs bind to one of 10 Frizzled (FZD) seven transmembrane domain cell surface receptors and bind with low-density lipoprotein receptor–related protein (LRP5/LRP6) coreceptors, thereby activating downstream intracellular signaling events (Fig. 21-6). β-Catenin plays an integral role in canonical WNT signaling. In the absence of WNT binding, in a protein complex with adenomatous polyposis coli (APC) and

axin, cytoplasmic β-catenin is phosphorylated by glycogen synthase kinase 3 (GSK3) and targeted for degradation. In the presence of Wnts, GSK3 is phosphorylated by Dishevelled (DVL) and inactivated; it cannot phosphorylate β-catenin. β-Catenin is stabilized, accumulates in the cytoplasm, and translocates to the nucleus, where it activates target gene transcription in a complex with T-cell factor (TCF) transcription factors. In mammals, the many β-catenin/TCF target genes include those of *vascular endothelial growth factor (VEGF), MYC,* and matrix metalloproteinases (e.g., *COMP, DMP1, ECM1*).

Some noncanonical WNT signaling pathways Frizzled receptors. However, all of these pathways are distinguished from the canonical WNT pathway by not involving β-catenin stabilization, degradation, and nuclear translocation. A well-known noncanonical Wnt signaling pathways is the WNT-cGMP/Ca²⁺ pathway. It acts through phospholipase C (PLC) to increase intracellular calcium concentrations, thereby activating protein kinase C (PKC) and calmodulin-dependent kinase II (CamKII) and resulting in myriad downstream effects.

In mammals, dysregulated WNT signaling is a prominent feature in many developmental disorders and cancer. A Frizzled gene *(FZD9)* occurs in the Williams-Beuren syndrome deletion region. *LRP5* mutations are found in

**FIGURE 21–6** WNT/β-catenin canonical signaling pathway in mammals. **A,** In the absence of Wnt ligand binding to the Frizzled *(FZD)* receptor, β-catenin is phosphorylated *(-P)* by a multiprotein complex and targeted for degradation. Target gene expression is repressed by T-cell factor *(TCF)*. **B,** When WNT binds to the FZD receptor, lipoprotein receptor–related protein *(LRP)* coreceptors are recruited, Dishevelled *(DVL)* is phosphorylated, and β-catenin then accumulates in the cytoplasm. Some β-catenin enters the nucleus to activate target gene transcription. *APC,* Adenomatous polyposis coli; *GSK3,* glycogen synthase kinase 3.

the osteoporosis-pseudoglioma syndrome. *Dvl2*-knockout mice have malformations of the cardiac outflow tract, abnormal somite segmentation, and neural tube defects. Similar to the Shh signaling pathway, canonical Wnt pathway mutations (in β-*catenin* [*CTNNB1*], *APC*, and *AXIN1* genes) have been described in children with medulloblastoma. Moreover, somatic *APC* mutations are common (>50%) in adults with sporadic colorectal carcinomas and germline *APC* mutations are a feature of familial adenomatous polyposis and Turcot syndrome (multiple colorectal adenomas and increased frequency of primary brain tumors).

## PROTEIN KINASES

### Receptor Tyrosine Kinases

#### Common Features

Growth factors include *insulin*, epidermal growth factor, nerve growth factor and other neurotrophins, and members of the platelet-derived growth factor family. They bind to cell surface transmembrane receptors found on target cells. These receptors are members of the RTK superfamily and have three domains: an extracellular ligand binding domain, a transmembrane domain, and an intracellular kinase domain (Fig. 21-7).

The receptors are found as monomers in the quiescent or unbound state, but on ligand binding, the receptor units dimerize. The process of dimerization brings the two intracellular kinase domains close enough that one

**FIGURE 21–7** Receptor tyrosine kinase *(RTK)* signaling. **A,** In the absence of ligand, the receptors are monomers and are inactive. **B,** On binding of ligand, the receptors dimerize and transphosphorylation occurs, which activates downstream signaling cascades. *P,* Phosphorylated.

kinase domain can phosphorylate and activate the other receptor (transphosphorylation). Transphosphorylation is required to fully activate the receptors, which initiate a series of intracellular signaling cascades. The mechanism of transphosphorylation requires both receptor subunits within a dimer to have functional kinase domains for signal transduction to occur. If there is an inactivating mutation of one receptor subunit's kinase domain, the functional consequence is to abolish signaling through a heterodimer resulting from the combination of wild-type and mutant receptor subunits (dominant negative mode of action). A mutation in the kinase domain of the VEGF receptor 3 (VEGFR3, now called FMS-related tyrosine kinase 4 [FLT4]) results in the autosomal dominant lymphatic disorder called Milroy disease.

### Regulation of Angiogenesis by Receptor Tyrosine Kinases

Growth factors promote cellular proliferation, migration, and survival (are antiapoptotic). Dysregulation of RTKs or their downstream signaling components are frequently found in human cancers. During embryogenesis, signaling through RTKs is crucial for normal development and affects many processes such as the growth of new blood vessels (see Chapter 4), cellular migration, and neuronal axonal guidance.

Endothelial cells are derived from a progenitor cell (hemangioblast) that can give rise to the hematopoietic cell lineage and endothelial cells. The early endothelial cells proliferate and eventually coalesce to form the first primitive blood vessels. This process is called **vasculogenesis**. After the first blood vessels are formed, they undergo intensive remodeling and maturation into the mature blood vessels in a process called **angiogenesis**. The maturation process involves the recruitment of vascular smooth muscle cells to the vessels that stabilize them. Vasculogenesis and angiogenesis depend on the function of two distinct RTK classes, members of the VEGF and TIE (tyrosine kinase with immunoglobulin-like and EGF-like domains) receptor families. VEGFA is essential for endothelial and blood cell development. *VegfA*-knockout mice fail to develop blood or endothelial cells and die at early embryonic stages. Heterozygous *VegfA-knockout* mice have severe defects in their vasculature, demonstrating that *VegfA* gene dose (haploinsufficiency) is important. A related molecule, VEGFC, is crucial for the development of lymphatic endothelial cells. VEGFA signals through two receptors, VEGFR1 and VEGFR2, that are expressed by endothelial cells. VEGFA signals predominantly through the VEGFR2 receptor for vasculogenesis to properly occur in the embryo.

The process of angiogenic refinement depends on the function of the Angiopoietin/TIE2 signaling pathway. TIE2 (also called TEK) is an RTK that is specifically expressed by endothelial cells, and Angiopoietin 1 and Angiopoietin 2 are its ligands that are expressed by the surrounding vascular smooth muscle cells. This represents a paracrine signaling system in which receptor and ligand are expressed in adjacent cells. The VEGF/VEGFR2 and Angiopoietin/TIE2 signaling pathways are co-opted by tumors to stimulate growth of new blood vessels, which stimulates their growth and metastasis. This

demonstrates how normal signaling pathways in the developing human can be reused for disease processes such as cancer.

### Hippo Signaling Pathway

Studies in *Drosophila* identified a set of kinases in the Hippo signaling pathway that when mutated resulted in increased organ size during development. The human orthologs of Hippo are called mammalian STE20-like protein kinase 1 (MST1) and MST2. Activated MST1 and MST2 phosphorylate the scaffold protein Salvador homolog 1 (SAV1) and the downstream kinases large tumor suppressor homolog 1 (LATS1) and LATS2 (Fig. 21-8). Similar to MST1M and ST2, LATS1 and LATS2 are bound to scaffold proteins MOB kinase activator 1A (MOB1A) and MOB1B, which are also phosphorylated by MST1 and MST2. The MST/MOB1 complex then phosphorylates the transcriptional coactivators yes-associated protein (YAP) and transcriptional coactivator with PDZ domain (TAZ). Phosphorylated YAP and TAZ proteins are retained in the cytoplasm, ubiquitinated, and degraded by the proteasome.

When the Hippo pathway is inactive, YAP and TAZ are localized to the nucleus and bind to the TEA domain–containing sequence-specific transcription factor (TEAD), which relieves repression mediated by the vestigial-like family member 4 (VGLL4) and activation of downstream target genes. The Hippo pathway is important in relaying signals received from adjacent cells and the ECM to the nucleus. For example, culturing mesenchymal stem cells on stiff matrices results in accumulation of YAP and TAZ in the nucleus and differentiation of these cells into bone cells. In contrast, culturing mesenchymal stem cells on softer matrices results in activation of the Hippo pathway, decreased nuclear YAP and TAZ levels, and differentiation into adipocytes. In the developing embryo, nuclear YAP and TAZ are essential for the determination of the trophoectodermal cells of the placenta. YAP and TAZ function is required to inhibit differentiation of human embryonic stem cells and for the generation of induced pluripotent stem cells (discussed later). Loss of Hippo signaling and increased YAP and TAZ nuclear localization has been implicated in several types of human cancer.

## NOTCH-DELTA PATHWAY

The NOTCH signaling pathway is integral for cell fate determination, including maintenance of stem cell niches, proliferation, apoptosis, and differentiation. These processes are essential for all aspects of organ development through regulation of lateral and inductive cell-cell signaling.

NOTCH proteins 1 through 4 are single transmembrane receptors that interact with membrane-bound NOTCH (see Chapter 5) ligands (e.g., Delta-like ligands DLL1, DLL3, DLL4) and Serrate-like ligands (e.g., Jagged 1 [JAG1], Jagged 2 [JAG2]) on adjacent cells (Fig. 21-9). Ligand-receptor binding triggers proteolytic events; some are mediated by secretases, leading to the release of the Notch intracellular domain (NICD). When the NICD

**FIGURE 21–8** Hippo signaling pathway in mammals. **A,** Activated mammalian STE20-like protein kinase 1 *(MST1)* phosphorylates its scaffolding protein Salvador homolog 1 *(SAV1)* and the downstream kinase large tumor suppressor homolog 1 *(LATS1)* and its scaffolding protein MOB kinase activator 1A *(MOB1A)*. On phosphorylation, LATS1 is activated and phosphorylates the yes-associated protein *(YAP)* 1 (YAP1), which results in YAP1 retention in the cytoplasm and degradation. The transcription of TEA domain–containing sequence-specific transcription factor 4 *(TEAD4)* is repressed due to binding of the vestigial-like family member 4 *(VGLL4)* transcriptional repressor. **B,** When the Hippo pathway is inactive, YAP1 translocates to the nucleus, displaces VGLL4 from TEAD4, and transcription of downstream target genes is activated, leading to increased cellular proliferation, increased "stemness," and increased pluripotency. *P,* Phosphorylated.

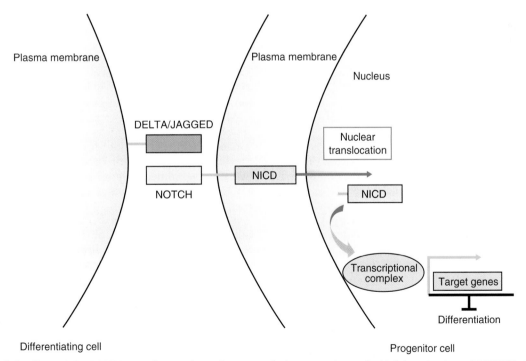

**FIGURE 21–9** NOTCH-DELTA signaling pathway in mammals. In progenitor cells *(right)*, activation of NOTCH signaling leads to cleavage of the NOTCH intracellular domain *(NICD)*. Proteases such as γ-secretase mediate this cleavage event. NICD translocates to the nucleus, binds to a transcriptional complex, and activates target genes, such as *HES1*, that inhibit differentiation. In differentiating cells *(left)*, NOTCH signaling is not active.

translocates to the nucleus, a series of intranuclear events induce expression of hairy enhancer of split (HES), an HLH transcription factor that maintains the progenitor state by repressing proneural basic HLH genes.

The process of lateral inhibition ensures that in a population of cells with equivalent developmental potential, there are the correct numbers of two distinct cell types. In the initial cell-cell interaction, the progenitor cell responding to the NOTCH-ligand DELTA through a negative feedback mechanism reduces its own expression of DELTA, with NOTCH receptor signaling maintaining the cell as an uncommitted progenitor. However, the adjacent cell maintains DELTA expression levels with reduced Notch signaling and differentiation, mediated by, for example, proneural HLH genes. Inductive signaling with other surrounding cells expressing morphogens may overcome the cell's commitment to a neural cell fate (default state) to produce an alternative glial cell fate.

Understanding the function of the NOTCH-DELTA signaling pathway in mammalian development has been assisted by loss-of-function studies in the mouse. Evidence of *JAG1* or *NOTCH2* mutations in Alagille syndrome (arteriohepatic dysplasia), with liver, kidney, cardiovascular, ocular, and skeletal malformations, and *NOTCH3* gene mutations in the CADASIL (*c*erebral *a*utosomal *d*ominant *a*rteriopathy with *s*ubcortical *i*nfarcts and *l*eukoencephalopathy) adult vascular degenerative disease, with a tendency to early-age onset of stroke-like events, support the importance of the Notch signaling pathway in embryonic and postnatal development, respectively.

Pharmacologic manipulation of the Notch signaling pathway may be a means to treat human diseases. For example, gamma secretase inhibitors (GSIs) have been studied in clinical trials for such diverse disorders as Alzheimer disease, pulmonary hypertension, and cancer. For the former, gamma secretase is also a protease required for the production of amyloid-β protein in the brain. Some of the GSIs under development are nonselective, whereas others spare the Notch signaling pathway.

## TRANSCRIPTION FACTORS

Transcription factors belong to a large class of proteins that regulate the expression of many target genes through activation or repression mechanisms. Typically, a transcription factor binds to specific nucleotide sequences in the promoter or enhancer regions of target genes and regulates the rate of transcription of its target genes by interacting with accessory proteins. Transcription factors can activate or repress target gene transcription, depending on the cell in which they are expressed, the specific promoter, the chromatin context, and the developmental stage. Some transcription factors do not need to bind to DNA to regulate transcription but may bind to other transcription factors already bound to the promoter DNA, thereby regulating transcription. They also may bind and sequester other transcription factors from their target genes, repressing their transcription.

The transcription factor superfamily is composed of many classes of proteins. The **Forkhead** (FOX) transcription factors include more than 40 members that play diverse roles in development and disease. These proteins contain a forkhead box of 80 to 100 amino acids (winged helix) that bind specific DNA sequences. Other examples of this diverse family of proteins include the HOX (homeobox), PAX, and bHLH transcription factors.

## HOX Proteins

*Hox* genes were first discovered in the fruit fly, *Drosophila melanogaster*. Mutations in these genes of the homeotic complex (HOM-C) lead to dramatic phenotypes (homeotic transformation), such as the *Antennapedia* gene in which legs instead of antennae sprout from the head. The order of the *Hox* genes along the anteroposterior axis is faithfully reproduced in their organization at the level of the chromosome. The order of the *HOX* genes along the anteroposterior axis and their chromosomal location is also conserved in humans. Defects in *HOXA1* have been shown to impair human neural development, and mutations in *HOXA13* and *HOXD13* result in limb malformations (see Chapter 16).

All of the *HOX* genes contain a 180–base pair sequence, the homeobox, which encodes a 60–amino-acid homeodomain composed of three α helices. The third (recognition) helix binds to DNA sites that contain one or more TAAT or ATTA tetranucleotide-binding motifs in the promoters of their target genes. The homeodomain is the most conserved region of the protein and is highly conserved across evolution, whereas other regions of the protein are not as well conserved. Mutations in the DNA-binding region of the homeobox gene *NKX2-5* are associated with cardiac atrial-septal defects, and mutations in *ARX* are associated with the central nervous system malformation syndrome lissencephaly (see Chapter 17).

## *PAX* Genes

All *PAX* genes contain conserved bipartite DNA-binding motifs called the Pax (or paired) domain, and most PAX family members also contain a homeodomain. PAX proteins can activate and repress transcription of target genes. The *D. melanogaster* ortholog of *Pax6*, *eyeless*, was shown to be essential for eye development because the homozygous mutant flies had no eyes. In gain-of-function experiments, ectopic expression of eyeless led to the formation of additional eyes. In fruit flies, *eyeless* is clearly a master regulator of eye development.

*Eyeless* shares a high degree of sequence conservation with its human ortholog *PAX6*. Mutant *PAX6* is associated with ocular malformations such as aniridia (absence of the iris) and Peter anomaly. In human eye diseases, the level of *PAX6* expression seems to be crucial because patients with only one functional copy (haploinsufficiency) have ocular defects and patients without *PAX6* function are anophthalmic (see Chapter 18). This concept of haploinsufficiency is a recurring theme for many transcription factors and corresponding human malformations.

*PAX3* and *PAX7* encode the homeodomain and DNA-binding domains. The human childhood cancer alveolar rhabdomyosarcoma results from a translocation that results in the formation of a chimeric protein in which PAX3 or PAX7 (including both DNA domains) is fused to the strong activating domains of the Forkhead family transcription factor FOXO1A. The autosomal dominant human disease Waardenburg syndrome type I results from mutations in the *PAX3* gene. Patients with this syndrome have hearing deficits, ocular defects (dystopia canthorum), and pigmentation abnormalities best typified by a white forelock.

## Basic Helix-Loop-Helix Transcription Factors

The basic helix-loop-helix (bHLH) genes produce a class of transcription factors that determine cell fate and regulate differentiation in many different tissues during development. At a molecular level, bHLH proteins contain a basic (positively charged) DNA-binding region that is followed by two α helices that are separated by a loop. The α helices have a hydrophilic and a hydrophobic side (amphipathic). The hydrophobic side of the helix is a motif for protein-protein interactions among different members of the bHLH family. This domain is the most conserved region of the bHLH proteins across different species. The bHLH proteins often bind other bHLHs (heterodimerize) to regulate transcription. These heterodimers are composed of tissue-specific bHLH proteins bound to ubiquitously expressed bHLH proteins.

The powerful pro-differentiation effect of bHLH genes can be repressed by several mechanisms. For example, inhibitors of differentiation (Id) proteins are HLH proteins that lack the basic DNA-binding motif. When Id proteins heterodimerize with specific bHLH proteins, they prevent binding of the bHLH proteins to their target gene promoter sequences, called E-boxes. Growth factors, which tend to inhibit differentiation, increase the level of Id proteins that sequester bHLH proteins from their target promoters. Growth factors also can stimulate phosphorylation of the DNA-binding domain of bHLH proteins, which inhibits their ability to bind to DNA.

Expression of bHLH genes is crucial for the development of tissues such as muscle (myogenin *[MYOD]*) and neurons (neurogenin *[NEUROD]*) in humans (see Chapter 15). *MYOD* expression was shown to be sufficient to transdifferentiate several cell lines into muscle cells, demonstrating that it is a master regulator of muscle differentiation. Studies of knockout mice confirmed that *MyoD* and another bHLH gene, *Myf5*, were crucial for

the differentiation of precursor cells into primitive muscle cells (myoblasts). Differentiation of these myoblasts into fully differentiated muscle cells is controlled by myogenin.

*Mash1* (*ASCL1* in humans) and *Neurogenin1* (*NEUROD3* in humans) are proneural genes that regulate the formation of neuroblasts from the neuroepithelium (see Chapter 17). Mouse models have shown that these genes are crucial for the specification of different subpopulations of precursors in the developing central nervous system. For example, *Mash1*-knockout mice had defects in forebrain development, whereas *Neurogenin1*-knockout mice had defects in cranial sensory ganglia and ventral spinal cord neurons. Specification of these neuroblasts is regulated by other proneural genes known as *NeuroD* and *Math5* (*ATOH7* in humans). Muscle and neuronal differentiation (see Chapters 15 and 17) are controlled by a cascade of bHLH genes that function at early and at late stages of cellular differentiation. Both differentiation pathways are inhibited by signaling through the Notch pathway.

## EPIGENETICS

Understanding of the role of epigenetic modifications in regulating embryonic development has greatly expanded in recent years. **Epigenetics** is different from genetics in that it represents the study of heritable changes in the function of genes that cannot be explained by underlying changes in DNA sequence. This classic definition of epigenetics has expanded to include the study of modifications such as histone acetylation and phosphorylation, in which although gene expression is impacted, the modifications are not necessarily inherited.

Four powerful mechanisms of epigenetic regulation are histone acetylation, histone methylation, DNA methylation, and miRNAs. These epigenetic marks (*epigenetic code*) are regulated by classes of enzymes that recognize the epigenetic marks (*readers*), add epigenetic markers to DNA or histone (*writers*), or remove the epigenetics marks (*erasers*). Examples of epigenetic regulators are discussed subsequently and shown in Table 21-2.

Disorders of chromatin remodeling include Rett, Rubinstein-Taybi, and α-thalassemia/X-linked mental retardation syndromes and various cancers. In the laboratory, **ChIPseq** (chromatin immunoprecipitation coupled with DNA sequencing) and **RNAseq** (RNA sequencing)

| Table 21–2 | Proteins Essential for the Regulation and Interpretation of Epigenetic Marks | | |
|---|---|---|---|
| **EPIGENETIC MODIFICATION** | **READER PROTEIN** | **WRITER PROTEIN** | **ERASER PROTEIN** |
| Histone acetylation | Chromatin remodeling enzymes: SMARCA4 (formerly BRG1) | Histone acetyltransferases (HATs): E1A binding protein, 300-KD (EP300) | Histone deacetylases (HDACs): HDAC1 |
| Histone methylation | Polycomb repressive complex: CBX2 | Histone methylases (HMTs): EZH2 | Histone demethylases: JARID1C |
| DNA methylation | MECP2 | DNA methylases: DNMT1 | Tet oncogene family members: methylcytosine dioxygenases (TET1) |

are powerful high-throughput means to identify specific gene targets of transcription factors throughout the genome and assess patterns of gene expression altered during stages of development or in diseases such as cancer.

## Histones

**Histones** are the positively charged nuclear proteins around which genomic DNA is coiled in units of approximately 140 base pairs to tightly pack it in structures known as *nucleosomes* within the nucleus. Histone octamers consist of histone 2A, 2B, 3, and 4 subunits. Modification of these proteins is a common pathway by which transcription factors regulate the activity of their target promoters. Examples of histone modifications include phosphorylation, ubiquitinylation, sumoylation, acetylation, and methylation. The latter two modifications are discussed in more depth in the following sections.

### Histone Acetylation

DNA is less tightly bound to acetylated histones, allowing more open access of transcription factors and other proteins to the promoters of their target genes. Histone acetylation status is controlled by genes such as histone acetyl transferases (HATs), which add acetyl groups (writers), and histone deacetylases (HDACs), which remove acetyl groups (erasers).

Transcription factors can modify histone acetylation by recruiting histone acetyl transferases or by recruiting histone deacetylases (Fig. 21-10). Reader proteins that bind to acetylated histones, such as the chromatin remodeling enzyme SMARCA4 (formerly BRG1), contain a protein structure called a *bromodomain*. Phosphorylation of histones also leads to an opening of the chromatin structure and activation of gene transcription.

## Histone Methylation

Histone methyltransferases (HMTs), which are writer enzymes, catalyze the addition of a methyl group to lysine residues on histone tails. This modification is removed by histone demethylases (HDMs), which are eraser enzymes. In contrast to histone acetylation, methylation of histones can result in the addition of one, two, or three methyl groups to an individual lysine residue and the activation or repression of gene expression, depending on the particular lysine residue that is modified. For example, trimethylation of lysine 9 on histone 3 (H3K9me3) is associated with repressed promoters, whereas trimethylation of lysine 4 on histone 3 (H3K4me3) is associated with active promoters.

Histone methylation status is read by many different classes of proteins. Mutations of histone modification readers, writers, and erasers can lead to diseases such as neurodevelopmental disorders and cancer.

## DNA Methylation

In contrast to the dynamic mechanism of histone modifications, DNA methylation is used for the long-term repression of genes. Cytosine residues are rapidly

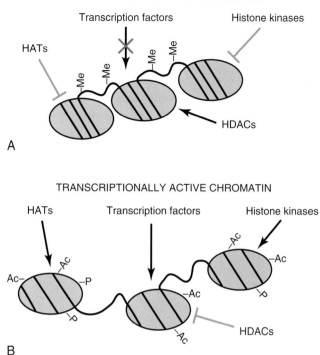

TRANSCRIPTIONALLY INACTIVE CHROMATIN

TRANSCRIPTIONALLY ACTIVE CHROMATIN

**FIGURE 21–10** Epigenetic modifications alter the transcriptional properties of chromatin. **A,** In areas of transcriptionally inactive chromatin, the DNA is tightly bound to the histone cores. The histones are not acetylated or phosphorylated. Histone deacetylases *(HDACs)* are active, whereas histone acetyl transferases *(HATs)* and histone kinases are inactive. DNA is highly methylated *(-Me)*. **B,** In areas of transcriptionally active chromatin, the DNA is not as tightly bound to the histone cores, and the DNA is unmethylated. The histone proteins are acetylated *(-Ac)* and phosphorylated *(-P)*. HDACs are inactive, whereas HATs and histone kinases are active.

methylated at GC dinucleotides after embryo implantation by DNA methyltransferases (writer enzymes). During embryonic development, pluripotency genes, which are expressed in embryonic stem cells, are repressed as the cells differentiate. Repression is maintained by methylation of these loci in differentiated cells. This methylation state is erased in the primordial germ cells to enable re-expression of pluripotency genes. DNA methylation is also used by the body for effective repression of viral genomes that are integrated into our own. The repressive marks are not reset in the primordial germ cells and inherited by the progeny.

In cancer, tumor suppressor genes are frequently inactivated by DNA methylation that allows uncontrolled cellular growth. Mutations in *MECP2*, which binds to methylated DNA (reader enzyme), result in the developmental disorder Rett syndrome. Several DNA demethylating agents, such as 5-azacytidine and decitabine, are being used clinically to treat various disorders, including cancer. These drugs, along with HDAC inhibitors such as valproic acid, are examples of epigenetic therapies.

## MicroRNAs

MicroRNAs (miRNA or miRs) are highly conserved, 22-nucleotide (short), noncoding RNAs that act post-transcriptionally to silence RNA. The biogenesis of miRNAs is complex and a highly regulated process. After exportation to the cytoplasm, pre-miRNAs require a ribonuclease known as Dicer to become processed into mature miRNA duplexes. One miRNA strand is included in the RNA-induced silencing complex (RISC).

The miRNAs target more than one half of the genes expressed during development, and each miRNA specifically targets hundreds of genes. Although they are not considered as a classic epigenetic means to modify gene expression, such as DNA methylation and histone modifications, miRNAs also modify gene expression without changing DNA sequence. The miRNAs fold over to form short hairpins, which can be distinguished from double-stranded RNA molecules.

Many diseases associated with miRNA dysregulation, including developmental syndromes and cancer, are included in the miR2Disease online database. Specific miRNAs associated with cancer are called *oncomirs*. Germline mutations of *DICER1* are associated with a familiar tumor predisposition syndrome that includes several rare cancers such as pleuropulmonary blastema, cystic nephroma, and medulloepithelioma.

miRNA profiling is being developed as a type of prognostic biomarker for disease outcomes. Biotechnology has adopted the power of RNA interference to knock down expression of specific RNA, and these methods are being introduced to the clinic as forms of miRNA therapy.

## STEM CELLS: DIFFERENTIATION VERSUS PLURIPOTENCY

Stem cells (Fig. 21-11) have the property of self-renewal through symmetric (vertical) or asymmetric (horizontal) cell divisions. Under specific conditions in the embryo and adult, these totipotent or pluripotent cells can give rise to all of the differentiated cell types in the body. Several types of stem cell populations have been characterized: embryonic stem cells (ESCs), adult stem cells, and cancer stem cells. ESCs, derived from the inner cell mass of the blastula, are **pluripotent** and can give rise to all differentiated cell types from the ectoderm, endoderm, and mesoderm (primary germ layers), but they do not contribute to extra-embryonic tissues. ESCs express several transcription factors, such as SOX2 and OCT4, which repress differentiation.

Adult stem cells are found in relative abundance in differentiated tissues and organs that undergo rapid regeneration, such as the bone marrow, hair follicles, and the intestinal mucosal epithelium. However, there are nests of adult stem cells in many other tissues, including those that have been previously considered nonregenerative, such as the central nervous system and retina. These stem cell populations are small and located in the subventricular zone and ciliary margins, respectively. Hematopoietic stem cells derived from bone marrow, peripheral blood, and umbilical cord sources are routinely used to

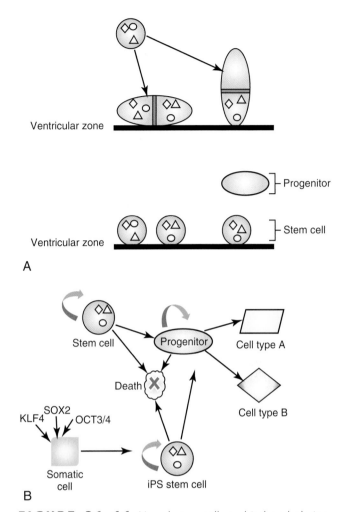

**FIGURE 21–11** Neural stem cells and induced pluripotent stem cells. **A,** Adult or embryonic stem cells can divide symmetrically, giving rise to two equivalent daughter stem cells (vertical cell division; the plane of mitosis is perpendicular to the ventricular surface) or asymmetrically, giving rise to a daughter stem cell and a nervous system progenitor cell (horizontal cell division; the plane of mitosis is parallel to the ventricular surface). In this example, the progenitor cell does not retain the nuclear or cytoplasmic factors (colored geometric shapes) that remain in the stem cell; however, the progenitor cell expresses new proteins (e.g., receptor tyrosine kinases) in its plasma membrane. **B,** Stem cells and induced pluripotent stem cells (*iPS*) have the capacity for self-renewal, cell death, and becoming progenitors. Progenitor cells have a more limited capacity for self-renewal, but they also can differentiate into various cell types or undergo cell death. Adult, differentiated somatic cells, such as skin fibroblasts, can be reprogrammed into iPS with the introduction of the master transcription factors SOX2, OCT3/4 (now called POU5F1), or KLF4.

treat primary immunodeficiencies and various inherited metabolic disorders and as a rescue strategy after myeloablative cancer treatments.

Cancer stem cells (CSCs) are under intense study since it became evident through the study of leukemias and solid tumors (e.g., colorectal cancer, malignant gliomas) that a small population of these cells, identified by various cell surface markers (e.g., CD133 in solid tumors), are often resistant to cancer treatments such as radiation or chemotherapy. Investigators are focusing their efforts on eradicating the CSC population in addition to standard therapies to produce higher cure rates.

The power of stem cells can be harnessed to repair degenerative disorders such as Parkinson disease and tissues severely damaged by ischemia (stroke) and trauma (spinal cord injury). Because researchers have been limited by the available sources of stem cells from embryos or adults, there has been tremendous interest in de-differentiating adult somatic cells (e.g., epithelial cells, fibroblasts) to induce pluripotent stem cells (iPS). Studies have identified several key master transcription factors (see Fig. 21-11*B*), such as *OCT4*, *SOX2*, *KLF4*, and *NANOG*, that can reprogram differentiated cells into pluripotent cells. Other studies have demonstrated the potential of **transdifferentiating** fibroblasts into neurons and cardiomyocytes in situ using tissue-specific combinations of transcription factors. These iPS cells can be manipulated using nonviral means of gene delivery, and they have the potential to treat most human diseases in which cell regeneration may restore structure and function.

## SUMMARY OF COMMON SIGNALING PATHWAYS USED DURING DEVELOPMENT

- There are marked differences between the various signaling pathways, but they share many common features: ligands, membrane-bound receptors and coreceptors, intracellular signaling domains, adapters, and effector molecules.
- Signaling pathways are co-opted at various times during development for stem cell renewal, cell proliferation, migration, apoptosis, and differentiation.
- Pathways have default settings that result in generation or maintenance of one cell fate rather than another.
- Many genes and signaling pathways are highly conserved throughout evolution. Orthologs of genes critical for invertebrate development (the nematode *Caenorhabditis elegans* and the fruit fly *D. melanogaster*) are found in vertebrates, including zebrafish, mice, and humans, often as members of multigene families.
- Knowledge of gene function has been acquired by reverse genetics using model systems with loss-of-function or gain-of-function transgenic approaches and by forward genetics beginning with the description of abnormal phenotypes arising spontaneously in mice and humans and subsequent identification of the mutant gene.
- There is evidence of cross-talk among pathways. Communication among various signaling pathways facilitates our understanding of the far-reaching consequences of single gene mutations that result in malformation syndromes affecting the development of multiple organ systems or in cancers.

## BIBLIOGRAPHY AND SUGGESTED READING

Alvarez-Buylla A, Ihrie RA: Sonic hedgehog signaling in the postnatal brain, *Semin Cell Dev Biol* 33:105, 2014.

Amakye D, Jagani Z, Dorsch M: Unraveling the therapeutic potential of the Hedgehog pathway in cancer, *Nat Med* 19:1410, 2013.

Andersson ER, Lendahl U: Therapeutic modulation of Notch signalling—are we there yet? *Nat Rev Drug Discov* 13:357, 2014.

Aster JC: In brief: notch signalling in health and disease, *J Pathol* 232:1, 2014.

Bahubeshi A, Tischkowitz M, Foulkes WD: miRNA processing and human cancer: DICER1 cuts the mustard, *Sci Transl Med* 3:111ps46, 2011.

Beets K, Huylebroeck D, Moya IM, et al: Robustness in angiogenesis: notch and BMP shaping waves, *Trends Genet* 29:140, 2013.

Benoit YD, Guezguez B, Boyd AL, et al: Molecular pathways: epigenetic modulation of wnt/glycogen synthase kinase-3 signaling to target human cancer stem cells, *Clin Cancer Res* 20:5372, 2014.

Berdasco M, Esteller M: Genetic syndromes caused by mutations in epigenetic genes, *Hum Genet* 132:359, 2013.

Berindan-Neagoe I, Monroig Pdel C, Pasculli B, et al: MicroRNAome genome: a treasure for cancer diagnosis and therapy, *CA Cancer J Clin* 64:311, 2014.

Blake JA, Ziman MR: Pax genes: regulators of lineage specification and progenitor cell maintenance, *Development* 141:737, 2014.

Castro DS, Guillemot F: Old and new functions of proneural factors revealed by the genome-wide characterization of their transcriptional targets, *Cell Cycle* 10:4026, 2011.

Das BC, Thapa P, Karki R, et al: Retinoic acid signaling pathways in development and diseases, *Bioorg Med Chem* 22:673, 2014.

De Robertis EM: Spemann's organizer and the self-regulation of embryonic fields, *Mech Dev* 126:925, 2009.

Dekanty A, Milán M: The interplay between morphogens and tissue growth, *EMBO Rep* 12:1003, 2011.

Dhanak D, Jackson P: Development and classes of epigenetic drugs for cancer, *Biochem Biophys Res Commun* 455:58, 2014.

Gaarenstroom T, Hill CS: TGF-β signaling to chromatin: how Smads regulate transcription during self-renewal and differentiation, *Semin Cell Dev Biol* 32:107, 2014.

Giannotta M, Trani M, Dejana E: VE-cadherin and endothelial adherens junctions: active guardians of vascular integrity, *Dev Cell* 26:441, 2013.

Goldman D: Regeneration, morphogenesis and self-organization, *Development* 141:2745, 2014.

Guillot C, Lecuit T: Mechanics of epithelial tissue homeostasis and morphogenesis, *Science* 340:1185, 2013.

Gutierrez-Mazariegos J, Theodosiou M, Campo-Paysaa F, et al: Vitamin A: a multifunctional tool for development, *Semin Cell Dev Biol* 22:603, 2011.

Hendriks WJ, Pulido R: Protein tyrosine phosphatase variants in human hereditary disorders and disease susceptibilities, *Biochim Biophys Acta* 1832:1673, 2013.

Hori K, Sen A, Artavanis-Tsakonas S: Notch signaling at a glance, *J Cell Sci* 126(Pt 10):2135, 2013.

Imayoshi I, Kageyama R: bHLH factors in self-renewal, multipotency, and fate choice of neural progenitor cells, *Neuron* 82:9, 2014.

Inoue H, Nagata N, Kurokawa H, et al: iPS cells: a game changer for future medicine, *EMBO J* 33:409, 2014.

Izzi L, Lévesque M, Morin S, et al: Boc and Gas1 each form distinct Shh receptor complexes with Ptch1 and are required for Shh-mediated cell proliferation, *Dev Cell* 20:788, 2011.

Jiang Q, Wang Y, Hao Y, et al: miR2Disease: a manually curated database for microRNA deregulation in human disease, *Nucleic Acids Res* 37:D98, 2009.

Kieran MW: Targeted treatment for sonic hedgehog-dependent medulloblastoma, *Neuro-Oncol* 16:1037, 2014.

Kim W, Kim M, Jho EH: Wnt/β-catenin signalling: from plasma membrane to nucleus, *Biochem J* 450:9, 2013.

Lam EW, Brosens JJ, Gomes AR, et al: Forkhead box proteins: tuning forks for transcriptional harmony, *Nat Rev Cancer* 13:482, 2013.

Lamouille S, Xu J, Derynck R: Molecular mechanisms of epithelial-mesenchymal transition, *Nat Rev Mol Cell Biol* 15:178, 2014.

Le Dréau G, Martí E: The multiple activities of BMPs during spinal cord development, *Cell Mol Life Sci* 70:4293, 2013.

Li CG, Eccles MR: PAX genes in cancer; friends or foes? *Front Genet* 3:6, 2012.

Lien WH, Fuchs E: Wnt some lose some: transcriptional governance of stem cells by Wnt/β-catenin signaling, *Genes Dev* 28:1517, 2014.

Lim J, Thiery JP: Epithelial-mesenchymal transitions: insights from development, *Development* 139:3471, 2012.

MacGrogan D, Luxán G, de la Pompa JL: Genetic and functional genomics approaches targeting the Notch pathway in cardiac development and congenital heart disease, *Brief Funct Genomics* 13:15, 2014.

Mallo M, Alonso CR: The regulation of Hox gene expression during animal development, *Development* 140:3951, 2013.

Mallo M, Wellik DM, Deschamps J: Hox genes and regional patterning of the vertebrate body plan, *Dev Biol* 344:7, 2010.

Manoranjan B, Venugopal C, McFarlane N, et al: Medulloblastoma stem cells: where development and cancer cross pathways, *Pediatr Res* 71(Pt 2):516, 2012.

Maze I, Noh KM, Soshnev AA, et al: Every amino acid matters: essential contributions of histone variants to mammalian development and disease, *Nat Rev Genet* 15:259, 2014.

Meijer DH, Kane MF, Mehta S, et al: Separated at birth? The functional and molecular divergence of OLIG1 and OLIG2, *Nat Rev Neurosci* 13:819, 2012.

O'Brien P, Morin P Jr, Ouellette RJ, et al: The Pax-5 gene: a pluripotent regulator of B-cell differentiation and cancer disease, *Cancer Res* 71:7345, 2011.

Park KM, Gerecht S: Harnessing developmental processes for vascular engineering and regeneration, *Development* 141:2760, 2014.

Pignatti E, Zeller R, Zuniga A: To BMP or not to BMP during vertebrate limb bud development, *Semin Cell Dev Biol* 32:119, 2014.

Rhinn M, Dollé P: Retinoic acid signalling during development, *Development* 139:843, 2012.

Ring A, Kim YM, Kahn M: Wnt/catenin signaling in adult stem cell physiology and disease, *Stem Cell Rev* 10:512, 2014.

Roussel MF, Robinson GW: Role of MYC in medulloblastoma, *Cold Spring Harb Perspect Med* 3:pii: a014308, 2013.

Sánchez Alvarado A, Yamanaka S: Rethinking differentiation: stem cells, regeneration, and plasticity, *Cell* 157:110, 2014.

Scadden DT: Nice neighborhood: emerging concepts of the stem cell niche, *Cell* 157:41, 2014.

Schlessinger J: Receptor tyrosine kinases: legacy of the first two decades, *Cold Spring Harb Perspect Biol* 6:pii: a008912, 2014.

Shah N, Sukumar S: The Hox genes and their roles in oncogenesis, *Nat Rev Cancer* 10:361, 2010.

Shearer KD, Stoney PN, Morgan PJ, et al: A vitamin for the brain, *Trends Neurosci* 35:733, 2012.

Sotomayor M, Gaudet R, Corey DP: Sorting out a promiscuous superfamily: towards cadherin connectomics, *Trends Cell Biol* 24:524, 2014.

Steffen PA, Ringrose L: What are memories made of? How Polycomb and Trithorax proteins mediate epigenetic memory, *Nat Rev Mol Cell Biol* 15:340, 2014.

Tee WW, Reinberg D: Chromatin features and the epigenetic regulation of pluripotency states in ESCs, *Development* 141:2376, 2014.

Thompson JA, Ziman M: Pax genes during neural development and their potential role in neuroregeneration, *Prog Neurobiol* 95:334, 2014.

Torres-Padilla ME, Chambers I: Transcription factor heterogeneity in pluripotent stem cells: a stochastic advantage, *Development* 141:2173, 2014.

Verstraete K, Savvides SN: Extracellular assembly and activation principles of oncogenic class III receptor tyrosine kinases, *Nat Rev Cancer* 12:753, 2012.

Wilkinson G, Dennis D, Schuurmans C: Proneural genes in neocortical development, *Neuroscience* 253:256, 2013.

Willaredt MA, Tasouri E, Tucker KL: Primary cilia and forebrain development, *Mech Dev* 130:373, 2013.

Wu MY, Hill CS: Tgf-beta superfamily signaling in embryonic development and homeostasis, *Dev Cell* 16:329, 2009.

Yang Y, Oliver G: Development of the mammalian lymphatic vasculature, *J Clin Invest* 124:888, 2014.

Zagozewski JL, Zhang Q, Pinto VI, et al: The role of homeobox genes in retinal development and disease, *Dev Biol* 393:195, 2014.

## CHAPTER 1

1. The secondary sexual characteristics develop, reproductive functions begin, and sexual dimorphism becomes more obvious during puberty. Consequently, the pubertal changes are not the same in males and females. In girls the ages of presumptive puberty are after age 8 years, with the process largely completed by age 16 years. In boys the ages of presumptive puberty are after age 9 years, with the process largely completed by age 18 years.

2. **Embryology** refers to the study of embryonic development; clinically, it refers to embryonic and fetal development and the study of prenatal development. **Teratology** refers to the study of abnormal embryonic and fetal development. It is the branch of embryology concerned with birth defects and their causes. Embryologic and teratologic studies are applicable to clinical studies because they indicate vulnerable prenatal periods of development.

3. All of the terms refer to female sexual cells. An **egg** refers to the cell of reptiles and birds, which is provided with a protective shell or membrane. The term **ovum** is imprecise because it has been used to apply to stages from the oocyte to the implanting blastocyst. The term **ovule** is used for the oocyte of mammals (e.g., vertebrate animals). A **gamete** refers to any germ cell, whether it is an oocyte or a sperm. The term **oocyte** is the international preferred term for humans.

## CHAPTER 2

1. Numeric changes in chromosomes arise chiefly from **nondisjunction** during a mitotic or meiotic cell division. Most clinically important abnormalities in chromosome number develop during the first meiotic division. Nondisjunction is the failure of double-chromatid chromosomes to dissociate during anaphase of cell division. As a result, both chromosomes pass to the same daughter cell and trisomy results. **Trisomy 21** (Down syndrome) is the most common numeric chromosomal disorder resulting in birth defects. This syndrome occurs approximately once in every 700 births in women 30 to 34 years of age; however, it is more common in older mothers.

2. A **morula** with an extra set of chromosomes in its cells is called a **triploid embryo**. This chromosome abnormality usually results from fertilization of an oocyte by two sperms (**dispermy**). A fetus could develop from a triploid morula and be born alive; however, this is unusual. Most triploid fetuses abort spontaneously; if born alive, triploid neonates die within a few days (see Chapter 20, Fig. 20-10).

3. Blockage of the uterine tubes resulting from infection is a major cause of infertility in women. Because occlusion prevents the oocyte from contacting the sperm, fertilization cannot occur. Infertility in men usually results from **defects in spermatogenesis**. Nondescent of the testes is one cause of **aspermatogenesis** (failure of sperm formation); however, normally positioned testes may not produce adequate numbers of actively motile sperms.

4. **Mosaicism** results from nondisjunction of double-chromatid chromosomes during early cleavage of a zygote rather than during gametogenesis. As a consequence, the embryo has two cell lines with different chromosome numbers. Persons who develop from these chromosomally abnormal embryos are **mosaics**. Approximately 1% of persons with Down syndrome are mosaics. They have relatively mild stigmata of the syndrome and are less mentally deficient than usual. Mosaicism can be detected before birth by cytogenetic studies after **amniocentesis** or **chorionic villus sampling**.

5. **Postcoital birth control pills** (morning-after pills) may be prescribed in an emergency (e.g., after sexual abuse). Ovarian hormones (e.g., estrogen) taken in large doses within 72 hours after sexual intercourse usually prevent implantation of a blastocyst, probably by altering tubal motility, interfering with corpus luteum function, or causing abnormal changes in the endometrium. *These hormones prevent implantation, not fertilization*; consequently, they should not be called contraceptive pills. Conception occurs, but the blastocyst does not implant. It would be more appropriate to call the pills "contraimplantation pills." Because the term **abortion** refers to premature stoppage of a pregnancy, it could be applied to early termination of pregnancy by prevention of blastocyst implantation.

6. Many early embryos are spontaneously aborted; the overall early spontaneous abortion rate is approximately 45%. The common cause of early spontaneous abortion is the presence of **chromosomal abnormalities**, such as those resulting from nondisjunction, failure of one or more pairs of chromosomes to separate.

7. It is estimated that between 12% and 25% of couples in North America are infertile. In one third to one half of these cases, the cause is male infertility. **Male**

**infertility** may result from endocrine disorders, abnormal spermatogenesis, or blockage of a genital duct. First, Jerry's semen should be evaluated (**sperm analysis**). The total number, motility, and morphologic characteristics of the sperms in the ejaculate are assessed in cases of male infertility. A man with fewer than 10 million sperms per milliliter of semen is likely to be sterile, especially when the specimen of semen contains immotile and morphologically abnormal sperms.

## CHAPTER 3

1. Yes, a chest radiograph may be taken because the patient's uterus and ovaries would not be directly in the x-ray beam. The only radiation that the ovaries would receive would be a negligible amount from scattering. Furthermore, this small amount of radiation would be highly unlikely to damage the products of conception if the patient happened to be pregnant.

2. Implantation is regulated by a delicate balance between estrogen and progesterone. The large doses of estrogen would upset this balance. Progesterone makes the endometrium grow thicker and more vascular so that the blastocyst may become embedded and nourished adequately. When media commentators refer to the "abortion pill," they are usually referring to RU486 (mifepristone). This drug interferes with implantation of a blastocyst by blocking the production of progesterone by the corpus luteum. A pregnancy can be detected at the end of the second week after fertilization using highly sensitive pregnancy tests. Most tests depend on the presence of an early pregnancy factor in the maternal serum. Early pregnancy can also be detected by **ultrasonography**.

3. More than 95% of ectopic pregnancies are in the uterine tube, and 60% of them are in the ampulla of the tube. **Endovaginal sonography** is often used to detect ectopic tubal pregnancies. The surgeon would likely perform a laparoscopic operation to remove the uterine tube containing the ectopic conceptus.

4. No, the surgery would not have produced the defect of the brain. Exposure of an embryo during the second week of development to the slight trauma that might be associated with abdominal surgery would not cause a birth defect. Furthermore, the anesthetics used during the operation would not induce a defect in the brain. Maternal exposure to teratogens during the first 2 weeks of development will not induce birth defects, but the conceptus may spontaneously abort.

5. Women older than 40 years of age are more likely to have a baby with a birth defect, such as Down syndrome; however, women older than 40 years may have normal children. Prenatal diagnosis (e.g., using **chorionic villus sampling** or amniocentesis) will tell whether the embryo has severe chromosomal

abnormalities (e.g., trisomy 13) that would cause its death shortly after birth. **Ultrasound examination of the embryo** may also be performed for the detection of certain morphologic anomalies (e.g., defects of the limbs and central nervous system). In most cases, the embryo is normal and the pregnancy continues to full term.

## CHAPTER 4

1. The hormones in contraceptive pills prevent ovulation and development of the luteal (secretory) stage of the menstrual cycle. Severe chromosomal abnormalities may have caused the spontaneous abortion. The incidence of birth defects in early abortions is high in women who become pregnant shortly after discontinuing the use of birth control pills. A pronounced increase in **polyploidy** (cells containing three or more times the haploid number of chromosomes) has been observed in embryos expelled during spontaneous abortions when conception occurred within 2 months after discontinuing oral contraception. *Polyploidy is fatal to developing embryos.* This information suggests that it is wise to use some other type of contraception for one or two menstrual cycles before attempting pregnancy. In the present case, the physician probably told the patient that her abortion was a natural screening process and that it was probably the spontaneous expulsion of an embryo that could not have survived because it likely had severe chromosomal abnormalities. Some women have become pregnant 1 month after discontinuing the use of contraceptive pills and have given birth to normal babies.

2. A highly sensitive **radioimmune test** would likely indicate that the woman was pregnant. The presence of embryonic and/or chorionic tissue in the endometrial remnants would be an absolute sign of pregnancy. By 5 days after the expected menses (approximately 5 weeks after the last normal menstrual period), the embryo would be in the third week of its development. The embryo would be approximately 2 mm in diameter and could be detected with **transvaginal ultrasound techniques**.

3. The central nervous system (brain and spinal cord) begins to develop during the third embryonic week. **Meroencephaly**, in which most of the brain and calvaria are absent, may result from environmental teratogens acting during the third week of development. This severe defect of the brain occurs because of failure of the cranial part of the neural tube to develop normally, which usually results from nonclosure of the rostral neuropore.

4. **Sacrococcygeal teratomas** arise from remnants of the primitive streak. Because cells from the primitive streak are pluripotent (may affect more than one organ or tissue), the tumors contain various types of tissue derived from all three germ layers. There is a clear-cut difference in the incidence of these tumors

with regard to gender; they are three to four times more frequent in females than in males.

5. **Endovaginal sonography** is an important technique for assessing pregnancy during the third week because the conceptus (embryo and membranes) can be visualized. It is, therefore, possible to determine whether the embryo is developing normally. A negative pregnancy test in the third week does not rule out an ectopic pregnancy, because ectopic pregnancies produce **human chorionic gonadotropin** at a slower rate than intrauterine pregnancies. This hormone is the basic element of pregnancy tests.

## CHAPTER 5

1. The physician would likely tell the patient that her embryo was undergoing a critical stage of its development and that it would be best for her baby if she would stop smoking. She would likely ask her to avoid taking any unprescribed medication throughout her pregnancy. The physician would also likely tell her that heavy cigarette smoking is known to cause **intrauterine growth restriction** and **underweight babies** and that the incidence of **prematurity** increases with the number of cigarettes that are smoked. The physician would also recommend that she not consume alcohol during her pregnancy, because of its known teratogenic effects (see Chapter 20, Fig. 20-17).

2. One cannot necessarily predict how a drug will affect the human embryo because human and animal embryos may differ in their response to drugs; for example, **thalidomide** is extremely teratogenic to human embryos but it has very little effect on some experimental animals, such as rats and mice. However, drugs known to be strong **teratogens** (agents that can produce birth defects) in animals should not be used during human pregnancy, especially during the embryonic period. The germ layers form during gastrulation. All tissues and organs of the embryo develop from the three germ layers: ectoderm, mesoderm, and endoderm. Formation of the primitive streak and notochord are important events during **morphogenesis** (development of the shape, size, and other features of a particular organ or part of the body).

3. Information about the starting date of a pregnancy may be unreliable because it depends on the patient's remembering an event (last menses) that occurred 2 or 3 months earlier. In addition, she may have had breakthrough bleeding at the time of her last normal menstrual period and may have thought that it was a light menses. **Endovaginal sonography** is reliable for estimating the probable starting date of a pregnancy and embryonic age.

4. Taking a sleeping pill may not harm the embryo, but a physician should be consulted about any medications. To cause severe limb defects, a known teratogenic drug would have to act during the critical period of limb development (24–36 days after fertilization). Teratogens interfere with differentiation of tissues and organs, often disrupting or arresting the embryo's development.

## CHAPTER 6

1. Physicians cannot always rely on information about the time of the last normal menstrual period provided by their patients, especially in cases in which determination of fertilization age is extremely important, for example, in **high-risk pregnancies** in which one might wish to induce labor as soon as possible. One can determine with reasonable accuracy the estimated date of confinement, or expected date of delivery, using **diagnostic ultrasonography** to estimate the size of the fetal head and abdomen. Normally, labor would be induced after 36 to 37 weeks, using hormones (e.g., prostaglandins and oxytocin), unless there is a good reason to do so earlier.

2. Chorionic villus sampling would likely be performed for the study of the fetal chromosomes. The most common chromosomal disorder detected in fetuses of women older than 40 years of age is trisomy 21 (Down syndrome). If the fetal chromosomes were normal but birth defects of the brain or limbs were suspected, **ultrasonography** would likely be performed. These methods allow one to look for **morphologic abnormalities** while scanning the entire fetus. The sex of the fetus could be determined by examining the sex chromosomes in cells obtained by chorionic villus sampling. At 10 or more weeks, the obstetric radiologist can determine fetal sex using ultrasonography.

3. There is considerable danger when uncontrolled drugs (over-the-counter drugs), such as aspirin and cough medicines, are consumed excessively or indiscriminately by pregnant women. **Withdrawal seizures** have been reported in infants born to mothers who are heavy drinkers. **Fetal alcohol syndrome** is present in some of these infants (see Chapter 20, Fig. 20-17). The physician would likely tell the patient not to take any drugs that are not prescribed. Drugs that are most detrimental to her fetus are under legal control and are dispensed with great care.

4. Many factors (fetal, maternal, and environmental) may reduce the rate of fetal growth (intrauterine growth retardation). Examples of such factors are intrauterine infections, multiple pregnancies, and chromosomal abnormalities. Cigarette smoking, narcotic addiction, and consumption of large amounts of alcohol are also well-established causes of intrauterine growth retardation. A mother interested in the growth and general well-being of her fetus consults her doctor frequently, eats a good-quality diet, and does not use illicit drugs, smoke, or drink alcohol.

5. *Amniocentesis is relatively devoid of risk.* The chance of inducing an abortion is estimated to be approximately 0.5%. Chorionic villus sampling can also be used for obtaining cells for chromosome study. In *percutaneous umbilical cord blood sampling*, a needle is inserted into the umbilical vein with the guidance of ultrasonography. Chromosome and hormone studies can be performed with the blood obtained.

6. **Neural tube defects** are indicated by *high levels of alpha fetoprotein.* Diagnostic studies would be done monitoring the levels of alpha fetoprotein. Further studies could be done using ultrasonography. *Low levels of alpha fetoprotein may indicate Down syndrome.* Chromosome studies may also be done to check the chromosome complement of the fetal cells.

## CHAPTER 7

1. **Polyhydramnios** is the accumulation of an excessive amount of amniotic fluid in the fetus. When it occurs over the course of a few days, there is an associated high risk of severe fetal birth defects, especially of the central nervous system (e.g., **meroencephaly** and **spina bifida cystica**). Fetuses with gross brain defects do not drink the usual amounts of amniotic fluid; hence, the amount of liquid increases. **Atresia** (blockage) of the esophagus is almost always accompanied by polyhydramnios because the fetus cannot swallow and absorb amniotic fluid. Twinning is also a predisposing cause of polyhydramnios.

2. There is a tendency for twins to "run in families." It appears unlikely that there is a genetic factor in monozygotic twinning, but a disposition to dizygotic twinning is genetically determined. The frequency of dizygotic twinning increases sharply with maternal age up to 35 years and then decreases; however, the frequency of monozygotic twinning is affected very little by the age of the mother. Determination of twin zygosity can usually be made by examining the placenta and fetal membranes. One can later determine zygosity by looking for genetically determined similarities and differences in a twin pair. Differences in DNA studies prove that twins are dizygotic.

3. A **single umbilical artery** occurs in approximately 1 of every 200 umbilical cords. This abnormality is accompanied by a 15% to 20% incidence of cardiovascular abnormalities.

4. Two zygotes were fertilized. The resulting blastocysts implanted close together and the placentas fused. The sample of chorionic villi was obtained from the chorionic sac of the female twin. If two chorionic sacs had been observed during ultrasonography, dizygotic twinning would have been suspected.

5. **Amniotic bands** form when the amnion tears and delaminates during pregnancy. The bands surround parts of the embryo's body and produce birth defects, such as absence of a hand or deep grooves in a limb. This constitutes the **amniotic band syndrome** or the amniotic band disruption complex. An alternative causative theory for amniotic band syndrome is vascular disruption.

## CHAPTER 8

1. A diagnosis of **congenital diaphragmatic hernia (CDH)** is most likely. The birth defect in the diaphragm that produces this hernia usually results from failure of the left pericardioperitoneal canal to close during the sixth week of development; consequently, herniation of abdominal organs into the thorax occurs. This compresses the lungs, especially the left one, and results in respiratory distress. The diagnosis can usually be established by a radiographic or sonographic examination of the chest. The defect can also be detected prenatally using ultrasonography. Characteristically, there are air- or fluid-filled loops of intestine in the left hemithorax of a neonate with CDH.

2. In retrosternal hernia, a rare birth defect, the intestine may herniate into the pericardial sac, or, conversely, the heart may be displaced into the superior part of the peritoneal cavity. Herniation of the intestine through the sternocostal hiatus causes this condition.

3. Congenital diaphragmatic hernia (CDH) occurs in approximately 1 of every 2200 births. A neonate diagnosed with CDH would immediately be positioned with the head and thorax higher than the abdomen to facilitate inferior displacement of the abdominal organs from the thorax. After a period of preoperative stabilization, an operation is performed with reduction of the abdominal viscera and closure of the diaphragmatic defect. Neonates with CDH may die because of severe respiratory distress from poor development of the lungs. However, most infants with this condition survive as a result of improvements in ventilator care.

4. Gastroschisis and epigastric hernias occur in the median plane of the epigastric region; these hernias are uncommon. The defect causing herniation results from failure of the lateral body folds to fuse in this region during the fourth week of gestation.

## CHAPTER 9

1. The most likely diagnosis is a cervical (branchial) sinus. When the sinus is infected, mucoid material is intermittently discharged. The external cervical (branchial) sinus is a remnant of the second pharyngeal groove or cervical sinus, or both. Normally, the groove and sinus disappear as the neck forms.

2. The position of the inferior parathyroid glands varies. They develop in close association with the thymus and are carried caudally with it during its descent through the neck. If the thymus fails to descend to

its usual position in the superior mediastinum, one or both inferior parathyroid glands may be located near the bifurcation of the common carotid artery. If an inferior parathyroid gland does not separate from the thymus, it may be carried into the superior mediastinum with the thymus.

3. The patient very likely has a thyroglossal duct cyst that arose from a small remnant of the embryonic thyroglossal duct. When complete degeneration of this duct does not occur, a cyst may form from it anywhere along the median plane of the neck between the foramen cecum of the tongue and the jugular notch in the manubrium of the sternum. A thyroglossal duct cyst may be confused with an ectopic thyroid gland, such as one that has not descended to its normal position in the neck.

4. Harelip is a misnomer because it refers to hares or rabbits that normally have partially median split upper lips. A median cleft lip in humans is a rare defect. Although some people still use the term *harelip*, it is improper. The two major groups of cleft lip in humans are unilateral and bilateral. Unilateral cleft lip results from failure of the maxillary prominence on the affected side to fuse with the medial nasal prominences. Clefting of the maxilla anterior to the incisive fossa results from failure of the lateral palatine process to fuse with the median palatine process (primary palate). Between 60% and 80% of persons who have a cleft lip with or without a cleft palate are male. When both parents are normal and have had one child with a cleft lip, the chance that the next infant will have the same lip defect is approximately 4%.

5. There is substantial evidence that anticonvulsant drugs such as phenytoin or diphenylhydantoin given to epileptic women during pregnancy increase the incidence of cleft lip and cleft palate by twofold to threefold compared with the incidence for the general population. Multiple genes with variable expression are thought to cause orofacial clefts.

## CHAPTER 10

1. Inability to pass a catheter through the esophagus into the stomach indicates **esophageal atresia**. Because this birth defect is commonly associated with tracheoesophageal fistula, the pediatrician would suspect this defect. A radiographic or sonographic examination would demonstrate the atresia. The presence of this defect would be confirmed by imaging the **nasogastric tube** arrested in the proximal esophageal pouch. If necessary, a small amount of air would be injected to highlight the image. When a certain type of tracheoesophageal fistula is present, there would also be air in the stomach that passed to it from a connection between the esophagus and the trachea. A combined radiographic, endoscopic, and surgical approach would usually be used to detect and remove a tracheoesophageal fistula.

2. An infant with **respiratory distress syndrome** or hyaline membrane disease tries to overcome the ventilatory problem by increasing the rate and depth of respiration. Intercostal, subcostal, and sternal retractions and nasal flaring are prominent signs of respiratory distress. *Hyaline membrane disease is a leading cause of respiratory distress syndrome* and death in live-born, premature neonates. A deficiency of pulmonary **surfactant** is associated with respiratory distress syndrome. Glucocorticoid treatment may be given during pregnancy to accelerate fetal lung development and surfactant production.

3. The most common type of tracheoesophageal fistula connects the trachea to the inferior part of the esophagus. This birth defect is associated with atresia of the esophagus superior to the fistula. A tracheoesophageal fistula results from incomplete division of the foregut by the tracheoesophageal septum into the esophagus and trachea.

4. In most types of tracheoesophageal fistula, air passes from the trachea through the tracheoesophageal fistula into the esophagus and stomach. **Pneumonitis** (pneumonia) resulting from the aspiration of oral and nasal secretions into the lungs is a serious complication of this birth defect. Giving the baby water or food by mouth is obviously contraindicated in such cases.

## CHAPTER 11

1. Complete absence of a lumen (**duodenal atresia**) may involve the second (descending) and third (horizontal) parts of the duodenum. The obstruction usually results from incomplete vacuolization of the lumen of the duodenum during the eighth week. The obstruction causes distention of the stomach and proximal duodenum because the fetus swallows amniotic fluid. The neonate swallows air, mucus, and milk. *Duodenal atresia is common in infants with Down syndrome*, as are other severe birth defects such as annular pancreas, cardiovascular abnormalities, malrotation of the midgut, and anorectal anomalies. **Polyhydramnios** occurs because the duodenal atresia prevents normal absorption of amniotic fluid from the fetal intestine distal to the obstruction. The fetus swallows amniotic fluid before birth; however, because of duodenal atresia, this fluid cannot pass along the intestine, be absorbed into the fetal circulation, and transferred across the placental membrane into the mother's circulation, from which it would enter her urine.

2. The **omphaloenteric duct** normally undergoes complete involution by the 10th week of development, at which time the intestines return to the abdomen. In 2% to 4% of people, a remnant of the duct persists as an **ileal diverticulum** (Meckel diverticulum); however, only a small number of these defects ever become symptomatic. In the present case, the entire duct persisted, so that the diverticulum was

connected to the anterior abdominal wall and umbilicus by a sinus tract. This defect is rare, and its external opening may be confused with a **granuloma** (inflammatory lesion) of the stump of the umbilical cord.

3. The fistula was likely connected to the blind end of the rectum. The defect, **imperforate anus** with a rectovaginal fistula, results from failure of the urorectal septum to form a complete separation of the anterior and posterior parts of the urogenital sinus. Because the inferior one third of the vagina forms from the anterior part of the urogenital sinus, it joins the rectum, which forms from the posterior part of the sinus.

4. This defect is an **omphalocele**. A small omphalocele, like the one described here, is sometimes erroneously called an *umbilical cord hernia*; however, it should not be confused with an umbilical hernia that occurs after birth and is covered by skin. The thin membrane covering the mass in the present case would be composed of peritoneum and amnion. The hernia would be composed of small intestinal loops. Omphalocele occurs when the intestinal loops fail to return to the abdominal cavity from the umbilical cord during the 10th week. In the present case, because the hernia is relatively small, the intestine may have entered the abdominal cavity and then herniated later when the rectus muscles did not approach each other close enough to occlude the circular defect in the anterior abdominal wall.

5. The ileum was probably obstructed (**ileal atresia**). Congenital atresia of the small intestine involves the ileum most frequently; the next most frequently affected region is the duodenum. The jejunum is involved least often. Some **meconium** (fetal feces) is formed from exfoliated fetal epithelium and mucus in the intestinal lumen. It is located distal to the obstructed area (atretic segment). During surgery, the atretic ileum would probably appear as a narrow segment connecting the proximal and distal segments of the intestine. The ileal atresia could have resulted from failure of recanalization of the lumen; however, more likely the atresia occurred because of a prenatal interruption of the blood supply to the ileum. Sometimes a loop of small bowel becomes twisted, interrupting its blood supply and causing **necrosis** of the affected segment. The atretic section of bowel usually becomes a fibrous cord connecting the proximal and distal segments of bowel.

## CHAPTER 12

1. Double renal pelves and ureters result from the formation of two ureteric buds on one side of the embryo. Subsequently, the primordia of these structures fuse. Both ureters usually open into the urinary bladder. Occasionally, the extra ureter opens into the urogenital tract inferior to the bladder. This occurs when the accessory ureter is not incorporated into the base of the bladder with the other ureter; instead, the extra ureter is carried caudally with the mesonephric duct and opens with it into the caudal part of the urogenital sinus. Because this part of the urogenital sinus gives rise to the urethra and epithelium of the vagina, the ectopic (abnormally placed) ureteric orifice may be located in either of these structures, which accounts for the continual dribbling of urine into the vagina. An **ectopic ureteral orifice** that opens inferior to the bladder results in urinary incontinence because there is no urinary bladder or urethral sphincter between it and the exterior. Normally, the oblique passage of the ureter through the wall of the bladder allows the contraction of the bladder musculature to act like a sphincter for the ureter, controlling the flow of urine from it.

2. **Accessory renal arteries** are common. Approximately 25% of kidneys receive two or more branches directly from the aorta; however, more than two is an exceptional finding. Supernumerary arteries enter either through the renal sinus or at the poles of the kidney, usually the inferior pole. Accessory renal arteries, more common on the left side, represent persistent fetal renal arteries that grow out in sequence from the aorta as the kidneys "ascend" from the pelvis to the abdomen. Usually, the inferior vessels degenerate as new ones develop. Supernumerary arteries are approximately twice as common as supernumerary veins. They usually arise at the level of the kidney. *The presence of a supernumerary artery is of clinical importance* in other circumstances because it may cross the ureteropelvic junction and hinder urine outflow, leading to dilation of the calices and pelvis on the same side (**hydronephrosis**). Hydronephrotic kidneys frequently become infected (**pyelonephritis**); infection may lead to destruction of the kidneys.

3. **Rudimentary horn pregnancies** are very rare; however, they are clinically important because it is difficult to distinguish between this type of pregnancy and a tubal pregnancy. In the present case, the uterine defect was the result *of retarded growth of the right paramesonephric duct* and incomplete fusion of this duct with its partner during development of the uterus. Most defects resulting from incomplete fusion of the paramesonephric ducts do not cause clinical problems; however, a rudimentary horn that does not communicate with the main part of the uterus may cause pain during the menstrual period because of distention of the horn by blood. Because most rudimentary uterine horns are thicker than uterine tubes, a rudimentary horn pregnancy is likely to rupture much later than a tubal pregnancy.

4. **Hypospadias of the glans penis** is the term applied to a defect in which the urethral orifice is on the ventral surface of the penis near the glans penis. The ventral curving of the penis is called **chordee**. Hypospadias of the glans penis results from failure of the urogenital folds on the ventral surface of the developing penis to fuse completely and establish

communication with the terminal part of the spongy urethra within the glans penis. Hypospadias may be associated with an inadequate production of androgens by the fetal testes, or there may be resistance to the hormones at the cellular level in the urogenital folds. *Hypospadias is thought to have a multifactorial etiologic basis* because close relatives of patients with hypospadias are more likely to have the defect than the general population. **Glanular hypospadias,** a common defect of the urogenital tract, occurs in approximately 1 in every 300 male infants.

5. This young woman is female, even though she has a 46,XY chromosome complement and small, nonfunctional testes. She has **androgen insensitivity syndrome.** Failure of masculinization to occur in these individuals results from a resistance to the action of testosterone at the cellular level in genitalia.

6. The embryologic basis of **indirect inguinal hernia** is persistence of the processus vaginalis, a fetal outpouching of peritoneum. This finger-like pouch evaginates the anterior abdominal wall and forms the inguinal canal. A **persistent processus vaginalis** predisposes to indirect inguinal hernia by creating a weakness in the anterior abdominal wall and a hernial sac into which abdominal contents may herniate if the intra-abdominal pressure becomes very high (as occurs during straining). The hernial sac would be covered by internal spermatic fascia, cremaster muscle, and cremasteric fascia.

## CHAPTER 13

1. **Ventricular septal defect** is the most common cardiac defect. It occurs in approximately 25% of children with congenital heart disease. Most patients with a large ventricular septal defect have a massive left-to-right shunt of blood, which causes cyanosis and congestive heart failure.

2. **Patent ductus arteriosus** is the most common cardiovascular defect associated with maternal rubella infection during early pregnancy. When the ductus arteriosus is patent in an infant, aortic blood is shunted into the pulmonary artery. One half to two thirds of the left ventricular output may be shunted through the patent ductus arteriosus. This extra work for the heart results in cardiac enlargement.

3. The tetrad of cardiac defects present in **tetralogy of Fallot** is pulmonary stenosis, ventricular septal defect, overriding aorta, and right ventricular hypertrophy. **Angiocardiography** or ultrasonography might be used to reveal the malpositioned aorta (straddling the ventricular septal defect) and the degree of pulmonary stenosis. **Cyanosis** occurs because of the shunting of unsaturated blood; however, it may not be present at birth. The main aim of therapy is to improve the oxygenation of the blood in the infant, usually by surgical correction of the pulmonary stenosis and closure of the ventricular septal defect.

4. **Cardiac catheterization** and ultrasonography would probably be performed to confirm the diagnosis of transposition of the great arteries. If this defect is present, a bolus (large quantity) of contrast material injected into the right ventricle would enter the aorta, whereas contrast material injected into the left ventricle would enter the pulmonary circulation. The infant was able to survive after birth because the ductus arteriosus remains open in these infants, allowing some mixing of blood between the two circulations. In other cases, there is also an **atrial septal defect** or ventricular septal defect that permits intermixing of blood. Complete transposition of the great arteries is incompatible with life if there are no associated septal defects or a patent ductus arteriosus.

5. This would probably be a **secundum type of atrial septal defect.** It would be located in the region of the oval fossa because this is the most common type of clinically significant atrial septal defect. Large defects, as in the present case, often extend toward the inferior vena cava. The pulmonary artery and its major branches are dilated because of the increased blood flow through the lungs and the increased pressure within the pulmonary circulation. In these cases, a considerable shunt of oxygenated blood flows from the left atrium to the right atrium. This blood, along with the normal venous return to the right atrium, enters the right ventricle and is pumped to the lungs. Large atrial septal defects may be tolerated for a long time, as in the present case, but progressive dilation of the right ventricle often leads to heart failure.

## CHAPTER 14

1. The common birth defect of the vertebral column is spina bifida occulta. This defect of the vertebral arch of the first sacral or last lumbar vertebra, or both, occurs in approximately 10% of people. The defect also occurs in cervical and thoracic vertebrae. The spinal cord and nerves are usually normal, and neurologic symptoms are usually absent. Spina bifida occulta does not cause back problems in most people.

2. A rib associated with the seventh cervical vertebra is clinically important because it may compress the subclavian artery or brachial plexus, or both, producing symptoms of artery and nerve compression. In most cases, cervical ribs produce no symptoms. These ribs develop from the costal processes of the seventh cervical vertebra and may fuse with the first rib, resulting in compressive symptoms, as in this patient. Cervical ribs occur in 0.5% to 1% of people.

3. A hemivertebra can produce a lateral curvature of the vertebral column (scoliosis). This birth defect of the vertebral column is composed of one half of a body, a pedicle, and a lamina. This defect results when the mesenchymal cells from the sclerotomes on one side fail to form the primordium of one half of a vertebra. There are more growth centers on the one side of the

vertebral column, and the imbalance causes the vertebral column to bend laterally.

4. Craniosynostosis indicates premature closure of one or more of the cranial sutures. This developmental abnormality results in malformations of the cranium. Scaphocephaly, a long narrow cranium, results from premature closure of the sagittal suture. This type of craniosynostosis accounts for approximately 50% of cases. Brain development is normal in these infants.

5. The features of Klippel-Feil syndrome are short neck, low hairline, restricted neck movements, fusion of one or more cervical motion segments, and abnormalities of the brainstem and cerebellum. In most cases, the number of cervical vertebral bodies is less than normal.

## CHAPTER 15

1. Absence of the sternocostal portion of the left pectoralis major muscle is the cause of the abnormal surface features observed. The costal heads of the pectoralis major and pectoralis minor muscles are usually present. Despite its numerous and important actions, absence of all or part of the pectoralis major muscle usually causes no disability; however, the defect caused by absence of the anterior axillary fold is striking, as is the inferior location of the nipple. The actions of other muscles associated with the shoulder joint compensate for the absence of part of the pectoralis major.

2. Approximately 13% of people lack a palmaris longus muscle on one or both sides. Its absence causes no disability.

3. The left **sternocleidomastoid muscle** was prominent when tensed. The left muscle is unaffected, and it does not pull the child's head to the right side. The short, contracted right sternocleidomastoid muscle tethers the right mastoid process to the right clavicle and sternum, and continued growth of the left side of the neck results in tilting and rotation of the head. **Congenital torticollis** (wry neck) is a relatively common condition that may occur because of injury to the muscle during birth. Some muscle fibers mighty have been torn, resulting in bleeding into the muscle. **Necrosis** of some fibers occurred over several weeks, and the muscle was replaced by fibrous tissue, which shortened the muscle and pulled the girl's head to the side.

4. Absence of striated musculature in the median plane of the anterior abdominal wall of the embryo is associated with **exstrophy of the urinary bladder**. This severe birth defect is caused by incomplete midline closure of the inferior part of the anterior abdominal wall and failure of mesenchymal cells to migrate from the somatic mesoderm between the surface ectoderm and the urogenital sinus during the fourth week of development. The absence of mesenchymal cells in the median plane results in failure of striated muscles to develop.

## CHAPTER 16

1. The number of female infants with dislocation of the hip is approximately eight times that of male infants. The hip joint is not usually dislocated at birth; however, the acetabulum is underdeveloped. Dislocation of the hip joint may not become obvious until the infant attempts to stand at approximately 12 months after birth. This condition is probably caused by deforming forces acting directly on the hip joint of the fetus.

2. Severe birth defects of the limbs (amelia and meromelia), similar to those produced by thalidomide, are rare and usually have a genetic basis. The **thalidomide syndrome** consists of absence of limbs (**amelia**); gross defects of the limbs (**meromelia**), such as attachment of the hands and feet to the trunk by small, irregularly shaped bones; intestinal atresia; and cardiac defects.

3. The most common type of clubfoot is **talipes equinovarus**, which occurs in approximately 1 of every 1000 neonates. In this deformation, the soles of the feet are turned medially and the feet are sharply plantar flexed. The feet are fixed in the tiptoe position, resembling the foot of a horse (Latin *equus*, horse).

4. **Syndactyly** (fusion of digits) is the most common type of limb defect. It varies from cutaneous webbing of the digits to **synostosis** (union of phalanges). Syndactyly is more common in the foot than in the hand. This defect occurs when separate digital rays fail to form in the fifth week of gestation or the webbing between the developing digits fails to break down between the sixth and eighth weeks. As a consequence, separation of the digits does not occur.

## CHAPTER 17

1. Ultrasound scanning of the fetus can detect absence of the neurocranium (acrania) as early as 14 weeks (see Fig. 17-35). Fetuses with meroencephaly (absence of part of the brain) do not drink the usual amounts of amniotic fluid, presumably because of impairment of the neuromuscular mechanism that controls swallowing. Because fetal urine is excreted into the amniotic fluid at the usual rate, the amount of amniotic fluid increases. Normally, the fetus swallows amniotic fluid, which is absorbed by its intestines and passed to the placenta for elimination through the mother's blood and kidneys. Meroencephaly, often inaccurately called anencephaly (absence of the brain), can be detected by a plain radiograph; however, radiographs of the fetus are not usually obtained. Instead, this severe defect is diagnosed by

ultrasonography or amniocentesis. An elevated level of alpha fetoprotein in the amniotic fluid indicates an open neural tube defect, such as acrania with meroencephaly or spina bifida with myeloschisis.

2. A neurologic defect is associated with meningomyelocele because the spinal cord or nerve roots, or both, are often incorporated into the wall of the protruding sac. This damages the nerves supplying various structures. Paralysis of the lower limbs often occurs, and there may be incontinence of urine and feces resulting from paralysis of the sphincters of the anus and urinary bladder.

3. The condition is called *obstructive hydrocephalus*. The block is most likely in the cerebral aqueduct of the midbrain. Obstruction at this site (stenosis or atresia) interferes with or prevents passage of ventricular fluid from the lateral and third ventricles to the fourth ventricle. Hydrocephalus is sometimes recognized using ultrasonography in the fetal period; however, most cases are diagnosed in the first few weeks or months after birth. Hydrocephalus can be recognized using ultrasonography of the mother's abdomen during the third trimester. Surgical treatment of hydrocephalus usually consists of shunting the excess ventricular fluid through a plastic tube to another part of the body (e.g., into the bloodstream or peritoneal cavity), from where it is excreted by the infant's kidneys.

4. Microencephaly (small brain) is usually associated with microcephaly (small calvaria). Because growth of the cranium largely depends on growth of the brain, arrest of brain development can cause microcephaly. During the fetal period, environmental exposure to agents such as cytomegalovirus, *Toxoplasma gondii*, herpes simplex virus, and high-level radiation induces microencephaly and microcephaly. Severe mental deficiency may occur as a result of exposure of the embryo or fetus to high levels of radiation during the 8- to 16-week period of development.

5. Partial or complete agenesis of the corpus callosum is associated with low intelligence in 70% of cases and seizures in 50% of patients. Some people are asymptomatic and lead normal lives. Agenesis of the corpus callosum may occur as an isolated defect; however, it is often associated with other central nervous system anomalies, such as holoprosencephalies, which are defects resulting from failure of cleavage of the prosencephalon (forebrain). As in this case, a large third ventricle may be associated with agenesis of the corpus callosum. The large ventricle exists because it is able to rise superior to the roofs of the lateral ventricles when the corpus callosum is absent. The lateral ventricles are usually moderately enlarged.

---

## CHAPTER 18

1. The mother had contracted **rubella** (German measles) during early pregnancy because her infant had the characteristic triad of defects resulting from infection of an embryo by the rubella virus. **Cataract** is common when severe infections occur during the first 6 weeks of pregnancy because the lens vesicle is forming. Congenital cataract is thought to result from invasion of the developing lens by the rubella virus. The most common cardiovascular lesion in infants whose mothers had rubella early in pregnancy is **patent ductus arteriosus**. Although a history of a rash during the first trimester of pregnancy is helpful for diagnosing the **congenital rubella syndrome**, embryopathy (embryonic disease) can occur after a subclinical maternal rubella infection (without a rash).

2. **Congenital ptosis** (drooping of superior eyelid) is usually caused by abnormal development or failure of development of the levator palpebrae superioris muscle. Congenital ptosis is usually transmitted by autosomal dominant inheritance; however, injury to the superior branch of the oculomotor nerve (CN III), which supplies the levator palpebrae superioris muscle, also can cause drooping of the upper eyelid.

3. The **protozoon** involved was *Toxoplasma gondii*, which is an intracellular parasite. The birth defects result from invasion of the fetal bloodstream and developing organs by *Toxoplasma* parasites. The parasites disrupt development of the central nervous system, including the eyes, which develop from outgrowths of the brain (optic vesicles). The physician should tell the woman about *Toxoplasma* cysts in meat and advise the woman to cook her meat well, especially if she decided to have more children. The physician should also tell her that *Toxoplasma* oocysts are often found in cat feces and that it is important for her to wash her hands with antibacterial soap after handling her cat and the litter box.

4. The infant had the characteristic phenotype of **trisomy 18**. Low-set, malformed ears associated with severe mental deficiency, prominent occiput, congenital heart defect, and failure to thrive suggest the trisomy 18 syndrome. This numeric chromosomal abnormality results from nondisjunction of the number 18 chromosome pair during gametogenesis. Its incidence is approximately 1 in 8000 neonates. Almost all of trisomy 18 fetuses abort spontaneously. Postnatal survival of these infants is poor, with 30% dying within a month of birth. The mean survival time is only 2 months. Less than 10% of these infants survive more than a year.

5. Detachment of the retina is a separation of the two embryonic retinal layers: the neural pigment epithelium derived from the outer layer of the optic cup and the neural retina derived from the inner layer of the cup. The intraretinal space, representing the cavity of the optic vesicle, normally disappears as the retina forms. The proximal part of the hyaloid artery normally persists as the central artery of the retina; however, the distal part of this vessel normally degenerates.

## CHAPTER 19

1. **Natal teeth** occur in approximately 1 in 2000 neonates. There are usually two teeth in the position of the mandibular medial incisors. They may be supernumerary teeth, but they are often prematurely erupted primary teeth. After it is established radiographically that they are supernumerary teeth, they usually are removed so that they do not interfere with eruption of the normal primary teeth. Natal teeth may cause maternal discomfort resulting from abrasion or biting of the nipple during nursing. They may also injure the infant's tongue, which lies between the alveolar processes of the jaws because the mandible is relatively small at birth.

2. Discoloration of the infant's teeth was likely caused by the administration of **tetracycline** to the mother during her pregnancy. Tetracyclines become incorporated into the developing enamel and dentine of the teeth and cause discoloration. **Dysfunction of ameloblasts** resulting from tetracycline therapy causes hypoplasia of the enamel (e.g., pitting). Most likely, the secondary dentition will be affected because enamel formation begins in the permanent teeth before birth (approximately 20 weeks in the incisors).

3. The birth defect of the skin is a capillary angioma or **hemangioma**. It is formed by an overgrowth of small blood vessels consisting mostly of capillaries, but there are also some arterioles and venules in it. The blotch is red because oxygen is not taken from the blood passing through it. This type of angioma is quite common, and the mother should be reassured that it has no clinical significance and requires no treatment. It will fade in a few years. This type of angioma was formerly called a *nevus flammeus* (flame-like birthmark). These names are sometimes applied to other types of angiomas, and to avoid confusion, it is better not to use them. *Nevus* is not a good term because it is derived from a Latin word meaning a mole or birthmark, which may or may not be an angioma.

4. A tuft of hair in the median plane of the back in the lumbosacral region usually indicates spina bifida occulta. It is the most common developmental defect of vertebrae, and it occurs in L5 or L1, or both, in approximately 10% of otherwise normal people. Spina bifida occulta usually has no clinical significance, but some infants with this vertebral defect may also have a birth defect of the underlying spinal cord and nerve roots.

5. The superficial layers of the epidermis of infants with lamellar **ichthyosis**, resulting from excessive keratinization, consist of fish-like, grayish brown scales that are adherent in the center and raised at the edges. Fortunately, the condition is rare; it is inherited as an autosomal recessive trait.

## CHAPTER 20

1. Between 7% and 10% of birth defects are caused by drugs, environmental chemicals, and infections. It is difficult for clinicians to assign specific defects to specific drugs for several reasons:

   - The drug may be administered as therapy for an illness that itself may cause the defect.
   - The fetal defect may cause maternal symptoms that are treated with a drug.
   - The drug may prevent the spontaneous abortion of an already malformed fetus.
   - The drug may be used with another drug that causes the birth defect.

   Women must understand that several drugs (e.g., **alcohol, cocaine**) cause severe defects if taken during early pregnancy (see Figs. 20-17 and 20-15) and that these drugs must be avoided.

2. Women older than the age of 41 years are more likely to have a child with Down syndrome or other chromosomal disorders than are younger women (25–29 years). Nevertheless, women older than age 41 have normal children. The physician caring for a pregnant 41-year-old woman will recommend chorionic villi sampling and amniocentesis to determine whether the fetus had a chromosomal disorder such as trisomy 21 or trisomy 13. A 41-year-old woman can have a normal baby; however, the chances of having a child with Down syndrome are 1 in 85 (see Table 20-2).

3. **Penicillin** has been widely used during pregnancy for more than 35 years without any suggestion of teratogenicity. Small doses of **aspirin** and other salicylates are ingested by most pregnant women, and when they are consumed as directed by a physician, the teratogenic risk is very low. *Chronic consumption of large doses of aspirin during early pregnancy may be harmful.* Alcohol and cigarette smoking should be avoided, and illicit drugs such as cocaine must be avoided.

4. The physician told the mother that there was no danger that her child would develop cataracts and cardiac defects because she has rubella infection (German measles). However, the physician also explained that cataracts often develop in embryos whose mothers contract the disease during early pregnancy. They occur because of the damaging effect the rubella virus has on the developing lens. The physician might have mentioned that contracting German measles before a girl's childbearing years would probably confer permanent immunity to rubella infection.

5. Cats that go outside may be infected with the parasite *Toxoplasma gondii*. It is prudent to avoid contact with cats and their litter during pregnancy. Oocysts of these parasites appear in the feces of cats and can be ingested during careless handling of litter. If the woman is pregnant, the parasite may cause severe fetal defects of the central nervous system, such as mental deficiency and blindness.

# Index

Page numbers followed by f indicate figures; b, boxes; t, tables.

**513**